I0056068

New Frontiers in Headache and Pain Research

New Frontiers in Headache and Pain Research

Edited by Sienna West

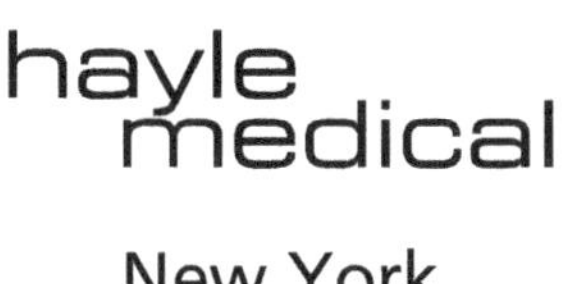

New York

Hayle Medical,
750 Third Avenue, 9th Floor,
New York, NY 10017, USA

Visit us on the World Wide Web at:
www.haylemedical.com

ISBN: 978-1-63241-686-5

Cataloging-in-Publication Data

New frontiers in headache and pain research / edited by Sienna West.
p. cm.
Includes bibliographical references and index.
ISBN 978-1-63241-686-5
1. Headache. 2. Pain--Treatment. 3. Neurology. I. West, Sienna.
RC392 .N48 2019
616.849 1--dc23

Table of Contents

Preface

Headache refers to the pain in the region of the head or neck. It is one of the most commonly experienced physical discomforts. There are more than 200 types of headaches, some benign while others are life-threatening. They are classified into primary and secondary headaches. Primary headaches are recurrent headaches, which are not caused by an underlying condition, whereas secondary headaches are caused due to a different condition such as an infection, vascular disorder, head injury, brain bleed or tumors. Although most headaches can be evaluated based on the clinical history itself, it can be challenging to differentiate between a low-risk and high-risk headache. Mild to moderate headaches are treated with NSAIDs or acetaminophen. The treatment of secondary headaches requires the treatment of the underlying condition, such as chemotherapy or surgery for a person with brain tumor. The topics included in this book on headache and pain research are of utmost significance and bound to provide incredible insights to readers. It presents researches and studies performed by experts across the globe. The extensive content of this book provides the readers with a thorough understanding of the subject.

Various studies have approached the subject by analyzing it with a single perspective, but the present book provides diverse methodologies and techniques to address this field. This book contains theories and applications needed for understanding the subject from different perspectives. The aim is to keep the readers informed about the progresses in the field; therefore, the contributions were carefully examined to compile novel researches by specialists from across the globe.

Indeed, the job of the editor is the most crucial and challenging in compiling all chapters into a single book. In the end, I would extend my sincere thanks to the chapter authors for their profound work. I am also thankful for the support provided by my family and colleagues during the compilation of this book.

Editor

1

The validation of the Hungarian version of the ID-migraine questionnaire

Éva Csépány[1,3], Marianna Tóth[2], Tamás Gyüre[1], Máté Magyar[1,3], György Bozsik[3], Dániel Bereczki[3], Gabriella Juhász[4,5] and Csaba Ertsey[3*]

Abstract

Background: Despite its high prevalence, migraine remains underdiagnosed and undertreated. ID-Migraine is a short, self-administrated questionnaire, originally developed in English by Lipton et al. and later validated in several languages. Our goal was to validate the Hungarian version of the ID-Migraine Questionnaire.

Methods: Patients visiting two headache specialty services were enrolled. Diagnoses were made by headache specialists according to the ICHD-3beta diagnostic criteria. There were 309 clinically diagnosed migraineurs among the 380 patients. Among the 309 migraineurs, 190 patients had only migraine, and 119 patients had other headache beside migraine, namely: 111 patients had tension type headache, 3 patients had cluster headache, 4 patients had medication overuse headache and one patient had headache associated with sexual activity also. Among the 380 patients, 257 had only a single type headache whereas 123 patients had multiple types of headache. Test-retest reliability of the ID-Migraine Questionnaire was studied in 40 patients.

Results: The validity features of the Hungarian version of the ID-Migraine questionnaire were the following: sensitivity 0.95 (95% CI, 0.92–0.97), specificity 0.42 (95% CI, 0.31–0.55), positive predictive value 0.88 (95% CI, 0.84–0.91), negative predictive value 0.65 (95% CI, 0.5–0.78), missclassification error 0.15 (95% CI, 0.12–0.19). The kappa coefficient of the questionnaire was 0.77.

Conclusion: The Hungarian version of the ID-Migraine Questionnaire had adequate sensitivity, positive predictive value and misclassification error, but a low specificity and somewhat low negative predictive value.

Keywords: ID-migraine questionnaire, Hungarian version, Validity features, Migraine

Background

Migraine is a common disease, which affects 14% of the population, and 18% of women [1] globally. In the USA, its lifetime prevalence is 25% in women [2]. It affects mainly the active, working, young adult population [3]. In Hungary, only one population based headache epidemiology study has been made to date [4]. This study reported 67% lifetime prevalence for any kind of headache: the one-year prevalence of migraine without aura was 7.6%, and the one-year prevalence of migraine with aura was 2%. Only 43% of migraineurs had ever consulted any physician because of their headache, and 15% of patients missed school or work because of their headache in the previous year.

According to the report of Global Burden of Disease studies, migraine is the third cause of disability in 15–49 years old men and women [5]. The disability, caused by migraine, affects many aspects of life, and leads to both physcial and emotional impairment [6]. In one Swedish study, researchers found that in migrainous patients, the health-releated quality of life is significantly worse, not only during the migraine attacks, but also between attacks, compared to healthy controls. In another study, 65% of migraine patients reported some degree of absenteeism from their workplace or school due to their headache [6]. The indirect costs of migraine are considerable: in the USA alone, approximately 13 billion dollars are spent each year for migrainre-related absenteeism from workplace and reduced ability to work

* Correspondence: csaba.ertsey@gmail.com
[3]Department of Neurology, Semmelweis University, Balassa u. 6, Budapest 1083, Hungary
Full list of author information is available at the end of the article

[7]. Despite migraine's serious negative effects on the individual, less than half of the patients ever recieve a medical diagnosis of headache [8, 9]. Furthermore, migraine is suboptimally treated, with only one-third receiving some kind of migraine-specific medication [10]. There are several factors of migraine being underdiagnosed and undertreated. The most important factor is that many migraine patients – even those with quite strong headaches – do not consult their doctors because of their headache, and therefore do not receive the diagnosis of migraine [8]. In the UK, 4.4% of the population would see a general practitioner because of a headache problem in a given year, 34% of whom (ie. 1.5% of the population) would be prescribed a migraine medication (acute or prophylactic), while only 2.1% of those who consult would be referred to a neurologist [11]. This compares to a 14.3% one-year prevalence of migraine in the UK [12]: the reason for the low consultation rates is not self-evident [11]. The severity of the attack may not be a decisive factor in consulting: an American survey found that 61% of those who had never consulted reported severe or very severe pain and 67% reported severe disability or the need for bed rest during their migraines [13]. A further difficulty in diagnosing migraine may be the duration of the doctor-patient meeting, which may not be enough to discuss the characteristics of the headaches. Furthermore, a number of primary care physicians may not have an adequate knowledge about headaches [14], and the IHS criteria are excessively complex and time-consuming for routine application in primary care [15, 16].

In order to facilitate the detection of migraine in primary care, Lipton et al. (2003) developed a brief, self-administered questionnaire, the ID-Migraine [17]. The questionnaire contains two pre-screening questions, one asking about headache-related disability, the other asking whether the patient would like to consult a doctor because of the headache. This is followed by three screening questions pertaining to the previous three months. These screening questions ask about headache-related disability, nausea and sensitivity of light. The ID-Migraine indicates migraine if a patient answered "yes" at least to two of the three screening questions. In the original study, the sensitivity of the ID-Migraine Questionnaire was 0.81, the specificity was 0.75, and the positive predictive value was 0.93. Test-retest reliability was good, with a kappa of 0.68. The ID-Migraine Questionnaire was therefore found to be a valid, reliable, and easy-to-use screening instrument to detect migraine, for patients presenting in primary care. The authors emphasized that the ID-Migraine Questionnaire is not a diagnostic instrument by itself, so a thorough evaluation of patients is necessary to make the diagnosis of migraine. Subsequently, the questionnaire was validated in Italian [18], Portuguese [19] and Turkish [20] languages with adequate results (Table 1). The questionnaire has been used in many specialty fields to screen migraine, not only in primary care [16, 21], but also in headache centers and neurology clinics [18, 19, 22]. Moreover, the questionnaire was successfully used for screening migraine patients in the emergency department [23], in a temporomandubular and orofacial pain clinic [24], and also in opthalamic and ear, nose and throat clinics [25]. The ID-Migraine Questionnaire proved to be reliable not only in adults, but also among adolescents [26]. It was also used in large-scale studies of migraine epidemiology [21] and genetic studies [27].

In this study we present the validity features of the Hungarian version of the ID-Migraine Questionnaire.

Methods

Patients between 18 and 65 years of age, presenting at the Headache Service of the Department of Neurology, Semmelweis University or the Headache Service of Esztergom Hospital, and reporting two or more headaches in the previous 3 months were involved. Both Services worked with the same methology. In order to include at least 300 patients in the study (ie. 100 patients per questionnaire item, which is a widely accepted and conservative way of assuring an adequate sample size in validation studies [28] we involved all patients visiting these Services in a two-year period who were willing to participate and gave informed consent to processing their results. The study protocol had been approved by the ethics committee of Semmelweis University. Patients completed the questionnaire at the occasion of their medical visit. Most of the patients filled in the questionnaire before the medical visit, ie. while they were waiting to be seen by the neurologist, who, on the other hand,

Table 1 Validation results of the ID-Migraine questionnaire in different languages

	Location of the research	Sensitivity (95% CI)	Specificity (95% CI)	PPV (95% CI)	NPV (95% CI)
English,2003[17]	primary care	0.81 (0.77 to 0.85)	0.75 (0.64 to 0.84)	0.93 (0.90 to 0.96)	NI
Italian, 2007[18]	headache centers	0.95 (0.91 to 0.98)	0.72 (0.62 to 0.82)	0.88 (0.82 to 0.93)	0.87 (0.78 to 0.95)
Turkish, 2007[19]	neurology outpatient clinics	0.92 (NI)	0.63 (NI)	0.72 (NI)	0.88 (NI)
Portuguese, 2008[20]	headache outpatient clinics	0.94 (0.87 to 0.97)	0.60 (0.46 to 0.73)	0.80 (0.71 to 0.87)	0.85 (0.70 to 0.94)

NI=no information, *PPV* = positive predictive value, *NPV* = negative predictive value, *CI* confidence interval

Note: NPV was not reported in the English study, classification errors were not reported in any of the studies, and no confidence intervals were reported in the Turkish study

did not use the questionnaire to ascertain the diagnosis that was based on the interview with the patient. A minority of the patients filled in the questionnaire while they were waiting for their written documentation, ie. after the medical visit. The patients also completed a 9-item Hungarian migraine screener (the MDX questionnaire), developed and validated by our group [29], which was used to collect information about the clinical characteristics of their headaches in more detail, but was not included as a reference tool in the validation process of ID-Migraine. All the patients underwent detailed internal medicine and neurological examination. The gold standard was the neurologists' clinical diagnosis, according to the International Classification of Headache Disorders (ICHD3-β). As in the original English version [17], the Hungarian version of the ID-Migraine was considered positive for migraine if a patient answered "yes" at least to two of the three screening questions. The responses to the ID-Migraine Questionnaire were then compared with the clinical diagnosis of migraine: if a patient had a diagnosis of migraine, she/he was considered a migraineur regardless of having other headaches beside migraine or not. Based on the primary diagnosis, the questionnaire's sensitivity, specificity, positive predictive value (PPV), negative predictive value (NPV), and classification error were calculated. These parameters were calculated for the individual items of the ID-Migraine Questionnaire, as well. Based on previously reported validation studies [18, 19] we also calculated these values in subgroups of patients according to sex, age (equal or below 44 years and above 44 years) and disease duration (equal or below 12 years and above 12 years) in order to have a more thorough vision of the Hungarian version's performance.

In addition, to evaluate the characteristics of the Hungarian ID-Migraine Questionnaire the receiver operating curve (ROC) was constructed among the 380 patients with different sensitivity (true positive rate) and 100-specificity (false positive rate) values according to the minimum number of positive answers to the ID-Migraine Questionnaire (0, 1, 2, and 3 positive answers).

Among the 380 headache sufferers, 40 patients completed the ID-Migraine Questionnaire twice, the second time was also during a follow-up visit. Test-retest reliability, using the Cohen's Kappa, was calculated in these 40 patients. The following values of Cohen's Kappa were used to evaluate the level of agreement [30]: < 0: no agreement; 0.0–0.20: slight agreement; 0.21–0.40: fair agreement; 0.41–0.60: moderate agreement; 0.61–0.80: substantial agreement; 0.81–1.0: perfect agreement.

We used an Excel spreadsheet for data input, and an online statistical package (VassarStats, http://vassarstats.net/) to calculate the ID-Migraine's validity features (sensitivity, specificity, PPV, NPV), the confidence intervals thereof, misclassification error and test-retest reliability.

Results

A total of 380 patients completed the Hungarian version of the ID-Migraine Questionnaire. Among the 380 patients, 80% were female and 20% were male. The median age was 36 years, the interquartile range was 19.8 years. The median disease duration was 10 years, the interquartile range was 16 years.

Table 2 summarizes the clinical headache diagnoses among the 380 patients. The number of clinically diagnosed migraineurs was 309; among them, 190 had only migraine, whereas 119 patients had another headache diagnoses beside migraine. The total number of non-migraine patients was 71; the primary diagnosis was tension type headache (TTH) in 45 patients, cluster headache in 19 patients, and other headache in 7 patients. Among the 380 patients, 257 had only one type headache, namely: 190 patients had only migraine, 44

Table 2 Clinical headache diagnoses among the 380 patients who completed the ID-Migraine questionnaire

Primary diagnosis	Number	Secondary diagnosis	Number
Migraine	309 (251 episodic and 58 chronic)	none	190
		tension type headache	111
		cluster headache	3
		medication overuse headache	4
		headache associated with sexual activity	1
Tension type headache	45 (12 episodic and 33 chronic)	none	44
		headache associated with sexual activity	1
Cluster headache	19 (18 episodic and 1 chronic)	none	16
		tension type headache	2
		SUNCT syndrome	1
Other headache	7	none	7

MOH medication overuse headache, *SUNCT* short-lasting unilateral neuralgiform headache with conjunctival injection and tearing

Table 3 The number of ID-Migraine Questionnaire positive patients in clinically diagnosed headache groups

Clinically diagnosed patients	ID-Migraine Questionnaire positive patients
total sample size: $n = 380$	$n = 334$
migraine group: $n = 309$	$n = 293$
tension type group: $n = 45$	$n = 23$
cluster type group: $n = 19$	$n = 16$
other headache group: $n = 7$	$n = 2$

had only TTH, 16 had only cluster headache and 7 had only other type of headache. The other 123 patients had more than one type of headache at the time of the study.

Among the 380 patients, 334 had a positive ID-Migraine score; 293 of them had a clinical diagnosis of migraine. Among the 45 patients, clinically diagnosed with TTH, 23 had a positive ID-Migraine score, as did 16 of the 19 patients, whose clinical diagnosis was cluster headache. Table 3 contains the number of positive ID-Migraine Questionnaires in the clinical headache groups.

Figure 1 shows the ROC curve with different cut off points (0, 1, 2, or 3 "yes" answere) to demonstrate the characteristics of the Hungarian ID-Migraine Questionnaire. To calculate validity measures we used the original cutoff value of at least two "yes" answers out of the three screening questions as reported by Lipton et al. [17].

Based on the whole sample ($n = 380$), the quality scores of the Hungarian version of the ID-Migraine Questionnaire were the following: sensitivity 0.95 (95%CI, 0.92–0.97), specificity 0.42 (95%CI, 0.31–0.55), positive predictive value (PPV) 0.88 (95%CI, 0.84–0.91), negative predictive value (NPV) 0.65 (95%CI, 0.5–0.78), misclassification error 0.15 (95%CI, 0.12–0.19).

Fourty of the 380 patients also completed the questionnaire during a follow-up visit. In this sample, the clinical diagnoses were as follows: 31 patients had migraine, 6 had TTH, 2 had cluster headache, and one had other (cervicogenic) headache. Two of the patients' clinical migraine diagnoses changed between the first and second ID-Migraine Questionnaire assessments: one had migraine as the initial diagnosis and TTH at follow-up, the other had TTH as the initial diagnosis and migraine at follow-up. The median interval between filling out the ID-Migraine Questionnaire for the first and second time was 90.5 days, the interquartile range was 475 days. At the time of the first completion, 36 of the 40 patients had a positive ID-Migaine Questionnaire. At the second time, 34 of the 40 patients had a positive test. The kappa coefficient of the questionnaire was 0.77, indicating a substantial agreement between the assesments. The overall percent of agreement was 0.95, the percent of positive agreement was 0.94.

Table 4 summarizes the quality scores for the separate items of the ID-Migraine Questionnaire using the data

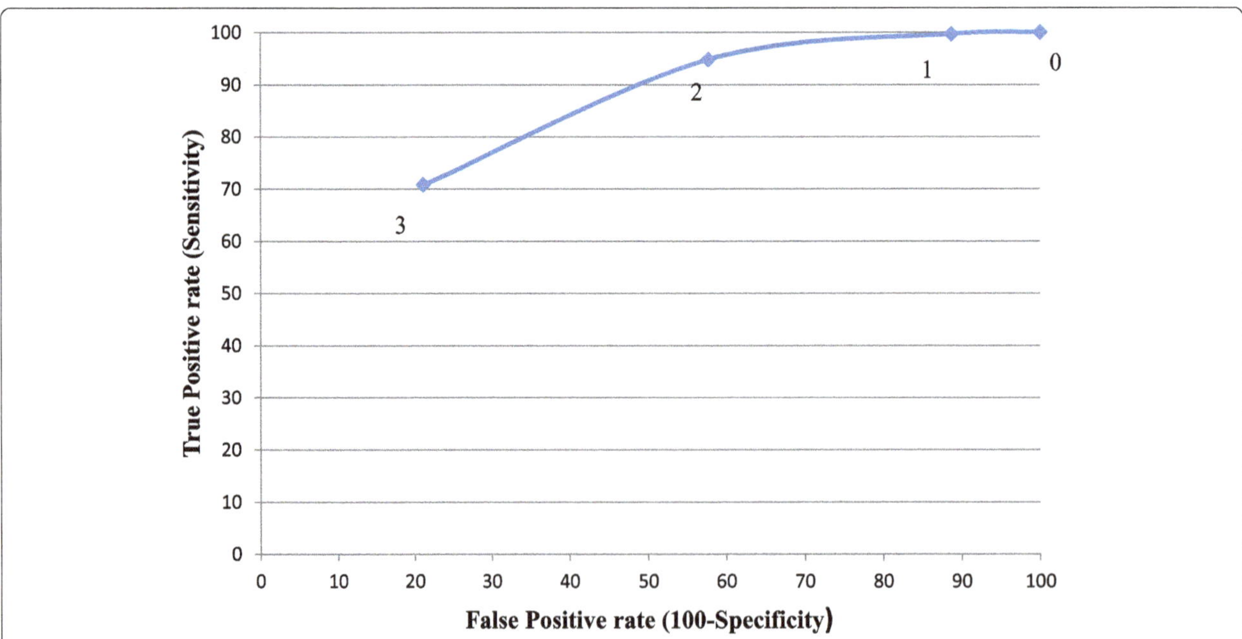

Fig. 1 The receiver operating curve of the ID-Migraine Questionnaire in the study population. The curve shows the sensitivity and specificity values according to the minimum number of positive answers for the ID-Migraine Questionnaire. Thresholds were determined according to the minimum number of positive answers to the ID-Migraine Questionnaire (0,1, 2 and 3 positive answers). 0: sensitivity: 1.00 (95% CI; 0.98–1.00); specificity: 0.00 (95% CI; 0.00–0.06). 1: sensitivity: 0.997 (95% CI; 0.98–1.00); specificity: 0.11 (95% CI; 0.05–0.22). 2: sensitivity: 0.95 (95% CI; 0.92–0.97); specificity: 0.42 (95% CI; 0.31–0.55). 3: sensitivity: 0.71 (95% CI; 0.65–0.76); specificity: 0.79 (95% CI; 0.67–0.87)

Table 4 Quality scores separately for the items of the Hungarian version of the ID-Migraine Questionnaire (n = 380)

	Sensitivity (95% CI)	Specificity (95% CI)	PPV (95% CI)	NPV (95% CI)	Classification error (95% CI)
Nausea	0.86 (0.82–0.90)	0.59 (0.47–0.70)	0.9 (0.86–0.93)	0.49 (0.38–0.60)	0.19 (0.15–0.23)
Photophobia	0.83 (0.78–0.86)	0.58 (0.45–0.69)	0.89 (0.85–0.93)	0.43 (0.33–0.54)	0.22 (0.18–0.27)
Disability	0.97 (0.94–0.98)	0.15 (0.08–0.26)	0.83 (0.79–0.87)	0.52 (0.3–0.74)	0.18 (0.15–0.23)
ID-migraine positive (≥2 "yes")	0.95 (0.92–0.97)	0.42 (0.31–0.55)	0.88 (0.84–0.91)	0.65 (0.5–0.78)	0.15 (0.12–0.19)

PPV = positive predictive value, *NPV* = negative predictive value, *CI* confidence interval

of 380 patients. All of the items (nausea, photophobia and disability) had high sensitivity and positive predictive value (> 0.8). We found the highest sensitivity for the disability (0.97), similarly to the Italian ID-Migraine Questionnaire. Nausea showed the highest positive predictive value (0.9). By contrast, we found signifcantly lower scores for the negative predictive value and specificity compared to sensitivity and positive predictive value.

Table 5 presents the quality scores of the questionnaire in the clinically relevant subgroups, namely according to sex, age (equal or below 44 years and above 44 years) and disease duration (equal or below 12 years and above 12 years). While the sensitivity and specificity of the ID-Migraine was the same in female and male patients, the PPV was noticeably higher, whereas the NPV and misclassification error were noticeably lower in females than males. There were no other substantial differences between the subgroups.

Given that the Hungarian version of the ID-Migraine had substantially lower specificity and NPV than the original and previous translations, we scrutinized those patients whose were diagnosed with nonmigraine headaches, especially whose ID-Migraine scores were positive, as was the case of 51% of TTH patients, 84% of cluster headache patients, and 29% of other headache patients, making use of the MDX questionnaire that contained the clinical characteristics of their headaches in more detail. Table 6 shows the clinical characteristics of these patients' headaches. All patients in all diagnostic groups reported an at least moderate severity of headache, regardless of their ID-Migraine score. In the TTH group, patients with a positive ID-Migraine score had an average of 3.3 migrainous features, compared to 2.0 in their ID-Migraine negative peers. In the cluster headache group, patients with a positive ID-Migraine score had, on average, 4.0 migrainous features, compared to 0.3 in ID-Migraine negative patients. In the group of other non-migraine headaches, patients with a positive ID-Migraine score had an average of 3.5 migrainous features, whereas the ID-Migraine negative patients had 2.0.

In the TTH group, 23 patients (4 episodic and 19 chronic) had a positive ID-Migraine score. Based on the clinical characteristics available from the MDX questionnaires, 14 patients (1 episodic and 13 chronic) could be considered as having migraines as well, whereas 3 episodic and 6 chronic TTH patients did not meet the criteria of migraine. The difference between the distribution of suspected migraine and no migraine was not significant (Chi square test: $p = 0.106$).

In the cluster headache group, 16 patients (15 episodic and 1 chronic) had a positive ID-Migraine score. As all of these patients were followed up at the Dept. of Neurology, and their clinical documentation was available, we performed a retrospective chart review to ascertain the diagnosis. Based on the clinical characteristics (strictly unilateral attacks; presence of ipsilateral autonomic features; periodicity) the diagnosis of cluster headace was confirmed in all of them. However, as 84% of cluster

Table 5 Quality scores of the Hungarian version of the ID-Migraine questionnaire in the clinically relevant subgroups

	N (%)	Sensitivity(95% CI)	Specificity (95% CI)	PPV (95% CI)	NPV (95% CI)	Classification error (95% CI)
Sex						
Women	304 (80%)	0.95 (0.92–0.97)	0.47 (0.30–0.65)	0.93 (0.90–0.96)	0.55 (0.36–0.73)	0.1 (0.07–0.14)
Men	76 (20%)	0.95 (0.81–0.99)	0.39 (0.24–0.56)	0.63 (0.49–0.75)	0.88 (0.60–0.98)	0.32 (0.22–0.44)
Age						
≤ 44 years	262 (69%)	0.96 (0.92–0.98)	0.44 (0.29–0.60)	0.89 (0.84–0.93)	0.69 (0.48–0.85)	0.13 (0.09–0.18)
> 44 years	118 (31%)	0.94 (0.86–0.98)	0.48 (0.27–0.69)	0.87 (0.78–0.93)	0.69 (0.41–0.88)	0.16 (0.10–0.24)
Duration of illness						
≤ 12 years	228 (60%)	0.96 (0.89–0.99)	0.41 (0.25–0.59)	0.82 (0.74–0.89)	0.78 (0.52–0.93)	0.18 (0.12–0.26)
> 12 years	152 (40%)	0.94 (0.85–0.98)	0.33 (0.09–0.69)	0.93 (0.84–0.97)	0.38 (0.10–0.74)	0.13 (0.06–0.21)

PPV = positive predictive value, *NPV* = negative predictive value, *CI* confidence interval

Table 6 The self-reported headache characteristics of the non-migraine patients versus their ID-Migraine status

Clinical diagnosis	ID-Migraine	Number of patients	Worse with movement	Nausea	Vomiting	Photophobia	Phonophobia
Tension type headache	positive	23	14	17	1	12	9
	negative	22	12	1	0	2	8
Cluster headache	positive	16	9	9	8	12	10
	negative	3	0	0	0	0	1
Other headache	positive	2	1	1	0	1	2
	negative	5	2	0	0	0	3

Note: All patients reported an at least moderate severity of pain so this was not included In Table 6

headache patients had a positive ID-Migraine score and they were overrepresented in the sample, we also calculated the quality scores excluding these patients. In this calculation, sensitivity was 0.95 (95%CI: 0.92–0.97), specificity was 0.52 (95% CI: 0.38–0.66), PPV was 0.92 (95% CI: 0.88–0.95), NPV was 0.63 (95% CI: 0.47–0.77) and misclassification error was 0.11 (95%CI: 0.08–0.15).

Finally the two patients who had other non-migrainous headaches and a positive ID-Migraine score could be considered as having migraines as well, based on the characteristics of their headaches.

Discussion

Our results demonstrated that the Hungarian version of the ID-Migraine Questionnaire is a reliable screening instrument for migraine based on data collected at specialist headache centres. The fact that all patients fully completed the questionnaire indicates that it is easy to understand and use, so it could be used as a screening tool in primary care, and also for research purposes. The sensitivity and positive predictive value of the Hungarian version of the ID-Migraine Questionnaire were quite similar to those of the original English version [17], with the Hungarian version having a higher sensitivity (0.95 vs. 0.81). The classification error (which had not been reported in the previous validation studies) was also acceptable. On the other hand, the specificity of the Hungarian version was markedly lower, and the negative predictive value was also somewhat lower than in the previous validation studies. It is important to note, that our sample was quite similar to other validation studies where the participants had also been recruited from headache centers [18–20, 29, 31–34].

All of the items (nausea, photophobia and disability) had high sensitivity and positive predictive value (> 0.8). This is in agreement with the Italian and Portugese versions of ID-Migraine Questionnaire [18, 19]. We found the highest sensitivity for the disability (0.97), similarly to the Italian ID-Migraine Questionnaire [18]. The nausea showed the highest positive predictive value (0.9), similarly to the portugese version of ID-Migraine Questionnaire [19], which supports the previous studies that headache-related nausea is an important accompaining symptom and has high impact on migraine [8, 35–39].

From the 309 clinically diagnosed migraine patients, 293 had positive ID-Migraine scores. This result supports the previous findings, that ID-Migraine Questionnaire has a high screening accuracy [17–19, 22, 25, 40–42].

In addition, the quality scores of the questionnaire showed no significant difference between clinically relevant subgroups, divided by sex, age and disease duration, similarly to the Portuguese and Italian versions of ID-Migraine Questionnaire [18, 19]. This suggests that the questionnaire may be used in the general population.

The cause of the lower specificity and NPV of the Hungarian version (0.42 vs 0.75 for the English version) may in part be due to the high number of false positive patients among the clinically diagnosed cluster headache and TTH patients. In particular, cluster headache was overrepresented in the sample (the prevalence of cluster headache patients in the sample was 5.0% versus a roughly 0.1% prevalence in the general population [43]. Sixteen of these 19 patients had a positive ID-Migraine score, which is not surprising considering the high incidence of nausea and photophobia occurring during cluster headache attacks, described first by Bahra et al. [44], and also corroborated by a Hungarian study [45] where the prevalence of nausea and photophobia during a cluster headache attacks were 43% and 68%, respectively. As shown in the Results section, eliminating the cluster headache patients resulted in a significant rise in the specificity, from 42% to 52%, while, interestingly, the NPV did not change much. Given the fact that the spontaneous occurrence of cluster headache in a similar sample from the general population would not be expected to be more than 1 patient, it may be safe to suggest that the specificity of the Hungarian version may be noticeably higher in representative samples.

Another issue affecting the specificity and NPV of the patients may have been a diagnostic error in chronic TTH patients. As outlined in the Results, 13 of the 19 chronic TTH patients with a positive ID-Migraine score could be considered migraineurs based on the characteristics of their headaches. As follow up data were not available for most TTH patients, this suggestion could neither be proved or disproved: however it is plausible that patients having chronic TTH and episodic migraines may not have had the latter diagnosis during their clinical visit. Our clinical experience with patients (not taking part in this study) who are followed up with a headache diary is that at least 20% of the patients who describe only migraine during the first visit would eventually be fund to have tension type headaches (TTH) as well, and a smaller percentage of patients originally diagnosed as 'pure' chronic TTH would also have attacks that fulfil the criteria of migraine. (This experience is not adequately reflected in the study as the number of patients included in the test-retest reliability part is still quite small.) These observations primarily affect the positive and negative predictive value and may increase the false positive test ratio, thus reducing the specificity of the questionnaire, and increasing its sensitivity and classification error.

A major limitation of our study is that our patients were recruited from patients visiting specialist headache services, so the sample is not representative of the general population. In particular, patients with episodic TTH were hugely underrepresented, and cluster headache patients were overrepresented. It is to be expected that, regardless of the diagnosis, patients with more severe head pain and accompanying symptoms would be overrepresented, and this may result in better quality indicators.

A further major limitation, that concerns the applicability of the ID-Migraine in the Hungarian population, is represented by the low specificity and low negative predictive value observed in our sample, the reasons of which are discussed above. The fact that test-retest reliability could only be tested in 10.5% of the patients represents a further limitation, although this percentage is actually slightly higher, than in the Portuguese validation study [19]. Finally, the fact that a minority of patients filled in the questionnaire after the medical visit is also a limitation, because the questions asked by the neurologist may have reinforced the patients' memories of the characteristics of headache that are the items in the ID-Migraine questionnaire.

Conclusion

Our validation study proved that the Hungarian version of the ID-Migraine Questionnaire is a reliable tool to screen migraine patients in Hungary, with a high sensitivity and positive predictive value. However, mainly because of the low specificity observed in the current study, using ID-Migraine as a standalone diagnostic tool in Hungarian patients is currently not feasible. Further testing of the instrument is required, preferably in a sample from the general population.

Abbreviations

CI: Confidence interval; ICHD3-β: International Classification of Headache Disorders; MOH: Medication overuse headache; NI: No information; NPV: Negative predictive value; PPV: Positive predictive value; ROC: Receiver operating curve; SUNCT: Short-lasting unilateral neuralgiform headache with conjunctival injection and tearing

Funding

No funding.

Authors' contributions

CE, EC, GB, TG, MM and MT made substantial contributions to conception and design, acquisition of data, analysis and interpretation of data, and drafted the manuscript. CE, DB and GJ revised it critically for important intellectual content, gived final approval of the version to be published, and agreed to be accountable for all aspects of the work in ensuring that questions related to the accuracy or integrity of any part of the work are appropriately investigated and resolved. All authors read and approved the final manuscript.

Competing interests

The authors declare that they have no competing interests.

Author details

[1]Szentágothai János Doctoral School of Neurosciences, Semmelweis University, Üllői u. 26, Budapest 1085, Hungary. [2]Department of Neurology, Vaszary Kolos Hospital, Petőfi Sándor u. 26-28, Esztergom 2500, Hungary. [3]Department of Neurology, Semmelweis University, Balassa u. 6, Budapest 1083, Hungary. [4]SE-NAP2 Genetic Brain Imaging Migraine Research Group, Semmelweis University, Nagyvárad tér 4, Budapest 1089, Hungary. [5]Department of Pharmacodynamics, Faculty of Pharmacy, Semmelweis University, Nagyvárad tér 4, Budapest 1089, Hungary.

References

1. Stovner L, Hagen K, Jensen R, Katsarava Z, Lipton R, Scher A et al (2007) The global burden of headache: a documentation of headache prevalence and disability worldwide. Cephalalgia 27(3):193–210
2. Diamond S, Bigal ME, Silberstein S, Loder E, Reed M, Lipton RB (2007) Patterns of diagnosis and acute and preventive treatment for migraine in the United States: results from the American migraine prevalence and prevention study. Headache 47(3):355–363
3. Osterhaus JT, Townsend RJ, Gandek B, Ware JE, Jr. Measuring the functional status and well-being of patients with migraine headache. Headache 1994; 34(6):337–343
4. Bank J, Marton S (2000) Hungarian migraine epidemiology. Headache 40(2): 164–169
5. Steiner TJ, Stovner LJ, Vos T (2016) GBD 2015: migraine is the third cause of disability in under 50s. J Headache Pain. 17(1):104
6. Linde M, Dahlof C (2004) Attitudes and burden of disease among self-considered migraineurs--a nation-wide population-based survey in Sweden. Cephalalgia 24(6):455–465
7. Hu XH, Markson LE, Lipton RB, Stewart WF, Berger ML. Burden of migraine in the United States: disability and economic costs. Arch Intern Med1999; 159(8):813–8
8. Lipton RB, Stewart WF, Diamond S, Diamond ML, Reed M (2001) Prevalence and burden of migraine in the United States: data from the American migraine study II. Headache 41(7):646–657
9. Lipton RB, Diamond S, Reed M, Diamond ML, Stewart WF (2001) Migraine diagnosis and treatment: results from the American migraine study II. Headache 41:638–645
10. Lipton RB, Scher AI, Kolodner K, Liberman J, Steiner TJ, Stewart WF (2002) Migraine in the United States: epidemiology and patterns of health care use. Neurology 58(6):885–894
11. Latinovic R, Gulliford M, Ridsdale L (2006) Headache and migraine in primary care: consultation, prescription, and referral rates in a large population. J Neurol Neurosurg Psychiatry 77(3):385–387

12. Steiner TJ, Scher AI, Stewart WF, Kolodner K, Liberman J, Lipton RB (2003) The prevalence and disability burden of adult migraine in England and their relationships to age, gender and ethnicity. Cephalalgia 23(7):519–527
13. Lipton RB, Stewart WF, Simon D (1998) Medical consultation for migraine: results from the American migraine study. Headache 38(2):87–96
14. Kobak KA, Katzelnick DJ, Sands G, King M, Greist JJ, Dominski M (2005) Prevalence and burden of illness of migraine in managed care patients. J Manag Care Pharm 11(2):124–136
15. Smetana GW (2000) The diagnostic value of historical features in primary headache syndromes: a comprehensive review. Arch Intern Med 160(18): 2729–2737
16. Khu JV, Siow HC, Ho KH (2008) Headache diagnosis, management and morbidity in the Singapore primary care setting: findings from a general practice survey. Singap Med J 49(10):774–779
17. Lipton RB, Dodick D, Sadovsky R, Kolodner K, Endicott J, Hettiarachchi J et al (2003) A self-administered screener for migraine in primary care: the ID migraine validation study. Neurology 61(3):375–382
18. Brighina F, Salemi G, Fierro B, Gasparro A, Balletta A, Aloisio A et al (2007) A validation study of an Italian version of the "ID migraine". Headache 47(6): 905–908
19. Gil-Gouveia R, Martins I (2010) Validation of the Portuguese version of ID-migraine. Headache 50(3):396–402
20. Karli N, Ertas M, Baykan B, Uzunkaya O, Saip S, Zarifoglu M et al (2007) The validation of ID migraine screener in neurology outpatient clinics in Turkey. J Headache Pain. 8(4):217–223
21. Di Piero V, Altieri M, Conserva G, Petolicchio B, Di Clemente L, Hettiarachchi J (2007) The effects of a sensitisation campaign on unrecognised migraine: the Casilino study. J Headache Pain 8(4):205–208
22. Cousins G, Hijazze S, Van de Laar FA, Fahey T (2011) Diagnostic accuracy of the ID migraine: a systematic review and meta-analysis. Headache 51(7): 1140–1148
23. Mostardini C, d'Agostino VC, Dugoni DE, Cerbo R (2009) A possible role of ID-migraine in the emergency department: study of an emergency department out-patient population. Cephalalgia 29(12): 1326–1330
24. Kim ST, Kim CY (2006) Use of the ID migraine questionnaire for migraine in TMJ and orofacial pain clinic. Headache 46(2):253–258
25. Ertas M, Baykan B, Tuncel D, Gokce M, Gokcay F, Sirin H et al (2009) A comparative ID migraine screener study in ophthalmology, ENT and neurology out-patient clinics. Cephalalgia 29(1):68–75
26. Zarifoglu M, Karli N, Taskapilioglu O (2008) Can ID migraine be used as a screening test for adolescent migraine? Cephalalgia 28(1):65–71
27. Juhasz G, Csepany E, Magyar M, Edes AE, Eszlari N, Hullam G et al (2017) Variants in the CNR1 gene predispose to headache with nausea in the presence of life stress. Genes Brain Behav 16(3):384–393
28. Anthoine E, Moret L, Regnault A, Sebille V, Hardouin JB (2014) Sample size used to validate a scale: a review of publications on newly-developed patient reported outcomes measures. Health Qual Life Outcomes 12:176
29. Csepany E, Bozsik G, Kellermann I, Hajnal B, Scheidl E, Palasti A, Toth M et al (2014) Examining the diagnostic accuracy of a new migraine screener. Ideggyogy Sz 67(7–8):258–268
30. Landis JR, Koch GG (1977) The measurement of observer agreement for categorical data. Biometrics 33(1):159–174
31. Diener HC, Dowson A, Whicker S, Bacon T (2008) Development and validation of a pharmacy migraine questionnaire to assess suitability for treatment with a triptan. J Headache Pain. 9(6):359–365
32. Iigaya M, Sakai F, Kolodner KB, Lipton RB, Stewart WF (2003) Reliability and validity of the Japanese migraine disability assessment (MIDAS) questionnaire. Headache 43(4):343–352
33. Zandifar A, Asgari F, Haghdoost F, Masjedi SS, Manouchehri N, Banihashemi M et al (2014) Reliability and validity of the migraine disability assessment scale among migraine and tension type headache in Iranian patients. Biomed Res Int 2014:978064
34. Manhalter N, Bozsik G, Palasti A, Csepany E, Ertsey C (2012) The validation of a new comprehensive headache-specific quality of life questionnaire. Cephalalgia 32(9):668–682
35. Lipton RB, Buse DC, Saiers J, Fanning KM, Serrano D, Reed ML (2013) Frequency and burden of headache-related nausea: results from the American migraine prevalence and prevention (AMPP) study. Headache 53(1):93–103
36. Pryse-Phillips W, Aube M, Bailey P, Becker WJ, Bellavance A, Gawel M et al (2006) A clinical study of migraine evolution. Headache 46(10):1480–1486
37. Holroyd KA, Drew JB, Cottrell CK, Romanek KM, Heh V (2007) Impaired functioning and quality of life in severe migraine: the role of catastrophizing and associated symptoms. Cephalalgia 27(10):1156–1165
38. Reed ML, Fanning KM, Serrano D, Buse DC, Lipton RB (2015) Persistent frequent nausea is associated with progression to chronic migraine: AMPP study results. Headache 55(1):76–87
39. Kelman L, Tanis D (2006) The relationship between migraine pain and other associated symptoms. Cephalalgia 26(5):548–553
40. Mattos A, Souza JA, Moreira PFF, Jurno ME, Velarde LGC (2017) ID-Migraine questionnaire and accurate diagnosis of migraine. Arq Neuropsiquiatr 75(7): 446–450
41. Wang X, San YZ, Sun JM, Zhou HB, Li X, Zhang ZM et al (2015) Validation of the Chinese version of ID-migraine in medical students and systematic review with meta-analysis concerning its diagnostic accuracy. J Oral Facial Pain Headache 29(3):265–278
42. Jurno M, Moreira Filho P, Ferreira A, Mattos AC, Souza J, Rezende D. Utility of ID-migraine as a screening tool in the specialty care (P04.253). Neurology 2012;78(1 Supplement):P04.253
43. Manzoni GC, Stovner LJ (2010) Epidemiology of headache. Handb Clin Neurol 97:3–22
44. Bahra A, May A, Goadsby PJ (2002) Cluster headache: a prospective clinical study with diagnostic implications. Neurology 58(3):354–361
45. Ertsey C, Vesza Z, Bangó M, Varga T, Nagyidei D, Manhalter N et al (2012) A prospective study evaluating the clinical characteristics of cluster headache. Ideggyogy Sz. 65(9–10):307–314

2

Headache disorder and the risk of dementia: a systematic review and meta-analysis of cohort studies

Jing Wang[1,2†], Weihao Xu[3,4†], Shasha Sun[3,4†], Shengyuan Yu[1,2*] and Li Fan[4*]

Abstract

Background: Until now, headache disorders have not been established as a risk factor for dementia. The aim of this study was to determine whether headache was associated with an increased risk of dementia.

Methods: We systematically searched electronic databases, including PubMed, Embase, and Web of Science, for studies investigating the association between headache and dementia. We then conducted a meta-analysis to determine a pooled-effect estimate of the association.

Results: We identified 6 studies (covering 291,549 individuals) to investigate the association between headache and the risk of all-cause dementia or Alzheimer's disease (AD). Pooled analyses showed that any headache was associated with a 24% greater risk of all-cause dementia (relative risk [RR] = 1.24; 95% confidential interval [CI]: 1.09–1.41; $P = 0.001$), and that any headache was not statistically significantly associated with an increased risk of AD (RR = 1.47; 95% CI: 0.82–2.63; $P = 0.192$).

Conclusions: Our results indicated that any headache was associated with an increased risk of all-cause dementia. However, additional studies are warranted to further confirm and understand the association.

Keywords: Headache, Dementia, Meta-analysis

Background

Dementia is the most common neurological disease in the elderly, with devastating impact on the quality-of-life of both the patients and their family members, apart from placing a huge economic burden on the society. Over the past 20 years, researchers have been working on finding a treatment for dementia, especially that associated with Alzheimer's disease (AD); however, results have been disappointing. Currently, there are no effective drugs that can significantly delay the progression of dementia [1]. In addition to drug treatment, researchers have also focused on the study of the risk factors for dementia in the effort that even if there is no effective treatment for the condition, the incidence thereof can still be reduced by effectively preventing and controlling the risk factors. The current identified risk factors for dementia include obesity, diabetes, hypertension, lipid metabolism disorders, coronary heart disease, and heart failure [2–5]. In addition, several studies have shown that treatment of hypertension, hyperlipidemia, and diabetes might reduce the risk of dementia [6–8].

Globally, about 45% of adults in the general population suffer from headache disorders [9]. These disorders are known to be risk factors for a variety of diseases, such as stroke, myocardial infarction and depression [10–12]. Previous studies have found migraine history to be significantly associated with cardiovascular disease and brain white-matter damage [13–15]. Non-migrainous headaches are also associated with some vascular risk factors [16, 17]. Such vascular risk factors and white-matter damage may increase the risk of dementia. Thus, headache disorders can be reasonably speculated to be associated with the increased risk of dementia. However, current evidence from longitudinal studies linking headache disorders to dementia is scarce, and study populations are often too small to detect clinically relevant associations. We therefore systematically reviewed and

* Correspondence: yusy1963@126.com; fanli301@hotmail.com
†Jing Wang, Weihao Xu and Shasha Sun contributed equally to this work.
[1]School of Medicine, Nankai University, Tianjin 300071, China
[4]National Clinical Research Center of Geriatric Diseases, Chinese PLA General Hospital, Fuxing Road 28, Haidian District, Beijing 100853, China
Full list of author information is available at the end of the article

meta-analyzed the available longitudinal population-based evidence to determine the association of headache disorders with risk of dementia.

Methods

Search strategy

We conducted our systematic review and meta-analysis in accordance with the Preferred Reporting Items for Systematic Reviews and Meta-Analyses (PRISMA) statement. We systematically searched the PubMed, Embase and Web of Science databases from their inceptions to June 1, 2018 for relevant studies. Our complete search strategy is presented in Additional file 1: Table S1. Additionally, we conducted a manual search of references in the included studies and of relevant reviews to find other relevant articles. We did not apply any language restrictions.

Selection criteria

Articles were included if they met the following criteria: [1] cohort studies; [2] report of incident dementia diagnosis as the outcome; and [3] investigation into the association of headache disorders with risk of incident all-cause dementia or of AD. Headache disorders included all types of headache. In this study, "any headache" was defined as "patient suffered from any type of headache in the past." We chose all-cause dementia as the primary outcome measure of interest, given that the syndrome diagnosis of dementia can be defined with high consistency across studies and is less dependent on advanced diagnostic testing, which is often not feasible in large population-based studies. Nevertheless, we acknowledged the importance of the various neuropathologies underlying the clinical manifestation of dementia. We chose AD as the secondary outcome measure to provide additional insight into the association of headache disorders with dementia. If more than 1 article reported data from 1 cohort or 1 health database, we included the study with the longest follow-up or largest number of participants. Studies were excluded if they did not provide a relative-risk (RR) estimate with corresponding 95% confidence interval (CI).

Two investigators independently assessed the eligibility of the literature. First, they identified eligible articles by title and abstract; next, each of them independently read the full text of each eligible article. Discrepancies between investigators were rechecked and, if necessary, discussed with a third investigator until consensus was achieved.

Data extraction and quality assessment

Two investigators independently extracted and summarized the relevant data of the included studies. The following information was extracted from each included study: author name, year of publication, country of study origin, population source, study design, sample size, years of follow-up, gender distribution, mean age and age range of study participants, headache type and dementia type.

We assessed the quality of the included articles using the Newcastle–Ottawa Quality Assessment Scale (NOS) [18]. Scores ranged from 0 to 9 points for cohort studies, with higher scores indicating higher study quality. We considered NOS scores of 0–3, 4–6, and ≥ 7 to indicate low, medium, and high quality, respectively.

Statistical analysis

We extracted the adjusted RR and 95% CI from each study and used them to assess the association between headache and risk of dementia. We used random-effects models, which included assumptions about potential differences between studies, for our pooled analysis [19]. Heterogeneity of included studies was assessed by chi-square test and I-squared (I^2) statistic. Statistical heterogeneity was considered significant when $P < 0.10$ for the χ^2 test or when $I^2 > 50\%$ [20]. We performed sensitivity analyses by excluding 1 study each time and re-running the analysis to verify the robustness of the overall results. We visually inspected the funnel plot to confirm publication bias. Egger's regression test [21] and Begg's test [22] were used to statistically assess publication bias. A 2-tailed *P*-value < 0.05 was considered statistically significant. We performed all analyses using Stata software version 12.0 (Stata Corp., College Station, Texas, US).

Results

We retrieved a total of 2871 studies from our database search. Out of those, we included 3 articles and 3 abstracts corresponding to 6 cohort studies in this meta-analysis. The study selection process is shown in Fig. 1.

Study characteristics

Overall, we included 6 studies covering 291,549 individuals in our meta-analysis. Two studies [23, 24] were retrospective in design, while the other 4 [25–28] were prospective. Three [23–25] had sample sizes > 50,000, and the other 3 [26–28] had sample sizes < 1500. The main characteristics of the included studies are shown in Table 1.

Quality assessment

We were able to assess the quality of the 3 full-length articles only. Specific assessments with NOS scores for these 3 studies are shown in Additional file 1: Table S2.

Any headache and risk of all-cause dementia

The 6 included studies all assessed the association between any headache and the risk of all-cause dementia. Overall, the history of any headache was associated with an increased risk of all-cause dementia (RR = 1.24; 95% CI: 1.09–1.41; $P = 0.001$; Fig. 2), but with considerable heterogeneity across studies ($I^2 = 63.5\%$; $P_{hetero} = 0.018$). Neither subgroup analysis by sample size (large or small) nor study

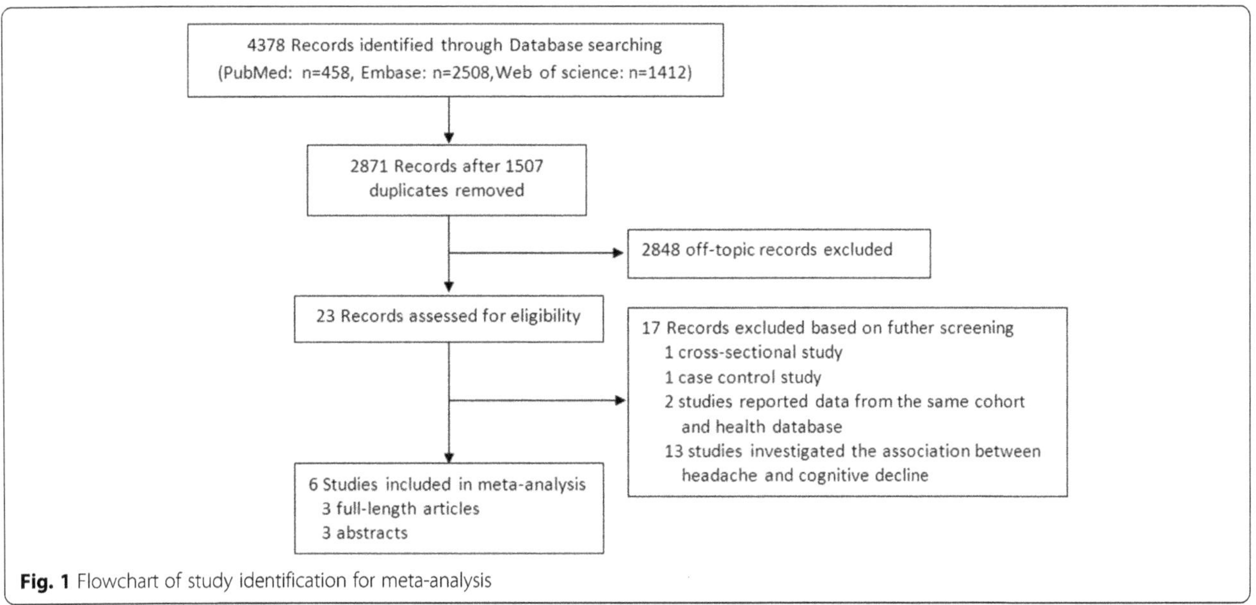

Fig. 1 Flowchart of study identification for meta-analysis

Table 1 The characteristics of included cohort studies in this meta-analysis

Author year	Country	Study design	Sample size	Follow-up years	Gender	Age	Headache type	Dementia type	Confounders adjusted
Chuang 2013	China	Retrospective cohort	Total: 167,340 Migraine: 33,468 No migraine: 133,872	12 (longest)	Male and Female	42.2 (mean)	Migraine	All-cause dementia	Age, sex, diabetes, hypertension, depression, head injury and CAD
Yang 2016	China	Retrospective cohort	Total: 69540 TTH: 13,908 No TTH: 55,632	8.14 (average)	Male and Female	≥20 48.9 (mean)	TTH	All-cause dementia; VaD; AD	Age, sex, diabetes, dyslipidemia, COPD, hypertension, IHD, AF, HF, stroke, depression, head injury, Parkinson's disease and migraine
Hagen 2013	Norway	Prospective cohort	Total: 51,859 Any headache: 21,871 No headache: 29,988	15 (average)	Male and Female	≥20 49.7 (mean)	Any headache Migraine Nonmigrainous headache	All-cause dementia; VaD; AD; Mixed dementia; VaD plus mixed dementia; Dementia with Lewy bodies; Frontotemp. dementia; Other types of dementia	Age, sex, education, total HADS score and smoking
Morton 2012	Canada	Prospective cohort	Total: 716	5 (average)	Male and Female	≥65	Migraine	All-cause dementia; VaD; AD	Age, sex, education, depression hypertension, diabetes, stroke, myocardial infarction and other heart conditions
Pavlovic 2013	USA	Prospective cohort	Total: 974 Migraine: 136 No migraine: 838	NA	Male and Female	≥70	Migraine	All-cause dementia	Age, sex, education, ethnicity, APOE-e4 carrier status, pain interference and pain intensity
Recchia 2016	Italy	Prospective cohort	Total: 1120	3.9 (average)	Male and Female	≥80	Any headache	All-cause dementia	Age, sex and education

CAD coronary artery disease, *TTH* tension-type headache, *VaD* vascular dementia, *AD* Alzheimer's disease, *COPD* chronic obstructive pulmonary disease, *IHD* ischemic heart disease, *AF* atrial fibrillation, *HF* heart failure, *HADS* hospital anxiety and depression scale, *NA* not available, *APOE* apolipoprotein E

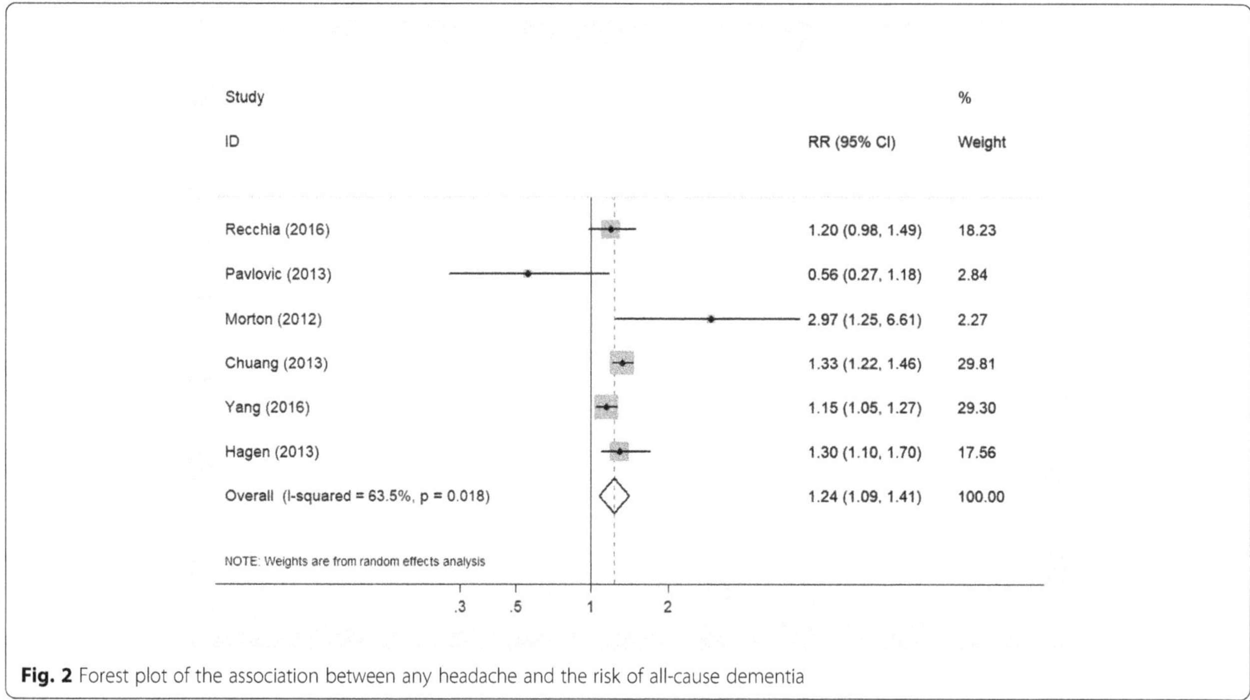

Fig. 2 Forest plot of the association between any headache and the risk of all-cause dementia

design (prospective or retrospective) could explain the origin of this heterogeneity. Sensitivity analysis (excluding 1 trial each time and recalculating the pooled RR for the remaining studies) showed that none of the individual studies had an evident influence on the pooled-effect size (Fig. 3). The analysis verified the robustness of the results. A visual inspection of the funnel plot showed no evidence of a significant publication bias (Fig. 4). Begg's ($P = 0.851$) and Egger's ($P = 0.089$) regression tests likewise indicated no publication bias in this meta-analysis.

Any headache and risk of AD

Three studies investigated the association between any headache and the risk of AD. Pooled results showed that any headache was not associated with an increased risk of AD (RR = 1.47; 95% CI: 0.82–2.63; $P = 0.192$; Fig. 5).

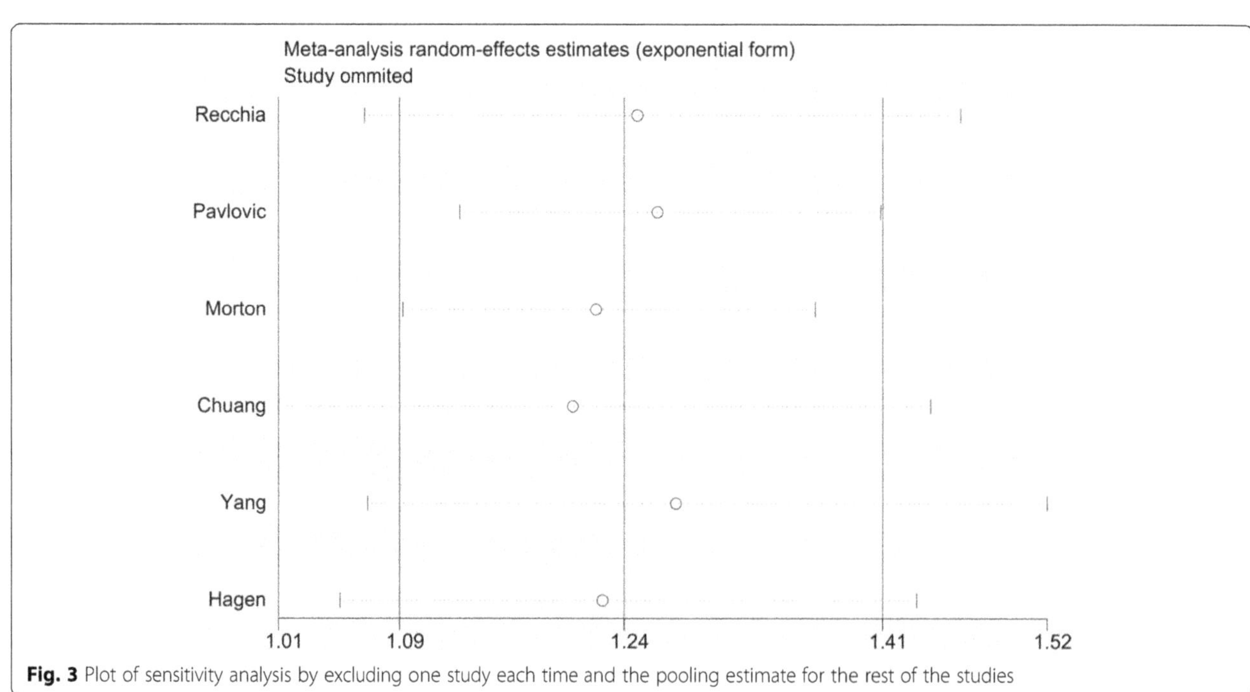

Fig. 3 Plot of sensitivity analysis by excluding one study each time and the pooling estimate for the rest of the studies

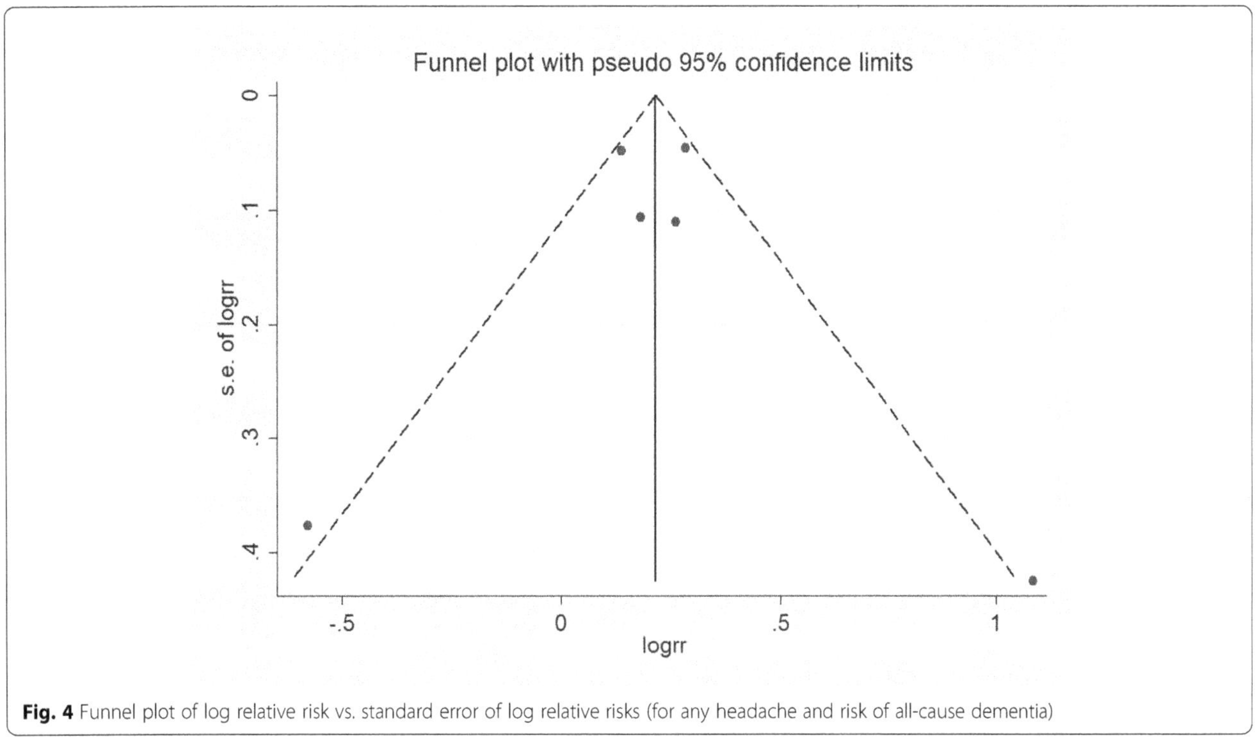

Fig. 4 Funnel plot of log relative risk vs. standard error of log relative risks (for any headache and risk of all-cause dementia)

Migraine and risk of dementia

Three studies reported the association between migraine and the risk of all-cause dementia. After pooling the reported effect estimates of these studies, we found an RR of 1.28 (95% CI: 0.64–2.54) for the association between history of migraine and risk of all-cause dementia. Only 1 study reported the association of migraine with the risk of AD, and its results showed that the history of migraine increased the risk of AD (RR = 4.22; 95% CI = 1.59–10.42; Additional file 1: Figure S1).

Discussion

In this systematic review and meta-analysis of cohort studies, we compiled current evidence on the association between headache disorders and the future risk of dementia in 291,549 individuals from 6 population-based studies. We

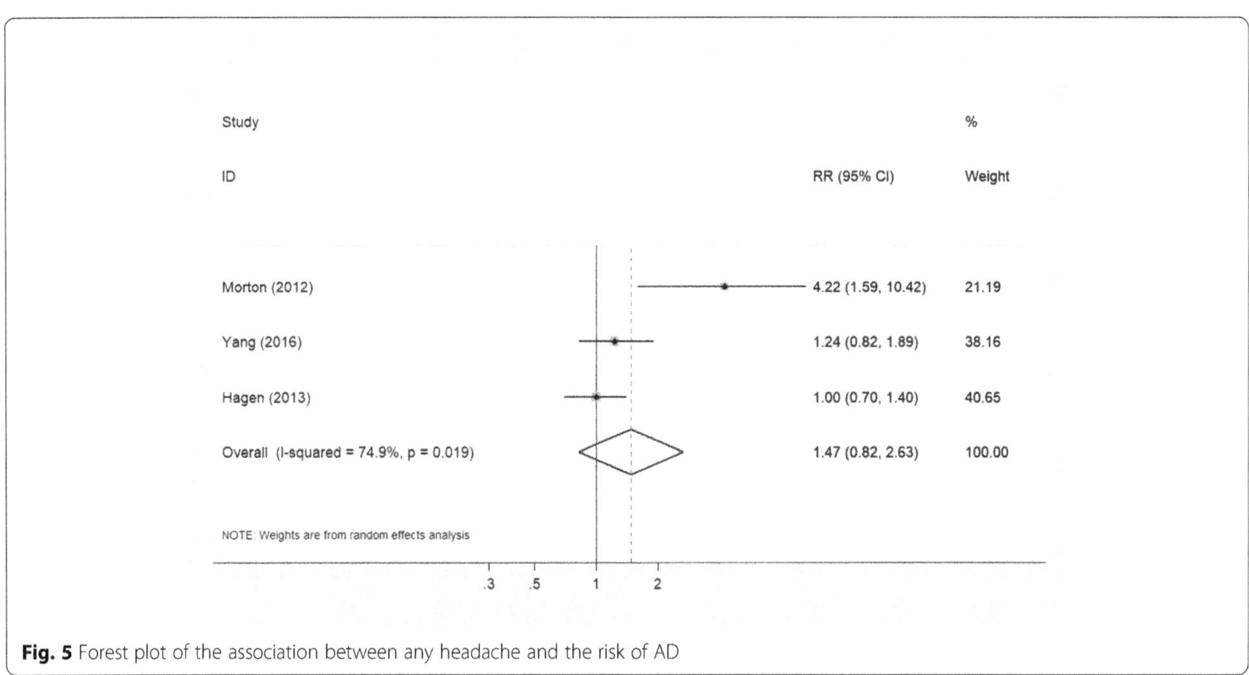

Fig. 5 Forest plot of the association between any headache and the risk of AD

found that any headache is a potential risk indicator for all-cause dementia.

Our results were further supported by findings of 2 other large population-based studies that we did not include in this meta-analysis (reasons for exclusion are shown in Additional file 1: Table S3). Stræte Røttereng et al. used data from Nord-Trøndelag Health Surveys conducted during 1995–1997 (HUNT2) and 2006–2008 (HUNT3), and found that both any headache and non-migrainous headache were more likely to be reported in dementia patients, when compared with the control group (any headache, odds ratio [OR] = 1.24; 95% CI: 1.04–1.49 and non-migrainous headache, OR = 1.49; 95% CI: 1.24–1.80) [29]. Tzeng et al. analyzed 10 years of follow-up data from the National Health Insurance Research Database of Taiwan and suggested that patients with primary headaches had twice the normal risk of developing dementia in the future (hazard ratio [HR] = 2.06; 95% CI: 1.72–2.46) [30]. All these findings indicated that headache disorders might be a potential predictor for dementia.

It should be noted that no statistically significant result was found in the pooled analysis of the association between migraine and all-cause dementia. However, the result of this analysis was based on only three studies with two were abstracts, and as such, should be interpreted with caution. The available data on migraine and risk of AD were also unsatisfactory. Although 1 study indicated that history of migraine was associated with increased risk of AD [25], there was insufficient evidence to draw any conclusion about this association. The current available evidence on migraine and dementia were scarce but could suggest us that the possible association might exist, and highlight the need for more population-based research on this association.

The pathological association between headache disorders and dementia remains largely unknown, but several mechanisms are speculated to be involved. First, headache is a common pain disorder. A previous study found that several brain structures involved in the pain network, such as the thalamus, insula, anterior cingulate, amygdalae, and temporal cortex, undergo morphometric changes during the disease process [31]. Interestingly, these brain regions also play important roles in the memory network [32]. In addition, a previous structural–neuroimaging study of chronic headache showed that the gray-matter volume of memory network structures, including the cingulate cortex, insula, prefrontal area, and parahippocampus, decreased significantly in individuals who suffered from headache compared with those who did not [33]. These significant changes in the overlapping pain and memory networks explain the potential correlation between chronic pain and memory impairment in headache patients. Second, a previous meta-analysis found an association of white-matter hyperintensity with an increased risk of dementia [34]. Incidentally, headache patients were reported to have an increased risk of white-matter hyperintensity [35]. Therefore, subtle changes in the brain white-matter might contribute to an increased risk of dementia in headache patients. Third, depression is common, with approximate 20% of the general population experiencing a depressive episode during their lifetime [36]. An association between depression and dementia has been suggested in previous studies. Headache, especially migraine, is often comorbid with depression [37]. Specifically, previous studies found that earlier-life depression or depressive symptoms were associated with a significantly increased risk of developing dementia [38, 39]. Vascular disease, alterations in the cortisol–hippocampal pathway, increased amyloid plaque formation, inflammatory changes, and deficits in nerve growth factors or neurotrophins are predicted to be the potential biological mechanisms linking depression to dementia [40]. Thus, an increased risk of dementia in headache patients might be partly due to comorbidity with depression. Finally, stress and mental tension have been identified as predictors of headache disorder [41]. A previous cohort study found an association between psychological stress in middle-aged women and the development of dementia, especially AD [42]. The underlying mechanism remained unclear, but the hypothalamic–pituitary–adrenal axis and the effects of glucocorticoids on the brain are thought to be behind the association [43].

To the best of our knowledge, our meta-analysis was the first to summarize the currently available evidence of the association between headache and the risk of dementia, and to indicate that any headache is a risk factor for developing all-cause dementia. Sensitivity analysis verified the stabilization of the results. However, there are some limitations as well. The number of studies included was small, and the meta-analysis of the association between any headache and the risk of AD included only 3 studies. As such, the results are likely to be imprecise [44], and, consequently, the conclusions drawn from this study should be considered preliminary. In addition, the studies included show quite high heterogeneity in terms of study design, population sizes and population age range. The potential effect of the heterogeneity should be taken into account when interpreting the findings of the review. Even so, our findings are still of great significance. The association we found might aid in identifying people prone to dementia or cognitive decline. This emphasizes the need to reveal the mechanisms underlying the link between headache and dementia, which may become all the more evident while improving the quality-of-life of patients with headache disorder. The information is critical to finding new preventive and treatment strategies for dementia. It is also of crucial importance that we figure out whether treatment for headache disorder might intervene in the overlapping pathways and subsequently reduce the risk of dementia.

Conclusions

We found that any headache was associated with an increased risk of all-cause dementia in the general population. Our results also highlighted that population-based data on the association of headache with incident dementia remains limited and that further study into the underlying mechanism of the association is warranted.

Abbreviations

AD: Alzheimer's disease; CI: confidence interval; HR: hazard ratio; NOS: Newcastle–Ottawa Quality Assessment Scale; OR: odds ratio; PRISMA: Preferred Reporting Items for Systematic Reviews and Meta-Analyses; RR: relative-risk

Acknowledgments

We thank LetPub (www.letpub.com) for its linguistic assistance during the preparation of this manuscript.

Funding

This work was supported by the National Key Research and Development Program (grant number 2017YFC1307701)

Authors' contributions

Study concept and design: JW, SYY. Acquisition of data: JW, SSS. Analysis and interpretation of data: JW, WHX, SSS. Drafting of the manuscript: JW, WHX. Critical revision of the manuscript for important intellectual content: SYY. All authors read and approved the final manuscript.

Competing interests

The authors declare that they have no competing interests.

Author details

[1]School of Medicine, Nankai University, Tianjin 300071, China. [2]Department of Neurology, Chinese PLA General Hospital, Fuxing Road 28, Haidian District, Beijing 100853, China. [3]Department of Geriatric Cardiology, Nanlou Division, Chinese PLA General Hospital, Beijing 100853, China. [4]National Clinical Research Center of Geriatric Diseases, Chinese PLA General Hospital, Fuxing Road 28, Haidian District, Beijing 100853, China.

References

1. Broadstock M, Ballard C, Corbett A (2014) Latest treatment options for Alzheimer's disease, Parkinson's disease dementia and dementia with Lewy bodies. Expert Opin Pharmacother 15(13):1797–1810
2. Anstey KJ, Cherbuin N, Budge M, Young J (2011) Body mass index in midlife and late-life as a risk factor for dementia: a meta-analysis of prospective studies. Obes Rev 12(5):e426–e437
3. Xu W, Qiu C, Gatz M, Pedersen NL, Johansson B, Fratiglioni L (2009) Mid- and late-life diabetes in relation to the risk of dementia: a population-based twin study. Diabetes 58(1):71–77
4. Sahathevan R, Brodtmann A, Donnan GA (2012) Dementia, stroke, and vascular risk factors; a review. Int J Stroke 7(1):61–73
5. Wolters FJ, Segufa RA, Darweesh SKL, Bos D, Ikram MA, Sabayan B, Hofman A, Sedaghat S (2018) Coronary heart disease, heart failure, and the risk of dementia: a systematic review and meta-analysis. Alzheimers Dementia
6. Jick H, Zornberg GL, Jick SS, Seshadri S, Drachman DA (2000) Statins and the risk of dementia. Lancet 356(9242):1627–1631
7. Skoog I (2009) Antihypertensive treatment and dementia. Pol Arch Med Wewn 119(9):524–525
8. Parikh NM, Morgan RO, Kunik ME, Chen H, Aparasu RR, Yadav RK, Schulz PE, Johnson ML (2011) Risk factors for dementia in patients over 65 with diabetes. Int J Geriatr Psychiatry 26(7):749–757
9. Stovner L, Hagen K, Jensen R, Katsarava Z, Lipton R, Scher A, Steiner T, Zwart JA (2007) The global burden of headache: a documentation of headache prevalence and disability worldwide. Cephalalgia 27(3):193–210
10. Jamieson DG, Cheng NT, Skliut M (2014) Headache and acute stroke. Curr Pain Headache Rep 18(9):444
11. Mahmoud AN, Mentias A, Elgendy AY, Qazi A, Barakat AF, Saad M, Mohsen A, Abuzaid A, Mansoor H, Mojadidi MK, Elgendy IY (2018) Migraine and the risk of cardiovascular and cerebrovascular events: a meta-analysis of 16 cohort studies including 1 152 407 subjects. BMJ Open 8(3):e020498
12. Blaauw BA, Dyb G, Hagen K, Holmen TL, Linde M, Wentzel-Larsen T, Zwart JA (2014) Anxiety, depression and behavioral problems among adolescents with recurrent headache: the young-HUNT study. J Headache Pain 15:38
13. Schurks M, Rist PM, Bigal ME, Buring JE, Lipton RB, Kurth T (2009) Migraine and cardiovascular disease: systematic review and meta-analysis. BMJ 339:b3914
14. Bigal ME, Kurth T, Santanello N, Buse D, Golden W, Robbins M, Lipton RB (2010) Migraine and cardiovascular disease: a population-based study. Neurology 74(8):628–635
15. Kruit MC, van Buchem MA, Launer LJ, Terwindt GM, Ferrari MD (2010) Migraine is associated with an increased risk of deep white matter lesions, subclinical posterior circulation infarcts and brain iron accumulation: the population-based MRI CAMERA study. Cephalalgia 30(2):129–136
16. Winsvold BS, Hagen K, Aamodt AH, Stovner LJ, Holmen J, Zwart JA (2011) Headache, migraine and cardiovascular risk factors: the HUNT study. Eur J Neurol 18(3):504–511
17. Winsvold BS, Sandven I, Hagen K, Linde M, Midthjell K, Zwart JA (2013) Migraine, headache and development of metabolic syndrome: an 11-year follow-up in the Nord-Trondelag health study (HUNT). Pain 154(8):1305–1311
18. Wells GA SB, O'Connell D, Peterson J, Welch V, Losos M, Tugwell P (2014) The Newcastle-Ottawa Scale (NOS) for assessing the quality of nonrandomised studies in meta-analyses. Available from: http://www.ohri.ca/programs/clinical_epidemiology/oxford.asp
19. Schurks M, Winter A, Berger K, Kurth T (2014) Migraine and restless legs syndrome: a systematic review. Cephalalgia 34(10):777–794
20. Higgins JP, Thompson SG, Deeks JJ, Altman DG (2003) Measuring inconsistency in meta-analyses. BMJ 327(7414):557–560
21. Egger M, Davey Smith G, Schneider M, Minder C (1997) Bias in meta-analysis detected by a simple, graphical test. BMJ 315(7109):629–634
22. Begg CB, Mazumdar M (1994) Operating characteristics of a rank correlation test for publication bias. Biometrics 50(4):1088–1101
23. Yang FC, Lin TY, Chen HJ, Lee JT, Lin CC, Kao CH (2016) Increased risk of dementia in patients with tension-type headache: a Nationwide retrospective population-based cohort study. PLoS One 11(6):e0156097
24. Chuang CS, Lin CL, Lin MC, Sung FC, Kao CH (2013) Migraine and risk of dementia: a nationwide retrospective cohort study. Neuroepidemiology 41(3–4):139–145
25. Hagen K, Stordal E, Linde M, Steiner TJ, Zwart JA, Stovner LJ (2014) Headache as a risk factor for dementia: a prospective population-based study. Cephalalgia 34(5):327–335
26. Morton R, Tyas S (2012) Does a historyof migraines increase the risk of Alzheimer's disease or vascular dementia? Alzheimers Dementia 8(4 Suppl 1):P504
27. Pavlovic J, Mowrey W, Hall CB, Katz MJ, Lipton RB (2013) Dementia outcomes in elderly with self-reported history of migraine. Cephalalgia 33(Suppl 1):139–140
28. Recchia A, Tettamanti M, Ammesso S, Garrì M, Mandelli S, Riva E, Lucca U (2016) Headaches and dementia in the oldest-old: the monzino 80-plus population-based study. Alzheimers Dementia 12(7 Suppl):P1120–P1121
29. Straete Rottereng AK, Bosnes O, Stordal E, Zwart JA, Linde M, Stovner LJ, Hagen K (2015) Headache as a predictor for dementia: the HUNT study. J Headache Pain 16:89
30. Tzeng NS, Chung CH, Lin FH, Yeh CB, Huang SY, Lu RB, Chang HA, Kao YC, Chiang WS, Chou YC, Tsao CH, Wu YF, Chien WC (2017) Headaches and risk of dementia. Am J Med Sci 353(3):197–206

31. Apkarian AV, Bushnell MC, Treede RD, Zubieta JK (2005) Human brain mechanisms of pain perception and regulation in health and disease. Eur J Pain 9(4):463–484
32. Svoboda E, McKinnon MC, Levine B (2006) The functional neuroanatomy of autobiographical memory: a meta-analysis. Neuropsychologia 44(12):2189–2208
33. Schmidt-Wilcke T, Leinisch E, Straube A, Kampfe N, Draganski B, Diener HC, Bogdahn U, May A (2005) Gray matter decrease in patients with chronic tension type headache. Neurology 65(9):1483–1486
34. Bos D, Wolters FJ, Darweesh SKL, Vernooij MW, de Wolf F, Ikram MA, Hofman A (2018) Cerebral small vessel disease and the risk of dementia: a systematic review and meta-analysis of population-based evidence. Alzheimers Dementia
35. Bell BD, Primeau M, Sweet JJ, Lofland KR (1999) Neuropsychological functioning in migraine headache, nonheadache chronic pain, and mild traumatic brain injury patients. Arch Clin Neuropsychol 14(4):389–399
36. Kessler RC, Berglund P, Demler O, Jin R, Merikangas KR, Walters EE (2005) Lifetime prevalence and age-of-onset distributions of DSM-IV disorders in the National Comorbidity Survey Replication. Arch Gen Psychiatry 62(6):593–602
37. Breslau N, Davis GC, Schultz LR, Peterson EL (1994) Joint 1994 Wolff award presentation. Migraine and major depression: a longitudinal study. Headache 34(7):387–393
38. Katon W, Pedersen HS, Ribe AR, Fenger-Gron M, Davydow D, Waldorff FB, Vestergaard M (2015) Effect of depression and diabetes mellitus on the risk for dementia: a national population-based cohort study. JAMA Psychiatry 72(6):612–619
39. Lin WC, Hu LY, Tsai SJ, Yang AC, Shen CC (2017) Depression and the risk of vascular dementia: a population-based retrospective cohort study. Int J Geriatr Psychiatry 32(5):556–563
40. Byers AL, Yaffe K (2011) Depression and risk of developing dementia. Nat Rev Neurol 7(6):323–331
41. Jensen R (2003) Diagnosis, epidemiology, and impact of tension-type headache. Curr Pain Headache Rep 7(6):455–459
42. Johansson L, Guo X, Waern M, Ostling S, Gustafson D, Bengtsson C, Skoog I (2010) Midlife psychological stress and risk of dementia: a 35-year longitudinal population study. Brain 133(Pt 8):2217–2224
43. Payne JD, Jackson ED, Hoscheidt S, Ryan L, Jacobs WJ, Nadel L (2007) Stress administered prior to encoding impairs neutral but enhances emotional long-term episodic memories. Learn Mem 14(12):861–868
44. IntHout J, Ioannidis JP, Rovers MM, Goeman JJ (2016) Plea for routinely presenting prediction intervals in meta-analysis. BMJ Open 6(7):e010247

3

Consistent effects of non-invasive vagus nerve stimulation (nVNS) for the acute treatment of migraine: additional findings from the randomized, sham-controlled, double-blind PRESTO trial

Paolo Martelletti[1], Piero Barbanti[2], Licia Grazzi[3], Giulia Pierangeli[4], Innocenzo Rainero[5], Pierangelo Geppetti[6], Anna Ambrosini[7], Paola Sarchielli[8], Cristina Tassorelli[9,10], Eric Liebler[11*], Marina de Tommaso[12]
and on Behalf of the PRESTO Study Group

Abstract

Background: Non-invasive vagus nerve stimulation (nVNS) has been shown to be practical, safe, and well tolerated for treating primary headache disorders. The recent multicenter, randomized, double-blind, sham-controlled PRESTO trial provided Class I evidence that for patients with episodic migraine, nVNS significantly increases the probability of having mild pain or being pain-free 2 h post stimulation. We report additional pre-defined secondary and other end points from PRESTO that demonstrate the consistency and durability of nVNS efficacy across a broad range of outcomes.

Methods: After a 4-week observation period, 248 patients with episodic migraine with/without aura were randomly assigned to acute treatment of migraine attacks with nVNS (n = 122) or a sham device (n = 126) during a double-blind period lasting 4 weeks (or until the patient had treated 5 attacks). All patients received nVNS therapy during the subsequent 4-week/5-attack open-label period.

Results: The intent-to-treat population consisted of 243 patients. The nVNS group (n = 120) had a significantly greater percentage of attacks treated during the double-blind period that were pain-free at 60 (P = 0.005) and 120 min (P = 0.026) than the sham group (n = 123) did. Similar results were seen for attacks with pain relief at 60 (P = 0.025) and 120 min (P = 0.018). For the first attack and all attacks, the nVNS group had significantly greater decreases (vs sham) in pain score from baseline to 60 min (P = 0.029); the decrease was also significantly greater for nVNS at 120 min for the first attack (P = 0.011). Results during the open-label period were consistent with those of the nVNS group during the double-blind period. The incidence of adverse events (AEs) and adverse device effects was low across all study periods, and no serious AEs occurred.

Conclusions: These results further demonstrate that nVNS is an effective and reliable acute treatment for multiple migraine attacks, which can be used safely while preserving the patient's option to use traditional acute medications as rescue therapy, possibly decreasing the risk of medication overuse. Together with its practicality and optimal tolerability profile, these findings suggest nVNS has value as a front-line option for acute treatment of migraine.

Trial registration: ClinicalTrials.gov identifier: NCT02686034.

Keywords: Neuromodulation, Vagus nerve stimulation, Migraine, Pain intensity, Double-blind, Open-label

* Correspondence: eric.liebler@electrocore.com
[11]electroCore, Inc., Basking Ridge, NJ, USA
Full list of author information is available at the end of the article

Background

Standard pharmacologic agents for the acute treatment of migraine can be limited by side effects, inconsistent efficacy, contraindications, risk of drug interactions, and their potential contribution to migraine chronification and medication overuse headache [1–5]. Opioids should be discouraged for the acute treatment of migraine due to significant safety concerns and lack of documented but remain frequently used in the emergency department setting, which significantly increases healthcare costs [6–9]. Practical alternatives are needed to address this healthcare challenge. Non-invasive neuromodulation therapies could represent a novel option for these patients [10, 11].

Non-invasive vagus nerve stimulation (nVNS; gammaCore®; electroCore, Inc., Basking Ridge, NJ, USA) demonstrated efficacy in studies of acute migraine treatment and has a strong safety and tolerability profile [12–15]. The multicenter, randomized, double-blind, sham-controlled PRESTO trial provided Class I evidence that for patients with an episodic migraine, acute treatment of migraine attacks with nVNS significantly increases the probability of having mild pain or being pain-free 2 h post stimulation [11]. The study also clearly demonstrated the practicality, safety, and tolerability of nVNS. Here, we report additional pre-defined secondary and other end points from the PRESTO study to illustrate the consistency and durability of nVNS effects across a broad range of outcomes.

Methods

Study design

Complete details of the methodology of the multicenter, randomized, double-blind, sham-controlled PRESTO trial have been reported previously [11]. The study was conducted across 10 Italian sites from January 11, 2016, through March 31, 2017, and consisted of an observational period, double-blind period, and open-label period (Fig. 1a). During the observational period, patients treated their migraine attacks with standard medications according to their individual prescriptions. Patients subsequently treated up to 5 migraine attacks with nVNS or sham stimulation during the double-blind period and up to 5 additional attacks with nVNS during the open-label period; only 1 attack could be treated in a 48-h period.

Patients

Study patients were 18 to 75 years of age, had a previous diagnosis of migraine with or without aura according to the International Classification of Headache Disorders, 3rd edition (beta version) criteria [16], were < 50 years of age at migraine onset, and had 3 to 8 migraine attacks per month with < 15 headache days per month during the last 6 months. Patients who were receiving preventive migraine medications at baseline (or other preventive medications determined to potentially interfere with the study) were required to have maintained a stable dose and frequency of these medications during the 2 months

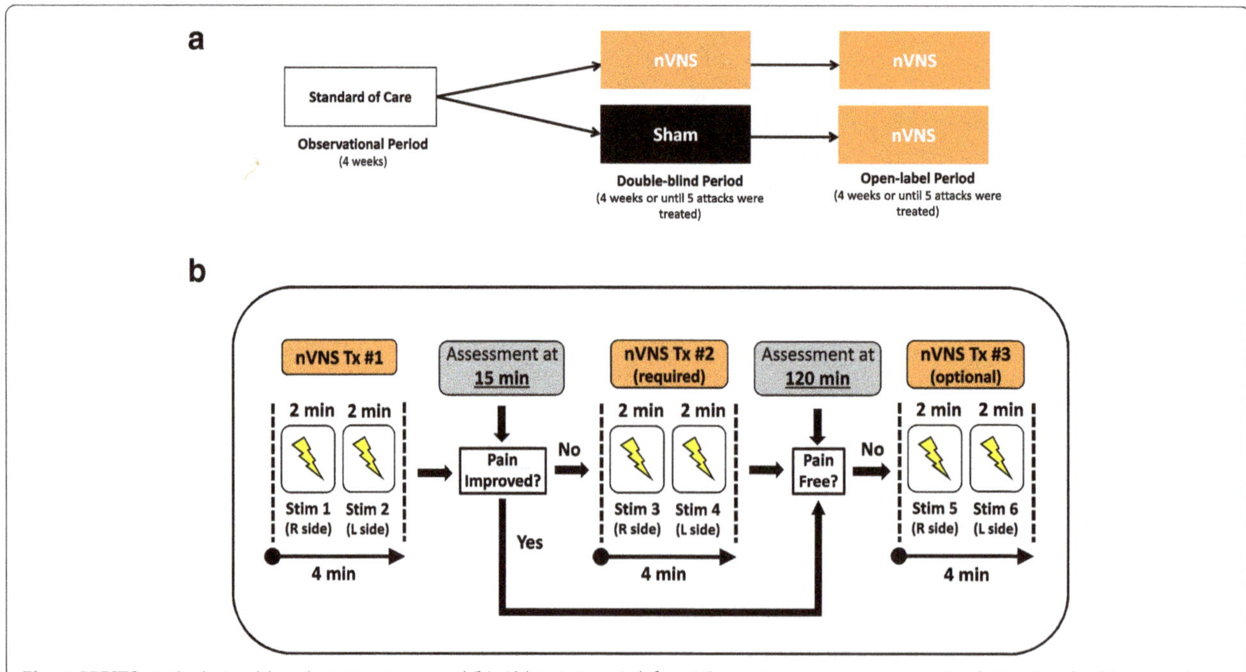

Fig. 1 PRESTO study design (**a**) and treatment protocol (**b**). Abbreviations: L, left; nvNS, non-invasive vagus nerve stimulation; R, right; Stim, stimulation; Tx, treatment

before enrollment and throughout the study; initiation of new preventive medications was not permitted during this period.

Interventions and study procedures

Patients were randomly assigned (1:1) to receive nVNS or sham (variable block design [4, 6], stratified by site). Full details of study randomization and blinding, as well as information about the active and sham devices, have been described previously [11].

Within 20 min of migraine pain onset, patients self-administered bilateral 120-s stimulations (ie, 1 stimulation each to the right and left sides of the neck) (Fig. 1b) and recorded post-treatment assessments in their study diaries 15, 30, 60, and 120 min and 24 and 48 h after completion of the initial bilateral stimulations. Patients were instructed to repeat the bilateral stimulations if pain had not improved at the 15-min assessment, and those who were not pain-free at the 120-min assessment had the option of administering an additional set of bilateral stimulations. Patients were asked to wait 120 min from the first set of stimulations before using acute rescue medication.

End points

Here, we present clinically relevant secondary and other end points not included in the original PRESTO publication to provide a more comprehensive depiction of the data set. *Pain-free* was defined as a score of 0 on the 4-point headache pain scale (with 0 indicating no pain and 3 indicating severe pain), and *pain relief* was defined as a score of 0 or 1 (both without use of rescue medication before 120 min) in a subject with pain of at least moderate severity at baseline. Attacks with mild pain (ie, a pain score of 1) at both baseline and the subsequent time point of interest were considered treatment failures. These definitions were used in assessment of the following end points:

- Percentages of all treated attacks that achieved pain freedom and pain relief at 30, 60, and 120 min for the double-blind period and at 120 min for the open-label period;
- Mean change in pain score from baseline to 30, 60, and 120 min for the first attack and for all attacks in the double-blind and open-label periods;
- Number of acute medications used per migraine attack during the observational, double-blind, and open-label periods;
- *Sustained treatment response* (defined as pain-free or pain relief [without use of rescue medication] at both 2 h and 24 h or at 2, 24, and 48 h) rates for the first attack and all attacks for the double-blind and open-label periods;
- Incidence of adverse events (AEs) and adverse device effects (ADEs).

Statistical methods

All efficacy end points were evaluated using the *intent-to-treat (ITT) population*, defined as all randomly assigned patients who treated at least 1 migraine attack in the double-blind period. Descriptive statistics were used to summarize continuous variables (means and 95% confidence intervals [CIs]) and categorical variables (frequency counts, percentages, and 95% CIs). Generalized linear mixed effects regression models were used to estimate the proportion of all attacks that were pain-free or had pain relief for the nVNS and sham groups, allowing for both subject-specific and population-averaged inferences in non-normally distributed data; *P* values were from resulting F tests. Mean change from baseline pain score was compared between treatment groups via 2-sample *t* tests for the first attack and via linear mixed effects regression models. Poisson regression was used to compare medication use per attack between treatment groups. For sustained treatment response (pain-free and pain relief), the nVNS and sham groups were compared via the chi-square test or Fisher exact test, as appropriate, for the first attack and via linear mixed effects regression models for all attacks. All data were analyzed using SAS®9.4 (SAS Institute Inc., Cary, NC, USA). Two-sided P values < 0.05 were considered statistically significant.

Results

Patients

Complete descriptions of patient disposition, demographics, and baseline characteristics in PRESTO are included in the original study publication [11]. The ITT population consisted of 243 patients (nVNS, n = 120; sham, n = 123). Two hundred thirty-nine patients entered the open-label period (nVNS, n = 117; sham, n = 122); among these, 238 patients (> 99%) completed this period (1 patient was lost to follow-up), with 220 (92%) treating at least 1 attack during the period. One patient who treated at least 1 attack in and completed the open-label period was not part of the ITT population. Table 1 summarizes key demographics and other key patient characteristics.

Efficacy: double-blind period

In the nVNS group, the percentage of all attacks that were pain-free at 60 min (16.3%) and 120 min (22.9%) was significantly greater than in the sham group (8.6% and 14.8%, respectively; $P < 0.05$ for both time points) (Fig. 2a). Similar significant results were seen for the

Table 1 Demographics and other key patient characteristics

Characteristic	nVNS (*n* = 120)	Sham (*n* = 123)	Total (*N* = 243)
Age, mean (SD), y	38.8 (11.0)	39.6 (11.8)	39.2 (11.4)
Female sex, No. (%)	95 (79.2)	91 (74.0)	186 (76.5)
Diagnosis, No. (%)			
Migraine with aura	8 (6.7)	9 (7.3)	17 (7.0)
Migraine without aura	112 (93.3)	114 (92.7)	226 (93.0)
Current preventive medication use, No. (%)	42 (35.0)	35 (28.5)	77 (31.7)
No. of acute medication days per mo,[a] mean (SD)	5.6 (1.7)	5.3 (1.7)	5.5 (1.7)
Attack severity at onset for all treated attacks in DB period, No. (%)	*n* = 359[b]	*n* = 329[b]	NA
Mild	113 (31.5)	105 (31.9)	
Moderate	156 (43.5)	166 (50.5)	
Severe	90 (25.1)	58 (17.6)	
Attack severity at onset for first treated attack in DB period, No. (%)	*n* = 119[b]	*n* = 119[b]	NA
Mild	40 (33.6)	46 (38.7)	
Moderate	51 (42.9)	55 (46.2)	
Severe	28 (23.5)	18 (15.1)	

© 2018 Tassorelli C, Grazzi L, de Tommaso M, Pierangeli G, Martelletti P, Rainero I, Dorlas S, Geppetti P, Ambrosini A, Sarchielli P, Liebler E, Barbanti P, PRESTO Study Group (2018) Non-invasive vagus nerve stimulation as acute therapy for migraine: the randomized PRESTO study [published online June 15, 2018]. Neurology:doi:https://doi.org/10.1212/WNL.0000000000005857. www.neurology.org. Adapted with permission
Abbreviations: *DB* Double-blind, *NA* Not applicable, *nVNS* Non-invasive vagus nerve stimulation, *SD* Standard deviation
[a]No. of days the patient typically takes acute migraine medication per month. [b]Patients with no reported baseline severity were excluded from this analysis

percentage of attacks with pain relief (Fig. 2b), which was 29.4% for the nVNS group and 20.3% for the sham group at 60 min (P = 0.025) and 35.2% for the nVNS group and 25.4% for the sham group at 120 min (P = 0.018).

For the first attack (Fig. 3a), the nVNS group had significantly greater decreases (vs the sham group) in mean pain score from baseline at 60 min (nVNS, 0.51; sham, 0.22; P = 0.029) and 120 min (nVNS, 0.62; sham, 0.23; P = 0.011). For all attacks (Fig. 3c), the mean decrease from baseline in pain score was significantly greater in the nVNS group (0.42) than in the sham group (0.22) at 60 min (P = 0.029) but not at 120 min (nVNS, 0.50; sham, 0.28; P = 0.057).

During the observational (run-in) period, study patients used a mean of 0.86 acute medications per attack. Acute medication use decreased during the double-blind period to 0.45 medications per attack in the nVNS group and 0.55 medications per attack in the sham group (P = 0.055).

Sustained pain-free and pain relief response rates were high in both the nVNS and sham groups at 24 h (≥75%) and 48 h (≥58%) for both the first attack and all attacks (Table 2).

Efficacy: open-label period

The percentages of all treated attacks that were pain-free (23.3%) or had pain relief (38.1%) at 120 min during the open-label period were similar to those of the nVNS group during the double-blind period (Fig. 2). Mean changes from baseline in pain score during the open-label period for the first attack (30 min, –or t; 60 min, – 0.56; 120 min, – 0.61) and for all treated attacks (30 min, – 0.38; 60 min, – 0.50; 120 min, – 0.57) were similar to those seen in the nVNS group during the double-blind period (Fig. 3). A mean of 0.46 acute medications per attack were used during the open-label period, which was similar to that of the

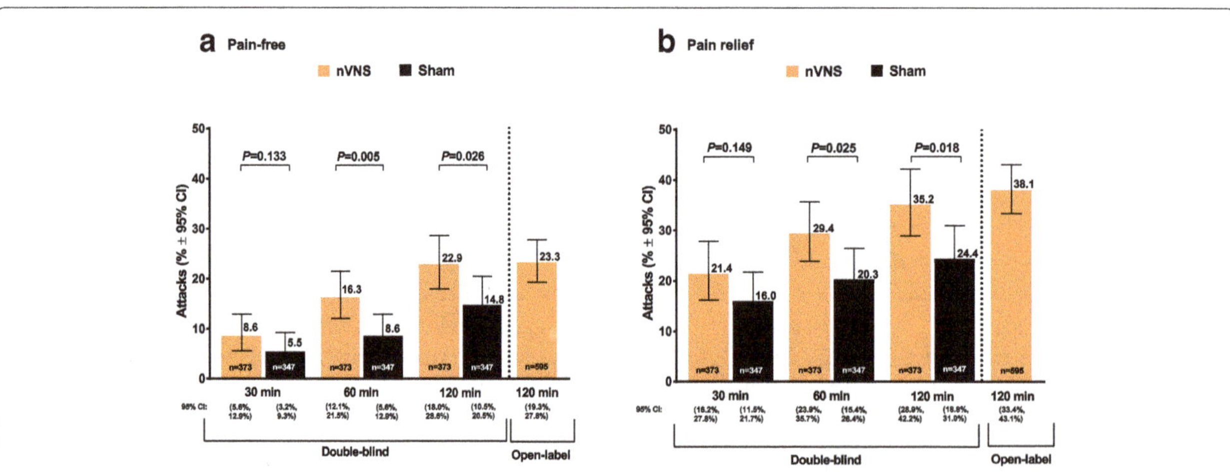

Fig. 2 Percentage of all treated attacks that were pain-free (**a**) or had pain relief (**b**) during the double-blind and open-label periods (ITT population, N = 243). Generalized linear mixed effects regression models were used to estimate the proportion of successful responses, allowing for both subject-specific and population-averaged inferences in non-normally distributed data. P values are from resulting F tests. Models were adjusted for subject's pain score at baseline, use of preventive therapies, and indicator or presence of aura. Abbreviations: CI, confidence interval; ITT, intent-to-treat; nVNS, non-invasive vagus nerve stimulation

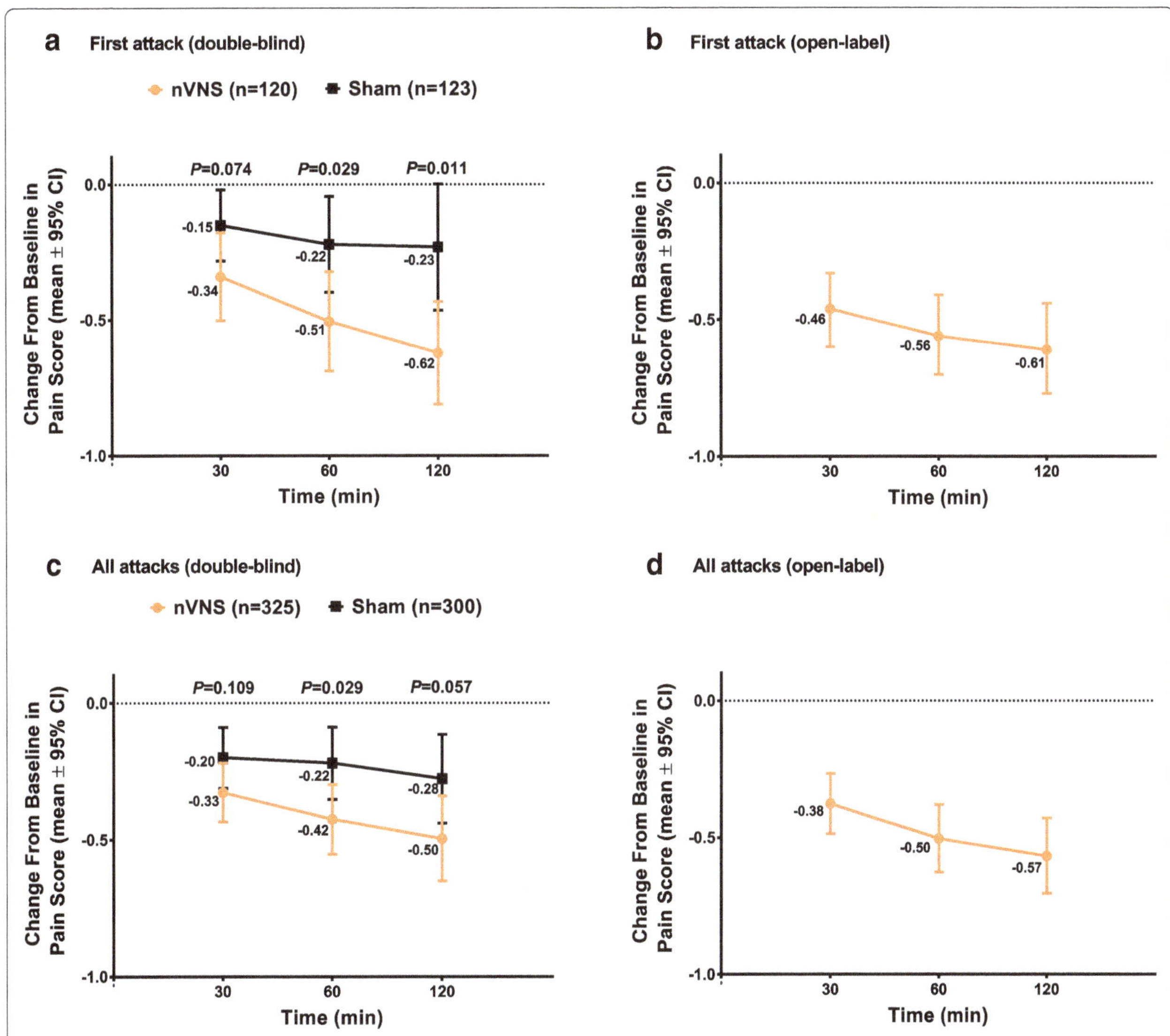

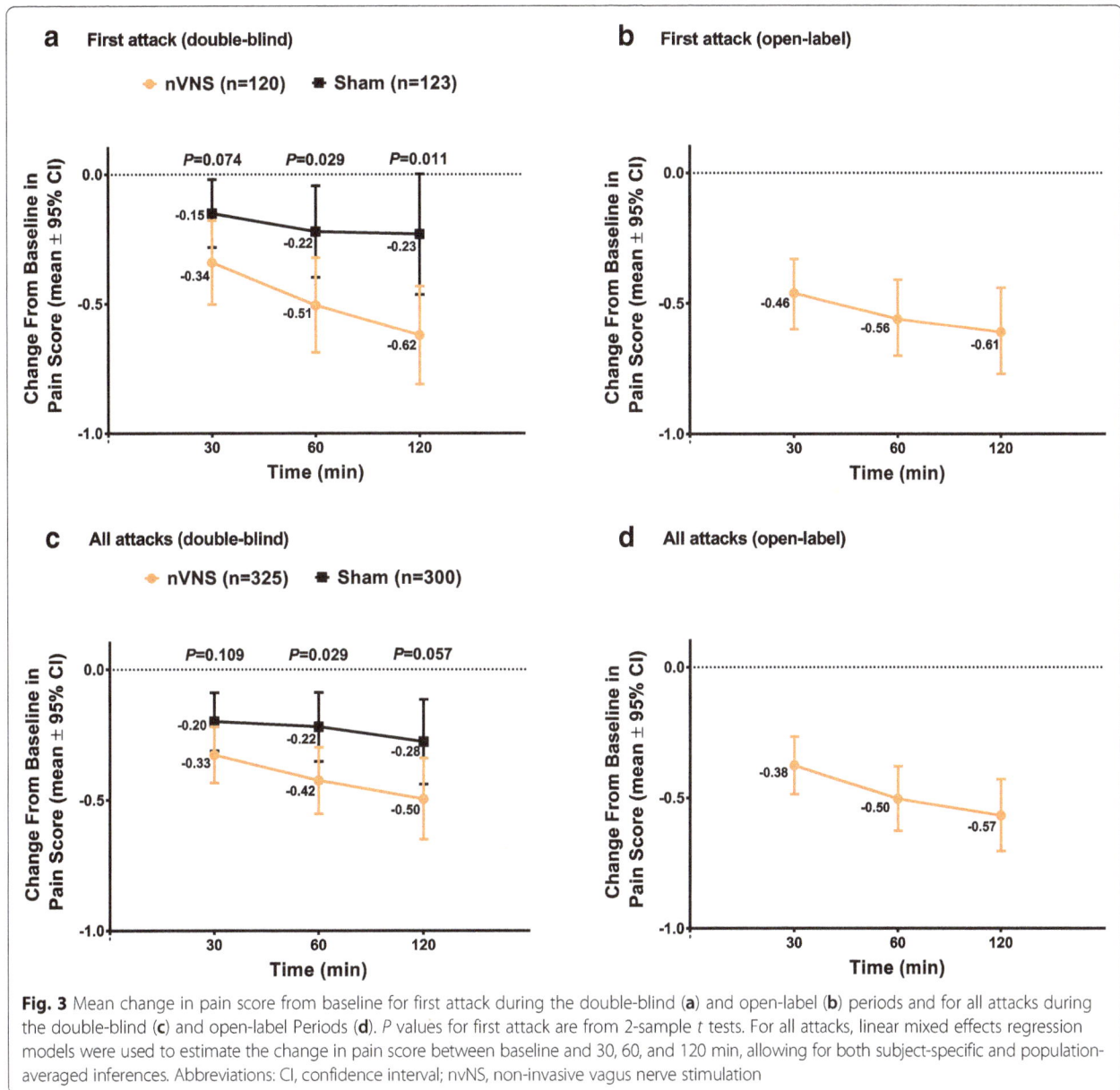

Fig. 3 Mean change in pain score from baseline for first attack during the double-blind (**a**) and open-label (**b**) periods and for all attacks during the double-blind (**c**) and open-label Periods (**d**). *P* values for first attack are from 2-sample *t* tests. For all attacks, linear mixed effects regression models were used to estimate the change in pain score between baseline and 30, 60, and 120 min, allowing for both subject-specific and population-averaged inferences. Abbreviations: CI, confidence interval; nvNS, non-invasive vagus nerve stimulation

nVNS group during the double-blind period (0.45 acute medications per attack) and was decreased from the observation period by 0.40 acute medications per attack. Sustained treatment response during the open-label period was generally similar to or greater than that seen in the nVNS group during the double-blind period (Table 2).

Safety

As previously reported [11], the incidence of AEs and ADEs was low across all study periods, and no serious AEs occurred. The only ADE reported by > 1 patient during the open-label period was vertigo, which was reported by 2 patients (1%).

Discussion

These additional results from the PRESTO study further demonstrate that nVNS is superior to sham across a broad range of relevant end points. In the nVNS group, significantly greater percentages of all attacks were pain-free or had pain relief at 60 and 120 min than in the sham group. The nVNS group also had significantly greater decreases from baseline in mean pain score for the first attack (60 and 120 min) and for all attacks (60 min). Among nVNS-treated attacks that were pain-free at 120 min, > 75% had a sustained response at 24 h. Ninety-eight percent of patients in the ITT population completed the open-label period, suggesting that the benefit from nVNS was maintained and that nVNS is a

Table 2 Sustained response at 24 and 48 h post-treatment

	Double-blind Period			Open-label Period
	nVNS	Sham	*P* Value	nVNS
	% (n/N) (95% CI)	% (n/N) (95% CI)		% (n/N) (95% CI)
All Attacks				
Pain-free				
24 h	79.0 (71/93) (67.9, 87.1)	83.7 (54/66) (69.9, 91.9)	0.532[a]	80.8 (118/146) (73.5, 86.6)
48 h	65.7 (59/93) (53.3, 76.3)	71.2 (46/66) (56.5, 82.5)	0.537[a]	70.3 (102/146) (61.6, 77.7)
Pain relief				
24 h	80.9 (109/138) (72.3, 87.3)	80.3 (78/99) (69.4, 87.9)	0.916[a]	80.5 (185/230) (74.5, 85.3)
48 h	74.1 (99/138) (64.0, 82.1)	72.1 (70/99) (60.7, 81.3)	0.775[a]	71.9 (165/230) (65.2, 77.7)
First Attack				
Pain-free				
24 h	75.0 (27/36) (57.8, 87.9)	84.6 (22/26) (65.1, 95.6)	0.359[b]	75.4 (46/61) (62.7, 85.5)
48 h	58.3 (21/36) (40.8, 74.5)	69.2 (18/26) (48.2, 85.7)	0.381[b]	65.6 (40/61) (52.3, 77.3)
Pain relief				
24 h	77.3 (58/75) (66.2, 86.2)	79.3 (46/58) (66.7, 88.8)	0.784[b]	78.8 (108/137) (71.0, 85.3)
48 h	69.3 (52/75) (57.6, 79.5)	71.0 (41/58) (57.3, 81.9)	0.866[b]	70.1 (96/137) (61.7, 77.6)

Abbreviations: *CI* Confidence interval, *nVNS* Non-invasive vagus nerve stimulation
[a]Generalized linear mixed effects regression models were used to estimate the proportion of successful responses, allowing for both subject-specific and population-averaged inferences in non-normally distributed data. [b]From chi-square test or Fisher exact test, as appropriate

durable acute therapy. The results for the total population during the open-label period were generally similar to those seen for the nVNS group during the double-blind period. Throughout the study, the incidence of AEs and ADEs was low, and no serious AEs were reported.

The findings from PRESTO are consistent with those from other clinical studies of acute nVNS use in migraine [12, 13]. They are supported by several potential mechanisms of action for the acute benefits of vagus nerve stimulation, including inhibition of central excitability through suppression of glutamate release, suppression of acute nociceptive activation of trigeminocervical neurons, and curbing expression of proteins associated with central sensitization of trigeminal neurons [17–19].

The high rates of sustained 24-h pain-free response to nVNS seen in PRESTO (> 75%) stand in contrast to the lower rates reported for oral triptans (10%–30%) and single-pulse transcranial magnetic stimulation (29%) [10, 20]. The protocol of the single-pulse transcranial magnetic stimulation study called for a study population restricted to patients with aura and a treatment time that was independent from the onset of pain (ie, within 1 h after aura onset), making comparison with the nVNS findings challenging [10]. The majority of patients enrolled in the PRESTO study had migraine without aura, and nVNS was delivered promptly after the onset of migraine pain (ie, within 20 min) [11]. In the majority of the triptan clinical trials, treatment was not initiated until migraine pain reached a moderate/severe level, partially due to the desire to avoid unnecessary adverse effects [20, 21]. Consistent with findings from PRESTO [22], rates of sustained response appear to be higher with the use of triptans during the early stages of migraine (34%–53%) than during the later stages (19%–31%) [21, 23]. These observations suggest that there are benefits to treating early in the course of migraine attacks—in a sense, intervening before the migraine process is fully activated. High rates of sustained pain-free response in both the nVNS and sham groups in PRESTO suggest that intervention early in the course of migraine might confer benefits, irrespective of the treatment.

Together with findings from multiple previous studies [12–15, 24–26], these results from PRESTO further highlight the clinical utility, practicality, and flexibility of nVNS. Across the double-blind and open-label periods, nVNS was used to treat > 900 migraine attacks, with data collected at multiple time points for each attack, demonstrating its consistent efficacy, safety, and tolerability as acute treatment for these attacks. nVNS can be used as monotherapy or in conjunction with other treatments without risk of pharmacologic interactions, offering a clinical versatility that other acute migraine treatments lack. These advantages, along with its convenience and ease of use, make nVNS an appealing and pragmatic option for early, adjunctive, and/or frequent use in the acute treatment of migraine. nVNS could also help minimize the risk of medication overuse associated with traditional acute treatments and reduce the frequency of opioid use for the acute treatment of migraine in the emergency department setting.

This study has a number of limitations. The selection of an appropriate sham device in neuromodulation studies is challenging. In accordance with previous recommendations to ensure maintenance of the study blind [27], the sham device used in PRESTO produced an active signal that could be perceived by the user but was not designed to stimulate the vagus nerve; recent data suggest that the strength of the sham device's signal may have inadvertently activated the vagus nerve and could have inflated the responses to sham treatment across all end points [28]. This phenomenon, which merits further investigation, may have been related to a psychobiological placebo effect but more likely resulted from the unanticipated physiologically active signal that may have decreased the difference in therapeutic gain seen between the nVNS and sham groups [11].

During both the double-blind and open-label periods, the mean number of acute medications used per migraine attack was substantially lower than that seen during the observational period. Such a decrease in medication use could be interpreted as evidence of treatment efficacy; however, these results must be interpreted with caution, as patients were encouraged to refrain from using acute medications for 120 min after stimulation with the study device. This study limitation most likely contributed to decreases in acute medication use in both the nVNS and sham groups during the double-blind period and may partially explain the lack of significance between treatment groups for this end point.

Conclusions

These results from clinically relevant secondary and other end points of the PRESTO study demonstrate the efficacy and reliability of nVNS for the acute treatment of migraine. nVNS provided dependable efficacy for the successful treatment of multiple attacks and can be used safely while preserving a patient's option to use additional acute medications as rescue therapy, thus potentially decreasing the risk of medication overuse. Together, these findings highlight the flexibility and practicality of nVNS as a front-line option for acute migraine attacks.

Abbreviations

ADE: Adverse device effect; AE: Adverse event; CI: Confidence interval; DB: Double-blind; ITT: Intent to treat; L: Left; NA: Not applicable; nVNS: Non-invasive vagus nerve stimulation; R: Right; SD: Standard deviation; Stim: Stimulation; Tx: Treatment

Acknowledgments

Medical writing support was provided by Elizabeth Barton, MS, of MedLogix Communications, LLC, in cooperation with the authors. Statistical analyses were conducted by Candace McClure, PhD, of North American Science Associates Inc.

Co-investigators:

The PRESTO Study Group

Coinvestigators are listed by study site: 1. Headache Science Centre, National Neurological Institute C. Mondino Fo undation and University of Pavia: **Cristina assorelli, MD, PhD (Principal Investigator)**; Vito Bitetto (Subinvestigator); Roberto De Icco, MD (Subinvestigator); Daniele Martinelli, MD (Subinvestigator); Grazia Sances, MD (Subinvestigator); Monica Bianchi, MD (Research Nurse); 2. Carlo Besta Neurological Institute and Foundation: **Licia Grazzi, MD (Principal Investigator)**; Anna Maria Padovan (Subinvestigator); 3. University of Bari Aldo Moro: **Marina de Tommaso, MD, PhD (Principal Investigator)**; Katia Ricci (Subinvestigator); Eleonora Vecchio, MD, PhD (Subinvestigator); 4. IRCCS Istituto delle Scienze Neurologiche di Bologna: **Pietro Cortelli, MD, PhD (Principal Investigator)**; Sabina Cevoli, MD, PhD (Subinvestigator); Giulia Pierangeli, MD, PhD (Subinvestigator); Rossana Terlizzi, MD (Subinvestigator); 5. Sapienza University of Rome: **Paolo Martelletti, MD, PhD (Principal Investigator)**; Andrea Negro, MD (Subinvestigator); Gabriella Addolorata Chiarillo (Research Nurse); 6. University of Turin: **Innocenzo Rainero, MD, PhD (Principal Investigator)**; Paola De Martino, MD, PhD (Subinvestigator); Annalisa Gai, MD (Subinvestigator); Flora Govone, MD (Subinvestigator); Federica Masuzzo, MD (Subinvestigator); Elisa Rubino, MD, PhD (Subinvestigator); Maria Claudia Torrieri, MD (Subinvestigator); Alessandro Vacca, MD (Subinvestigator); 7. University Hospital of Careggi: **Pierangelo Geppetti, MD, PhD (Principal Investigator)**; Alberto Chiarugi, MD, PhD (Subinvestigator); Francesco De Cesaris (Subinvestigator); Simone Li Puma (Subinvestigator); Chiara Lupi (Subinvestigator); Ilaria Marone (Subinvestigator); 8. IRCCS Neuromed: **Anna Ambrosini, MD, PhD (Principal Investigator)**; Armando Perrotta, MD, PhD (Subinvestigator); 9. Santa Maria della Misericordia Hospital: **Paola Sarchielli, MD, PhD (Principal Investigator)**; Laura Bernetti, MD (Subinvestigator); Ilenia Corbelli, MD, PhD (Subinvestigator); Michele Romoli, MD (Subinvestigator); Simone Simoni, MD (Subinvestigator); Angela Verzina, MD (Subinvestigator); 10. IRCCS San Raffaele Pisana: **Piero Barbanti, MD, PhD (Principal Investigator)**; Cinzia Aurilia, MD (Subinvestigator); Gabriella Egeo, MD, PhD (Subinvestigator); Luisa Fofi, MD (Subinvestigator). electroCore Study Team: **Eric Liebler (Senior Vice President, Neurology)**; Annelie Andersson (Senior Director, Clinical Director); Lia Spitzer (Senior Director, Clinical/Study Manager); Juana Marin, MD (Clinical Advisor, Safety Monitor); Candace McClure, PhD (North American Science Associates Inc., Statistician); Lisa Thackeray, MS (North American Science Associates Inc., Statistician), Maria Giovanna Baldi (Monitor); Daniela Di Maro (Monitor).

Funding

This study was sponsored by electroCore, Inc.

Authors' contributions

LG, EL, and CT contributed to the PRESTO study design. All primary investigators were involved in participant recruitment and treatment for the PRESTO study. All authors participated in data collection, interpretation, and validation and had full access to all study data. CT and EL were involved in data analysis. EL drafted and revised the manuscript for content in cooperation with all authors. All authors reviewed, critiqued, and contributed to revision of the manuscript content and provided approval of the final manuscript draft to be submitted to the *Journal of Headache and Pain*. The principal author, PM, takes responsibility for all aspects of the work and for ensuring that questions related to the accuracy or integrity of any part of the work were appropriately investigated and resolved.

Competing interests

P. Martelletti has received research grants, advisory board fees, or travel fees from ACRAF; Allergan S.p.A.; Amgen Inc.; electroCore, Inc.; Novartis AG; and Teva Pharmaceutical Industries Ltd.

L. Grazzi has received consultancy and advisory fees from Allergan S.p.A. and electroCore, Inc.

G. Pierangeli has nothing to disclose.

I. Rainero has received consultancy fees from electroCore, Inc., and Mylan N.V. and research grants from the European Commission – Horizon 2020. He is also a principal investigator for RCTs sponsored by Axovant Sciences Ltd. and TauRx Pharmaceuticals Ltd.

P. Geppetti has received consultancy fees from Allergan S.p.A.; electroCore, Inc.; Evidera; Novartis AG; Pfizer Inc.; and Sanofi S.p.A. and research grants from Chiesi Farmaceutici S.p.A. He is also a principal investigator for RCTs sponsored by Eli Lilly and Company; Novartis AG; and Teva Pharmaceutical Industries Ltd.

A. Ambrosini has received consultancy fees from Almirall, S.A., and travel grants from Allergan S.p.A., Almirall, S.A., and Novartis.

P. Sarchielli has received clinical study fees from Allergan S.p.A.

P. Barbanti has received consultancy fees from Allergan S.p.A.; electroCore, Inc.; Janssen Pharmaceuticals, Inc.; Lusofarmaco; and Visufarma and advisory fees from Abbott Laboratories; Merck & Co., Inc.; Novartis AG; and Teva Pharmaceutical Industries Ltd. He is also a principal investigator for RCTs sponsored by Alder BioPharmaceuticals Inc.; Eli Lilly and Company; GlaxoSmithKline Pharmaceuticals Ltd.; and Teva Pharmaceutical Industries Ltd.

C. Tassorelli has consulted for Allergan S.p.A.; electroCore, Inc.; Eli Lilly and Company; and Novartis AG and has received research grants from the European Commission and the Italian Ministry of Health. She is also a principal investigator or collaborator for RCTs sponsored by Alder BioPharmaceuticals Inc.; Eli Lilly and Company; Novartis; and Teva Pharmaceutical Industries Ltd.
E. Liebler is an employee of electroCore, Inc., and receives stock ownership.
M. de Tommaso has received advisory fees from Allergan S.p.A.; Neopharmed; and Pfizer Inc.

Author details
[1]Department of Clinical and Molecular Medicine, Sapienza University, Rome, Italy. [2]Headache and Pain Unit, Istituto di Ricovero e Cura a Carattere Scientifico (IRCCS) San Raffaele Pisana, Rome, Italy. [3]Neuroalgology Unit, Carlo Besta Neurological Institute and Foundation, Milan, Italy. [4]IRCCS Istituto delle Scienze Neurologiche di Bologna, Bologna, Italy. [5]Department of Neuroscience, University of Turin, Turin, Italy. [6]Headache Centre, University Hospital of Careggi, Florence, Italy. [7]IRCCS Neuromed, Pozzilli, IS, Italy. [8]Neurologic Clinic, Santa Maria della Misericordia Hospital, Perugia, Italy. [9]Headache Science Centre, IRCCS C. Mondino Foundation, Pavia, Italy. [10]Department of Brain and Behavioral Sciences, University of Pavia, Pavia, Italy. [11]electroCore, Inc., Basking Ridge, NJ, USA. [12]Neurophysiology and Pain Unit, University of Bari Aldo Moro, Bari, Italy.

References

1. Lopes M, Dunn JD, Calhoun AH, Rapoport AM (2012) Concepts in acute migraine management: clinical and managed care perspectives. Am J Pharm Benefits 4(5):201–206
2. Negro A, Koverech A, Martelletti P (2018) Serotonin receptor agonists in the acute treatment of migraine: a review on their therapeutic potential. J Pain Res 11:515–526. https://doi.org/10.2147/JPR.S132833
3. Puledda F, Messina R, Goadsby PJ (2017) An update on migraine: current understanding and future directions. J Neurol 264(9):2031–2039. https://doi.org/10.1007/s00415-017-8434-y
4. Rolan PE (2012) Drug interactions with triptans: which are clinically significant? CNS Drugs 26(11):949–957. https://doi.org/10.1007/s40263-012-0002-5
5. Bigal ME, Lipton RB (2009) Overuse of acute migraine medications and migraine chronification. Curr Pain Headache Rep 13(4):301–307
6. Bonafede M, Sapra S, Shah N, Tepper S, Cappell K, Desai P (2018) Direct and indirect healthcare resource utilization and costs among migraine patients in the United States. Headache 58(5):700–714. https://doi.org/10.1111/head.13275
7. Friedman BW, Irizarry E, Solorzano C, Latev A, Rosa K, Zias E, Vinson DR, Bijur PE, Gallagher EJ (2017) Randomized study of IV prochlorperazine plus diphenhydramine vs IV hydromorphone for migraine. Neurology 89(20): 2075–2082. https://doi.org/10.1212/WNL.0000000000004642
8. Friedman BW, West J, Vinson DR, Minen MT, Restivo A, Gallagher EJ (2015) Current management of migraine in US emergency departments: an analysis of the National Hospital Ambulatory Medical Care Survey. Cephalalgia 35(4):301–309. https://doi.org/10.1177/0333102414539055
9. Orr SL, Friedman BW, Christie S, Minen MT, Bamford C, Kelley NE, Tepper D (2016) Management of Adults with Acute Migraine in the emergency department: the American headache society evidence assessment of parenteral pharmacotherapies. Headache 56(6):911–940. https://doi.org/10.1111/head.12835
10. Lipton RB, Dodick DW, Silberstein SD, Saper JR, Aurora SK, Pearlman SH, Fischell RE, Ruppel PL, Goadsby PJ (2010) Single-pulse transcranial magnetic stimulation for acute treatment of migraine with aura: a randomised, double-blind, parallel-group, sham-controlled trial. Lancet Neurol 9(4):373–380. https://doi.org/10.1016/S1474-4422(10)70054-5
11. Tassorelli C, Grazzi L, de Tommaso M, et al. (2018) Non-invasive vagus nerve stimulation as acute therapy for migraine: the randomized PRESTO study. Neurology 91(4):e364–e373.
12. Barbanti P, Grazzi L, Egeo G, Padovan AM, Liebler E, Bussone G (2015) Non-invasive vagus nerve stimulation for acute treatment of high-frequency and chronic migraine: an open-label study. J Headache Pain 16:61. https://doi.org/10.1186/s10194-015-0542-4
13. Goadsby PJ, Grosberg BM, Mauskop A, Cady R, Simmons KA (2014) Effect of noninvasive vagus nerve stimulation on acute migraine: an open-label pilot study. Cephalalgia 34(12):986–993. https://doi.org/10.1177/0333102414524494
14. Kinfe TM, Pintea B, Muhammad S, Zaremba S, Roeske S, Simon BJ, Vatter H (2015) Cervical non-invasive vagus nerve stimulation (nVNS) for preventive and acute treatment of episodic and chronic migraine and migraine-associated sleep disturbance: a prospective observational cohort study. J Headache Pain 16:101. https://doi.org/10.1186/s10194-015-0582-9
15. Silberstein SD, Calhoun AH, Lipton RB, Grosberg BM, Cady RK, Dorlas S, Simmons KA, Mullin C, Liebler EJ, Goadsby PJ, Saper JR, Group ES (2016) Chronic migraine headache prevention with noninvasive vagus nerve stimulation: the EVENT study. Neurology 87(5):529–538. https://doi.org/10.1212/WNL.0000000000002918
16. (2013) The International Classification of Headache Disorders, 3rd edition (beta version). Cephalalgia 33(9):629–808. https://doi.org/10.1177/0333102413485658
17. Akerman S, Simon B, Romero-Reyes M (2017) Vagus nerve stimulation suppresses acute noxious activation of trigeminocervical neurons in animal models of primary headache. Neurobiol Dis 102:96–104. https://doi.org/10.1016/j.nbd.2017.03.004
18. Hawkins JL, Cornelison LE, Blankenship BA, Durham PL (2017) Vagus nerve stimulation inhibits trigeminal nociception in a rodent model of episodic migraine. Pain Rep 2(6):e628. https://doi.org/10.1097/PR9.0000000000000628
19. Oshinsky ML, Murphy AL, Hekierski H Jr, Cooper M, Simon BJ (2014) Noninvasive vagus nerve stimulation as treatment for trigeminal allodynia. Pain 155(5):1037–1042. https://doi.org/10.1016/j.pain.2014.02.009
20. Ferrari MD, Roon KI, Lipton RB, Goadsby PJ (2001) Oral triptans (serotonin 5-HT(1B/1D) agonists) in acute migraine treatment: a meta-analysis of 53 trials. Lancet 358(9294):1668–1675. https://doi.org/10.1016/S0140-6736(01)06711-3
21. Cady R, Elkind A, Goldstein J, Keywood C (2004) Randomized, placebo-controlled comparison of early use of frovatriptan in a migraine attack versus dosing after the headache has become moderate or severe. Curr Med Res Opin 20(9):1465–1472. https://doi.org/10.1185/030079904X2745
22. Grazzi L, Tassorelli C, de Tommaso M, Pierangeli G, Martelletti P, Rainero I, Geppetti P, Ambrosini A, Sarchielli P, Liebler E, Barbanti P (2018) Practical and clinical utility of non-invasive vagus nerve stimulation (nVNS) for the acute treatment of migraine: post hoc assessment of the randomized, sham-controlled, double-blind PRESTO trial [abstract MTIS2018-059]. Cephalalgia 38(1S):42. https://doi.org/10.1177/0333102418789865
23. Cady RK, Sheftell F, Lipton RB, O'Quinn S, Jones M, Putnam DG, Crisp A, Metz A, McNeal S (2000) Effect of early intervention with sumatriptan on migraine pain: retrospective analyses of data from three clinical trials. Clin Ther 22(9):1035–1048
24. Gaul C, Diener HC, Silver N, Magis D, Reuter U, Andersson A, Liebler EJ, Straube A, Group PS (2016) Non-invasive vagus nerve stimulation for prevention and acute treatment of chronic cluster headache (PREVA): a randomised controlled study. Cephalalgia 36(6):534–546. https://doi.org/10.1177/0333102415607070
25. Goadsby PJ, de Coo IF, Silver N, Tyagi A, Ahmed F, Gaul C, Jensen RH, Diener HC, Rabe K, Straube A, Liebler E, Marin J, Ferrari MD, Group AS (2018) Non-invasive vagus nerve stimulation for the acute treatment of episodic and chronic cluster headache: findings from the randomized, double-blind, sham-controlled ACT2 study. Cephalalgia 38(5):959–969. https://doi.org/10.1177/0333102417744362
26. Silberstein SD, Mechtler LL, Kudrow DB, Calhoun AH, McClure C, Saper JR, Liebler EJ, Rubenstein Engel E, Tepper SJ, Group AS (2016) Non-invasive vagus nerve stimulation for the acute treatment of cluster headache: findings from the randolnnocenzo Raineromized, double-blind, sham-controlled ACT1 study. Headache 56(8):1317–1332. https://doi.org/10.1111/head.12896
27. Asano E, Goadsby PJ (2013) How do we fashion better trials for neurostimulator studies in migraine? Neurology 80(8):694. https://doi.org/10.1212/WNL.0b013e3182825174
28. Moeller M, Schroeder CF, May A (2018) Comparison of active and "sham" non-invasive vagal nerve stimulation on lacrimation in healthy volunteers [abstract PS76]. Headache 58(suppl 2):135–136. https://doi.org/10.1111/head.13306

4

Polarity-specific modulation of pain processing by transcranial direct current stimulation – a blinded longitudinal fMRI study

Steffen Naegel[1*], Josephine Biermann[1], Nina Theysohn[2], Christoph Kleinschnitz[1], Hans-Christoph Diener[1], Zaza Katsarava[1,3,5,6], Mark Obermann[1,4] and Dagny Holle[1]

Abstract

Background: To enrich the hitherto insufficient understanding regarding the mechanisms of action of transcranial direct current stimulation (tDCS) in pain disorders, we investigated its modulating effects on cerebral pain processing using functional magnetic resonance imaging (fMRI).

Methods: Thirteen right-handed healthy participants received 20 min of 1.5 mA tDCS applied over the primary motor cortex thrice and under three different stimulation pattern (1.anodal-tDCS, 2.cathodal-tDCS, and 3.sham-tDCS) in a blinded cross-over design. After tDCS neural response to electric trigeminal-nociceptive stimulation was investigated using a block designed fMRI.

Results: Pain stimulation showed a distinct activation pattern within well-established brain regions associated with pain processing. Following anodal tDCS increased activation was detected in the thalamus, basal ganglia, amygdala, cingulate, precentral, postcentral, and dorsolateral prefrontal cortex, while cathodal t-DCS showed decreased response in these areas ($p_{FWE} < 0.05$). Interestingly the observed effect was reversed in both control conditions (visual- and motor-stimulation). Behavioral data remained unchanged irrespective of the tDCS stimulation mode.

Conclusions: This study demonstrates polarity-specific modulation of cerebral pain processing, in reconfirmation of previous electrophysiological data. Anodal tDCS leads to an activation of the central pain-network while cathodal tDCS does not. Results contribute to a network-based understanding of tDCS's impact on cerebral pain-processing.

Keywords: Neuromodulation, Nociception, Pain, fMRI, tDCS, Transcranial direct current stimulation

Background

Experimental and non-experimental pain causes activation in a complex neuronal network previously reported as pain neuromatrix, reflecting the multidimensionality of pain [1]. Sensory-discriminative components of pain are processed by primary (S1) and secondary (S2) somatosensory cortices, the thalamus, and posterior part of the insula in the lateral pain system [2], while affective-motivational components are processed in the medial pain-system including the anterior cingulate cortex (ACC), and anterior parts of the insula [3–6]. Several other brain areas are involved in motor, cognitive and autonomic aspects of pain, as well as pain modulation [2, 3, 7–10].

Some pain and headache disorders appear to be caused by a dysbalanced network [11], and neuromodulatory approaches are increasingly used therapies. Transcranial direct current stimulation (tDCS) is a non-invasive, safe, and painless technique which is applied in various chronic pain disorders such as fibromyalgia [12], spinal cord injury pain [13] and menstrual migraine [14]. TDCS modulates activity in brain regions specific to the site of application and stimulation parameters. For anodal stimulation a raised and for cathodal stimulation a

* Correspondence: steffen.naegel@uk-essen.de
[1]Department of Neurology, University of Duisburg-Essen, University Hospital Essen, Hufelandstr. 55, 45122 Essen, Germany
Full list of author information is available at the end of the article

decreased level of cortical excitability at the targeted brain area was previously shown [4, 15]. Pain reduction caused by stimulation of the primary motor-cortex may result from modulation of the pain processing network, but so far is only insufficiently understood.

Methods

The aim of this study was to assess the effect of tDCS on cerebral pain processing using functional magnetic resonance imaging (fMRI) and to identify the brain areas involved in this neuro-modulation.

Thirteen (6 women) healthy subjects were investigated using functional resonance magnetic imaging (fMRI). Inclusion criteria were age over 18 years and right-handedness. Exclusion criteria were primary headache-syndromes and other pain conditions as well as psychiatric or other somatic illnesses. All thirteen participants did not experience any pain or injuries during the study period and four weeks prior to study inclusion, and all were advised to prevent sleep-deprivation before study participation and to not take any alcohol, central acting drugs or pain medication for at least 24 h before each experiment.

All participants gave their written informed consent according to the Declaration of Helsinki prior to study inclusion. The local ethics committee of the University of Duisburg-Essen approved the study protocol.

Due to the small number of fMRI studies and tDCS no formal power calculation was performed. The sample size was estimated corresponding to previous tDCS studies using fMRI.

Study design and fMRI-data acquisition

Imaging was performed using a 3 Tesla MRI scanner (Magnetom Skyra, Siemens Healthcare, Erlangen, Germany) equipped with a standard 20-channel head/neck coil. All participants underwent the standardized scanning procedure three times. The order of the DC-Stimulation (sham, anodal, and cathodal) was pseudo-randomly preassigned for each subject and subjects were blinded regarding stimulation type at any time. Between the scanning time points a two-month interval was kept to prevent carryover-effects. Imaging included T1 (magnetization prepared rapid acquisition gradient echo, MPRAGE), and functional magnetic resonance imaging (EPI, 3x3x3mm, 52 Slices, FOV-read = 240 mm, TR =3020 ms TE = 26 ms flip-angle 90°). Order of sequences including DC-stimulation was equal on every appointment and is illustrated in Fig. 1.

Prior to analysis all images were rated regarding image quality and pathologies. This was double-checked by an experienced neuro-radiologist (N.T.) and found to be unremarkable in all subjects.

FMRI was performed using a block-design with 7 images per task/stimulus-epoch (=21,14 s), and baseline periods with a duration 13 images (=39,26 s). Three different conditions (A, B, C) were investigated.

A: Nociceptive stimuli (11 blocks/epochs per session) were applied to the right forehead by a special copper platinum planar concentric electrode (Walter Graphtek, Luebeck, Germany, http://www.walter-graphtek.com/) 10 mm above the entry zone of the supraorbital nerve. It was previously shown that this setup is able to specifically depolarize C-Fibers and thereby, is pain specific [16]. In each epoch 7 nociceptive stimuli (=one per image) were administered. Each stimulus was applied as pulse-train of five pules (temporal summation, monopolar square wave, duration 0.5 ms, pulse interval 5 ms, pulse length: 1000 μs, V_{max}: 400 V). Pulses were generated by a commercially available high voltage constant current stimulator (DS7AH, Digitimer Ltd., Welwyn Garden City, England, UK). Stimulus intensity was adjusted to a numeric rating scale (NRS) of 5/10 by setting the amperage before MRI and tDCS procedure. During fMRI subjects noted the experienced pain intensity after every stimulation block applying NRS (0–10) within a 6 s rating period.
B: Visual stimulation (2 blocks/epochs per session) using a build in projection-system rearwards the MRI was applied with a 20 × 15 square checkerboard matrix alternation (frequency of 4 Hz over 7 consecutive images) projected with a size of 100cmx75cm covering the complete field of view out of the 70 cm MR-Bore.
C: The third condition was a motor task (3 blocks per session). Subjects were instructed to tap the left index and thumb a frequency of 1 Hz. Visual instruction was

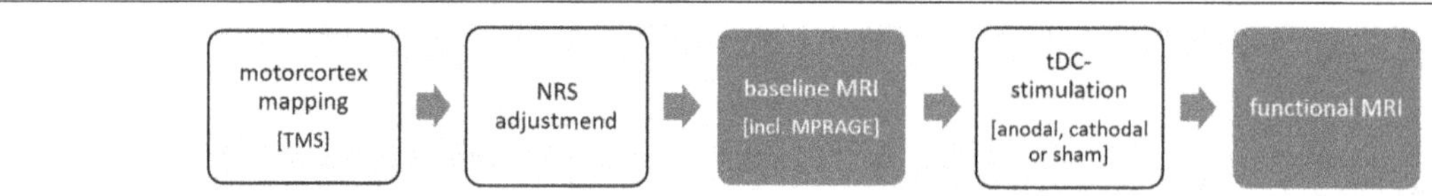

Fig. 1 Study sequence per appointment. Illustration of the study sequence for each appointment (3 per subject), white boxes represent activity outside the scanner including motorcortex mapping using transcranial magnetic stimulation, pre DCS stimulus intensity adjustment (NRS = 5), and DC Stimulation (anodal, cathodal or sham in pseudorandomized order). Grey boxes represent MRI measurements including anatomical and functional MRI)

given for 7 consecutive images and subjects were advised to quickly re-close eyes during these blocks and to stop tapping when scanner room darkens again. Accuracy was controlled from scanners anteroom.

Functional MRI data processing and analysis

Functional MRI data processing and analysis was performed using SPM8 (Wellcome Trust Centre for Neuroimaging, UCL, London, UK [https://www.fil.ion.ucl.ac.uk/spm/]) and MATLAB (Matlab R2015a, The MathWorks, Natick, MA, USA). First four scans were excluded to prevent tampering due to general scanner drift. Preprocessing included "realign and unwarp", co-registration of the structural and mean functional image, normalization into the Montreal Neurological Institute (MNI)-space by segmentation of the anatomical image, and normalization of the co-registered EPI images. Spatial smoothing was performed with an isotropic Gaussian kernel of 8 mm full-width at half maximum [17].

First level statistics was performed using a general linear model with repeated box-cars convolved with a hemodynamic response function provided with SPM8. In that model all three conditions as well as the 6 s rating period were considered. To compensate for the presence of movement artefacts, movement parameters were included as covariates.

To assess activation pattern of the conditions (trigeminal nociception, visual stimulation, and motor activity) a primary, explorative random-effects group analysis was performed averaging all DC-stimulation types with a whole brain family wise error corrected (FWE) threshold of $p < 0.05$.

To investigate effects of the tDC-stimulation on cerebral activation a definite second level statistic was performed using a longitudinal random-effects model feed with the results from first level for trigeminal nociception, visual, and motor-tasks. To investigate the maximum effect on BOLD (blood oxygen level depended)-signal changes induced by the applied tDC-stimulation, a direct comparison of anodal and cathodal stimulation was calculated. For the evaluation of trigeminal nociception, we a priori identified regions generally accepted to be involved in pain processing as described previously [18]. Anatomical regions of interest (ROIs) were derived from "automated anatomic labeling toolbox"-templates (AAL) for the thalamus, amygdala, basal ganglia (combined AAL template: caudate + pallidum + putamen), dorsolateral prefrontal, insular, supplementary motor, primary somatosensory, cingulate cortex (combined AAL template: cingulum_ant + cingulum_mid), and the cerebellum (combined AAL template: Cerebelum_Crus1 + 2, Cerebelum3–10, and Vermis_1–10) using marsbar [19, 20]. As the left primary motorcortex was directly targeted by tDCS this (combined AAL template: paracentral_Lobule_L + precentral_L) was additionally added as ROI. Significance level for exploratory analysis was set to $p_{unc} < .0005$. Region of interest analysis was applied using Family-Wise-Error correction with a significance level of $p_{FWE} < .05$.

For all fMRI data, only results surviving corrected thresholding with $p_{FWE} < 0.05$ are reported and discussed (Exception: Table 2 additionally presenting results from the exploratory analysis, $p_{unc} < .0005$).

Statistical analysis on clinical and demographic data

For demographics and behavioral data ANOVA ($p < 0.05$) with post-hoc Bonferroni analysis was performed with IBM SPSS Statistics Version 22 (International Business Machines Corporation, Armonk, New York, USA).

DC-stimulation

After pre-imaging (e.g. MPRAGE) subjects left the scanner and received DC-Stimulation of the left primary motor cortex (M1) applied by HDCstim (Newronika s.r.l., Milan, Italy) equipped with two saline-soaked sponge covered electrodes (anode: 5x5cm^2; cathode: 6 × 8.4cm^2). Stimulation was performed for 20 min with an intensity of 1,5 mA and a current ramp of 7 s. The opposite electrode was placed over the contralateral supraorbital region. The primary motor-cortex was mapped using transcranial magnetic stimulation (TMS) (MagPro X100, MagVenture Inc., Atlanta, GA, USA) identifying the representation of the right first dorsal interosseous muscle (IOD1) one hour before MR-recording. TMS was performed using a figure-of-eight coil (handle directed rearwards) and superficial MEP recording. Three tDCS application modes were used: 1.) anodal (a-tDCS), 2.) cathodal (c-tDCS) and 3.) sham (s-tDCS). For s-tDCS 30 s of anodal stimulation was delivered and afterwards ceased without participants knowledge, which is an established blinding method [21, 22]. The M1 was targeted as in the current literature it is the most convincing stimulation-region regarding clinical and experimental pain [23–25].

Results

Demographic and behavioral data

We investigated 13 healthy subjects (6 female). All subjects were right-handed and average age was 23,92 (± 1.98 SD) years. No subject suffered from any relevant illnesses, including pain and headache disorders. Analysis of collected behavioral data did not show any significant differences in pain ratings on a verbal rating scale of zero to ten (0 = no pain, 10 = worst imaginable pain; $p = 0.377$, NRS anodal 6.81 ± 1.58, cathodal 5.99 ± 1.53, sham 6.55 ± 1.43) nor in applied nociceptive stimulus intensity ($p = 0.995$, anodal 1.31 ± 0.97 mA, cathodal 1.28 ± 0.98 mA, sham 1.28 ± 0.98 mA).

Functional magnetic resonance imaging (fMRI)

Explorative data assessment

Single subject activations (not provided) and explorative primary group analyses showed cerebral activation pattern consistent with anatomical knowledge and previously reported results for pain-, motor- and visual-processing (Table 1).

BOLD-modulation by DC-stimulation

Comparison of the different stimulation modalities revealed stimulation mode dependent activation/BOLD-response differences for trigeminal nociception, motor and visual stimulation.

Modulation of nociceptive processing

Comparing anodal with cathodal stimulation a BOLD response increase for anodal stimulation was detected in multiple pain processing areas including bilateral amygdala and basal ganglia, left sided thalamus, cingulate cortex, premotor and motor cortex and right sided dorsolateral prefrontal and postcentral cortex (Table 2; Fig. 2). No decrease of BOLD-response was seen in this comparison (post-anodal < post-cathodal). Investigating the contrast estimates of the regions represented by peak voxels it becomes obvious that cathodal DC-stimulation leads to a decreased and anodal DCS to an increased BOLD response in the investigated pain processing areas, while BOLD-signal-intensities after sham-stimulation were found to be in between of those two conditions (Fig. 2). When directly contrasting active (anodal and cathodal) to sham stimulation the modulation of the BOLD response did not reach the defined significance threshold.

Modulation of control conditions

In both control conditions (visual- and motor-paradigm) the observed effect was antipodal to the effect on trigeminal nociception showing a decrease of the BOLD-response in the calcarine- (for visual stimulation) and right precentral-gyrus (for left hand motor activation) comparing post-anodal vs. post-cathodal activation (Table 3, Fig. 3). As in nociception no voxels showing the opposite modulatory patterns of activity could be identified.

Discussion

This study aimed to explore the underling mechanism of the previously described antinociceptive effects of tDCS targeting the primary motor cortex, and demonstrates polarity-specific effects of tDCS on specific brain regions associated with trigeminal pain processing.

Anodal tDCS increased BOLD-response in the thalamus, basal ganglia, cingulate cortex, dorsolateral prefrontal cortex and amygdala, whereas cathodal tDCS lead to a decrease of activation in these regions. These areas are involved in human trigeminal pain processing and were described to play a role in several pain disorders as well as experimental pain studies, with different contributions to pain perception and processing. Irrespectively of polarity behavioral data were not altered after tDCS. Cerebral activations for control paradigms (motor task and visual stimulation) were in the expected range and located within expected brain areas.

It is well-known that anodal tDCS leads to increased cortical excitability, while cathodal tDCS induces the opposite effect. Investigating the effects of tDCS Vaseghi et al. demonstrated that anodal tDCS over M1 enhances brain excitability for at least 30 min using motoric evoked potentials (MEP) [26]. Several other studies confirmed increased MEP after application of a-tDCS over M1 [4, 15, 27–29]. Our nociceptive data mesh with these results conclusively, showing increased activation BOLD signal after anodal stimulation.

More supporting evidence is coming from electrophysiological pain studies, showing that tDCS also modulates pain-related evoked potentials recorded after painful electrical stimulation of the forehead and the hand in healthy volunteers [30]. Cathodal tDCS generates inhibition of trigeminal and extracranial pain processing while a-tDCS leads to excitation. Similar results were observed investigating laser evoked potentials. After c-tDCS N2 amplitude and P2 components were significantly reduced compared with anodal and sham stimulation [31].

Only few data exist for functional imaging of pain processing after tDCS. Ihle et al. investigated 16 healthy volunteers in a randomized, cross-over sham controlled study using fMRI with an acute heat pain paradigm [32]. No significant polarity-specific changes of brain activation were observed comparing active with sham stimulation. When directly contrasting anodal and cathodal stimulation a decrease of activation in the hypothalamus, inferior parietal cortex, inferior parietal lobe, anterior insula, and precentral gyrus was observed in an uncorrected analysis. This changes interestingly were mainly observed on the contra-stimulus side (changes of activation mainly in the right hemisphere following right sided heat stimulation and left sided tDCS, $p_{unc} < 0.001$). Although anatomic structures similar to our study were affected, the effects showed opposite behaviour with a decrease of activation after anodal stimulation. It remains speculative, but as duration and site of stimulation was comparable in both studies, differences might be caused by differing current intensities and type of pain (heat stimulus vs. electrical stimulation). And

Table 1 Average fMRI activation

MNI X Y Z		Anatomical area	k_E	T
		A – Nociceptive processing		
-30–58 -26	L	Cerebellar hemisphere	6763	10.22
26–58 -24	R	Cerebellar hemisphere		9.47
6–64 -16	BL	Cerebellar vermis		9.47
-38–12 56	L	Motor cortex	11,434*	9.09
-2 2 56		Suppl. Motor area /SMA		9.02
-62–20 18		Somatosensory cortex (head)		8.94
64–16 20	R	Somatosensory cortex (head)	7887†	8.82
60 12 0		Rolandic operculum		8.80
58 12 18		Frontal inf. Operculum		7.03
42 46 18	R	Dorsolateral-prefrontal-cortex	331	5.67
36 50 24				5.24
-34 44 28	L	Dorsolateral-prefrontal-cortex	45	5.08
-10–22 48	L	Cingulum	48	5.07
40–14 -6	R	Posterior insula	35	4.95
46–26–4		Superior temporal gyrus		4.90
52–38 -16	R	Middle temporal gyrus	46	4.89
56–48 -18		Inferior temporal gyrus		4.83
		B – Visual processing		
-8–88 0	BL	Calcarine gyrus	32,000‡	18.86
4–88 -2		Lingual gyrus		17.93
6–80 -2				17.31
0–54 -36	BL	Cerebellar vermis	91	7.34
50–4 54	R	Middle Frontal Gyrus	53	5.30
		C – Motor processing		
38–18 58	R	M1/Precentral Gyrus	2438	20.67
50–16 52				12.48
-16–50 -20	L	Cerebellar hemisphere	1502	15.62
-58–18 48	L	Pre- + Postcentral Gyrus	113	6.61
8–4 54	R	Suppl. motor cortex	226	6.52
6 0 66				5.39
-8–88 0	BL	Calcarine gyrus	800	6.47
8–98 -4				5.82
10–82 4				5.23
16–20 6	R	Thalamus	42	5.77

Averaged BOLD responses (respecting all three tDC-stimulation paradigms to a third) to A nociceptive stimulation, B visual stimulation and C motor activation (incl. visual instruction); All results are whole brain Family-Wise-Error corrected ($p_{FWE} < 0.05$). Fused blobs: *including activation in the thalamus, anterior and posterior insular cortex, † including activation in the thalamus, anterior insular cortex and basal ganglia. ‡ widespread bilateral activation of V1, visual thalami and downstream visual cortices. R = right, L = left, BL = bilateral, k_E = cluster extend; MNI = Montreal Neurological Institute

Table 2 Effect of tDCS on trigeminal nociceptive processing

MNI X Y Z		Anatomical area	k_E	T	p_{FWE} cluster	p_{FWE} peak
−22 8–16	L	Amygdala[a]	107	4.48	.005	.001
−12 2 4	L	Basal ganglia[a]	208	4.24	.033	.006
26 0–20	R	Amygdala[a]	125	4.18	.002	.001
56–30 -8	R	Mid. temporal gyrus	74	4.17	NA	NA
−10 -28 70	L	M1 and premotor cortex[a]	162	4.11	.010	.012
−14 -10 18	L	Thalamus[a]	39	3.99	.015	.008
56–18 6	R	Superior temporal gyrus	86	3.97	NA	NA
14 4 6	R	Basal ganglia[a]	94	3.93	.027	.029
−50 -32 12	L	Superior temporal gyrus	49	3.85	NA	NA
66–8 18	R	Postcentral gyrus[a]	24	3.81	.042	.025
−40 -2 -18	L	Posterior Insular cortex	27	3.77	NS	NS
−6 -4 44	L	Cingulate cortex[a]	47	3.77	.03	.027
10–24 74	R	Suppl. motor/premotor cortex	25	3.73	NS	NS
4 14 0	R	Basal ganglia / Caudate ncl.[a]	59	3.68	.027	.032
38 2 54	R	DLPFC[a]	44	3.67	.044	.047
44 42 4	R	DLPFC	42	3.58	NS	NS

Areas with significant DC-stimulation induced alterations (postcathodal vs. postanodal). Illustration in Fig. 2. Exploratory significance level $p_{unc} < .0005$. Additional region of interest analysis (ROI) with applied Family-Wise-Error correction for the neuropain-matrix as indicated in the materials and method section ([a]$p_{FWE} < 0.05$)
R = right, L = left, BL = bilateral, Ke = cluster extend, MNI = Montreal Neurological Institute: NA = not applicable, NS = not significant. M1 = primary motorcortex, DLPFC = dorsolateral prefrontal cortex

indeed, there is evidence that different stimulation intensities may lead to antipodal cortical reaction regarding excitability [33].

As other experimental studies, we were not able to demonstrate a significant modulation of the recorded behavioral data. A meta-analysis including eight studies showed that c-tDCS of the primary motor-cortex leads to significant sensory threshold but not pain threshold alterations in healthy volunteers. Interestingly in chronic pain, pain-levels were significantly reduced [34]. No modulation of behavioral data caused by tDCS was detected by several other studies [31, 32] investigating acute pain. Taking this together TDCs may be able to modulate chronic but not acute and experimental pain.

Interpreting the results of motor processing our data are perfectly in line with the concept of intercortical/ transcalosal inhibition [35] as tDCS was applied to the contralateral hemisphere (left M1) of the task based activation of the primary motor cortex (right M1, left hand), which was decreased after anodal stimulation.

The observed alterations in the visual system are difficult to interpreted and remain speculative. Recent evidence supports a complex relationship and influence between the here targeted nociceptive and the also affected visual central processing [36].

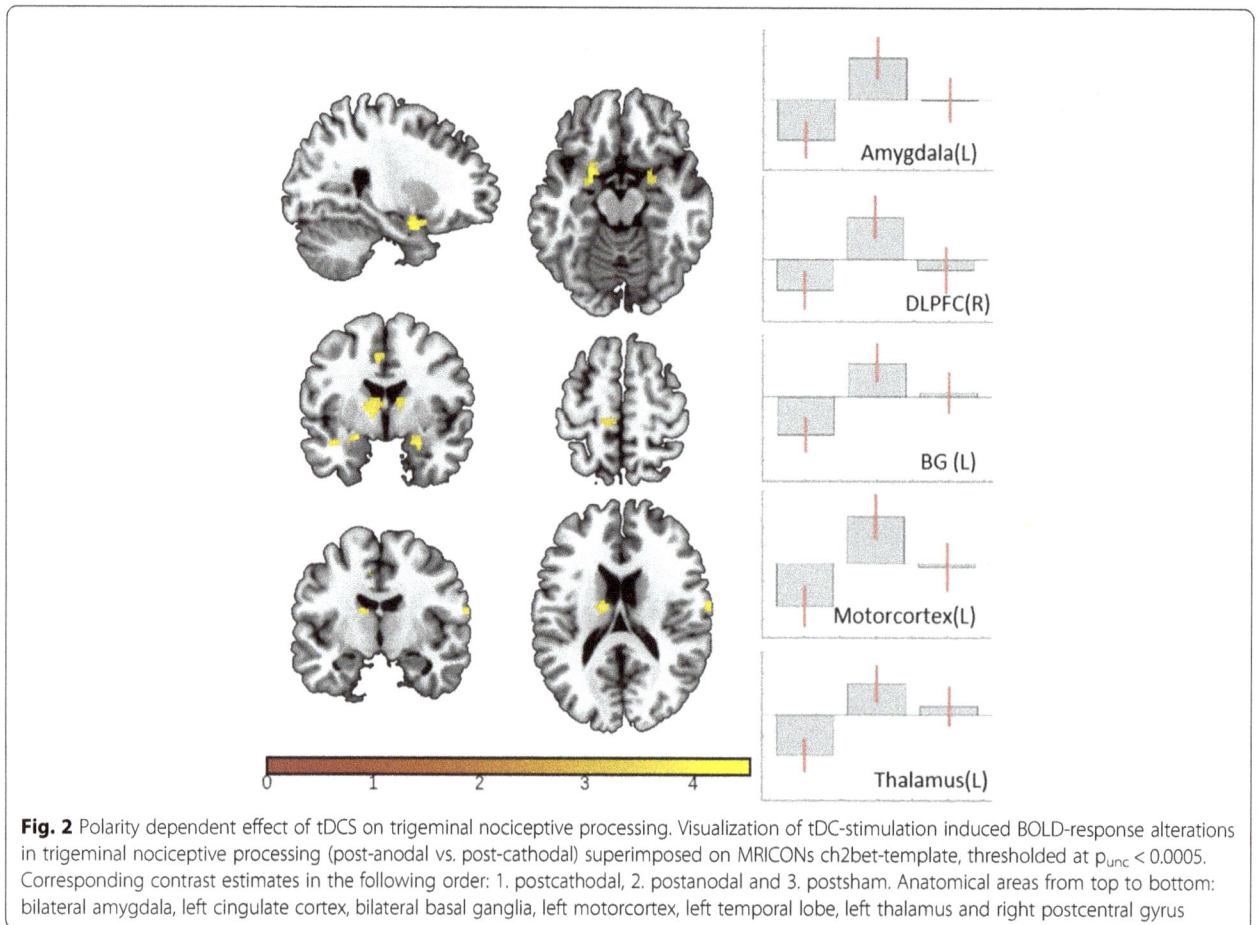

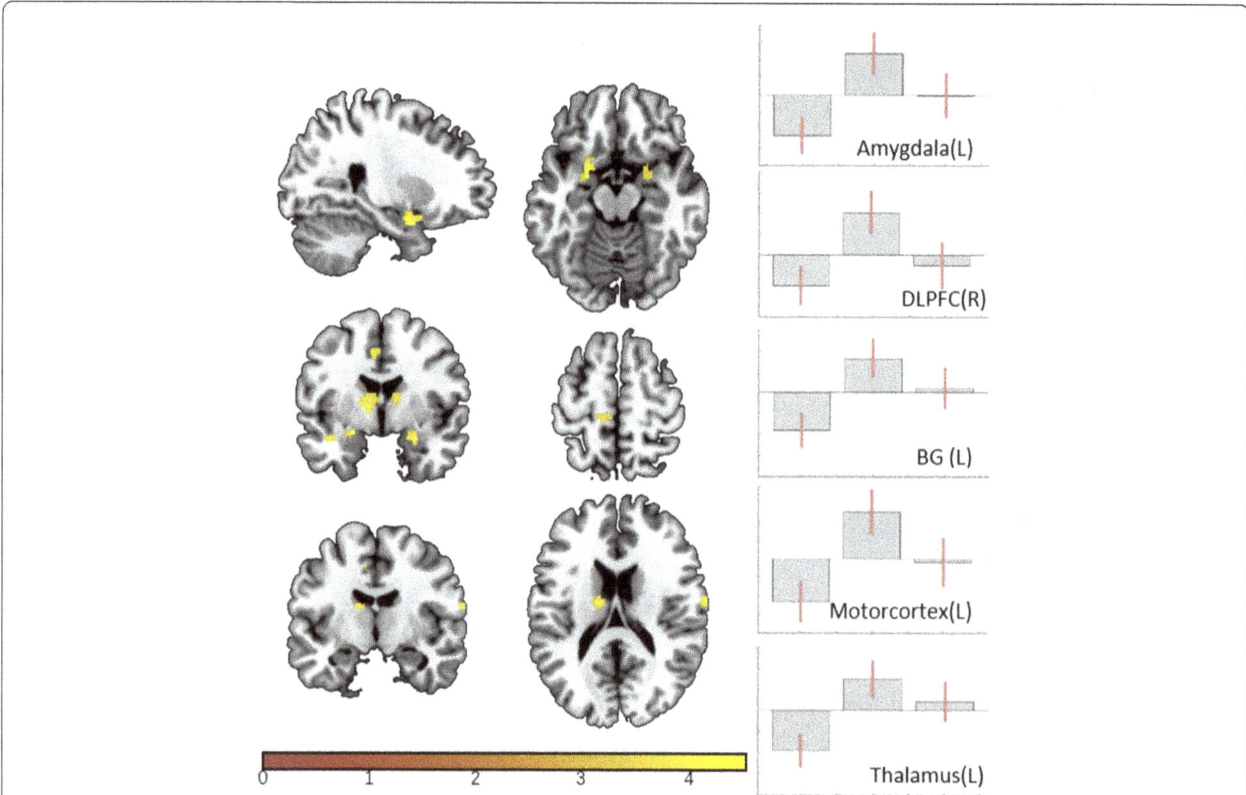

Fig. 2 Polarity dependent effect of tDCS on trigeminal nociceptive processing. Visualization of tDC-stimulation induced BOLD-response alterations in trigeminal nociceptive processing (post-anodal vs. post-cathodal) superimposed on MRICONs ch2bet-template, thresholded at $p_{unc} < 0.0005$. Corresponding contrast estimates in the following order: 1. postcathodal, 2. postanodal and 3. postsham. Anatomical areas from top to bottom: bilateral amygdala, left cingulate cortex, bilateral basal ganglia, left motorcortex, left temporal lobe, left thalamus and right postcentral gyrus

The underlying neurobiological mechanisms of tDCS are still unclear. Different mechanisms were previously discussed involving a cascade of events at cellular and molecular levels [37]. Local and distant neuroplastic changes were described [37]. Several neurotransmitters such as dopamine, acetylcholine, and serotonin are involved in this process [38, 39]. GABAergic neurotransmission via interneurons is modulated by tDCS [40]. Animal studies showed that anodal stimulation causes depolarization while cathodal stimulation causes hyperpolarization of neurons [41, 42] inducing an alteration of neural activity not only during tDCS but also hours later [41]. Pharmacological studies suggest that NMDA and GABAergic systems are involved in the underlying neurobiological mechanisms [40, 43, 44]. Additionally, spectroscopic data showed that cerebral GABA and glutamate concentrations were altered after tDCS application [45, 46].

Table 3 Effect of tDCS on motor and visual processing

MNI X Y Z	Anatomical area		k_E	T
Visual				
20–64 4	BL	Calcarine gyrus	1848	6.62
-14–40 -4	L	Lingual gyrus	15	4.74
18–62 -10	R	Lingual gyrus	6	4.47
Motor				
40–18 62	R	M1/Precentral Gyrus	15	4.82

Areas with significant DC-stimulation induced alterations (postcathodal vs. postanodal) in both control paradigms. Illustration in Fig. 3. All results whole brain Family-Wise-Error corrected ($p_{FWE} < 0.05$). R = right, L = left, BL = bilateral, Ke = cluster extend, MNI = Montreal Neurological Institute

Regarding the effect of tDCS on pain processing immediate after-effects and long-lasting effects have to be differentiated [47, 48]. TDCS-induced alterations of the acid-base balance of neuronal membranes were thought to play an important role for direct modulation of central pain processing leading to a reduction of NMDA receptor activity [49]. Long-lasting effects were thought to be mediated at a synaptic level by NMDA receptors in terms of long-term-potentiation (LTP) and depression (LTD) respectively [43, 44]. Further research suggested that also non-synaptic mechanisms might be involved in long-lasting effects of tDCS [47]. As a result of these molecular and cellular processes, modulation of functions of brain areas related to pain processing may occur. Previous animal experiments suggested that tDCS regulates neuronal activity by top-down modulation not only in the brain but also in the spinal cord. tDCS

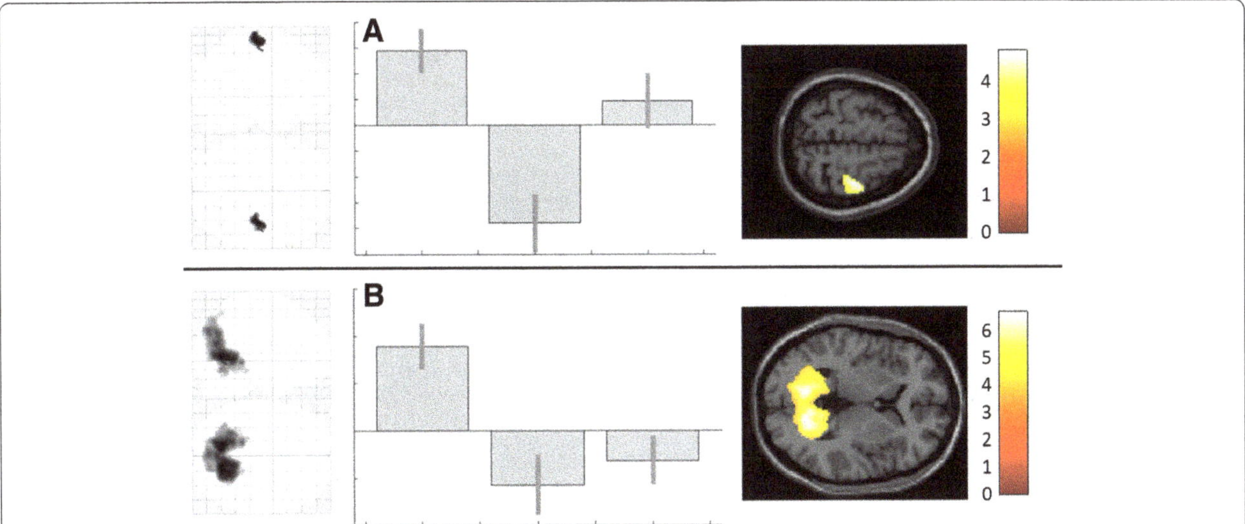

Fig. 3 Polarity dependent effect of tDCS on visual and motor processing. Significant ($p_{FWE} < .05$) alterations of BOLD-response after DCS (postcathodal vs. postanodal) for A. motor- (precentral-gyrus), and B visual-processing (calcarine-gyrus). Illustrated as SPM generated glass-brain and T1-overlay; for better visualization both displayed with a threshold of $p_{unc} < .0005$. Corresponding contrast estimates in the following order: 1. postcathodal, 2. postanodal and 3. postsham. For coordinates and further details see Table 3

decreased brain-derived neurotrophic factor (BDNF) levels within the spinal cord and brainstem in areas involved in the descending pain processing system thereby decreasing pain sensitivity [50].

Hence, tDCS dependent pain reduction might be the result of combined modulation of the pain processing network and facilitation of descending pain inhibitory mechanisms. The widespread alterations in the central nociceptive processing identified in this study support this network based hypothesis. Until now it remains unclear whether the observed effects are different in patients suffering from pain as most of the studies investigated healthy volunteers. Animal data indicate that chronic stress might influence brain reaction to tDCS [50]. BDNF levels were only reduced by tDCS in unstressed animals. Therefore, the impact of DCS in patients might be significantly different from healthy subjects. Additionally, disorder-specific effects might be conceivable and contribute to the current heterogeneity of study results.

The here observed effects of tDCS may be of particular interest in the context of migraine, as anodal tDCS was previously shown to have alleviating effect on chronic and episodic courses of migraineurs [51–55]. At first glance this may be counterintuitive as migrainous brains, especially interictally, were proven to have a lack of habituation regarding multiple sensory modalities [56]. The current study demonstrates an even higher pain related activation immediate after single session a-tDCS. However treatment effects in clinical studies were only detected with delay and after several sessions. Furthermore, brains of migraineurs may react different from those of healthy controls, and migraine hyperresponsiveness is yet not fully understood as there is an ongoing debate, whether this is the result of a decreased inhibition, or a decreased pre-activation [56, 57]. To treat this hyperresponsiveness simply by means of inhibitory neuromodulation is probably too simply thought, as in fact treatment studies using DCS or TMS favor excitatory over inhibitory stimulation [51, 53–55, 58–61]. Demonstrating modulation not only localized cortical, but also subcortical and in remote structures hint towards a more complex and network wide modulation, which is further supported by our findings for motor activity and visual stimulation demonstrating tDCS's reversed influence on even more remote networks.

A limitation of the study is that data were obtained from healthy young volunteers without any history of pain. Pain was artificially induced and not caused by a genuine pain disorder. Therefore, activation as well as modulation might be different in pain patients who may respond differently to tDCS. Additionally, only pain modulation after tDCS of M1 was investigated. Further research is needed regarding optimal tDCS application time, site of stimulation, current intensity and electrode size.

Conclusion

We hereby demonstrate polarity-specific modulation of specific brain regions associated with cerebral pain processing using tDCS. Anodal tDCS led to an increase of activation within the cerebral pain-network while cathodal tDCS led to a decrease of activation. These findings support previous electrophysiological findings detecting an increase of cortical excitability after a-tDCS and a decrease after c-tDCS. The results enrich the understanding of the antinociceptive capabilities of tDCS as they point towards a network wide modulation of this system. Furthermore, the observations for motor activity and visual stimulation improve the knowledge regarding tDCS's influence on even more remote networks, as for these the modulatory effect was reversed in the contralateral M1 and bilaterally in the visual cortices. Further studies need to evaluate whether these data can be transferred to patients with pain and headache disorders.

Abbreviations

AAL: Automated anatomic labeling; ACC: Anterior cingulate cortex; a-tDCS: Anodal transcranial direct current stimulation; BDNF: Brain derived neurotrophic factor; BOLD: Blood oxygen level dependent; c-tDCS: Cathodal transcranial direct current stimulation; FWE: Family wise error correction; fMRT: Functional magnetic resonance imaging; LTD: Long term depression; LTP: Long term potentiation; M1: Primary motor cortex; MNI: Montreal neurological institute; MPRAGE: Magnetization prepared rapid acquisition gradient echo; NRS: Numeric rating scale; ROI: Region of interest; S1: Primary somatosensory cortex; S2: Secondary somatosensory cortex; SPM: Statistical parametric mapping; s-tDCS: Sham transcranial direct current stimulation; tDCS: Transcranial direct current stimulation; TMS: Transcranial magnetic stimulation

Acknowledgments

We would like to thank all study participants for their patience and endurance that allowed us to collect these results without any loss of follow up.

Funding

This project was funded by the Medical Faculty of the University of Duisburg-Essen (IFORES grand for Steffen Naegel) and the Grünenthal scientific grand (Dagny Holle), none of which resulted in competing interests.

Author's contributions

SN: Study conception and design; Acquisition of data; Analysis of data; Interpretation of data; Drafting of manuscript. JB: Acquisition of data; Analysis of data; Interpretation of data. NT: Acquisition of data; Analysis of data; Drafting of manuscript. CK: Interpretation of data; Critical revision of the manuscript. HCD: Study conception and design; Interpretation of data; Critical revision of the manuscript. ZK: Study conception and design; Interpretation of data; Critical revision of the manuscript. MO: Study conception and design; Interpretation of data; Critical revision of the manuscript. DH: Study conception and design; Acquisition of data; Analysis of data; Interpretation of data; Critical revision of the manuscript. All authors read and approved the final manuscript.

Competing interests

The author declare that they have no competing interests

Author details

[1]Department of Neurology, University of Duisburg-Essen, University Hospital Essen, Hufelandstr. 55, 45122 Essen, Germany. [2]Institute of Diagnostic and Interventional Radiology and Neuroradiology, University of Duisburg-Essen, University Hospital Essen, Hufelandstr. 55, 45122 Essen, Germany. [3]Department of Neurology, Evangelical Hospital Unna, Holbeinstr. 10, 59423 Unna, Germany. [4]Center for Neurology, Asklepios Hospitals Schildautal, Karl-Herold-Straße 1, 38723 Seesen, Germany. [5]EVEX Medical Corporation, 40 Vazha-Pshavela Avenue, Tbilisi 0177, Georgia. [6]Sechenov University Moscow, 8-2 Trubetskaya str., Moscow 119991, Russian Federation.

References

1. Iannetti GD, Mouraux A (2010) From the neuromatrix to the pain matrix (and back). Exp Brain Res 205:1–12. https://doi.org/10.1007/s00221-010-2340-1
2. Chen JL, Carta S, Soldado-Magraner J et al (2013) Behaviour-dependent recruitment of long-range projection neurons in somatosensory cortex. Nature 499:336–340. https://doi.org/10.1038/nature12236
3. Kulkarni B, Bentley DE, Elliott R et al (2005) Attention to pain localization and unpleasantness discriminates the functions of the medial and lateral pain systems. Eur J Neurosci 21:3133–3142. https://doi.org/10.1111/j.1460-9568.2005.04098.x
4. Lang N, Nitsche MA, Paulus W et al (2004) Effects of transcranial direct current stimulation over the human motor cortex on corticospinal and transcallosal excitability. Exp Brain Res 156:439–443. https://doi.org/10.1007/s00221-003-1800-2
5. O'Connell NE, Wand BM, Marston L et al (2011) Non-invasive brain stimulation techniques for chronic pain. A report of a Cochrane systematic review and meta-analysis. Eur J Phys Rehabil Med 47:309–326
6. Vaseghi B, Zoghi M, Jaberzadeh S (2014) Does anodal transcranial direct current stimulation modulate sensory perception and pain? A meta-analysis study. Clin Neurophysiol Off J Int Fed Clin Neurophysiol 125:1847–1858. https://doi.org/10.1016/j.clinph.2014.01.020
7. Apkarian AV, Bushnell MC, Treede R-D, Zubieta J-K (2005) Human brain mechanisms of pain perception and regulation in health and disease. Eur J Pain Lond Engl 9:463–484. https://doi.org/10.1016/j.ejpain.2004.11.001
8. Peyron R, Laurent B, García-Larrea L (2000) Functional imaging of brain responses to pain. A review and meta-analysis (2000). Neurophysiol Clin Clin Neurophysiol 30:263–288
9. Luedtke K, Rushton A, Wright C et al (2012) Transcranial direct current stimulation for the reduction of clinical and experimentally induced pain: a systematic review and meta-analysis. Clin J Pain 28:452–461. https://doi.org/10.1097/AJP.0b013e31823853e3
10. Ostrowsky K, Magnin M, Ryvlin P et al (2002) Representation of pain and somatic sensation in the human insula: a study of responses to direct electrical cortical stimulation. Cereb Cortex N Y N 1991 12:376–385
11. Naegel S, Holle D, Desmarattes N et al (2014) Cortical plasticity in episodic and chronic cluster headache. NeuroImage Clin 6:415–423. https://doi.org/10.1016/j.nicl.2014.10.003
12. Fagerlund AJ, Hansen OA, Aslaksen PM (2015) Transcranial direct current stimulation as a treatment for patients with fibromyalgia: a randomized controlled trial. Pain 156:62–71. https://doi.org/10.1016/j.pain.0000000000000006
13. Ngernyam N, Jensen MP, Arayawichanon P et al (2015) The effects of transcranial direct current stimulation in patients with neuropathic pain from spinal cord injury. Clin Neurophysiol Off J Int Fed Clin Neurophysiol 126:382–390. https://doi.org/10.1016/j.clinph.2014.05.034
14. Wickmann F, Stephani C, Czesnik D et al (2015) Prophylactic treatment in menstrual migraine: a proof-of-concept study. J Neurol Sci 354:103–109. https://doi.org/10.1016/j.jns.2015.05.009
15. Nitsche MA, Paulus W (2001) Sustained excitability elevations induced by transcranial DC motor cortex stimulation in humans. Neurology 57: 1899–1901
16. Kaube H, Katsarava Z, Käufer T et al (2000) A new method to increase nociception specificity of the human blink reflex. Clin Neurophysiol 111: 413–416
17. Ashburner J, Friston KJ (2005) Unified segmentation. Neuroimage 26: 839–851
18. May A (2009) New insights into headache: an update on functional and structural imaging findings. Nat Rev Neurol 5:199–209. https://doi.org/10.1038/nrneurol.2009.28
19. Tzourio-Mazoyer N, Landeau B, Papathanassiou D et al (2002) Automated anatomical labeling of activations in SPM using a macroscopic anatomical parcellation of the MNI MRI single-subject brain. NeuroImage 15:273–289. https://doi.org/10.1006/nimg.2001.0978
20. Brett M, Anton J-L, Valabregue R, Poline J-B (2002) Region of interest analysis using an SPM toolbox. NeuroImage Vol 16; no 2.: [abstract] presented at the 8th international conference on functional mapping of the human brain, June 2–6, 2002, Sendai, Japan
21. Gandiga PC, Hummel FC, Cohen LG (2006) Transcranial DC stimulation (tDCS): a tool for double-blind sham-controlled clinical studies in brain stimulation. Clin Neurophysiol 117:845–850. https://doi.org/10.1016/j.clinph.2005.12.003

22. Ambrus GG, Antal A, Paulus W (2011) Comparing cutaneous perception induced by electrical stimulation using rectangular and round shaped electrodes. Clin Neurophysiol Off J Int Fed Clin Neurophysiol 122:803–807. https://doi.org/10.1016/j.clinph.2010.08.023
23. Boggio PS, Zaghi S, Lopes M, Fregni F (2008) Modulatory effects of anodal transcranial direct current stimulation on perception and pain thresholds in healthy volunteers. Eur J Neurol 15:1124–1130. https://doi.org/10.1111/j.1468-1331.2008.02270.x
24. Fregni F, Gimenes R, Valle AC et al (2006) A randomized, sham-controlled, proof of principle study of transcranial direct current stimulation for the treatment of pain in fibromyalgia. Arthritis Rheum 54:3988–3998. https://doi.org/10.1002/art.22195
25. Lefaucheur J-P, Antal A, Ayache SS et al (2017) Evidence-based guidelines on the therapeutic use of transcranial direct current stimulation (tDCS). Clin Neurophysiol Off J Int Fed Clin Neurophysiol 128:56–92. https://doi.org/10.1016/j.clinph.2016.10.087
26. Vaseghi B, Zoghi M, Jaberzadeh S (2015) How does anodal transcranial direct current stimulation of the pain neuromatrix affect brain excitability and pain perception? A randomised, double-blind, sham-control study. PLoS One 10:e0118340. https://doi.org/10.1371/journal.pone.0118340
27. Nitsche MA, Paulus W (2000) Excitability changes induced in the human motor cortex by weak transcranial direct current stimulation. J Physiol 527(Pt 3):633–639
28. Uy J, Ridding MC (2003) Increased cortical excitability induced by transcranial DC and peripheral nerve stimulation. J Neurosci Methods 127:193–197
29. Fricke K, Seeber AA, Thirugnanasambandam N et al (2011) Time course of the induction of homeostatic plasticity generated by repeated transcranial direct current stimulation of the human motor cortex. J Neurophysiol 105: 1141–1149. https://doi.org/10.1152/jn.00608.2009
30. Hansen N, Obermann M, Poitz F et al (2011) Modulation of human trigeminal and extracranial nociceptive processing by transcranial direct current stimulation of the motor cortex. Cephalalgia Int J Headache 31:661–670. https://doi.org/10.1177/0333102410390394
31. Csifcsak G, Antal A, Hillers F et al (2009) Modulatory effects of transcranial direct current stimulation on laser-evoked potentials. Pain Med Malden Mass 10:122–132. https://doi.org/10.1111/j.1526-4637.2008.00508.x
32. Ihle K, Rodriguez-Raecke R, Luedtke K, May A (2014) tDCS modulates cortical nociceptive processing but has little to no impact on pain perception. Pain 155:2080–2087. https://doi.org/10.1016/j.pain.2014.07.018
33. Batsikadze G, Moliadze V, Paulus W et al (2013) Partially non-linear stimulation intensity-dependent effects of direct current stimulation on motor cortex excitability in humans. J Physiol 591:1987–2000. https://doi.org/10.1113/jphysiol.2012.249730
34. Vaseghi B, Zoghi M, Jaberzadeh S (2015) A meta-analysis of site-specific effects of cathodal transcranial direct current stimulation on sensory perception and pain. PLoS One 10:e0123873. https://doi.org/10.1371/journal.pone.0123873
35. Perez MA, Cohen LG (2009) Interhemispheric inhibition between primary motor cortices: what have we learned? J Physiol 587:725–726. https://doi.org/10.1113/jphysiol.2008.166926
36. Torta DME, Van Den Broeke EN, Filbrich L, et al (2017) Intense pain influences the cortical processing of visual stimuli projected onto the sensitized skin. PAIN. 158:691. https://doi.org/10.1097/j.pain.0000000000000816
37. Medeiros LF, de Souza ICC, Vidor LP, et al (2012) Neurobiological effects of transcranial direct current stimulation: a review. Front Psychiatry 3:110 . doi: https://doi.org/10.3389/fpsyt.2012.00110
38. Kuo M-F, Grosch J, Fregni F et al (2007) Focusing effect of acetylcholine on neuroplasticity in the human motor cortex. J Neurosci 27:14442–14447. https://doi.org/10.1523/JNEUROSCI.4104-07.2007
39. Monte-Silva K, Kuo M-F, Thirugnanasambandam N et al (2009) Dose-dependent inverted U-shaped effect of dopamine (D2-like) receptor activation on focal and nonfocal plasticity in humans. J Neurosci 29:6124–6131. https://doi.org/10.1523/JNEUROSCI.0728-09.2009
40. Nitsche MA, Liebetanz D, Schlitterlau A et al (2004) GABAergic modulation of DC stimulation-induced motor cortex excitability shifts in humans. Eur J Neurosci 19:2720–2726. https://doi.org/10.1111/j.0953-816X.2004.03398.x
41. Bindman LJ, Lippold OC, Redfearn JW (1964) The action of brief polarizing currents on the cerebral cortex of the rat (1) during current flow and (2) in the production of long-lasting after-effects. J Physiol 172:369–382
42. Purpura DP, JG MM (1965) Intracellular activities and evoked potential changes during polarization of motor cortex. J Neurophysiol 28:166–185
43. Liebetanz D, Nitsche MA, Tergau F, Paulus W (2002) Pharmacological approach to the mechanisms of transcranial DC-stimulation-induced after-effects of human motor cortex excitability. Brain J Neurol 125:2238–2247
44. Nitsche MA, Fricke K, Henschke U et al (2003) Pharmacological modulation of cortical excitability shifts induced by transcranial direct current stimulation in humans. J Physiol 553:293–301. https://doi.org/10.1113/jphysiol.2003.049916
45. Stagg CJ, Best JG, Stephenson MC et al (2009) Polarity-sensitive modulation of cortical neurotransmitters by transcranial stimulation. J Neurosci 29:5202–5206. https://doi.org/10.1523/JNEUROSCI.4432-08.2009
46. Clark VP, Coffman BA, Trumbo MC, Gasparovic C (2011) Transcranial direct current stimulation (tDCS) produces localized and specific alterations in neurochemistry: a ^{1}H magnetic resonance spectroscopy study. Neurosci Lett 500:67–71. https://doi.org/10.1016/j.neulet.2011.05.244
47. Ardolino G, Bossi B, Barbieri S, Priori A (2005) Non-synaptic mechanisms underlie the after-effects of cathodal transcutaneous direct current stimulation of the human brain. J Physiol 568:653–663. https://doi.org/10.1113/jphysiol.2005.088310
48. Nitsche MA, Jaussi W, Liebetanz D et al (2004) Consolidation of human motor cortical neuroplasticity by D-cycloserine. Neuropsychopharmacol Off Publ Am Coll Neuropsychopharmacol 29:1573–1578. https://doi.org/10.1038/sj.npp.1300517
49. Chesler M (2003) Regulation and modulation of pH in the brain. Physiol Rev 83:1183–1221. https://doi.org/10.1152/physrev.00010.2003
50. Spezia Adachi LN, Quevedo AS, de Souza A et al (2015) Exogenously induced brain activation regulates neuronal activity by top-down modulation: conceptualized model for electrical brain stimulation. Exp Brain Res 233:1377–1389. https://doi.org/10.1007/s00221-015-4212-1
51. Przeklasa-Muszyńska A, Kocot-Kępska M, Dobrogowski J et al (2017) Transcranial direct current stimulation (tDCS) and its influence on analgesics effectiveness in patients suffering from migraine headache. Pharmacol Rep PR 69:714–721. https://doi.org/10.1016/j.pharep.2017.02.019
52. Auvichayapat P, Janyacharoen T, Rotenberg A et al (2012) Migraine prophylaxis by anodal Transcranial direct current stimulation, a randomized. Placebo-Controlled Trial 95:10
53. Andrade SM, de Brito Aranha REL, de Oliveira EA et al (2017) Transcranial direct current stimulation over the primary motor vs prefrontal cortex in refractory chronic migraine: a pilot randomized controlled trial. J Neurol Sci 378:225–232. https://doi.org/10.1016/j.jns.2017.05.007
54. DaSilva AF, Mendonca ME, Zaghi S et al (2012) tDCS-induced analgesia and electrical fields in pain-related neural networks in chronic migraine. Headache J Head Face Pain 52:1283–1295. https://doi.org/10.1111/j.1526-4610.2012.02141.x
55. Viganò A, D'Elia TS, Sava SL et al (2013) Transcranial direct current stimulation (tDCS) of the visual cortex: a proof-of-concept study based on interictal electrophysiological abnormalities in migraine. J Headache Pain 14. https://doi.org/10.1186/1129-2377-14-23
56. Coppola G, Pierelli F, Schoenen J (2007) Is the cerebral cortex hyperexcitable or hyperresponsive in migraine? Cephalalgia Int J Headache. 27:1427–439. https://doi.org/10.1111/j.1468-2982.2007.01500.x.
57. Chadaide Z, Arlt S, Antal A et al (2007) Transcranial direct current stimulation reveals inhibitory deficiency in migraine. Cephalalgia Int J Headache 27:833–839. https://doi.org/10.1111/j.1468-2982.2007.01337.x
58. Antal A, Kriener N, Lang N et al (2011) Cathodal transcranial direct current stimulation of the visual cortex in the prophylactic treatment of migraine. Cephalalgia 31:820–828. https://doi.org/10.1177/0333102411399349
59. Chen P-R, Lai K-L, Fuh J-L et al (2016) Efficacy of continuous theta burst stimulation of the primary motor cortex in reducing migraine frequency: a preliminary open-label study. J Chin Med Assoc 79:304–308. https://doi.org/10.1016/j.jcma.2015.10.008
60. Rocha S, Melo L, Boudoux C et al (2015) Transcranial direct current stimulation in the prophylactic treatment of migraine based on interictal visual cortex excitability abnormalities: a pilot randomized controlled trial. J Neurol Sci 349:33–39. https://doi.org/10.1016/j.jns.2014.12.018
61. Teepker M, Hötzel J, Timmesfeld N et al (2010) Low-frequency rTMS of the vertex in the prophylactic treatment of migraine. Cephalalgia 30:137–144. https://doi.org/10.1111/j.1468-2982.2009.01911.x

5

Using the child behavior checklist to determine associations between psychosocial aspects and TMD-related pain in children and adolescents

Amal Al-Khotani[1,2,3*], Mattias Gjelset[1], Aron Naimi-Akbar[4], Britt Hedenberg-Magnusson[1,3,5], Malin Ernberg[1,3] and Nikolaos Christidis[1,3]

Abstract

Background: Since children and adolescents are frequently experiencing emotional and behavioral consequences due to pain, their parents should be aware of this emotional and behavioral status. Therefore, the aim of this study was to analyze and describe the parents' reports of the emotional and behavioral status of children and adolescents with different types of temporomandibular disorders using the Child Behavior Checklist.

Methods: This Cross-sectional study comprises of 386 randomly selected children and adolescents that ages between 10 and 18 years in Jeddah. One day prior the clinical examination according to Research Diagnostic Criteria for temporomandibular disorders (TMD) Axis I and II, Arabic version of the Child Behavior Checklist scale was distributed to the parents of participant. According to the diagnosis, the participants were divided into three groups; non-TMD group, TMD-pain group, and TMD-painfree group.

Results: In regard to internalizing problems, the parents to the children and adolescents in the TMD-pain group rated a higher frequency of anxiety, depression and somatic complaints in their children than the parents of children in the non-TMD group ($p < 0.05$). Only one significant association regarding the externalizing problems was found for the aggressive behavior in the TMD-pain group.

Conclusion: The parents rated that their children with TMD-pain suffer from emotional, somatic and aggressive behavior to a higher degree than healthy control subjects. Also, the parents believed that TMD-pain influenced their children's physical activities but not social activities.

Keywords: Pain, Psychology, Children, Adolescents, Child behaviour checklist

Background

During the last decades, pain among children and adolescents has been recognized as a significant health problem. As the practice of pediatric pain has progressed a lot, also the impact that chronic pain has on the children's daily living has been documented. This includes limitations in both social and physical functioning as well as their family's well-being [1]. It has been shown that children and adolescents are frequently experiencing emotional and behavioral consequences due to pain [2]. Therefore, it is of great importance that the emotional and behavioral status of the children is not just evaluated but also known by their parents.

One way to assess parents' knowledge regarding their children's emotional and behavioral status is by using questionnaires handed to the parents. One of those is the Child Behavior Checklist (CBCL) [3] that has been used to describe the psychosocial status of nurture children and adolescents. It should be completed by the child's parent or child's caregiver who has had the child for a period equal to or more than six months. CBCL measures not only the emotional, behavior and physical problems in school-age

* Correspondence: aalkhotani@yahoo.com; http://ki.se/dentmed
[1]Division of Oral Diagnostics and Rehabilitation, Department of Dental Medicine, Karolinska Institutet, Box 4064, SE-141 04 Huddinge, Sweden
[2]East Jeddah Hospital, Ministry of health, Jeddah, Saudi Arabia
Full list of author information is available at the end of the article

children from 6 to 18 years old, but it also reports the child's social competence such as social and peer relationships, as well as family relationships [3]. CBCL has been used in previous studies to explore the emotional and behavior problems in children and adolescents and to correlate these psychometric measures to different pain conditions such as juvenile chronic arthritis (JIA), pediatric cancer, and hematological conditions (4, 5). In one study, CBCL showed that children with cancer and hematological condition suffered from internalizing symptoms such as anxiety, depression and somatic problems [4], while another study reported no association between pain and child psychosocial functioning [5]. Other studies have also used CBCL to assess the psychosocial profile of children with sleep disorders, headache, abdominal pain and irritable bowel syndrome. Those studies showed that children reported at least one emotional and/or behavioral disorder [6–8]. Furthermore, CBCL was used to evaluate the mental health of children living with a mother suffering from chronic pain [9].

Temporomandibular disorders (TMD) in children and adolescents seem to be a more significant problem than previously believed with a prevalence reaching up to 27.2% [10]. Earlier studies have shown prevalences that range between 4.2% and 27% [10, 11]. Recent studies have used different psychometric measures in children and adolescents suffering from TMD [2, 12–14]. These methodological differences between studies are present since it until recently was no suitable instrument measuring the TMD-associated problems for youngsters suffering from emotional and somatic pain. Similar to other conditions, TMD is accompanied by comorbid and somatization disorders (psychological suffering that felt like a real somatic pain) [15]. Also, in psychological studies, a comorbidity with psychiatric conditions and psychological distress has been shown to significantly and negatively modify the outcome of patients with chronic conditions like headache, making it a reliable predictor of suicidal risk [16]. Therefore, there is a great need to use a proper psychometric approach to analyze all possible TMD-related problems. Most of the studies have used the questionnaires from the Research Diagnostic Criteria for Temporomandibular Disorders (RDC/TMD) Axis II [13, 14], which are validated for adults. Other studies have used specially constructed questionnaires to ask the parents about their children's emotional status when they complain of TMD [12]. Further, just a few studies have used the Youth self-report (YSR) [17], which is a "child-rating scale" analogous to CBCL, to evaluate emotional and behavioral functioning in children and adolescents [2, 15]. A recent study from our research group used YSR to assess the emotional, behavior and somatic functioning among children and adolescents with various TMD condition (2). The same study found a significant association between TMD-pain and anxiety, depression, somatic problems, aggressive behavior as well as thought problems. Until now, the emotional effects on children with different TMD-pain conditions have not been assessed using the "parent- rating scale", i.e. the CBCL.

Taken together, we hypothesized that psychosocial problems in children and adolescents are associated with a diagnosis of TMD with pain (TMD-pain) but not with a diagnosis of TMD without pain (TMD-pain-free) when CBCL is used. Therefore, the purpose of the present study was to analyze and describe the parents' reports of the emotional and behavioral status of children and adolescents with different types of temporomandibular disorders (TMD) using the Child Behavior Checklist (CBCL).

Methods

This study is part of a larger project from our research group. This cross-sectional study followed the guidelines of the Declaration of Helsinki and was approved by the local ethics committee at the Department of Medical Study and Research, Ministry of Health, Jeddah, Saudi Arabia. Before inclusion, all participants or their parents gave both verbal and written consent, after receiving written information. An extended verbal explanation was further provided upon request.

In the current study, a total of 633 children and adolescents of both sexes, aged between 10 and 18 years were asked to participate, 509 of them agreed to participate. The sample consisted of children among the general population of Jeddah; a major and cosmopolitan city in Saudi Arabia. A total of 386 parents completed the questionnaire. The flow-chart (Fig. 1) illustrates not just the participation-rate from the different areas of Jeddah, but also how many completed forms were handed in, among boys and girls separately. However, we do not have the information on why the forms were not handed in, neither why some children did not participate at the clinical examination.

Study setting

The city of Jeddah was divided into five regions (North, South, East, West, and Central). Because the education in Saudi Arabia is based on single-sex schools: two schools with boys and two schools with girls were randomly selected from the predefined list of schools from each region as grouped by the ministry of education, with children aged 10–18. The randomization was performed by the principal investigator (NC), who did not participate in the data collection, with an internet-based application (www.randomization.com) [10]. One class from each school was chosen, using stratified selction based on age for the randomization in order to get the most representative and homogenous matrerial as possible. This randomization was also performed by NC, with an average of 28 pupils. A dental assistant who did not participate in

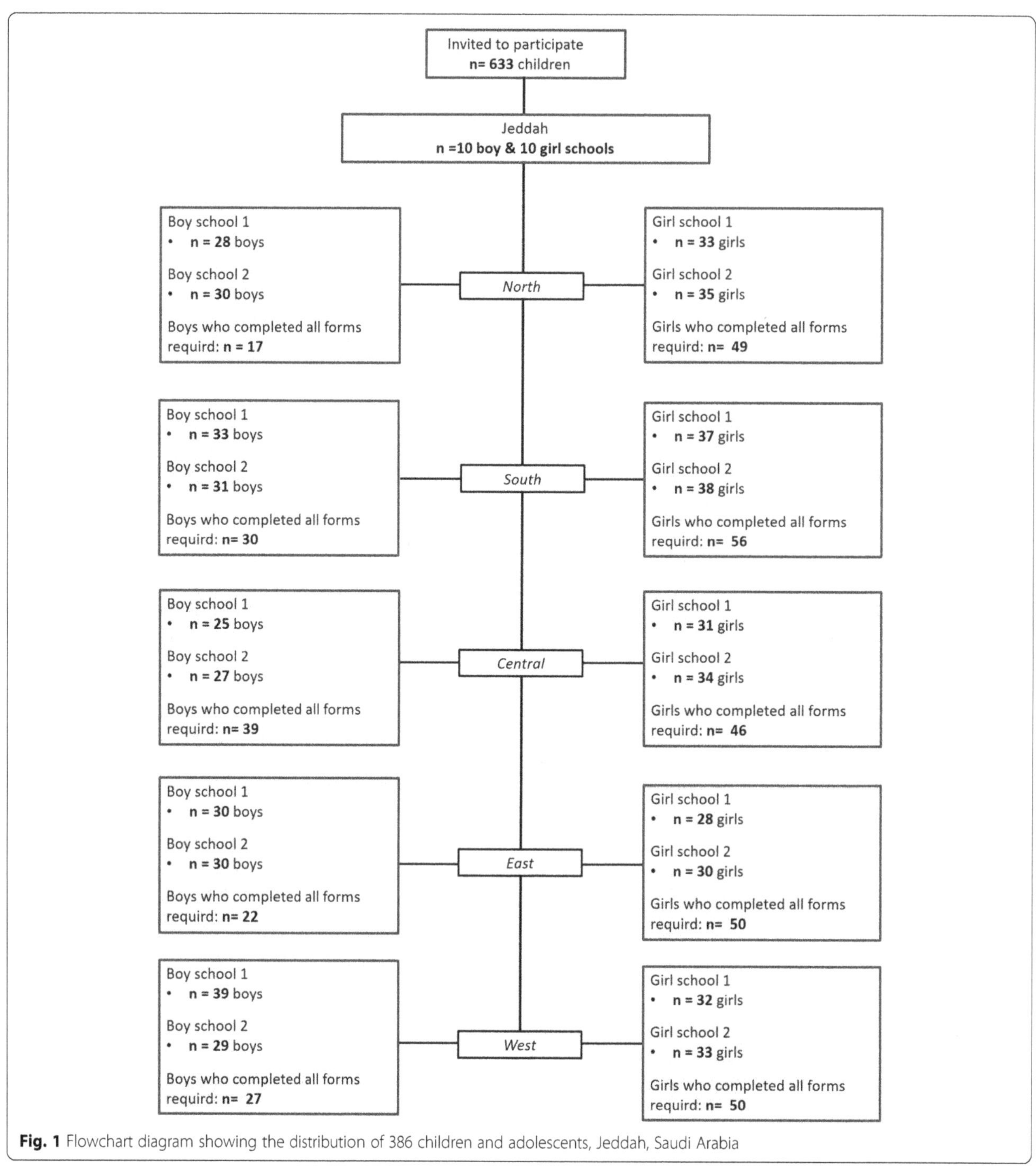

Fig. 1 Flowchart diagram showing the distribution of 386 children and adolescents, Jeddah, Saudi Arabia

the project drew the school classes' titles from a bucket by using simple sampling method. One day before visiting each school, a sealed envelope containing proper information about the study, questions regarding demographic data (including ethnic, socioeconomic background information, and medical history), the CBCL questionnaires, as well as the consent form, was distributed to the parents through their children. Due to cultural considerations, boys were invited to be examined in the dental clinic of the primary health care center in each region, while girls' examination was performed in girls' school at the school nurse's room.

On the day of the examination, all envelopes that were sent to the parents were collected, followed by a verbal explanation about the aim of the study by one examiner (AA-K). Each participant was asked two validated questions about the presence of orofacial pain (TMD-pain) [11]; 1) "Do you have pain in the temple, face, temporomandibular joint, or jaws once a week or more?" 2) "Do you have pain when you open your mouth wide or chew once a week or more?". The clinical examination was performed according to the RDC/TMD (Axis I) protocol by one examiner (A A-K), who was trained by an orofacial pain specialist (ME; calibrated to a gold-standard examiner (Thomas List)). The RDC/TMD protocol was chosen since it is reliable as an examination protocol for children with TMD [11, 18], while the newer DC/TMD [19] was not used on children at that time.

Measures

Research diagnostic criteria for temporomandibular disorders Axis I The RDC/TMD is a standardized dual diagnostic method for TMD [20]. It was developed to increase the strength and reliability of the results of multicenter projects, e.g. when various specialties from different countries collaborate, but also to enable comparison of results between studies. This diagnostic tool consists of Axis I, a clinical examination, and Axis II, a biobehavioral questionnaire. In Axis I, the TMJ and orofacial muscles are examined to diagnose the presence of one of the following clinical clusters: muscle disorders, internal derangement, or degenerative joint disorders. In the Axis II, the biobehavioral section is divided into four primary domains: the GCPS, the Jaw Disability Checklist (JDC), the Depression and Non-specific Physical Symptoms scales (SCL-90-R), and patient characteristics. Axis I has been shown to be reliable in children and adolescents [11]. However, the SCL-90-R of the Axis II has not been validated for children and adolescents younger than 13 years of age [21]. Therefore, the SCL-90-R was replaced with both the YSR and CBCL in the current project.

Child behavior checklist (CBCL) The emotional, behavior and somatic functioning, as well as social competence, were assessed by using the Arabic version of the CBCL questionnaires, licensed from the ASEBA/Research Center for Children, Youth & Families, University of Vermont, Burlington, VT USA. Of note, three statements about sexual problems were removed from the questionnaires due to cultural considerations.

CBCL is a validated questionnaire that assesses emotional and behavior problems in children age between 6 and 18 years [3, 22]. It consists of two main domains: 1) Problem Checklist, and 2) Social Competence. The Problem Checklist contains 112 statements which are grouped into three subscales; a) broad-band internalizing and externalizing problems, b) eight narrow-band syndromes, and c) Diagnostic and Statistical Manual of Mental Disorders (DSM)-oriented scales.

The second domain: the Social competence comprises seven statements that cover three areas; social relations, physical activities, and the mean of self-reported academic performance. Each statement is rated as 0 (not true), 1 (somewhat or sometimes true), or 2 (very true or often true).

Statistics

The proper data grouping into the subscales was performed by using the licensed software scoring program (ASEBA version 9.1). As a result, percentiles and T-scores are presented for all subscales and syndromes. The normal T-score range for all syndromes is 50–64, the borderline clinical range is 65–69, while the clinical range is 70–100. In regards to Social competence, the normal T-score range is 36–65, the borderline clinical range is 32–35, and the clinical range is 20–31.

The 386 participants were divided into three groups; non-TMD, TMD-pain and TMD-pain-free depending on the diagnoses presented in our previous study [10]. The mean and standard deviation (SD), median and (IQR) and also frequencies (%) are presented as descriptive statistics. To analyze differences in T-scores between the groups, the median score was modeled using quantile regression. In the unadjusted model TMD groups were included as dichotomous dummy variables with non-TMD pain as the reference group. The multivariate model adjusted for potential confounding factors included sex (male/female), age (10–13 years/14–18 years), and Saudi Arabian nationality (yes/no) as dichotomous variables. Also, the family income was modeled as dichotomous dummy variables that included three categories (below average/average/above average). Those categories were based on the average income in Saudi Arabia for the year 2013 (15,000 SR/month) (https://www.stats.gov.sa/). Subgroup analyses stratified by sex and age groups separately were performed with the non-TMD group as reference and with the stratification variable excluded from the model. *P*-values were based on 100 bootstrap samples. P-values lower than 0.05 and confidence intervals not including 0 were considered statistically significant. All analyzes were performed in STATA 12 SE.

Results

Demographic characteristics

Table 1 presents children and adolescents categorized into three groups; a) the non-TMD group; i.e. children and adolescents with no definite TMD diagnosis and no orofacial pain, b) the TMD-pain-free group; children and adolescents diagnosed with osteoarthrosis and/or disc displacement with or without reduction, and c) TMD-pain group; children and adolescents diagnosed with myofascial pain with or without limited mouth opening and/or arthralgia and/or osteoarthritis. As presented in our previous studies, there were no significant differences between the groups in regards to demographic characteristics [2, 10].

Table 1 Patient characteristics for 386 participants in Jeddah, Saudi Arabia

	Non-TMD n (%)	TMD-pain-free n (%)	TMD-pain n (%)
Individuals	279 (72.3)	22 (5.7)	85 (22)
Age (years)			
Mean (SD)	13.7 (2.2)	14.6 (2.3)	14 (2.2)
Median	13	14	13
Min-max	10–18	12–18	11–18
10–13 years	156 (55.9)	9 (40.9)	43 (50.6)
14–18 years	123 (44.1)	13 (59.1)	42 (49.4)
Sex			
Boys	101 (36.2)	9 (40.9)	25 (29.4)
Girls	178 (63.8)	13 (59.1)	60 (70.6)
Birth place			
Saudi Arabia	261 (93.5)	20 (90.9)	79 (92. 9)
Non-Saudi[a]	18 (6.5)	2 (9.1)	6 (7.1)
Nationality			
Saudi Arabia	177 (63.4)	10 (45.5)	49 (57.6)
Non-Saudi[a]	102 (36.6)	12 (54.5)	36 (42.4)
Family income			
Below average	152 (55.9)	11 (52.4)	46 (54.8)
Average	93 (34.2)	9 (42.9)	26 (31)
Above average	27 (9.9)	1 (4.8)	12 (14.3)

[a]Middle East, Gulf Area and Africa

All results presented below concerns the parents' reports of their child's status. To simplify reading, this has been omitted.

Physical activities and social competence

The mean values of the children's physical activities and social competence were within normal range for all three groups (Table 2). In this respect, there were no significant differences between the TMD-pain group and the TMD-pain-free group or the non-TMD group. When only the pain-free groups were compared, the adjusted and unadjusted analysis showed significantly higher ratings for physical activity in the TMD-pain-free group.

When we stratified for sex, the adjusted analysis presented significantly higher scores for physical activities for boys in the TMD-pain-free group (Coefficient = 8; 95% CI: 2.0–14.0), but not for boys with TMD-pain (Coefficient = – 1; 95% CI: -5.7- 3.7).

Unadjusted analysis revealed significantly higher T-score for physical activities in the younger age group (10–13 years) with TMD-pain. Adjusted analysis showed significantly higher T-scores in the TMD-pain-free group (Coefficient = 5.5; 95% CI: 0.84–10.2) in the older age group (14–18 years).

Table 2 The parents' reports of children's physical activities and social competence in 386 randomly selected children and adolescents in the general population of the city of Jeddah, Saudi Arabia

	Non-TMD	TMD-pain-free	TMD-pain
Activites (scale range)			
Mean (SD)	35.2 (8)	37.6 (9.4)	37.9 (8.8)
Median (IQR)	34 (44)	40 (36)	37 (41)
Min-max	20–64	20–56	20–61
Unadjusted	ref.	6*	3
95% CI		0.7–11.3	(−0.1)-6.1
Adjusted		5*	3
95% CI		0.8–9.2	(− 0.1)- 6.0
Social (scale range)			
Mean (SD)	40 (6.5)	40.8 (6.5)	40.5 (6.9)
Median (IQR)	39 (38)	41 (23)	39 (37)
Min-max	24–62	29–52	25–62
Unadjusted	ref.	2	0
95% CI		(−3.1)-7.1	(−2.6)-2.6
Adjusted		2	0
95% CI		(−2.7)-6.7	(−2.2)-2.2

The regression analysis of TMD-pain and TMD-pain-free were calculated with Non-TMD as reference group (ref.) in the quantile regression model
*significant association

In respect to social competence, unadjusted analysis revealed significantly higher T-scores in the TMD-pain-free group (Coefficient = 4; 95% CI: 0.20–7.8) than in the other groups, but this was not found in the adjusted analysis.

Broadband internalizing and externalizing scale and narrow-band syndrome scale

For all narrow-band syndromes, the mean and median range of T-scores were within normal range in all three groups (50–64). In the unadjusted analysis, the TMD-pain-free group showed significantly higher T-scores for one externalizing problem (Rule-Breaking Behavior syndrome). Both the unadjusted and adjusted analyses showed higher T-scores for all internalizing problems and for one externalizing problem (Aggressive Behavior) in the TMD-pain group, as shown in Table 3. When we stratified for sex, girls in the TMD pain group showed significantly higher scores for Anxious/Depressed (Coefficient = 7; 95% CI: 3.0–11), Withdraw/Depressed (Coefficient = 3; 95% CI: 0.004–6.0), and Somatic complaints (Coefficient = 4; 95% CI: 0.7–7.3), in the unadjusted analyses. These findings remained almost the same in the adjusted analysis; Anxious/Depressed (Coefficient = 7; 95% CI: 3.8–10.2), Withdraw/Depressed (Coefficient = 3; 95% CI: -0.13-6.0, no longer significant), and Somatic complaints (Coefficient = 6; 95% CI: 3.0–9.0). Boys with TMD-pain showed significantly higher scores for

Table 3 Associations between TMD and eight narrow-band syndromes extracted from the child behavior checklist (CBCL)

	Syndromes	Non-TMD	TMD-pain-free	TMD-pain
Internalizing problems	Anxious/Depressed			
	Unadjusted Coeff.	ref	2	5*
	95% CI		(−2.3)-6.3	1.3–8.7
	Adjusted Coeff.	ref	2	6*
	95% CI		(−1.6)-5.6	1.8–10.2
	Withdrawn/Depressed			
	Unadjusted Coeff.	ref	-1	3*
	95% CI		(−5.7)-3.7	0.3–5.7
	Adjusted Coeff.	ref	−1.5	3.5*
	95% CI		(−5.1)-2.1	0.6–6.4
	Somatic Complaints			
	Unadjusted Coeff.	ref	0	5*
	95% CI		(−4)-4	(1.3)-8.7
	Adjusted Coeff.	ref	0	6*
	95% CI		(−2.8)-2.8	3–9.1
Externalizing problems	Social Problems			
	Unadjusted Coeff.	ref	0	2
	95% CI		(−4.4)-4.4	−1.7-5.7
	Adjusted Coeff.	ref	0	3
	95% CI		(−5.2)-5.2	(−0.6)-6.6
	Thought Problems			
	Unadjusted Coeff.	ref	−1	1
	95% CI		(−3.4)-1.4	(−2)-4
	Adjusted Coeff.	ref	−0.7	0.7
	95% CI		(−1.7)-0.4	(−2)-3.3
	Attention Problem			
	Unadjusted Coeff.	ref	0	1
	95% CI		(−2.9)-2.9	(−0.9)-3
	Adjusted Coeff.	ref	1	1
	95% CI		(−1.4)-3.4	(−0.7)-2.7
	Rule-Breaking Behavior			
	Unadjusted Coeff.	ref	3*	1
	95% CI		0.2–5.8	(−1.5)-3.5
	Adjusted Coeff.	ref	2.5	1
	95% CI		(−0.3)-5.3	(−1.1)-3.1
	Aggressive Behavior			
	Unadjusted Coeff.	ref	0	3*
	95% CI		(−2.7)-2.7	0.2–5.8
	Adjusted Coeff.	ref	0	4*
	95% CI		(−3.3)-3.3	1.3–6.7

The regression analysis of TMD-pain and TMD-pain-free were calculated with Non-TMD as reference group (ref.) in the quantile regression model
Unadjusted analysis and analysis adjusted for age, sex, ethnic origin and parental income is presented. Regression coefficients are presented with 95% confidence intervals retrieved from quantile regression analysis
*significant association

somatic complaints in both the unadjusted (Coefficient = 11; 95% CI: 5.0–17.0) and adjusted analyses (Coefficient = 8; 95% CI: 2.8–13.2). Younger children with TMD-pain scored significantly higher for internalizing disorders in both the unadjusted and adjusted analyses; Anxious/Depressed (Coefficient = 6; 95% CI: 0.8–11 and Coefficient = 6; 95% CI: 1.5–10.5), Withdraw/Depressed (Coefficient = 3; 95% CI: -0.13-6.13 and Coefficient = 4; 95% CI: 0.9–7.1), and Somatic complaints (Coefficient = 6; 95% CI: 1.9–10.1 and Coefficient = 8; 95% CI: 4.5–11.5).

In regards to externalizing disorders, the score for rule breaking syndrome was significantly higher in girls with TMD-pain (Coefficient = 3; 95% CI: 0.5–5.5) Adjusted analysis showed higher score in the older age group with TMD-pain for rule breaking syndrome (Coefficient = 3; 95% CI: 0.2–5.8). Further, the score for aggressive syndrome was significantly higher in boys with TMD-pain in the adjusted analysis (Coefficient = 5; 95% CI: 0.13–9.9). Both the unadjusted and adjusted analysis showed significantly higher T-scores for younger children with TMD-pain for aggressive syndrome (Coefficient = 5; 95% CI: 1.4–8.6 and 5; 95% CI: 1.5–8.5, respectively).

DSM-oriented scales

In unadjusted and adjusted analyses, the TMD-pain group differed significantly from the non-TMD group regarding affective, anxiety, and somatic problems in the DSM-oriented scales (Table 4).

When the DSM-oriented scales were analyzed separately for age and sex, significantly higher Anxiety Problems in both the unadjusted and adjusted analysis (Coefficient = 6; 95% CI: 0.5–11.5 and Coefficient = 5.5; 95% CI: 1.1–9.8), Somatic Problems (Coefficient = 9; 95% CI: 4.4–13.6 and Coefficient = 6; 95% CI: 1.2–10.8) and Conduct Problems (Coefficient = 4; 95% CI: 0.5–7.5 and Coefficient = 4; 95% CI: 0.4–7.6) were found among girls with TMD-pain. Boys with TMD-pain showed significantly higher score in both the unadjusted and adjusted analysis for Somatic Problems (Coefficient = 9; 95% CI: 4.4–13.6 and Coefficient = 6; 95% CI: 1.2–10.8, respectively).

In the younger age group (10–13 years) TMD-pain was associated with significantly higher score in the unadjusted and adjusted analysis for Affective Problems (Coefficient = 6; 95% CI: 0.4–11.6 and Coefficient = 5; 95% CI: 1.0–9.0), Anxiety Problems (Coefficient = 5; 95% CI: 0.2–9.8 and Coefficient = 5.5; 95% CI: 1.1–9.8), Somatic Problems (Coefficient = 9; 95% CI: 4.4–13.6 and Coefficient = 5; 95% CI: 1.1–8.9) and Conduct Problems (Coefficient = 4; 95% CI: 0.5–7.5 and Coefficient = 3; 95% CI: 0.3–5.7) .

Table 4 Associations between TMD and DSM-Oriented scale: Regression coefficients are presented with 95% confidence intervals retrieved from quantile regression analysis

	Non-TMD	TMD-pain-free	TMD-pain
Affective Problems			
Unadjusted Coeff.	ref	−1	5*
95% CI		(−4.5) – 2.5	(1.2)-8.8
Adjusted Coeff. ref		-2	4*
95% CI		(−6.2)-2.5	0.83–7.2
Anxiety Problems			
Unadjusted Coeff.	ref	0	5*
95% CI		(−5.7)-5.7	0.7–9.3
Adjusted Coeff. ref		0	5*
95% CI		(−6.0)-6.0	1.8–8.2
Somatic Problems			
Unadjusted Coeff.	ref	0	9*
95% CI		(−2.7)-2.7	4.6–13.4
Adjusted Coeff. ref		0	9*
95% CI		(−3.2)-3.2	4.8–13.2
Attention Deficit/Hyperactivity Problems			
Unadjusted Coeff.	ref	−1	0
95% CI		(−4.7)-2.7	(−3.4)-3.4
Adjusted Coeff. ref		0	1
95% CI		(−2.7)-2.7	(−2)-4
Oppositional Defiant Problems			
Unadjusted Coeff.	ref	0	1
95% CI		(−1)-1	(−0.5)-2.5
Adjusted Coeff. ref		0	1
95% CI		(−0.6)-0.6	(−0.4)-2.4
Conduct Problems			
Unadjusted Coeff.	ref	2	2
95% CI		(−2.2)-6.2	(−1.2)-5.2
Adjusted Coeff. ref		2	2
95% CI		(−3.4)-7.4	(−0.9)-4.9

The regression analysis of TMD-pain and TMD-pain-free were calculated with Non-TMD as reference group (ref.) in the quantile regression model
Both unadjusted analysis and adjusted for age, sex, ethnic origin and parental income are presented
*significant association

Discussion

The main finding of the current study is that parents of children suffering from painful TMD conditions, as indicated by the CBCL, reported that their children have emotional problems, somatic problems, and aggressive behavior. Parents of children/adolescents with painful TMD conditions also reported that their children have internalizing problems, such as Anxious/Depressed, Withdrawn/Depressed, Somatic Complaints, in contrast to parents of children/adolescents with non-painful TMD conditions. These findings are not surprising and coincide well with the results from our previous study assessing the same psychometric variables but from the children/adolescents themselves using YSR [2]. Also, other studies using

CBCL to evaluate psychometric variables of children and adolescents suffering from pain due to different health conditions have shown similar findings in this study. Those studies reported that parents rated children complaining of pain with a higher degree internalizing problems such as withdrawn, somatic complaints, and anxious/depressed, than parents of children with no pain [4, 6, 7, 23]. Among those studies, one study highlighted the importance of multidimensional assessment models, such as CBCL, to be used for children with chronic musculoskeletal pain [23].

In regards to externalizing problems, the parents of children and adolescents who suffered from TMD-pain rated the children and adolescents as aggressive. Similar results were reported by children and adolescents, who suffered from TMD-pain when they asked about their emotional functioning in our previous study [2]. List et al. (2001) found the aggressive behavior among adolescents with TMD-pain, when children-rating scale (YSR) were used, compared to healthy controls [15]. Unlike the current study, our previous study showed that social as well as thought problems were associated with children and adolescents having TMD-related pain [2]. However, the parents in the current study did not indicate that they were aware of their children social and thought problems. An explanation for this difference is that YSR is a child-rating scale that subjectively measures the child's real perception regarding their feelings. Whereas, the parent rating scale (CBCL) was shown to efficiently measure the externalizing problems in their offspring rather than internalizing problems [24].

While the DSM-oriented scale was analyzed in the current study, the parents of children and adolescents in the TMD-pain group revealed that their children complain of anxiety, affective, and somatic problems. This finding ascertained similar results with the previous study from our group, in which children and adolescents with TMD-pain reported that they suffered from anxiety, affective, and somatic problems as well [2]. This indicates that parents are aware of their children's problems and therefore they can help their children to manage those problems early in life. This recommendation is to prevent the emotional and behavioral problems that meet the criteria of DSM-VI from being sustained to adulthood as suggested in one longitudinal study [25]. One explanation for the continuation of the emotional and behavioral problems into the adulthood is that TMD-pain and its associated emotional problems share memories from early pain experiences, then it is easy to recall these associations later in life [18, 26]. With respect to physical activities the parents of children and adolescents with non-painful TMD rated that their children were reasonably physically active. This finding is a contrast to the findings from our previous study in which children and adolescents in the TMD-pain-free group reported a lower rate of sports activities [2] and might confirm the importance of using self-report measures among youth who suffer from different pain conditions.

Consistent with our previous study, the parents' report revealed that social relations were within the normal range in all groups [2]. However, parents indicated that the risk of having depressive and somatic symptoms was higher among girls than boys with TMD-pain. Although this finding is in contrast to our previous study, studies indicate that girls with TMD-pain report higher degree of depressive and somatic problems than boys [1, 15]. Further, the parents' report that their girls with TMD-pain possess rule breaking behavior to a higher degree than boys with TMD-pain, while aggressive behavior is more common in boys with TMD-pain. However, these associations were not found in our previous study when the child-self rating scale was used. This difference in the findings between our two studies can be explained by the notion that the YSR is subjectively measuring the perception of the child's own behavior, while CBCL measures the parent opinion about their off-spring. Nevertheless, many other studies showed that parents reported fewer or more problems than their children/adolescents do [27–29]. This might indicate the importance of using the YSR in evaluating the emotional and behavior problems especially for adolescents with painful TMD conditions. The YSR may therefore be recommended in children that are mature enough to include all possible internalizing and externalizing problems precisely, especially during diagnosing, whereas the CBCL seems useful in young children with painful TMD conditions. Especially in children that are too young to fill in a questionnaire by themselves. With this in mind, and the fact that children and adolescents are frequently experiencing emotional and behavioral consequences due to pain [2], one has to consider if there is a need to also have the parents' view point (using for instance the CBCL). Also, since it has been shown that a comorbidity with psychiatric conditions and psychological distress has a significant and negative outcome for patients with chronic conditions like headache [16], one can assume that the CBCL also could be used as reliable predictor for the outcome of TMD.

One of the strengths of the current study is that the one examiner performed the RDC/TMD examination. This examiner was trained and calibrated with a gold standard clinician who is specialized in Orofacial Pain and Jaw Function. Another strength is the use of a reliable examination method (RDC/TMD) for children and adolescents and also a validated questionnaire, which has been used in many previous studies among children [11, 30, 31]. The random enrollment of participants is another strength.

One limitation of the current study could be the high drop-out rate among boys. Despite the settings for boys and girls were equal, the higher drop-out rate among boys was difficult to avoid as the place of examination were not the same among boys and girls. While the boys were invited to visit the nearest primary health care center, the girls were examined in the nurse room inside each school. A second reason to the higher drop-out rate in boys could be that Saudi girls are showing more dental care awareness than boys [32]. Another limitation of the study is the lack of information on the parents answering, i.e. sex, age, educational level, income, etc. Thus, we cannot be certain that the children and parents understood and interpreted the questions correctly.

Conclusion

In conclusion, the present study revealed that the parents rated that their children with TMD-pain suffer from emotional, somatic and aggressive behavior to a higher degree than healthy control subjects. The main outcome from the present study emphasizes the importance of using self-reported measures among youth suffering from pain conditions. For children that are too young to fill in a questionnaire by themselves parent-reported scales are suggested.

Abbreviations

CBCL: Child Behaviour Checklist; RDC/TMD: Research Diagnostic Criteria for Temporomandibular disorders; TMD: Temporomandibular disorders; TMJ: Temporomandibular joint; YSR: Youth Self Report Scale

Acknowledgments

The authors would like to thank Dr. Emad Albadawi, Jeddah Dental Speciality Centre, Ministry of Health, Jeddah, Saudi Arabia for his support in the clinical part of the research study. Also, the author would like to thank Miss Joudi Bathallath in helping with the examination of the students.

Funding

The current study was financially supported by a grant from Ministry of health, Saudi Arabia. The authors declare no potential conflicts of interest concerning publication of this article.

Authors' contributions

All authors have read and approved the final version of the manuscript. AAK, designed and performed the research, analyzed the data and wrote the manuscript. MG, processed data and participated in manuscript editing. ANA, designed the research, analyzed the data, and participated in the draft the manuscript. BHM, participated in the design and participated in manuscript editing ME, participated in the design and planning of the research and participated in manuscript editing. NC, designed the research, analyzed the data, and participated in manuscript editing.

Competing interests

The authors declared no conflicts of interest. The authors alone are responsible for the content and writing of the paper. All authors have read and approved the final version of the manuscript.

Author details

[1]Division of Oral Diagnostics and Rehabilitation, Department of Dental Medicine, Karolinska Institutet, Box 4064, SE-141 04 Huddinge, Sweden. [2]East Jeddah Hospital, Ministry of health, Jeddah, Saudi Arabia. [3]Scandinavian Center for Orofacial Neurosciences (SCON), Huddinge, Sweden. [4]Oral and maxillofacial surgery, Department of Dental Medicine, Karolinska Institutet, Huddinge, Sweden. [5]Department of Clinical Oral Physiology at the Eastman Institute, Stockholm Public Dental Health, Stockholm, Sweden.

References

1. Nilsson IM, Drangsholt M, List T (2009) Impact of temporomandibular disorder pain in adolescents: differences by age and gender. J Orofac Pain 23(2):115–122
2. Al-Khotani A, Naimi-Akbar A, Gjelset M, Albadawi E, Bello L, Hedenberg-Magnusson B et al (2016) The associations between psychosocial aspects and TMD-pain related aspects in children and adolescents. J Headache Pain 17:30
3. Achenbach T, Edelbrock C (1991) The child behavior checklist manual. The University of Vermont, Burlington, VT
4. Baker AM, Raiker JS, Elkin TD, Palermo TM, Karlson CW (2017) Internalizing symptoms mediate the relationship between sleep disordered breathing and pain symptoms in a pediatric hematology/oncology sample. Children's Health Care 46(1):34–48
5. Vandvik IH, Eckblad G (1990) Relationship between pain, disease severity and psychosocial function in patients with juvenile chronic arthritis (JCA). Scand J Rheumatol 19(4):295–302
6. Galli F, D'Antuono G, Tarantino S, Viviano F, Borrelli O, Chirumbolo A et al (2007) Headache and recurrent abdominal pain: a controlled study by the means of the child behaviour checklist (CBCL). Cephalalgia 27(3):211–219
7. Gulewitsch MD, Weimer K, Enck P, Schwille-Kiuntke J, Hautzinger M, Schlarb AA (2017) Stress reactivity in childhood functional abdominal pain or irritable bowel syndrome. Eur J Pain 21(1):166–177
8. Kohyama J, Furushima W, Hasegawa T (2003) Behavioral problems in children evaluated for sleep disordered breathing. Sleep and Hypnosis 5:89–94
9. Evans S, Keenan TR, Shipton EA (2007) Psychosocial adjustment and physical health of children living with maternal chronic pain. J Paediatr Child Health 43(4):262–270
10. Al-Khotani A, Naimi-Akbar A, Albadawi E, Ernberg M, Hedenberg-Magnusson B, Christidis N (2016) Prevalence of diagnosed temporomandibular disorders among Saudi Arabian children and adolescents. J Headache Pain. 17:41
11. Nilsson IM, List T, Drangsholt M (2005) Prevalence of temporomandibular pain and subsequent dental treatment in Swedish adolescents. J Orofac Pain 19(2):144–150
12. Alamoudi N (2002) Correlation between oral parafunction and temporomandibular disorders and emotional status among Saudi children. J Clin Pediatr Dent 26(1):71–80
13. Pereira LJ, Pereira-Cenci T, Pereira SM, Cury AA, Ambrosano GM, Pereira AC et al (2009) Psychological factors and the incidence of temporomandibular disorders in early adolescence. Braz Oral Res. 23(2):155–160
14. Pizolato RA, Freitas-Fernandes FS, Gaviao MB (2013) Anxiety/depression and orofacial myofacial disorders as factors associated with TMD in children. Braz Oral Res 27(2):156–162
15. List T, Wahlund K, Larsson B (2001) Psychosocial functioning and dental factors in adolescents with temporomandibular disorders: a case-control study. J Orofac Pain 15(3):218–227
16. Serafini G, Pompili M, Innamorati M, Gentile G, Borro M, Lamis DA et al (2012) Gene variants with suicidal risk in a sample of subjects with chronic migraine and affective temperamental dysregulation. Eur Rev Med Pharmacol Sci 16(10):1389–1398
17. Achenbach T, Rescorla L (2001) The manual for the ASEBA School-age Forms & Profiles. University of Vermont, Research Center for Children, Youth, and Families, Burlington
18. Wahlund K, List T, Ohrbach R (2005) The relationship between somatic and emotional stimuli: a comparison between adolescents with temporomandibular disorders (TMD) and a control group. Eur J Pain 9(2):219–227
19. Schiffman E, Ohrbach R, Truelove E, Look J, Anderson G, Goulet JP et al (2014) Diagnostic criteria for temporomandibular disorders (DC/TMD) for clinical and research applications: recommendations of the international RDC/TMD consortium network* and orofacial pain special interest Groupdagger. J Oral Facial Pain Headache 28(1):6–27

20. Dworkin SF, LeResche L (1992) Research diagnostic criteria for temporomandibular disorders: review, criteria, examinations and specifications, critique. J Craniomandib Disord 6(4):301–355
21. Goldfinger K, Pomerantz AM (2014) Psychological assessment and report writing, 2nd edn. SAGE Publications, Inc., California
22. Achenbach TM (1966) The classification of children's psychiatric symptoms: a factor-analytic study. Psychol Monogr 80(7):1–37
23. Varni JW, Wilcox KT, Hanson V, Brik R (1988) Chronic musculoskeletal pain and functional status in juvenile rheumatoid arthritis: an empirical model. Pain 32(1):1–7
24. Phares V, Compas BE, Howell DC (1989) Perspectives on child behavior problems: comparisons of children's self-reports with parent and teacher reports. Psychological Assessment: A Journal of Consulting and Clinical Psychology 1(1):68
25. Hofstra MB, Van Der Ende J, Verhulst FC (2001) Adolescents' self-reported problems as predictors of psychopathology in adulthood: 10-year follow-up study. Br J Psychiatry 179:203–209
26. Lane RD, Reiman EM, Bradley MM, Lang PJ, Ahern GL, Davidson RJ et al (1997) Neuroanatomical correlates of pleasant and unpleasant emotion. Neuropsychologia 35(11):1437–1444
27. Rescorla LA, Ginzburg S, Achenbach TM, Ivanova MY, Almqvist F, Begovac I et al (2013) Cross-informant agreement between parent-reported and adolescent self-reported problems in 25 societies. J Clin Child Adolesc Psychol 42(2):262–273
28. Herjanic B, Reich W (1997) Development of a structured psychiatric interview for children: agreement between child and parent on individual symptoms. J Abnorm Child Psychol 25(1):21–31
29. Kolko DJ, Kazdin AE (1993) Emotional/behavioral problems in clinic and nonclinic children: correspondence among child, parent and teacher reports. J Child Psychol Psychiatry 34(6):991–1006
30. Matijasevich A, Murray E, Stein A, Anselmi L, Menezes AM, Santos IS et al (2014) Increase in child behavior problems among urban Brazilian 4-year olds: 1993 and 2004 Pelotas birth cohorts. J Child Psychol Psyc 55(10):1125–1134
31. Mesman J, Koot HM (2000) Child-reported depression and anxiety in preadolescence: II. Preschool predictors. J Am Acad Child Adolesc Psychiatry 39(11):1379–1386
32. Al Subait A, Alousaimi M, Geeverghese A, Ali A, El Metwally A (2016) Oral health knowledge, attitude and behavior among students of age 10–18 years old attending Jenadriyah festival Riyadh; a cross-sectional study. Saudi J Dental Res 7(1):45–50

6

Impact of migraine on the clinical presentation of insomnia: a population-based study

Jiyoung Kim[1], Soo-Jin Cho[2], Won-Joo Kim[3], Kwang Ik Yang[4], Chang-Ho Yun[5] and Min Kyung Chu[6*]

Abstract

Background: Insomnia and migraine are closely related; insomnia aggravates migraine symptoms. This study was conducted to investigate the impact of migraine on the clinical presentation of insomnia symptoms.

Methods: The data of the Korean Headache-Sleep Study (KHSS) were used in the present study. The KHSS is a nation-wide cross-sectional population-based survey regarding headache and sleep in Korean adults aged 19 to 69 years. If a participant's Insomnia Severity Index (ISI) score ≥ 10, she/he was classified as having insomnia. The clinical presentation of insomnia symptoms was assessed using total and subcomponent scores of the ISI.

Results: Of 2695 participants, 290 (10.8%) and 143 (5.3%) individuals were assigned as having insomnia and migraine, respectively. The proportions of migraine (12.8% vs. 4.4%, $p < 0.001$) and non-migraine headache (59.0% vs. 39.9%, $p < 0.001$) were higher among individuals with insomnia compared to those without insomnia. Among participants with insomnia, total ISI scores were not significantly different among participants with migraine, non-migraine, and non-headache [median and interquartile range: 13.0 (11.0–17.5) vs. 13.0 (11.0–17.5) vs. 12.0 (11.0–16.0), $p = 0.245$]. ISI scores for noticeability of sleep problems to others were significantly higher among participants with migraine [3.0 (2.0–4.0) vs. 2.0 (2.0–3.0), $p = 0.011$] and non-migraine headache [3.0 (2.0–4.0) vs. 2.0 (2.0–3.0), $p = 0.001$] compared to those without headache history. Other ISI subcomponent scores did not significantly differ between headache status groups.

Conclusions: Participants with insomnia had an increased risk of migraine and non-migraine headache compared to those without insomnia. Among participants with insomnia, overall insomnia severity was not significantly influenced by the headache status.

Keywords: Clinical presentation, Headache, Insomnia, Insomnia symptom, Migraine

Background

Migraine is a common neurological disorder and affects 5–15% of the general population [1]. Owing to its disabling symptoms, migraineurs encounter disability and decreased quality of life [2]. Even in periods without migraine symptoms, migraineurs may have a fear of developing a headache because migraine attacks often cause a failure to perform social obligations at school, the workplace, or at home [3]. Sleep disturbances are common complaints among migraineurs [4–6]. Individuals with migraine or headache with sleep disturbances often encounter more severe symptoms and decrease quality of life [5, 7, 8].

Insomnia is another disorder with high prevalence, affecting 10–30% of the general population [9]. Insomnia is associated with hypertension, coronary heart disease, and diabetes, among others [10]. Furthermore, insomnia in the working age population is one of the factors that cause a decrease in productivity [11]. Therefore, insomnia is an important public health problem like migraine.

Migraine and insomnia exhibit a strong relationship. Cross-sectional studies have persistently demonstrated a significant comorbidity for these two disorders in clinical and population-based studies [12]. Two longitudinal

* Correspondence: chumk@yonsei.ac.kr
[6]Department of Neurology, Severance Hospital, Yonsei University College of Medicine, 50-1 Yonsei-ro, Seodaemoon-gu, Seoul, Republic of Korea
Full list of author information is available at the end of the article

studies using a single dataset show a bidirectional comorbidity of migraine and insomnia. Individuals have an increased risk of developing migraine 11 years after the onset of insomnia and vice versa [13, 14]. The risk for developing insomnia increases in patients with an increased migraine headache frequency, and the risk for developing migraine was positively correlated with severe insomnia. Such a strong bidirectional comorbidity suggests shared pathophysiological mechanisms [15].

According to previous studies, migraineurs have an increased risk of developing insomnia compared to patients suffering from non-migraine headache and healthy subjects. Furthermore, migraineurs with insomnia present with a higher headache frequency and increased headache intensity compared to those without insomnia [8]. Nevertheless, information about the impact of migraine on the prevalence and clinical presentation of insomnia in a population-based sample is currently limited. We hypothesized that migraine affects the prevalence and clinical presentation of insomnia symptoms. The purposes of the present study were to investigate 1) the prevalence of migraine and insomnia, 2) the impact of migraine on the prevalence of insomnia, and 3) the impact of migraine on the clinical presentation of insomnia in a general population-based sample.

Methods

Study population and survey process

The data of the Korean Headache-Sleep Study (KHSS) were used in the present study. The KHSS was a nation-wide, cross-sectional survey regarding headache and sleep disorder among Korean adults aged 19 to 69 years. It also included items regarding symptoms of anxiety and depression. The study design, methods, and process were described in detail previously [6]. In brief, the KHSS adopted a two-stage clustered random sampling method for all Korean territories except Jeju-do. This method sampled participants proportionally to the population distribution and socioeconomic status. Trained interviewers conducted the survey by face-to-face interviews using a questionnaire. All trained interviewers were employees of Gallup Korea and had previous experience in social surveys. Data collection of the KHSS was performed from November 2011 to January 2012. The KHSS was approved by the Institutional Review Board and Ethics Committee of Hallym University Sacred Heart Hospital (IRB No. 2011-I077). Written informed consent was obtained from all participants.

Migraine assessment

Diagnosis of migraine was based on criteria A to D for migraine without aura in the third edition beta version of the International Classification of Headache Disorders (ICHD-3 beta; code 1.1: A, 5 or more attacks in a lifetime; B, attack duration of 4–72 h; C, any 2 of the 4 typical headache characteristics [i.e., unilateral pain, pulsating quality, moderate-to-severe pain intensity, and aggravation by routine physical activity]; and D, attacks associated with at least one of the following: nausea, vomiting, or both photophobia and phonophobia) [16]. We did not distinguish between migraine without aura (code 1.1) and migraine with aura (code 1.2). Therefore, migraine included both migraine with aura and migraine without aura. Our survey method has been reported to have a sensitivity of 75.0% and a specificity of 88.2% [17].

Non-migraine headache assessment

Participants that experienced more than one minute of headache in the last twelve months but did not satisfy the criteria for migraine diagnosis were classified as a distinct non-migraine headache group.

Insomnia assessment

Insomnia was evaluated by using the Insomnia Severity Index (ISI), which is a self-report questionnaire with the following seven items: difficulties in sleep onset, difficulties in sleep maintenance, early awakening in the morning, sleep dissatisfaction, interference of sleep problems with daily functioning, noticeability of sleep problems to others, and worries caused by the sleep problems. This index measures the individual's perceptions of their sleep problem by evaluating the severity of the insomnia problems within the last two weeks. The total ISI score ranges from 0 to 28 [18]. Participants with a total ISI score of 10 or more were classified in our study as suffering from insomnia according to a previous epidemiological study [19]. Additionally, we investigated whether the sleep was usually non-refreshing. We asked participants to choose from the categories none, mild, moderate, severe, and very severe and graded each response as 0, 1, 2, 3, and 4, respectively.

Statistical analyses

The Kolmogorov-Smirnov test was used to evaluate the normality of the distribution. After normality was confirmed, Student's t-test or analysis of variance was used to compare continuous variables. If normality was not confirmed, the Mann-Whitney *U* test was used to compare differences between two independent groups. For comparison of ordinal variables among more than three groups, we used Kruskal-Wallis test. To adjust for multiple testing, *p-values* were calculated using the Bonferroni post hoc test. Categorical variables were compared using the chi-square test. The significance level was set at $p < 0.05$ for all analyses. Statistical analyses were performed using the Statistical Package for Social Sciences 22.0 (SPSS 22.0; IBM, Armonk, NY, USA).

Results

Survey

During the survey, interviewers contacted 7430 individuals, and 3144 permitted to participate. Of those, 449 individuals waived participation, and thus 2695 participants completed the whole survey (cooperation rate of 36.3%; Fig. 1). The distributions of age, sex, size of the residential area, and education level of KHSS participants was not significantly different from those of the Korean general population (Table 1).

Prevalence of insomnia and migraine

Of the 2695 participants, 290 (10.8%) participants reported an ISI score ≥ 10 and were classified as having insomnia. The ISI score of all participants was [2.0 (1.0–5.0), median and interquartile range]. Of the 1273 (47.2%) participants, who reported that they experienced at least one attack of headache during the last year, 143 (5.3%) participants were classified as having migraine. Therefore, 1130 (41.9%) were classified as having non-migraine headache (Table 1).

Prevalence of migraine and non-migraine headache according to the presence of insomnia

Among the 290 participants with insomnia, 37 (12.8%), 171 (59.0%), and 82 (28.3%) participants were classified as having migraine, non-migraine headache, and non-headache, respectively. The prevalence of migraine (12.8% vs. 4.4%, $p < 0.001$) and non-migraine headache (59.0% vs. 39.9%, $p < 0.001$) was significantly higher among participants with insomnia compared to that in participants without insomnia (Fig. 2).

Total and subcomponent ISI scores among participants with insomnia according to the headache status

In the 290 participants with insomnia, the total ISI score was not significantly different among migraine, non-migraine headache, and non-headache groups. A further analysis of the seven ISI subcomponent scores revealed that only the categories interference with daily functioning and noticeability of sleep problems to others exhibited significantly different scores among the three headache groups. Furthermore, our additional parameter non-refreshing sleep showed significant score differences among these groups. Post hoc analyses revealed that the scores for noticeability of sleep problems to others, and non-refreshing sleep were significantly higher in participants of the non-migraine headache group than those in the non-headache group and score for noticeability of sleep problems to others was significantly higher in participants of the migraine group than those in the non-headache group. However, subcomponent for interference with daily functioning did not show significance in post hoc analysis (Table 2).

Prevalence of insomnia according to the headache status

Insomnia prevalence among participants with migraine, non-migraine headache, and non-headache was 25.9%, 15.1%, and 5.8%, respectively (Fig. 3). The prevalence of insomnia among migraineurs was significantly higher compared to participants with non-migraine headache ($p = 0.001$) and non-headache ($p < 0.001$).

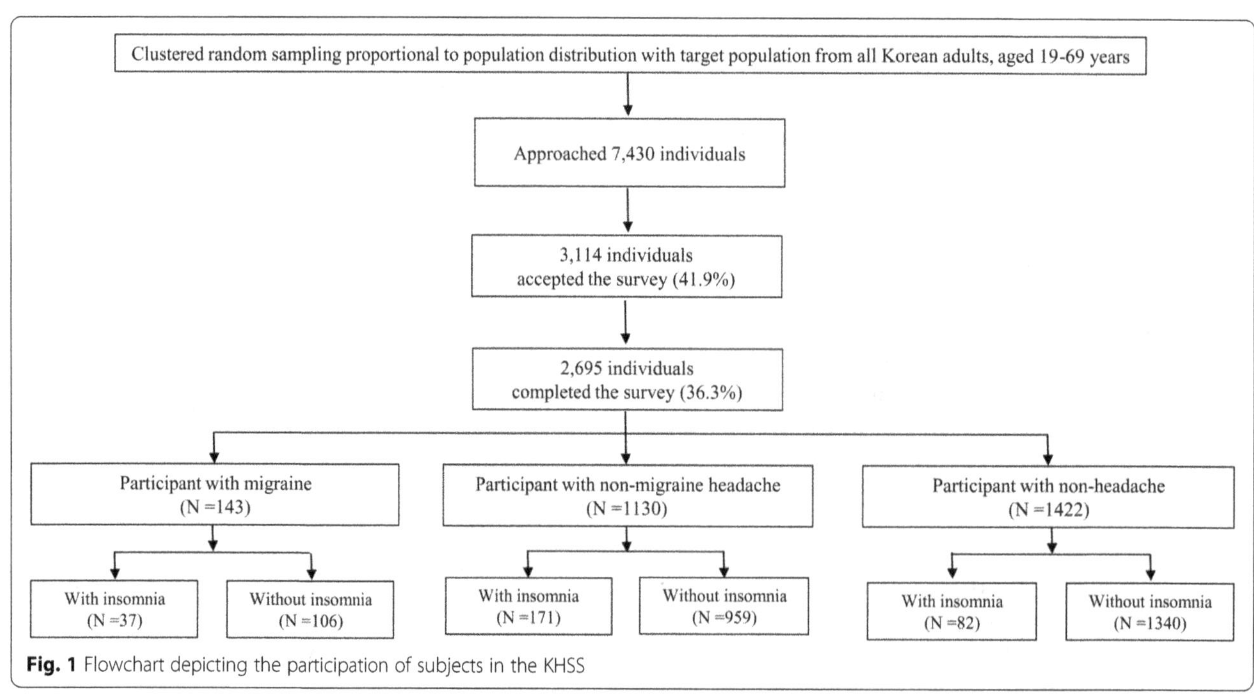

Fig. 1 Flowchart depicting the participation of subjects in the KHSS

Table 1 Sociodemographic characteristics of survey participants, the total Korean population, and cases identified as having migraine, non-migraine headache, and insomnia

	Survey participants N (%)	Total population N (%)	*P*	Migraine N, % (95% CI)	Non-migraine headache N, % (95% CI)	Insomnia N, % (95% CI)
Gender						
Men	1345 (49.3)	17,584,365 (50.6)	*0.854*[a]	36, 2.7 (1.8–3.5)	471, 35.0 (32.5–37.6)	117, 8.7 (7.2–10.2)
Women	1350 (50.7)	17,198,350 (49.4)		107, 7.9 (6.5–9.4)	659, 48.8 (46.2–51.5)	173, 12.8 (11.0–14.6)
Age						
19–29	542 (20.5)	7,717,947 (22.2)	*0.917*[a]	25, 4.5 (2.7–6.2)	231, 42.6 (38.4–46.8)	59, 10.9 (8.3–13.5)
30–39	604 (21.9)	8,349,487 (24.0)		42, 7.0 (4.9–9.1)	269, 44.5 (40.6–48.5)	53, 8.8 (6.5–11.0)
40–49	611 (23.1)	8,613,110 (24.8)		39, 6.5 (4.5–8.4)	277, 45.3 (41.4–49.3)	66, 10.8 (8.3–13.3)
50–59	529 (18.9)	6,167,505 (17.7)		22, 4.1 (2.4–5.9)	204, 38.6 (34.4–42.7)	63, 11.9 (9.1–14.7)
60–69	409 (15.6)	3,934,666 (11.3)		15, 3.9 (2.0–5.7)	149, 36.4 (31.7–41.1)	49, 12.0 (8.8–15.1)
Size of residential area						
Large city	1248 (46.3)	16,776,771 (48.2)	*0.921*[a]	76, 6.1 (4.8–7.5)	525, 42.1 (39.3–44.8)	136, 10.9 (9.2–12.6)
Medium-to-small city	1186 (44.0)	15,164,345 (43.6)		48, 4.0 (2.9–5.2)	488, 41.1 (38.3–44.0)	125, 10.5 (8.8–12.3)
Rural area	261 (9.7)	2,841,599 (8.2)		19, 7.4 (4.2–10.6)	117, 44.8 (38.8–50.9)	29, 11.1 (7.3–14.9)
Education level						
Middle school or less	393 (14.9)	6,608,716 (19.0)	*0.752*[a]	22, 5.5 (4.2–7.7)	156, 42.0 (37.1–46.9)	62, 15.8 (12.2–19.4)
High school	1208 (44.5)	15,234,829 (43.8)		60, 5.0 (3.8–6.3)	502, 41.6 (38.8–44.4)	116, 9.6 (7.9–11.3)
College or more	1068 (39.6)	12,939,170 (37.2)		60, 5.6 (4.3–7.0)	457, 42.8 (40.0–45.8)	109, 10.2 (8.4–12.0)
Not responded	26 (1.0)			1, 3.8 (0.0–11.8)	6, 23.1 (5.7–40.4)	3, 11.5 (0.0–24.7)
Total	2695 (100.0)	34,782,715 (100.0)		143, 5.3 (4.5–6.2)	1130, 41.9 (40.0–43.8)	290, 10.8 (9.6–11.9)

[a]Comparison of sex, age group, size of residential area, and educational level distributions between the sample in the present study and the total population of Korea
N, number; *CI*, confidence interval

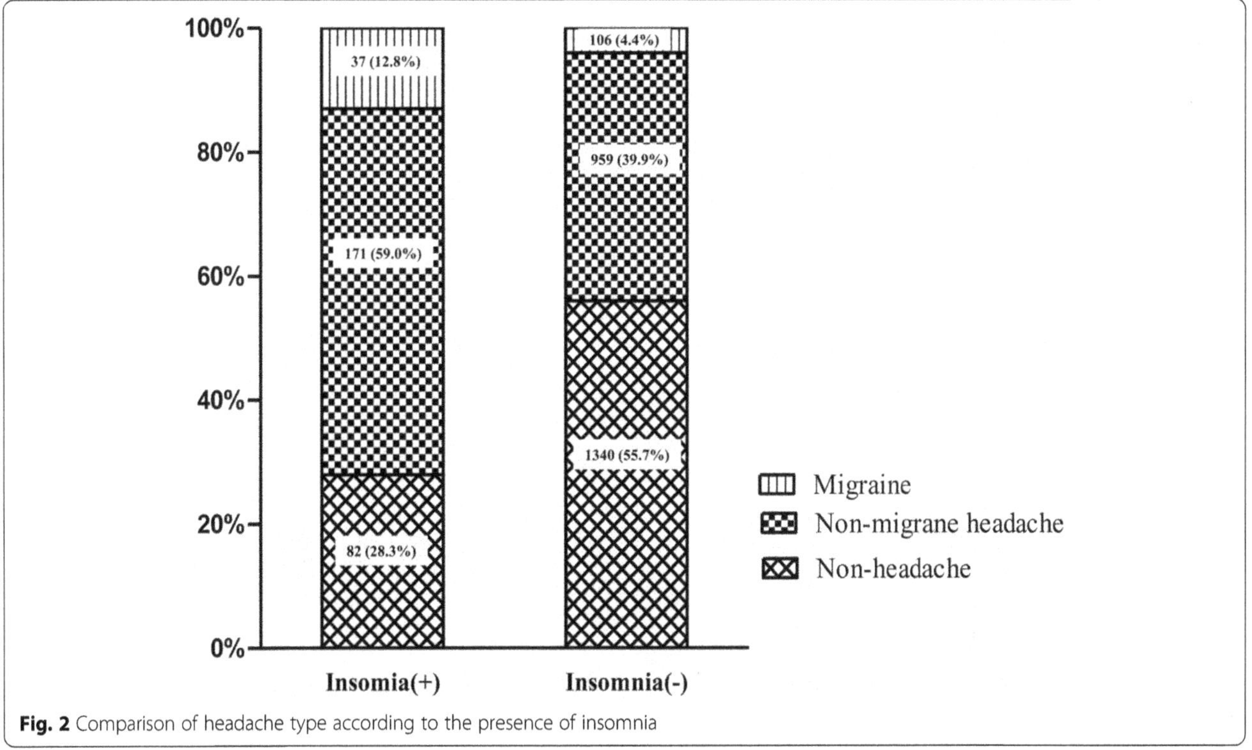

Fig. 2 Comparison of headache type according to the presence of insomnia

Table 2 Total ISI and its subcomponent scores among participants with insomnia in relation to the headache status

	Migraine ($N = 37$)	Non-migraine headache ($N = 171$)	Non-headache ($N = 82$)	*P*
Total ISI score	13.0 (11.0–17.5)	13.0 (11.0–17.0)	12.0 (11.0–16.0)	*0.245*
Falling asleep	2.0 (1.0–3.0)	2.0 (1.0–3.0)	2.0 (1.0–3.0)	*0.796*
Staying asleep	2.0 (1.0–3.0)	2.0 (1.0–3.0)	2.0 (1.0–3.0)	*0.671*
Early awakening	2.0 (1.0–3.0)	2.0 (1.0–3.0)	2.0 (1.0–3.0)	*0.303*
Satisfaction	4.0 (3.5–4.0)	4.0 (3.0–5.0)	4.0 (3.0–4.0)	*0.245*
Interference	3.0 (3.0–4.0)	3.0 (2.0–4.0)	3.0 (2.0–3.0)	*0.032*
Noticeability	3.0 (2.0–4.0)[a]	3.0 (2.0–4.0)[a]	2.0 (2.0–3.0)	*0.002*
Worry	3.0 (2.0–4.0)	3.0 (2.0–4.0)	3.0 (2.0–3.0)	*0.364*
Non-refreshing sleep[b]	2.0 (2.0–3.0)	3.0 (2.0–4.0)[a]	2.0 (1.0–3.0)	*0.001*

Variables are presented as median (interquartile range)
Kurskal-Wallis test was used to compare among three groups
[a]Significantly higher in the post hoc analysis compared to the non-headache group
[b]Non-refreshing sleep score is not included in the total ISI score

Headache frequency, headache intensity, and impact of headache according to the presence of insomnia among participants with migraine and non-migraine headache

The Visual Analogue Scale (VAS) score for headache intensity (median [interquartile range], 7.0 [5.0–9.0] vs. 6.0 [5.0–7.0]; $p = 0.003$) and the Headache Impact Test-6 (HIT-6; 60.0 ± 9.5 vs. 52.3 ± 8.4; $p < 0.001$) score were significantly higher in migraineurs with insomnia compared to those in migraineurs without insomnia. Headache frequency per month was discernibly different according to the presence of insomnia without reaching statistical significance (5.7 ± 8.2 vs. 3.2 ± 5.4, $p = 0.093$). Among participants with non-migraine headache, headache frequency per month, VAS score for headache intensity, and HIT-6 score were significantly higher when insomnia was present (Table 3).

Discussion

The key findings of the present study were as follows: 1) The prevalence of migraine and non-migraine headache was significantly higher among participants with insomnia compared to those without insomnia; 2) Among participants with insomnia, the total ISI score was not significantly different among migraine, non-migraine headache, and non-headache groups and 3) Among participants with migraine, the prevalence of insomnia was

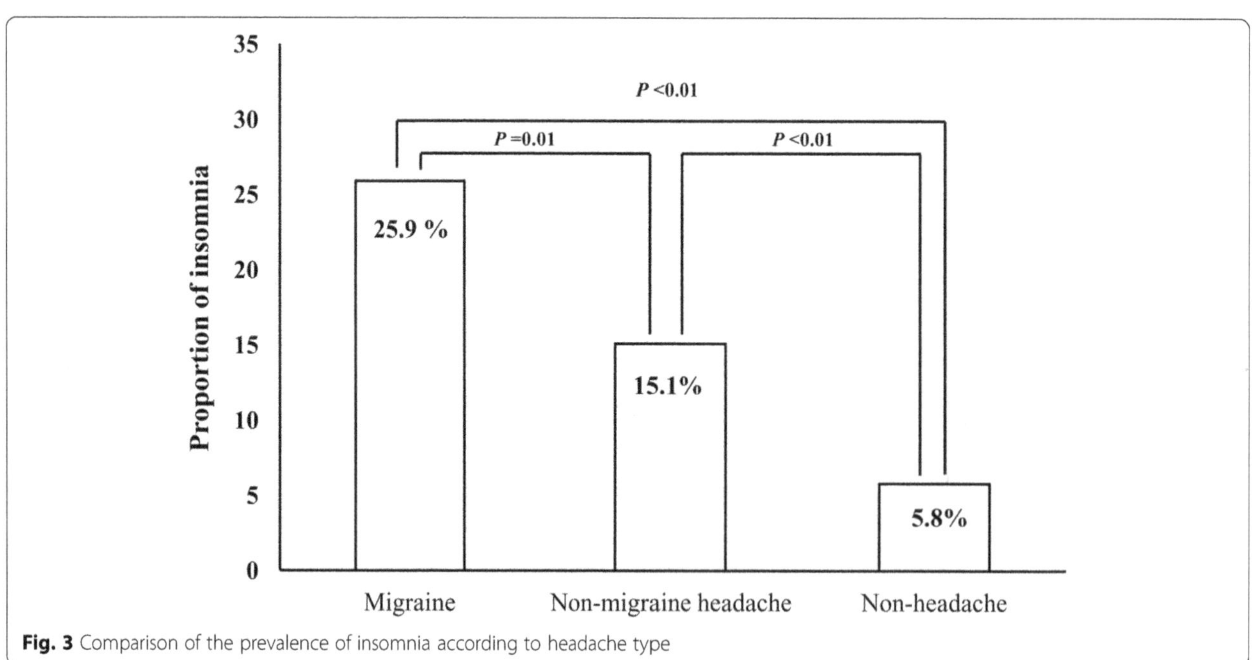

Fig. 3 Comparison of the prevalence of insomnia according to headache type

Table 3 Headache frequency, VAS score of headache intensity, and impact of headache in relation to the presence of insomnia among participants with migraine and non-migraine headache

	Migraine with insomnia (*N* = 37)	Migraine without insomnia (*N* = 106)	*P*	Non-migraine headache with insomnia (*N* = 171)	Non-migraine headache without insomnia (*N* = 959)	*P*
Headache frequency	5.7 ± 8.2	3.2 ± 5.4	*0.093*	3.7 ± 6.8	2.1 ± 4.9	*0.004*
VAS score[a]	7.0 (5.0–9.0)	6.0 (5.0–7.0)	*0.003*	5.0 (4.0–7.0)	5.0 (3.0–6.0)	*< 0.001*
HIT-6 score	60.0 ± 9.5	52.3 ± 8.4	*< 0.001*	50.1 ± 8.6	44.4 ± 6.7	*< 0.001*

VAS Visual Analogue Scale, *HIT-6* Headache Impact Test-6
[a]Variable is analyzed by Mann–Whitney U test and shown as a median (interquartile range)

higher than participants with non-migraine headache and non-headache. Migraine symptoms exacerbated with the presence of insomnia.

There is limited information available about the impact of insomnia on the clinical presentation of headache. It has been reported that in individuals with headache or migraine, those with insomnia present an increased symptom severity compared to those without [13]. Nevertheless, information regarding the impact of headache or migraine on the clinical presentation of insomnia is currently scarce. Our study is the first report in a population-based setting that individuals with insomnia have an increased risk of suffering from migraine and non-migraine headache. Furthermore, the insomnia severity as reflected by the total ISI score did not differ among headache status groups in individuals with insomnia (Table 2). These findings suggest that the headache status does not influence the overall severity of insomnia among affected individuals. In contrast, insomnia has a significant impact on the clinical presentation of migraine. Migraineurs with insomnia experienced a higher headache intensity and impact of headache (HIT-6 score) compared to migraineurs without insomnia (Table 3).

What could be the underlying mechanism for the difference between the impact of migraine on insomnia severity and the impact of insomnia on migraine severity? It is possible that their distinct anatomy and pathophysiology contribute to the contrast findings. Hypothalamus has been understood to play key regulatory roles both for migraine and sleep controls. The supraoptic nucleus in anterior region plays a key role in the regulation of sleep and arousal. Pain perception was regulated by arcuate nucleus in tuberal region [20]. Although supraoptic nucleus and arcuate nucleus are located nearby in hypothalamus, they have distinctive anatomical locations. A recent functional magnetic resonance imaging study showed that posterior hypothalamic activation was noted during the acute migraine stage [21]. Orexinergic system acts a regulatory role both in sleep and pain. Orexin-A and orexin-B were synthesized in hypothalamus and promote arousal. Nevertheless, they do different roles in pain modulation. Orexin-A is able to inhibit neurogenic dural vasodilation via activation of the orexin receptor type 1, resulting in inhibition of prejunctional release of calcitonin-gene related peptide from trigeminal neurons [22]. In contrast, orexin-B increases the A and C-fibre responses to dural electrical stimulation as well as spontaneous activity [23].

Among the ISI subcomponents, the score for noticeability of sleep problems to others was significantly higher among participants with migraine and non-migraine headache compared to participants without headache. Furthermore, the score for non-refreshing sleep were significantly higher among participants with non-migraine headache compared to participants without headache (Table 2). In contrast, other subcomponent scores including difficulties in sleep onset, difficulties in sleep maintenance, early awakening, sleep dissatisfaction, and worries caused by the current sleep problems were not significantly different. The distinct association of the headache status with only certain subcomponents of insomnia suggests that certain subcomponents are distinctive from other subcomponents. Further, our findings are in agreement with the previous findings that nonrestorative sleep (NRS) is a distinctive subtype of insomnia from other subtypes of insomnia. These studies showed that individuals with NRS was more frequently associated with daytime impairment than individuals with difficulty initiation of sleep (DIS), difficulty maintaining sleep (DMS) and early morning awakening (EMA) [24–27]. While NRS is reported to be associated with longer sleep latency, shorter sleep duration, increased alpha activity during non-rapid eye movement sleep, longer duration of cyclic alternating patterns and chronic pain condition, information on the differences in pathophysiology of NRS from other subtypes of insomnia is currently sparse [25, 28–30]. Therefore, more research on pathophysiology of NRS is needed for better management of NRS.

In the present study, we used the ISI to assess insomnia. This psychometric scale includes items for difficulty in falling asleep, difficulty in staying asleep, and early awakening which enables the classification of insomnia subtypes [18]. Although we did not identify insomnia cases by interviews based on International Classification of Sleep Disorders, 3rd edition or the Diagnostic and Statistical Manual of Mental Disorders, 5th edition criteria which are the 'gold standard' for the evaluation of insomnia, we are convinced that we successfully evaluated insomnia because the insomnia prevalence in the present study is in a similar range found in Asian countries by previous studies [29, 31, 32].

The present study has some limitations. First, we could not evaluate whether participants of this study underwent pharmacological or non-pharmacological treatment for insomnia. Second, as this is a cross-sectional study, we could not investigate changes in insomnia symptoms before and after migraine treatment. Third, the overall response rate was not high in our study. However, we used a two-stage clustered random sampling, proportional to the population distribution of Korea. Therefore, the distribution of age, sex, size of residential area, and educational level of our participants was similar to those of the Korean general population. In addition, the prevalence of migraine, non-migraine and insomnia in the KHSS were similar to that of previous studies [17, 33]. Despite these limitations, there are several strengths in the present study. First, the impact of migraine on the severity and clinical presentation of insomnia symptoms as well as on the prevalence of insomnia was evaluated. Second, the present study also evaluated the impact of insomnia on the clinical presentation migraine. Third, the distributions of age, sex, size of the residential area, and education level in this study's participants were not significantly different from the general population in Korea. The results of this study seem to appropriately reflect the characteristics of the general Korean population.

Conclusions

Subjects with insomnia have an increased prevalence of migraine and vice versa in a population-based setting. Although insomnia is associated with increased headache frequency and severity among migraineurs, insomnia severity is, apart from some subcomponents, not significantly influenced by the presence of migraine. Our findings indicate that migraine and insomnia affect each other but their asymmetric causal relationship needs further investigation in future studies.

Abbreviations

CI: Confidence Interval; DIS: Difficulty Initiating Sleep; DMS: Difficulty Maintaining Sleep; DSM: Diagnostic and Statistical Manual of Mental Disorders; EMA: Early Morning Awakening; HIT-6: Headache Impact Test-6; ICHD: International Classification of Headache Disorders; ICSD: International Classification of Sleep Disorders; ISI: Insomnia Severity Index; KHSS: Korean Headache-Sleep Study; NRS: Non-Restorative Sleep; VAS: Visual Analogue Scale

Acknowledgements

The authors would like to thank Gallup Korea for providing technical support for the Korean Headache-Sleep Study.

Funding

This study was supported by a 2011 grant from the Korean Academy of Medical Sciences.

Authors' contributions

JYK conceptualized and designed the study, analysed the data and wrote the manuscript. SJC, WJK, KIY, and CHY conceptualized the study and collected the data. MKC conceptualized and designed the study, collected and analysed the data, and wrote the manuscript. All authors read and approved the final manuscript.

Competing interests

Jiyoung Kim has no potential conflicts of interest.
Soo-Jin Cho was a site investigator of multicenter trial sponsored by Otsuka Korea, Eli Lilly and Company, Korea BMS, and Parexel Korea Co., Ltd.. Soo-Jin Cho also worked as an advisory member for Teva. Soo-Jin Cho received research support from Hallym University Research Fund 2016 and Academic award of Myung In Pharm. Co. Ltd. Soo-Jin Cho also received lecture honoraria from Yuyu Pharmaceutical Company and Allergan Korea.
Won-Joo Kim has no potential conflicts of interest.
Kwang Ik Yang has no potential conflicts of interest.
Chang-Ho Yun has no potential conflicts of interest.
Min Kyung Chu was a site investigator for a multi-center trial sponsored by Otsuka Korea, Novartis International AG and Eli Lilly and Company. Min Kyung Chu worked an advisory member for Teva, and received lecture honoraria from Allergan Korea and Yuyu Pharmaceutical Company in the past 24 months.

Author details

[1]Department of Neurology, BioMedical Research Institute, Pusan National University Hospital, Pusan National University School of Medicine, Busan, South Korea. [2]Department of Neurology, Dongtan Sacred Heart Hospital, Hallym University College of Medicine, Hwaseong, South Korea. [3]Department of Neurology, Gangnam Severance Hospital, Yonsei University College of Medicine, Seoul, South Korea. [4]Sleep Disorders Center, Department of Neurology, Soonchunhyang University College of Medicine, Cheonan Hospital, Cheonan, South Korea. [5]Clinical Neuroscience Center, Department of Neurology, Seoul National University Bundang Hospital, Seongnam, South Korea. [6]Department of Neurology, Severance Hospital, Yonsei University College of Medicine, 50-1 Yonsei-ro, Seodaemoon-gu, Seoul, Republic of Korea.

References

1. Stovner L, Hagen K, Jensen R, Katsarava Z, Lipton R, Scher A, Steiner T, Zwart JA (2007) The global burden of headache: a documentation of headache prevalence and disability worldwide. Cephalalgia 27(3):193–210
2. Lipton RB, Stewart WF, Diamond S, Diamond ML, Reed M (2001) Prevalence and burden of migraine in the United States: data from the American migraine study II. Headache 41(7):646–657
3. Lampl C, Thomas H, Stovner LJ, Tassorelli C, Katsarava Z, Lainez JM, Lanteri-Minet M, Rastenyte D, Ruiz de la Torre E, Andree C, Steiner TJ (2016) Interictal burden attributable to episodic headache: findings from the Eurolight project. J Headache Pain 17:9
4. Kim J, Cho SJ, Kim WJ, Yang KI, Yun CH, Chu MK (2017) Insufficient sleep is prevalent among migraineurs: a population-based study. J Headache Pain 18(1):50
5. Kim J, Cho SJ, Kim WJ, Yang KI, Yun CH, Chu MK (2016) Excessive daytime sleepiness is associated with an exacerbation of migraine: a population-based study. J Headache Pain 17(1):62
6. Cho SJ, Chung YK, Kim JM, Chu MK (2015) Migraine and restless legs syndrome are associated in adults under age fifty but not in adults over fifty: a population-based study. J Headache Pain 16:554

7. Chung PW, Cho SJ, Kim WJ, Yang KI, Yun CH, Chu MK (2017) Restless legs syndrome and tension-type headache: a population-based study. J Headache Pain 18(1):47
8. Kim J, Cho SJ, Kim WJ, Yang KI, Yun CH, Chu MK (2016) Insomnia in probable migraine: a population-based study. J Headache Pain 17(1):92
9. Ohayon MM (2002) Epidemiology of insomnia: what we know and what we still need to learn. Sleep Med Rev 6(2):97–111
10. Morin CM, Jarrin DC (2013) Epidemiology of insomnia: prevalence, course, risk factors, and public health burden. Sleep Med Clin 8(3):281–297
11. Daley M, Morin CM, LeBlanc M, Gregoire JP, Savard J (2009) The economic burden of insomnia: direct and indirect costs for individuals with insomnia syndrome, insomnia symptoms, and good sleepers. Sleep 32(1):55–64
12. Uhlig BL, Engstrom M, Odegard SS, Hagen KK, Sand T (2014) Headache and insomnia in population-based epidemiological studies. Cephalalgia 34(10): 745–751
13. Odegard SS, Sand T, Engstrom M, Stovner LJ, Zwart JA, Hagen K (2011) The long-term effect of insomnia on primary headaches: a prospective population-based cohort study (HUNT-2 and HUNT-3). Headache 51(4):570–580
14. Odegard SS, Sand T, Engstrom M, Zwart JA, Hagen K (2013) The impact of headache and chronic musculoskeletal complaints on the risk of insomnia: longitudinal data from the Nord-Trondelag health study. J Headache Pain 14:24
15. Yang CP, Wang SJ (2017) Sleep in patients with chronic migraine. Curr Pain Headache Rep 21(9):39
16. Headache Classification Subcommittee of the International Headache S (2004) The international classification of headache disorders: 2nd edition. Cephalalgia : an international journal of headache 24 Suppl 1:9–160
17. Kim BK, Chu MK, Lee TG, Kim JM, Chung CS, Lee KS (2012) Prevalence and impact of migraine and tension-type headache in Korea. J clin neurol 8(3): 204–211
18. Bastien CH, Vallieres A, Morin CM (2001) Validation of the insomnia severity index as an outcome measure for insomnia research. Sleep Med 2(4):297–307
19. Morin CM, Belleville G, Belanger L, Ivers H (2011) The insomnia severity index: psychometric indicators to detect insomnia cases and evaluate treatment response. Sleep 34(5):601–608
20. Sun YG, Gu XL, Lundeberg T, Yu LC (2003) An antinociceptive role of galanin in the arcuate nucleus of hypothalamus in intact rats and rats with inflammation. Pain 106(1–2):143–150
21. Schulte LH, Allers A, May A (2017) Hypothalamus as a mediator of chronic migraine: evidence from high-resolution fMRI. Neurology 88(21):2011–2016
22. Holland PR, Akerman S, Goadsby PJ (2005) Orexin 1 receptor activation attenuates neurogenic dural vasodilation in an animal model of trigeminovascular nociception. J Pharmacol Exp Ther 315(3):1380–1385
23. Bartsch T, Levy MJ, Knight YE, Goadsby PJ (2004) Differential modulation of nociceptive dural input to [hypocretin] orexin a and B receptor activation in the posterior hypothalamic area. Pain 109(3):367–378
24. Roth T, Jaeger S, Jin R, Kalsekar A, Stang PE, Kessler RC (2006) Sleep problems, comorbid mental disorders, and role functioning in the national comorbidity survey replication. Biol Psychiatry 60(12):1364–1371
25. Ohayon MM (2005) Prevalence and correlates of nonrestorative sleep complaints. Arch Intern Med 165(1):35–41
26. Roth T, Zammit G, Lankford A, Mayleben D, Stern T, Pitman V, Clark D, Werth JL (2010) Nonrestorative sleep as a distinct component of insomnia. Sleep 33(4):449–458
27. Stone KC, Taylor DJ, McCrae CS, Kalsekar A, Lichstein KL (2008) Nonrestorative sleep. Sleep Med Rev 12(4):275–288
28. Terzano MG, Parrino L, Spaggiari MC, Palomba V, Rossi M, Smerieri A (2003) CAP variables and arousals as sleep electroencephalogram markers for primary insomnia. Clin Neurophysiol 114(9):1715–1723
29. Ohayon MM, Hong SC (2002) Prevalence of insomnia and associated factors in South Korea. J Psychosom Res 53(1):593–600
30. White KP, Speechley M, Harth M, Ostbye T (1999) The London fibromyalgia epidemiology study: comparing the demographic and clinical characteristics in 100 random community cases of fibromyalgia versus controls. J Rheumatol 26(7):1577–1585
31. Li K, Sun X, Cui L (2008) A survey on sleep quality of the people aged over 18-years-old in Hebei Province. Chin Ment Health J 22(4):302
32. Yeo BK, Perera IS, Kok LP, Tsoi WF (1996) Insomnia in the community. Singap Med J 37(3):282–284
33. Suh S, Yang HC, Fairholme CP, Kim H, Manber R, Shin C (2014) Who is at risk for having persistent insomnia symptoms? A longitudinal study in the general population in Korea. Sleep Med 15(2):180–186

7

Accuracy of the painDETECT screening questionnaire for detection of neuropathic components in hospital-based patients with orofacial pain: a prospective cohort study

Daniyal J Jafree[1*], Joanna M Zakrzewska[2], Saumya Bhatia[2] and Carolina Venda Nova[2]

Abstract

Background: Better tools are required for the earlier identification and management of orofacial pain with different aetiologies. The painDETECT questionnaire is a patient-completed screening tool with utility for identification of neuropathic pain in a range of contexts. 254 patients, referred from primary care for management of orofacial pain and attending a secondary care centre, were prospectively recruited, and completed the painDETECT prior to consultation. The aim of this study was to determine the accuracy of the painDETECT to detect neuropathic components of orofacial pain, when compared to a reference standard of clinical diagnosis by experienced physicians, in a cohort of hospital-based patients.

Results: For the 251 patients included in the analysis, the painDETECT had a modest ability to detect neuropathic components of orofacial pain (AUROC, 0.63; 95% CI, 0.58–0.70; $p = 0.001$). Patients with orofacial pain diagnoses associated with neuropathic components had higher painDETECT scores than those with non-neuropathic components. However, the painDETECT was weaker at distinguishing patients with mixed pain types, and multiple diagnoses were associated with poor accuracy of the painDETECT.

Conclusion: In secondary care settings, the painDETECT performed modestly at identifying neuropathic components, and underestimates the complexity of orofacial pain in its mixed presentations and with multiple diagnoses. Prior to clinical applications or research use, the painDETECT and other generic screening tools must be adapted and revalidated for orofacial pain patients, and separately in primary care, where orofacial pain is considerably less common.

Keywords: Screening tool, Orofacial pain, Trigeminal neuralgia, Temporomandibular disorder, Neuropathic pain, Questionnaire, Diagnosis

Introduction

Accurate diagnosis of orofacial pain (OFP) is essential for appropriate patient management in primary and secondary care. Acquisition of a detailed pain history and examination directs diagnoses and treatment [1]. However, diagnosis of OFP is complex. Certain types of OFP are musculoskeletal in origin, such as temporomandibular disorders (TMD), others are neuropathic, such as trigeminal neuralgia (TN) and nerve injury-post dental extraction, whereas some have an unknown aetiology, such as chronic (persistent) idiopathic facial pain (CIFP). Mixed pain syndromes may also exist, where, rather than a binary distinction, pain may exist on a continuum of 'more or less neuropathic' [2, 3]. Due to a limited understanding of the pathophysiology of these processes, and the possibility of multiple OFP diagnoses occurring within the same patient, misdiagnosis and inappropriate referral of these patients is common, particularly for non-specialist clinicians [4, 5]. The management of musculoskeletal compared to neuropathic origin varies. For example, though commonly prescribed in primary and secondary care, non-steroidal anti-inflammatory medications are not recommended for neuropathic pain [6].

* Correspondence: daniyal.jafree.13@ucl.ac.uk
[1]Faculty of Medical Sciences, University College London, London, UK
Full list of author information is available at the end of the article

Moreover, the management of neuropathic pain is challenging, as patients are frequently unresponsive to drug treatment [7]. Earlier recognition and distinction of the aetiology of OFP in patients is needed, particularly due to the substantial patient burden and interference with daily living that some diagnoses may have [8].

Patient-completed screening questionnaires may supplement the recognition and clinical diagnosis of OFP in a variety of settings. These are paper-based or electronic tools that are easily administered to patients. In differentiating between common dental conditions and unknown OFP diagnoses [9], screening questionnaires may be useful for the earlier triaging of OFP patients to appropriate secondary or tertiary care pathways. However, it is important that these tools are validated for use in different settings, including primary or secondary care and epidemiological surveys. Such screening questionnaires may also be available to patients to complete and score over the internet, with no input from health care professionals, which adds to the importance of determining if they can accurately recognise different OFP diagnoses.

One such tool developed in 2006, the painDETECT screening questionnaire (PD-Q), uses a scoring method between – 1 and 38 to estimate the likelihood of a neuropathic pain component in patients. The PD-Q was originally designed to identify neuropathic components in back pain [10]. Since its conception, the PD-Q has been validated and translated into multiple languages, it is easy for patients to use, and has been shown to identify neuropathic pain components in different contexts, including lower back pain, arthritis, fibromyalgia, thoracotomy and malignancy [11]. Compared to other screening tools for neuropathic pain, the PD-Q does not require clinical examination, inquires about pain evoked by mild pressure and heat or cold [12] and thus has the potential to be used as a rapid pre-consultation tool to differentiate between aetiologies of OFP. To date, the PD-Q has been tested in populations of patients with specific OFP diagnoses. Elias and colleagues found that 34% of patients with post-traumatic trigeminal nerve injury at their centre obtained a PD-Q score of at least 19 [13]. More recently, Heo and colleagues applied the PD-Q to patients with burning mouth syndrome (BMS), and found a low sensitivity and high specificity for the identification of neuropathic pain components in this population [14]. Testing the PD-Q across a broad range of facial pain diagnoses is required to determine whether this tool would have utility as a screening tool for neuropathic pain in OFP. Our centre receives a heterogeneous group of patients with OFP [5], providing an opportunity to assess the PD-Q in a secondary care setting. The aim of this study was to determine the utility of the PD-Q to detect neuropathic pain in a hospital-based cohort of patients with OFP.

Methods

Design and setting

Given its diagnostic nature, this prospective, single-centre cohort study was conducted in concordance with the latest version of the STARD checklist for reporting studies of diagnostic accuracy [15]. Ethical approval was gained for the study from the South East London REC 3 Proportionate Review Sub Committee (Reference: 10/H0808/84). Patients were recruited at a London academic facial pain centre, which sees over 700 new patients a year, referred by primary care practitioners or specialists and in the oral surgery unit [5]. Prior to their appointment at our centre, patients routinely complete a series of questionnaires [16].

Participants

Recruitment was conducted by three specialty dentists between 2010 and 2015, each completing their postgraduate studies. During the project phase of the dentists' postgraduate studies, all patients referred from primary care, and attending OFP clinics and one oral surgery clinic, were consecutively recruited. Participants were excluded from the study if they: were below 18 years of age at consultation, had declined participation, were unable to complete the questionnaire without assistance. Participants with acute pain and those with more than one OFP diagnosis were recruited. From each participant, the following characteristics were planned, prior to PD-Q completion or consultation, and collected for each participant: age in years, gender, any secondary clinical diagnoses and the presence of anxiety or depression based on Hospital Anxiety and Depression Scale scores [17].

Test methods

Participants completed a paper-based copy of the PD-Q prior to their consultation with the clinician. The questionnaires were collected by the specialty dentists, and not shown to the assessing clinicians. Uncompleted questionnaires were returned to the patient before consultation to encourage completion, but questionnaires remaining incomplete were excluded from analyses. The clinical diagnosis of each patient, serving as the reference standard of diagnosis, was obtained after a full assessment by an expert in pain medicine by means of a consultation, with a detailed pain history and clinical examination. Secondary diagnoses, classified as either orofacial pain or an alternative pre-existing non-orofacial diagnosis, were assigned to patient if necessary, but the primary diagnosis was classified as the predominant pain experienced. An independent clinician reviewed the initial diagnoses and confirmed these after initiation of a management plan. Clinical diagnosis was selected as a reference test, as it is presently the gold standard for diagnosis; based on the requirement of a detailed pain history and examination for differential diagnosis of OFP [18]. Clinical diagnoses were then grouped according to The International Classification of Headache Disorders [19], with a separate and specific classification applied for TMD [20]. Prior to analysis, clinical diagnoses were grouped into predominantly neuropathic, pain of a mixed aetiology with both neuropathic and non-neuropathic components, or non-neuropathic. At this stage, participants with a diagnosis not confirmed by an independent clinician were excluded from analysis.

The completed questionnaires were scored according to the methodology described in the original reports of the PD-Q [10]. Cut-offs were applied for analysis of the PD-Q as previously described. A PD-Q score ≤ 12 indicates a neuropathic component is not likely, whereas a score ≥ 19 indicates that a neuropathic component is likely. Between PD-Q scores of 12 and 19, neuropathic pain can be present, but is uncertain. Cut-offs were not applicable for the reference standard of clinical diagnosis. As the questionnaires were completed by each participant prior to consultation, clinicians were blinded to the results of the index test. Independent study investigators received clinical information, the results of the index test and reference standard.

Analysis and statistics

As a previous study found the PD-Q to have an AUC of approximately 0.8 to distinguish BMS from nociceptive pain [14], it was anticipated that the PD-Q would have an accuracy of 80%, and it is required to estimate this figure to within 5% of the true population value. With a 95% confidence interval (CI), it was calculated that 246 patients were required for the study. The primary outcome of the study was the accuracy of the PD-Q for recognition of neuropathic pain components, compared with clinical diagnosis made by senior staff. This was determined using: sensitivity, specificity, predictive values, and receiver operating characteristics (ROC). For ROC analysis, the 'test' state was defined as patients with neuropathic pain or pain of mixed aetiology, whereas patients with non-neuropathic pain served as the 'control' state. ROC curves were drawn and the area under the curve (AUC) was calculated. The accuracy of the PD-Q was further analysed by comparing the PD-Q scores for patients with neuropathic, non-neuropathic or mixed pain using a Kruskal-Wallis test. Where a significant difference in PD-Q was observed across diagnoses, pairwise multiple comparisons with Bonferroni correction were used to calculate adjusted p values between individual diagnoses. The secondary outcome of the study related to factors influencing correct diagnosis of the PD-Q. This included determining Pearson's correlation co-efficient (r) between PD-Q scores and each patient characteristic, and a stepwise multivariate logistic regression to independently determine the adjusted effect (using normalised β values) of each patient characteristic and PD-Q scores.

All continuous variables, where parametric, are presented as means with standard deviations (SD), and where non-parametric, are presented as medians with interquartile range (IQR). Categorical variables are presented numerically and as a percentage of the sample. p values less than or equal to 0.05 were considered statistically significant. 95% CIs were applied to all continuous outcomes, and percentages were calculated for categorical outcomes. All data were managed, analysed and graphed using IBM SPSS Statistics for Macintosh, Version 25.0 (IBM Corp., Armond, NY) and Prism for Macintosh, Version 7 (GraphPad Software Inc., San Diego, CA).

Results

Participants and characteristics

254 participants attended the facial pain clinic during recruitment periods between 2010 and 2015, and were given the PD-Q to complete prior to their appointment with the clinician (Fig. 1). All participants were subsequently seen by the facial pain team, who took the history and performed the examination to ascertain the clinical diagnosis. From the 254 patients, one patient was excluded due to non-completion of the questionnaire. From the remaining 253 patients, a further two were excluded due to discrepancy in the clinical diagnosis. Therefore, 251 out of 254 (98.8%) of patients were included in the analysis. Patient characteristics are presented in Table 1, stratified by the aetiology of OFP. The overall characteristics of the cohort of 251 participants were as follows: mean age, 47.3 (SD, 15.7); proportion of females, 191/251 (76.1%); proportion with a secondary diagnosis, 74/251 (29.4%, see Additional file 1: Table S1) and proportion with anxiety or depression, 48/250 (19.2%). The numbers of patients for each clinical diagnosis are shown in Table 2.

Accuracy of the PD-Q for recognition of neuropathic pain components in orofacial pain

The PD-Q scores were calculated for each of the 251 participants, stratified by neuropathic, non-neuropathic or mixed aetiology. There was minimal time between administration of the PD-Q and subsequent appointment with a clinician. No participants experienced adverse events during the study period.

ROC curve analysis was performed to determine the accuracy of the PD-Q in detection of neuropathic pain components. The AUC was calculated and compared to an identity line, with an area of 0.50, and sensitivities and specificities were derived for each cut-off of the PD-Q (Fig. 2). The AUC of the PD-Q was significantly higher than that of the identity line (AUC, 0.63; 95% CI,

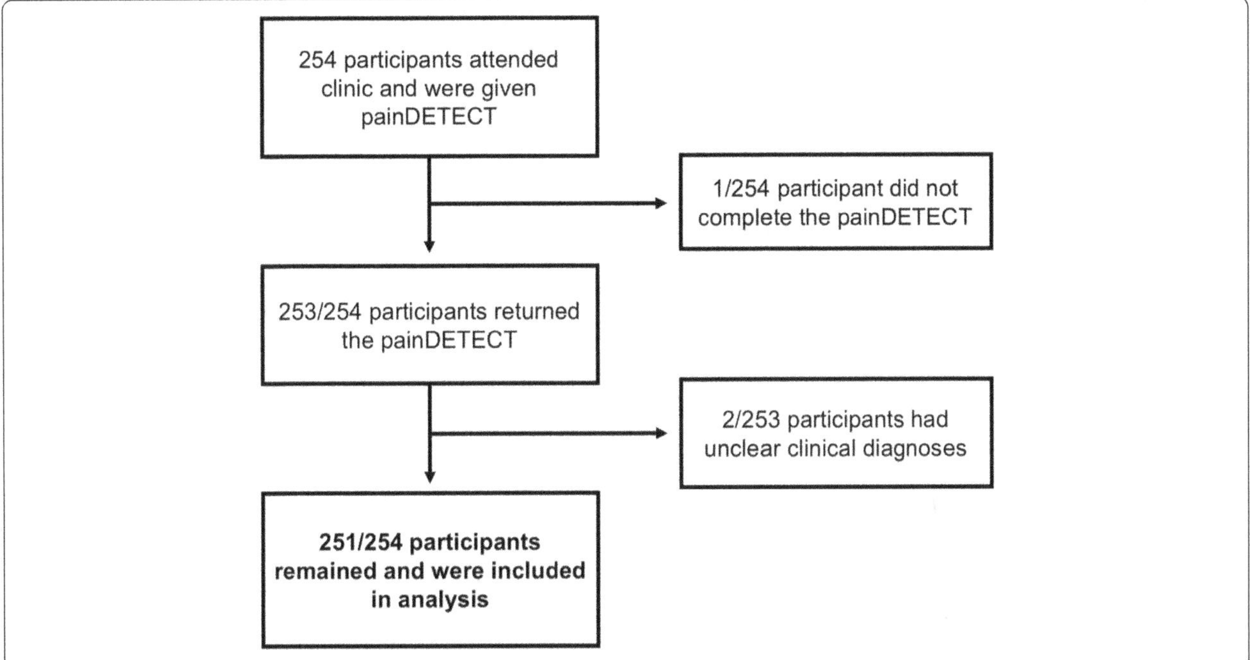

Fig. 1 Participant flow diagram. One patient who did not complete the questionnaire had difficulty reading the questionnaire. The two patients with unclear clinical diagnoses were categorised as having orofacial pain of mixed aetiology

0.58–0.70; $p = 0.001$). Our statistical model derived sensitivities and specificities corresponding to the PD-Q scores, and predictive values were calculated from these, given the prevalence of neuropathic or non-neuropathic pain within the patient cohort. At a cut-off of 11.5, given a prevalence of 54.6% patients without neuropathic pain components in the cohort, the PD-Q had a sensitivity of 59.6%, specificity of 56.9%, PPV of 62.4% and NPV of 53.5%. At a cut-off of 19.5, given a prevalence of 45.4% patients with some neuropathic pain components in the cohort, the PD-Q had a sensitivity of 28.9%, specificity of 83.2%, PPV of 58.9% and NPV of 58.5%.

PD-Q scores were compared between the five most common OFP diagnoses within the cohort, using a Kruskal-Wallis test (Fig. 3). Overall, there was a significant difference ($p < 0.001$) between median PD-Q scores of patients with neuropathic pain (median, 17.0; IQR, 10.0–24.0), non-neuropathic pain (median, 11.0; IQR, 6.0–17.0) or mixed pain (median, 10.0; IQR, 7.0–17.0) aetiologies of OFP. Pairwise comparisons revealed statistically significant differences in median PD-Q score between neuropathic and non-neuropathic pain ($p < 0.001$) and between neuropathic and mixed pain ($p = 0.008$), but not between non-neuropathic and mixed pain ($p > 0.5$). The median PD-Q scores for the 12 most common clinical diagnoses, containing five or more patients per group and accounting for 212/251 (84.5%) of the cohort, are shown in Table 3.

Table 1 Patients characteristics grouped by pain type

Patient characteristics	Neuropathic ($n = 72$)	Non-neuropathic ($n = 137$)	Mixed ($n = 42$)
Mean age in years (± SD)	54.0 ± 13.1	42.6 ± 15.6	51.1 ± 15.0
Female (%)	51 (70.8)	107 (78.1)	33 (78.6)
Secondary clinical diagnosis (%)	23 (31.9)	34 (24.8)	17 (40.5)
Anxiety or depression[a] (%)	12 (16.7)	29 (21.2)	7 (16.7)
Anxiety only	*5*	*12*	*6*
Depression only	*5*	*10*	*0*
Both anxiety and depression	*2*	*7*	*1*

[a]: Anxiety or depression as determined by HADS scores

Patient factors associated with PD-Q score in orofacial pain

We performed a multivariate linear regression to determine whether any of the patient characteristics including: age, gender, secondary diagnosis or presence of anxiety or depression had an influence on the PD-Q score independently. There was a significant correlation between the PD-Q score and a secondary diagnosis ($r = -0.20$; $p = 0.001$) and also anxiety or depression ($r = -0.15$; $p = 0.009$). However, when adjusted in the regression model, only a secondary diagnosis contributed significantly to the PD-Q score ($\beta = -0.18$; $p = 0.006$) when adjusted for patient age, gender and presence of anxiety or depression. Anxiety or depression, when adjusted for other patient characteristics, did not reach significance ($\beta = -0.12$; $p = 0.055$).

Table 2 Classification and frequency of OFP diagnoses

Neuropathic (*n*)	Non-neuropathic (*n*)	Mixed pain (*n*)
Trigeminal neuralgia (27)	Temporomandibular disorder (88)	Atypical odontalgia (20)
Trigeminal neuropathic pain (22)	Pericoronitis (8)[a]	Chronic idiopathic facial pain (13)
Burning mouth syndrome (6)	Psychosomatic pain (8)	Chronic post-dental treatment (6)
Trigeminal neuralgia with concomitant pain (5)	Migraine (5)	Post-radiotherapy (1)
Short unilateral neuralgiform headache attacks with autonomic features (5)	Pulpitis (4)[a]	Post-stroke (1)
Short-lasting unilateral neuralgiform headache with conjunctival injection and tearing (1)	Acute post-dental treatment (3)[a]	Post-brain surgery (1)
Post-herpetic neuralgia (2)		
Hemicrania continua (2)	Unspecified muscular (3)	
	Periodontitis (3)[a]	
Neuropathic post-trauma (1)	Tension headache (2)	
Facial pain with multiple sclerosis (1)	Hypervigilance (2)	
Tumour-associated neuropathic (1)	Temporal arteritis (1)	
	Non-odontogenic, persistent orofacial muscle pain (1)	
	Denture granuloma (1)[a]	
	Rheumatoid arthritis (1)	
	Parotitis (1)[a]	
	Dental abscess (1)[a]	
	Erythema migrans (1)	
	Post apicectomy (1)[a]	
	Insertion of dental implant (1)[a]	
	Fibromyalgia (1)	

[a]: Pain is dental in origin

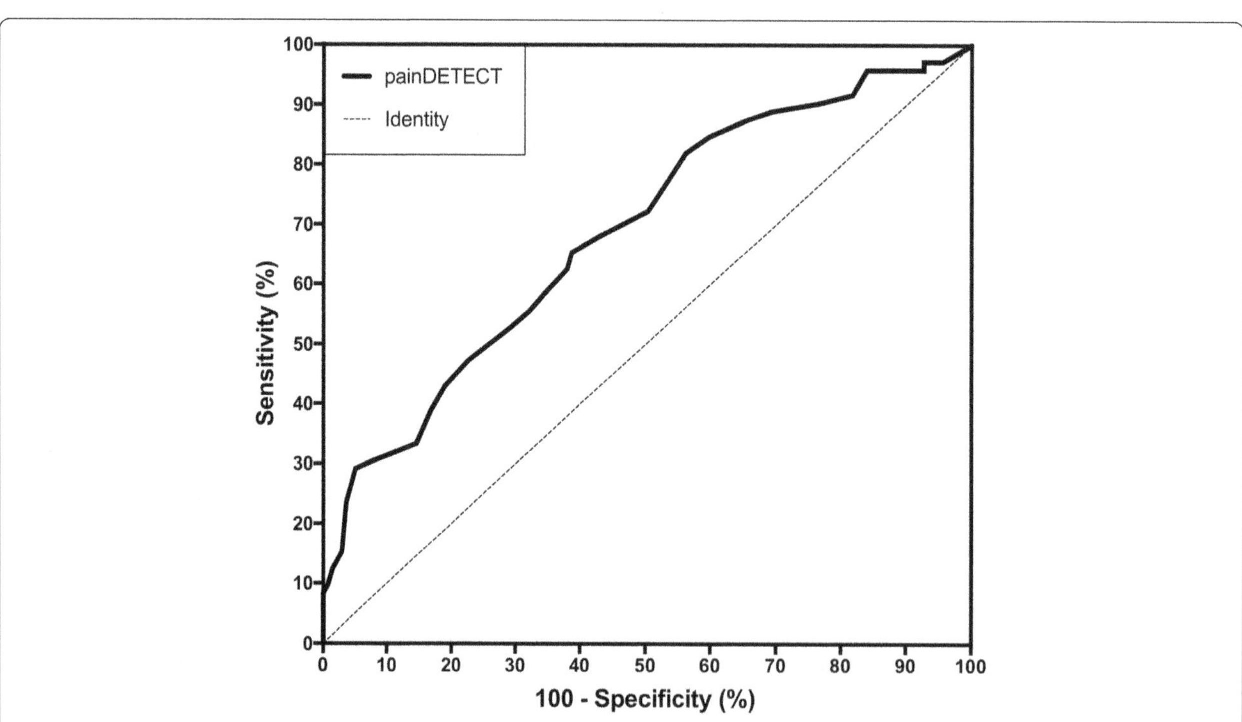

Fig. 2 AUROC analysis of the PD-Q for detecting neuropathic pain components in the cohort. The AUC is compared to that of an identity line, with an area of 0.5. The difference in areas between the curve and the identity line was significant ($p = 0.001$)

Discussion

This prospective study tested the accuracy of the PD-Q in identifying neuropathic pain components in a hospital-based cohort, with a broad range of orofacial pain diagnoses. At the PD-Q score above which neuropathic components are likely, the PD-Q had a low sensitivity and high specificity. Conversely, at the lower PD-Q cut-off, the PD-Q has a modest sensitivity and specificity. The PPVs and NPVs were modest at both cut-offs, indicating a reasonable likelihood that patients with a score above 19 would have a neuropathic pain component, and that patients with a score below 12 would not. PD-Q scores were significantly different between clear neuropathic OFP diagnoses, such as TN or TNP, compared to non-neuropathic diagnoses, such as TMD, whereas mixed diagnoses such as CIFP were more ambiguous. Together, these data suggest that the PD-Q identifies neuropathic components when clear-cut, but unsurprisingly, performs less well in patients with a complex, mixed diagnosis, particularly when multiple diagnoses are present.

Previous studies have examined the utility of the PD-Q for OFP diagnoses in tertiary centres, and suggest the PD-Q may not be an appropriate tool in this context. Elias and colleagues found that only 34% of patients with post-traumatic trigeminal nerve injury obtained a PD-Q score of at least 19 [13]. Heo and colleagues applied the PD-Q to patients with BMS, and found a low sensitivity (16.7%) and high specificity (97.4%) at a cut-off of 19 [14]. These studies, with smaller sample sizes, include patients with predominantly neuropathic pain, and their findings may reflect the low sensitivity of the PD-Q at the higher cut-off value in the present study. In contrast, our ROC analysis suggested that the PD-Q has potential for recognition of neuropathic pain in this hospital-based cohort, likely because our patient population is more heterogeneous and representative of secondary care.

Unlike other questionnaires for neuropathic pain, the PD-Q does not involve clinical examination. Such examination, including changes in sensory perception, is critical for making a diagnosis of a neuropathic pain [12]. The PD-Q was originally designed to identify neuropathic components in lower back pain [10]. Though response rates in this study reflect the ease of completing the questionnaire, the design of the PD-Q makes it difficult for patients to highlight and draw areas where pain predominates and radiates to, particularly considering as the size of the head is very small in the figure within the PD-Q. Questions in the PD-Q referring to possible pain triggers do not account for specific face pain triggers such as washing the face, showering compared to bathing, or the cold wind; all of which are clues towards orofacial pain of a neuropathic aetiology, such as classic TN [21].

Despite the strengths of this study, including its prospective nature, blinding of the clinician to the questionnaire results and the confirmation of the reference standard of clinical diagnosis by an independent clinician, our data should be interpreted with caution. Firstly, the study was conducted in a secondary care centre, receiving population of orofacial pain patients not representative of primary care or non-specialist settings. Data previously published from this centre indicated that up to 46% of the patients seen have a diagnosis of TMD [5], whereas its estimated prevalence in the general population is between 2 and 6% in developed countries [22]. Given this prevalence, the rarity of conditions such as TMD and TN would make a prospective study in primary care extremely challenging. Another difficulty in translating these results to primary care is the possibility of changes to the way the questionnaire is filled out in different settings. In different settings, patients may rate their pain variably, dependent on their expectations and desired outcomes of their consultation. Other factors differ between centres, such as the person administering the measure, be they clinician, family member or study investigator. Moreover, only a small number of patients with acute dental pain were recruited, which contrasts with primary dental care in which acute dental pain is predominant. However, the inclusion of these patients demonstrated that acute dental pain is not classified as neuropathic, and demonstrate that patients who score highly in primary dental care should be referred to a specialist centre for appropriate management of neuropathic pain. A second limitation is the difficulty in accommodating for the large proportion of patients in each group with a secondary diagnosis. This is representative of the complexity of orofacial pain presentations, and considerably influences the ability of the PD-Q to accurately identify OFP aetiology, independent of other patient factors, but likely influences non-adjusted analyses. To accommodate for this, study clinicians made a primary diagnosis based on patient history and examination, to determine the predominant type of pain. The study is further limited by characteristics not recorded, such as the pain intensity or educational level of patients, both of which could influence PD-Q scores. Though patients were recruited consecutively over individual study periods, the nature of the study, namely the periods of time during which patients were not recruited due to absence of postgraduate students, may have introduced selection bias to the sample. Re-test validity was not included in this study. Finally, the clinician confirming the diagnosis, though independent, was not blinded to diagnosis made at first consultation, and may be biased by this information or by treatment response. The time between diagnosis made at first consultation and independent confirmation was not recorded.

The accuracy of the PD-Q is only one of the considerations when determining a screening tool for OFP. The PD-Q appears a valid tool, in its effectiveness in

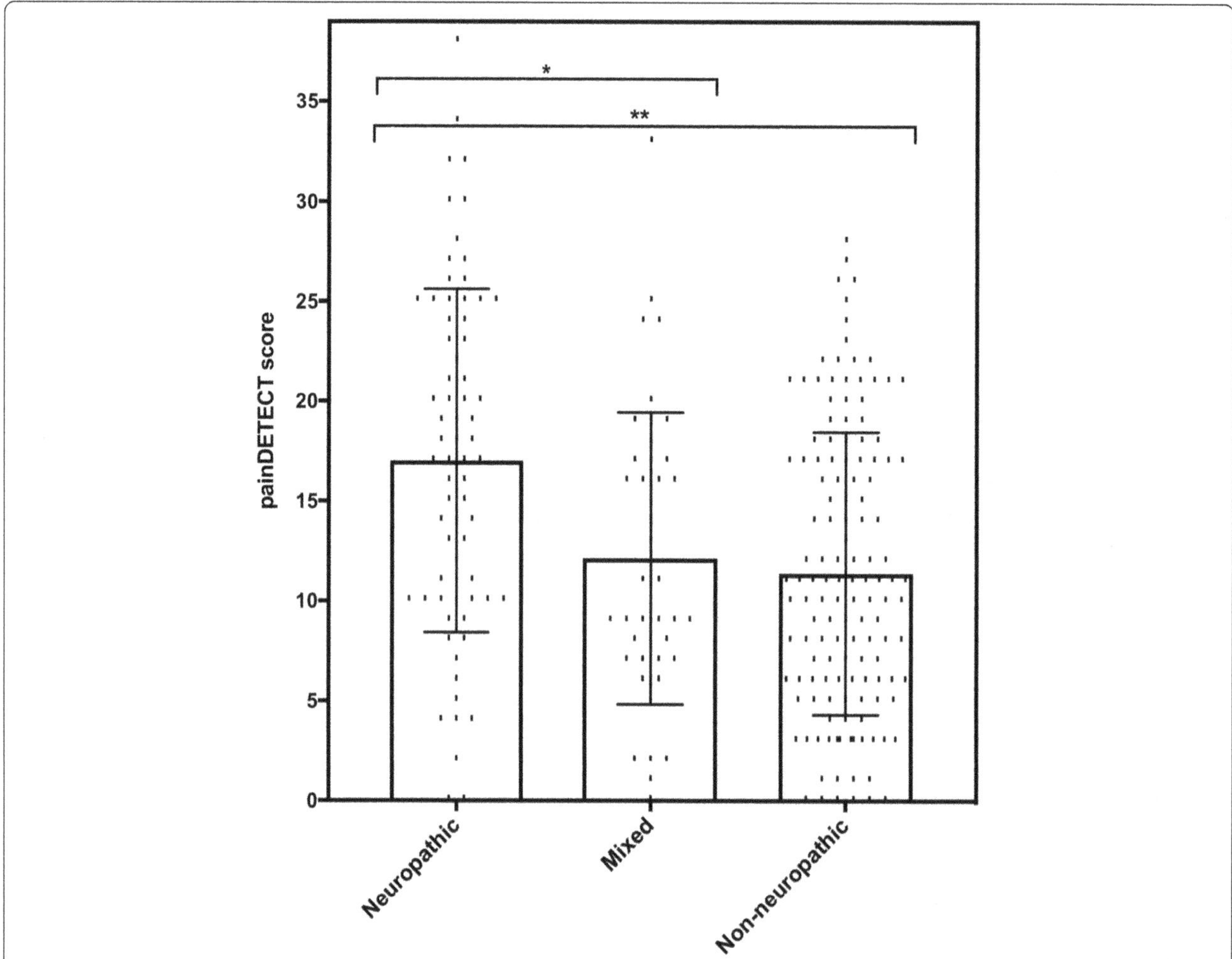

Fig. 3 Scatterplot representing median PD-Q scores for each type of pain in the OFP cohort. Error bars indicate IQR. Brackets and asterisks represent statistically significant differences between median PD-Q scores. *: $p < 0.05$, **: $p < 0.01$

Table 3 painDETECT scores grouped by clinical diagnosis

Type of pain	Clinical diagnosis	*n*	Median painDETECT score	IQR
Neuropathic	Trigeminal neuralgia	27	17.0	11.0–21.0
	Trigeminal neuropathic pain	21	17.0	10.0–26.5
	Burning mouth syndrome	6	9.5	8.3–16.8
	Trigeminal neuralgia with concomitant pain	5	17.0	8.0–18.0
	Short unilateral neuralgiform headache attacks with autonomic features	5	27.0	25.0–31.0
Non-neuropathic	Temporomandibular disorder	88	10.5	5.0–17.0
	Pericoronitis	8	11.0	10.3–14.0
	Psychosomatic	8	17.5	6.8–21.0
	Migraine	5	12.0	3.0–21.0
Mixed	Atypical odontalgia	20	8.0	5.3–14.0
	Chronic idiopathic facial pain	13	16.0	8.5–18.0
	Chronic post-dental treatment	6	12.5	5.3–24.0

distinguishing neuropathic from non-neuropathic pain in other contexts [11], the continuous score of the PD-Q reflecting the spectrum of neuropathic pain presentations [3] and its availability and validation in different languages. What has not been compared is the ultimate treatment and outcome of patients and how these relate to the initial PD-Q scores, which could be considered its criterion validity. Moreover, the reliability of the PD-Q in patients with OFP needs to be ascertained prior to its implementation in practice. Preliminary data at our centre indicates a strong concordance in PD-Q score before and after consultation with a facial pain clinician, but larger sample sizes are needed to validate this. The utility and performance of the PD-Q could also be compared to other screening tools for neuropathic pain [12], and more specific screening tools for OFP diagnoses, such as those available for TMD and TN [23, 24]. Finally, the differences between settings prompt a revalidation of the PD-Q in primary care [25], given the considerably lower prevalence of specific OFP diagnoses in general clinical and dental practice.

Conclusions

Patient-completed screening tools, such the PD-Q, have promise in both primary care and hospital practice, given their ease of use, high completion rate and the potential to aid the triaging of patients with OFP prior to consultation. Such tools may help to identify patients in primary care who need a specialist referral, those in dentistry who have a non-odontogenic origin of their pain or may help to inform clinicians as to the aetiology of pain to make earlier decisions about management and therapy. However, the PD-Q performed modestly in our centre given the complexity of presentation and as many patients have more than one co-existing diagnosis. Prior to clinical and further research applications, the PD-Q must be adapted and revalidated for orofacial pain patients, and separately in primary care, where orofacial pain is considerably less common. Ultimately, either patient-completed screening tools should only be implemented within settings they were designed, or pre-existing general screening tools needs to be optimised in different settings to reflect the variety of clinical situations for which such tools may be applicable.

Abbreviations

AUC: area under the curve; BMS: burning mouth syndrome; CI: confidence interval; CIFP: chronic idiopathic facial pain; IQR: interquartile range.; OFP: orofacial pain; PD-Q: painDETECT screening questionnaire; ROC: receiver operating characteristics; SD: standard deviation; TMD: temporomandibular disorder; TN: trigeminal neuralgia

Acknowledgements

The authors would like to thank the UCL AcaMedics scheme, for linking DJ to the Orofacial Pain Unit, and Sarah Tonks and Abdouldaim Ukwas; postgraduate students who contributed to the ethics approval and PD-Q data collection.

Funding

This work was undertaken by JZ at University College London Hospitals NHS Foundation Trust, who receive a proportion of funding from the Department of Health's NIHR Biomedical Research Centre funding scheme. The funder had no role in study design, data collection, analysis, data interpretation or writing the manuscript.

Authors' contributions

All authors contributed to the planning and design of the study, and SB with the collection of data. DJ, SB, JMZ and CVN analysed the data and DJ wrote the first draft of the manuscript. Subsequently, all authors were involved in the critical revision and acceptance of the final manuscript for publication.

Competing interests

The author declares that he has no competing interests.

Author details

[1]Faculty of Medical Sciences, University College London, London, UK.
[2]Eastman Dental Institute, UCLH NHS Foundation Trust, London, UK.

References

1. Zakrzewska JM (2013) Differential diagnosis of facial pain and guidelines for management. Br J Anaesth 111:95–104
2. Treede RD, Jensen TS, Campbell JN, Cruccu G, Dostrovsky JO, Griffin JW, Hansson P, Hughes R, Nurmikko T, Serra J (2008) Neuropathic pain: redefinition and a grading system for clinical and research purposes. Neurology 70:1630–1635
3. Jensen TS, Baron R, Haanpää M, Kalso E, Loeser JD, Rice AS, Treede RD (2011) A new definition of neuropathic pain. Pain 52:2204–2205
4. Zakrzewska JM (2013) Multi-dimensionality of chronic pain of the oral cavity and face. J Headache Pain 14:37
5. Lang M, Selvadurai T, Zakrzewska JM (2016) Referrals to a facial pain service. Brit Dent J 220:345–348
6. Moore RA, Chi CC, Wiffen PJ, Derry S, Rice AS (2015) Oral nonsteroidal anti-inflammatory drugs for neuropathic pain. Cochrane Database Syst Rev 10. https://doi.org/10.1002/14651858.CD010902.pub2
7. Finnerup NB, Attal N, Haroutounian S, McNicol E, Baron R, Dworkin RH, Gilron I, Haanpää M, Hansson P, Jensen TS, Kamerman PR, Lund K, Moore A, Raja SN, Rice AS, Rowbotham M, Sena E, Siddall P, Smith BH, Wallace M (2015) Pharmacotherapy for neuropathic pain in adults: a systematic review and meta-analysis. Lancet Neurol 14:162–173
8. Tölle T, Dukes E, Sadosky A (2006) Patient burden of trigeminal neuralgia: results from a cross-sectional survey of health state impairment and treatment patterns in six European countries. Pain Pract 6:153–160

9. Aggarwal VR, McBeth J, Zakrzewska JM, Macfarlane GJ (2008) Unexplained orofacial pain - is an early diagnosis possible? Br Dent J 205:140–141
10. Freynhagen R, Baron R, Gockel U, Tölle TR (2006) painDETECT: a new screening questionnaire to identify neuropathic components in patients with back pain. Curr Med Res Opin 22:1911–1920
11. Freynhagen R, Tölle TR, Gockel U, Baron R (2016) The painDETECT project – far more than a questionnaire on neuropathic pain. Curr Med Res Opin 32: 1033–1057
12. Bennett MI, Attal N, Backonja MM, Baron R, Bouhassira D, Freynhagen R, Scholz J, Tölle TR, Wittchen HU, Jensen TS (2007) Using questionnaires to identify neuropathic pain. Pain 127:199–203
13. Elias LA, Yilmaz Z, Smith JG, Bouchiba M, van der Valk RA, Page L, Barker S, Renton T (2013) PainDETECT: a suitable questionnaire for neuropathic pain in patients with painful post-traumatic trigeminal nerve injuries? Int J Oral Maxillofac Surg 43:120–126
14. Heo J, Ok S, Ahn Y, Ko M, Jeong S (2015) The application of neuropathic pain questionnaires in burning mouth syndrome patients. J Oral Facial Pain Headache 29:177–182
15. Bossuyt PM, Reitsma JB, Bruns DE, Gatsonis CA, Glasziou PP, Irwig L, Lijmer JG, Moher D, Rennie D, HCW d V, Kressel HY, Rifai N, Golub RM, Altman DG, Hooft L, Korevaar DA, Cohen JF, For the STARD Group (2015) STARD 2015: an updated list of essential items for reporting diagnostic accuracy studies. BMJ 351:h5527. https://doi.org/10.1136/bmj.h5527
16. Napeñas JJ, Nussbaum ML, Eghtessad M, Zakrzewska JM (2011) Patients' satisfaction after a comprehensive assessment for complex chronic facial pain at a specialised unit: results from a prospective audit. 211:e24 doi: https://doi.org/10.1038/sj.bdj.2011.1054
17. Snaith RP (2003) The hospital anxiety and depression scale. Health Qual Life Outcomes 1:29
18. Renton T, Durham J, Aggarwal VR (2012) The classification and differential diagnosis of orofacial. Pain 12:569–576
19. Headache Classification Committee of the International Headache Society (2013) The international classification of headache disorders, 3rd edition. Cephalgia 33:629–808
20. Schiffman E, Ohrbach R, Truelove E, Look J, Anderson G, Goulet JP, List T, Svensson P, Gonzalez Y, Lobbezoo F, Michelotti A, Brooks SL, Ceusters W, Drangsholt M, Ettlin D, Gaul C, Goldberg LJ, Haythornthwaite JA, Hollender L, Jensen R, John MT, De Laat A, de Leeuw R, Maixner W, van der Meulen M, Murray GM, Nixdorf DR, Palla S, Petersson A, Pionchon P, Smith B, Visscher CM, Zakrzewska J, Dworkin SF, International RDC/TMD Consortium Network, International association for Dental Research; Orofacial Pain Special Interest Group, International Association for the Study of Pain (2014) Diagnostic criteria for temporomandibular disorders (DC/TMD) for clinical and research applications: recommendations of the international RDC/TMD consortium network and orofacial pain special interest group. J Oral Facial Pain Headache 28:6–27
21. Zakrzewska JM, Linskey ME (2015) Trigeminal neuralgia. BMJ 350:h1238. https://doi.org/10.1136/bmj.h1238
22. Durham J, Newton-John TRO, Zakrzewska JM (2015) Temporomandibular disorders. BMJ 350:h1154. https://doi.org/10.1136/bmj.h1154
23. Gonzalez YM, Schiffman E, Gordon SM, Seago B, Truelove EL, Slade G, Ohrbach R (2011) Development of a brief and effective temporomandibular disorder pain screening questionnaire: reliability and validity. J Am Dent Assoc 142:1183–1191
24. McCartney S, Weltin M, Burchiel KJ (2014) Use of an artificial neural network for diagnosis of facial pain syndromes: an update. Stereotact Funct Neurosurg 92:44–52
25. Crombie IK, Davies HT (1998) Selection bias in pain research. Pain 74:1–3

8

Long-term follow-up of a community sample of adolescents with frequent headaches

Bo Larsson*, Johannes Foss Sigurdson and Anne Mari Sund

Abstract

Background: Several outcome studies have reported on the short- and long-term effects of migraine in selected clinical samples of children and adolescents. However, current knowledge of the course, incidence, and outcome predictors of frequent headaches in early adolescents in community populations is limited, and little is known about the long-term effects. Headache remains untreated in most of these young people. Here we examined the course, incidence, and outcome predictors of frequent headaches (at least once a week) over the long term (14 years) using previously assessed data at the baseline and 1-year follow-up of early adolescents.

Methods: Out of an original sample of 2440 who participated in the first two assessments, a sample of 1266 participants (51.9% response rate) aged 26–28 years (mean = 27.2 years) completed an electronic questionnaire comprising questions about their headache frequency and duration at the long-term follow-up. These headache characteristics together with gender, age, parental divorce, number of friends, school absence, impairment of leisure-time activities and seeing friends, pain comorbidity, and emotional (in particular, depressive symptoms) and behavioral problems were analyzed.

Results: In these young people, 8.4% reported frequent headaches (at least once a week) at the extended follow-up, while 19% of the participants having such headaches at baseline again reported such levels with a negligible gender difference. Over the follow-up period, 7.4% had developed frequent headaches, and a higher percentage of females reported such headaches (11.3% in females, 1.5% in males). In a multivariate model, frequent headaches at the baseline, gender (worse prognosis in females), impairment of leisure-time activities and seeing friends, and higher level of depressive symptoms significantly predicted headache frequency at the long-term follow-up.

Conclusions: Our findings suggest that gender, greater social impairment, and comorbid depressive symptoms are important indicators for both the short- and long-term prognosis of frequent headaches in early adolescents in community populations.

Keywords: Adolescence, Headache, Prevalence, Incidence, Long-term follow-up

Background

Headache is one of the most common health and somatic complaints reported by adolescents in the general population [1–5]. In two reviews of epidemiological surveys conducted in various countries and cultures, the estimated mean prevalence rates of unspecified headaches among children and adolescents were 54.4% [4] and 58.4% [4, 5]. A striking increase in the prevalence of unspecified headaches and migraine occurs at the onset of puberty among girls but not boys [4–8]. Such complaints can negatively affect the quality of life and lead to impairments in daily functioning such as school performance, absence and recreational activities [9]. Severe or frequent headaches in children and adolescents are also related to emotional problems; in particular, anxiety, depression, behavioral problems [10, 11], other somatic symptoms, social impairment, problems interacting with peers, pain comorbidity, and parental headache [12, 13].

* Correspondence: bo.larsson@ntnu.no
Regional Center for Child and Youth Mental Health and Child Welfare – Central Norway, NTNU, Klostergat. 46/48, N-7489 Trondheim, Norway

The persistence of headaches among children and adolescents experiencing unspecified headaches or migraine is an important aspect and burden of these complaints. Several retrospective and prospective follow-up studies of clinical samples of children and adolescents experiencing primarily migraine have reported on both the short-term and longer perspectives [14–17]. However, such samples typically include young people with more complicated neurological symptoms, frequent attacks, or impairment compared with those who are not referred [18].

In community surveys conducted in Scandinavia and Germany, the course of unspecified headaches in these age groups has been investigated primarily over the short term covering 1–3-year periods [14, 19–25] for which the overall persistence of headaches in the general population has been found to be high. For example, at the 1-year follow-up evaluation, slightly more than half (57%) of children and adolescents with headaches still experienced such complaints, as reported by parents [19]. In another similar longitudinal study, one-third of early adolescents reported frequent headaches (at least once a week) [20]. In a 3-year follow-up of school children, most of those with headaches (80%) still reported headaches, and female gender and the frequency of headaches predicted the persistence of these complaints [22].

To date, the existing information on the long-term prognosis of headaches in children and adolescents in community populations is limited. In a pioneering survey conducted in the 1950s, Bille followed a subsample of school-aged children with non migrainous headaches for a 6-year period [26] and another group with pronounced migraine at various time points for an extended period up to 40 years [27, 28]. Although about half of the children with migraine still had attacks around the age of 50 years, the prognosis was better for men than for women. In a school-based sample, Özge and collaborators followed 1155 children for a 6-year period up to mid-adolescence [29]. The overall headache prevalence increased from 45.2 to 78.7%, and most students had stable headaches, although the headache diagnoses showed a high transition rate over time. In this sample, female gender and having a parent with headaches predicted headache stability. In a 5- and 10-year follow-up of 8-year old children in a community study, Schmidt and colleagues found a high stability of headaches across the two reassessment points up to late adolescence (73 and 47%, respectively) [30].

In a 13-year follow-up of a sample of 335 school children into young adulthood (21–27 years of age), Brattberg [31] reported that about one-quarter still had headaches, while the same percentage represented incident cases. A headache frequency of at least once a week predicted the persistence of headaches. A longitudinal 15-year study of headaches severe enough to disturb daily life in the past 6 months collected data for children starting school (age 7 years) and again at the ages of 13–14 and 22 years [32]. The overall headache prevalence was virtually unchanged during and after puberty in this study. However, these estimates were surprisingly low, probably because of the conservative definition of recurrent headaches associated with impairment used in the study. In a general population study of migraine and other headaches among children starting school from the same research group in Turku, Finland, Anttila and collaborators examined long-term trends at two separate time points in adulthood when the participants were 22 and 35 years of age in separate cohorts [33]. They found an increase in the incidence of frequent headache and migraine in both boys and girls over a 30-year period. In another extensive longitudinal study of a large sample ($N = 11,407$) from the general population in the UK, parent-reported headaches among children starting school were associated with the frequency of headaches, multiple somatic symptoms, and psychiatric morbidity at the age of 33 years [8].

We have previously reported on the incidence, course, and 1-year outcomes of frequent headaches among early adolescents in a representative sample of the general population [19].We also assessed the influence of several potential predictors of outcomes: gender, age, relationships with peers, parental divorce, pain comorbidity and impairment related to disease or pain, and behavioral and emotional problems; in particular, depressive symptoms. In the present study, we investigated these aspects further in a long-term (14-year) study of the participants in our original sample.

Methods

Study design

The Youth and Mental Health Study is a longitudinal study conducted in Mid-Norway that assesses risk and protective factors in the development of mental health in adolescents aged 12–15 years [34]. In a first phase in 1998, a representative sample of 2813 students (98.5% attending public schools) from 22 schools in two counties of Mid-Norway (South and North Trøndelag), which included urban and rural areas, was drawn with a probability according to size (proportional allocation) from a total population of 9292 children.

Sample and assessment points

Baseline data (T1) were collected from 2464 adolescents with an 88.3% response rate and a mean age of 13.7 years (SD 0.58, range 12.5–15.7); 50.8% were girls. One year later (T2), 2432 respondents were reassessed at a mean age of 14.9 years (SD 0.6, range 13.7–17.0; 50.4% girls). Other details of the sample selection are presented elsewhere [31].

Individuals participating at T1 or T2 ($N = 2532$) were again asked to participate in a long-term follow-up study in young adulthood during the spring of 2012 (T3) about 14 years after T1 when they were a mean age of 27.2 years (SD 0.59, range 26.0–28.2). At this time, 92 of the participants were not eligible because of death ($n = 13$) or no identifiable home address ($n = 79$). Thus, 2440 young adults were invited to participate in this follow-up study, of which 1266 (51.9%) participated (56.7% females) (see Fig. 1 for details of participant flow). The headache frequency at the baseline did not differ significantly between participants and nonparticipants at T3.

In the first two waves, data were collected through questionnaires completed during two school hours. In the long-term follow-up study in adulthood, all assessment data were collected electronically.

Assessment measures

Background factors and predictors

In addition to gender and age, the following psychosocial factors were included because they were identified by an extensive review of risk factors as being important predictors in children and adolescents experiencing migraine or tension-type headaches referred to a clinic compared with headache-free controls [35]: *parental divorce, low number of friends (more common among children with tension-type*

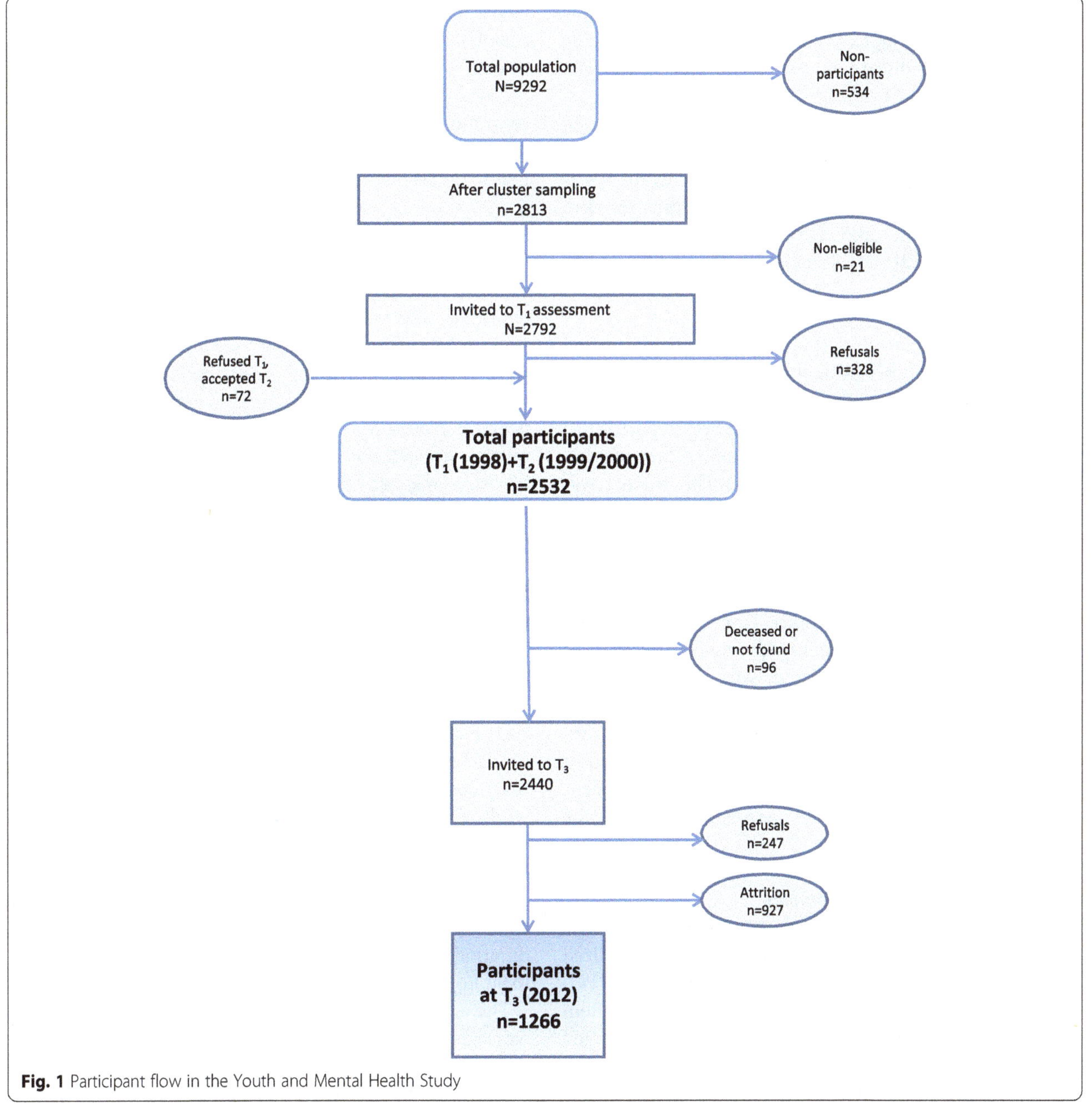

Fig. 1 Participant flow in the Youth and Mental Health Study

headaches), and school absence (more common among children with migraine [9]. Adolescents had provided information about parental divorce before T1. The number of friends at the assessment point was subgrouped into "0 to 1" and "2 or more friends" categories. At T1, 27.7% ($N = 684$) of the adolescents had divorced parents, and 4% of the students reported having a low number of friends (0 to 1).

Impairment

At T1, the adolescents were asked whether they had been absent from school because of disease, injury, or pain during the past 12 months. The possible answers were "No," "A few days," "1–3 weeks," "1–3 months," and "More than 3 months". They were also asked whether they had decreased or stopped leisure-time activities or seeing friends because of disease, injury, or pain during the past 12 months ("No" or "Yes").

Because various types of internalizing problems, such as anxiety, depression, somatic symptoms, and behavioral problems are often associated with recurrent headaches in children and adolescents, these domains were included as baseline predictors in our previous 1-year follow-up study [20] as well as in the present long-term follow-up evaluation.

Youth self-report

To provide a broad assessment of the adolescents' emotional and behavioral problems, a Norwegian version of the widely used and standardized Youth Self-Report (YSR) problem scale was used [36]. The instrument includes 103 items and 16 socially desirable items. The subject was asked to rate each item on a three-point scale (0 = "Not true"; 1 = "Somewhat or sometimes true"; and 2 = "Very true or often true") for the past 6 months. In addition to a total problem score, two broadband dimensions—internalizing and externalizing syndromes—can be formed from the subscales. The internalizing syndrome comprises three narrow-band syndromes—Withdrawn, Somatic complaints, and Anxious/depressed—and the externalizing syndrome comprises Aggression and Delinquent subscales. All of these subscales were included in this study. Three pain items (aches or pains, headaches, stomachaches) in the somatic subscale were excluded from the sum score.

The mood and feelings questionnaire

To assess specifically depressive symptoms among the adolescents using a comprehensive and standardized measure, the Mood and Feelings Questionnaire (MFQ) was completed by participants [37]. This is a 34-item questionnaire designed for children and adolescents aged 8–18 years to report depressive symptoms as specified by the DSM-III-R diagnostic system. The individual is asked to report on his or her feelings during the preceding 2 weeks. Responses are made to statements on a 3-point scale ("Not true," "Sometimes true," and "True"), and total scores range from 0 to 68. The MFQ has been shown to have high internal consistency, test–retest stability, and convergent validity in the present research project [34].

Headache and other pain

On all three test occasions (T1–T3), the adolescents/ young adults were asked whether they had regular and troublesome pain complaints (except for menstrual pain). If they answered positively, they were asked to rate the frequency of pain ("1–3 times a month," "1–3 times a week," or "Daily or almost daily") for headache, stomach pains, back pains, and pains in the arm or leg (hereafter called limb pain). They were also asked about the duration of pain ("Less than an hour," "1–4 h," and "More than 4 hours"). Those who reported at least weekly pains were regarded as experiencing frequent pain, a criterion also used here as our prime outcome variable in the long-term follow-up evaluation at T3.

Statistical analyses

Descriptive statistics included percentage, mean, and standard deviation (SD) for continuous variables. The chi-square test was used to analyze bivariate correlations between categorical variables. Analyses of percentages were conducted using the z-distribution. Student's *t*-test was used to examine differences in means between independent groups for continuous variables. To examine the relative importance of significant explanatory factors in bivariate analyses, logistic regression analyses using the enter method were performed. In all analyses, $p < .05$ was considered to be significant.

Results

Headache prevalence

At the long-term follow-up and ages 26–28 years (T3), 82.5% of the participants reported having headaches rarely or not at all, 9% had headaches 1–3 times a month, 6% had headaches 1–3 times per week, and 2.4% had headaches occurring daily or almost daily. Thus, 8.4% of participants reported frequent headaches at least once a week. Of the participants who experienced headaches, 43.3% reported a duration of 1–4 h, 29% had a shorter duration, and 27.6% had a longer duration. The association between headache frequency and duration was significant and was strongest for those with the longest duration and headaches occurring daily or almost daily (6.9%), [χ^2 (4) = 16.14, $p < .001$].

The association between gender and headache frequency was significant, [χ^2 (3) = 46.55, $p < .001$] females reported a higher frequency than males; in particular, for frequent headaches (12.7% versus 2.8%, respectively). Similarly, headache duration was significantly related to gender, [χ^2 (2) = 15.53, $p < .001$]. Gender was not significantly associated with the longest duration, but about half of the females (51.2%) experienced headaches lasting 1–4 h, whereas only about one-quarter of the males (23.5%) experienced headaches of this duration.

Pain comorbidity

At the long-term follow-up, 6.6% of participants reported frequent headaches only, whereas 1.8% of the participants with such headaches also had another frequent comorbid pain (in the stomach, back, or limbs: 14, 5.6 and 1.9%, respectively). This was significantly higher than for those with no such headache, [χ^2 (1) = 8.11, $p < .001$].

Course and incidence of headaches

Of those participants who had frequent weekly headaches at T1, 19.1% also reported such headaches at the long-term follow-up. Having weekly headaches at T1 or T2 or both occasions was significantly associated with reporting frequent headaches at T3, [χ^2 (3) = 26.53, $p < .001$] as compared with not having weekly headaches at T1 (17.1 and 6.7%, respectively). A slightly but not significantly higher stability between T1 and T3 was found for females than for males with frequent headaches (18.1 and 15.7%, respectively). Headache duration at T1 did not predict duration or frequency of headaches at T3, and age at T1 was not significantly related to the occurrence of headaches at T3.

At the long-term follow-up, 7.4% of participants not having frequent headaches at T1 reported frequent headaches (incident cases). The difference in incidence rates between gender was highly significant, (Z = 6.81, $p < .001$): 11.3% of the females but only 1.5% of the males had reported frequent headaches at T3.

Predictors of long-term outcome

The bivariate analyses showed that, besides gender (see above), parental divorce, pain comorbidity at T1, and impairment during leisure-time activities or seeing friends because of disease, injury, or pain were significantly associated with reports of frequent versus infrequent versus headaches at T3, [χ^2 (1) = 11.32, $p < .001$, χ^2 (1) = 8.11, $p < .001$, and χ^2 (1) = 5.13, $p < .05$, respectively]. The percentages reporting frequent versus infrequent headaches at T3 for each variable were as follows: for parental divorce, affirmed vs not: 13.1% vs 7.0%; for pain comorbidity at T1, affirmed vs not: 14.4% vs 7.6%; and impairment during leisure-time activities or seeing friends because of disease, injury, or pain, affirmed vs not: 13.9% vs 7.6%, respectively). However, the number of friends and school absence were not significantly related to long-term outcome. Further analyses showed that all internalizing problem subscales on the YSR and the total mean scores on the MFQ significantly predicted outcome—reporting frequent or infrequent headaches at T3. However, the mean total values for the two externalizing subscales (aggressive and delinquent behavior) at T1 did not predict headache frequency at T3.

Multivariate analysis

The significant explanatory factors in our bivariate analyses (except for the anxious/depressed subscale on the YSR, which was excluded because of the high correlation with the MFQ sum score; $r = .68$) were entered into a logistic regression analysis to examine their relative importance. The results ($n = 1087$) showed that the following explanatory baseline factors significantly predicted frequent headache (vs infrequent) at T3: gender (B = 1.64, SE = 0.34, $p < .001$, odds ratio (OR) = 5.14, 95% confidence interval (CI) = 2.65, 9.95); frequent headaches (B = 0.74, SE = 0.32, $p < .05$, OR = 2.10, 95% CI = 1.12, 3.94); impairment of leisure-time activities and seeing friends (B = 0.80, SE = 0.33, $p < .05$, OR = 2.22, 95% CI = 1.17, 4.20); and sum scores of depressive symptoms on the MFQ (B = 0.22, SE = 0.11, $p < .05$, OR = 1.02, 95% CI = 1.00, 1.05). The Hosmer–Lemeshow test was nonsignificant, which indicated a goodness of fit for the model.

Discussion

In the present long-term follow-up study, early adolescents (aged 12–15 years) in a representative general population sample were reassessed about 14 years later in adulthood (mean age 27.2 years) with a focus on the prevalence, incidence, course, and outcome predictors of frequent versus infrequent headaches.

Our prevalence estimates for these young adults and a report of headaches at least once a month at the extended follow-up was low—17.5%—and only 8.4% of participants reported frequent headaches occurring once a week or more. These relatively low estimates of headache frequency may reflect our introductory phrasing of the question, "Do you suffer from regular pain?" This item was used to allow comparisons of prevalence estimates and changes across the follow-up period with the rates reported by early adolescents at the baseline and our previous 1-year follow-up evaluation [20]. The present prevalence estimates are similar to those of a large epidemiological survey of adults conducted in one of the counties and the same health region as included in the present baseline study. In the previous study, 11.6% of females and 4.4% of males reported frequent headaches ("Have you suffered from headaches during the past year?") [38]. Furthermore, our estimate of daily or almost daily headaches (2.4%) was identical to that reported in the previous survey of adults. Although this latter survey was conducted some years before our present follow-up evaluation, our estimates seem to be reliable and are likely to reflect the true prevalence rates of headaches in this age group of young adults.

Over a short-term perspective of 1–3 years, the persistence of headaches has been shown to be high; that is, between 33% and nearly 80% of children and adolescents still experienced headaches at reassessment; in particular, frequent headaches [19, 20, 22, 23]. High persistence rates have also been reported in follow-up studies for longer periods (5–10 years) in which half to most (47–83.5%) of the school children still had headaches in adolescence [29, 30], whereas about one-quarter of young adults still reported headaches in longer follow-up evaluations (13–15 years) [31, 32]. To date, the longest follow-up studies of school-aged children were performed by Bille, who examined the course of pronounced migraine over 30–40-year intervals when about 50% of the participants were about 50 years of age and still experienced migraines [28].

In the present study of early adolescents with frequent headaches, who were followed for about 14 years, 19% of the participants reported such headaches, but there was a negligible gender difference. Our findings seem to be similar to those of Aromaa and colleagues, who performed a 15-year follow-up study of frequent headaches in school children as they became young adults [32]. However, their definition of frequent headaches during the past 6 months also included impairment of the child and specific areas in daily life, which may have contributed to very low prevalence rates and smaller numbers in subgroups.

While annual incidence rates of headaches were reported for children and early adolescents in two community-based surveys [19, 20], our previous study estimated the 1-year incidence for frequent headaches as 6.5%. In a reassessment of school children with no headache at baseline, Özge and colleagues [29] reported that three-quarters had developed some form of headache disorder at the 6-year follow-up. In longer follow-up studies of 14 and 26 years, 25.1% [8] and 12.2% [29] of school children had developed unspecified headaches, respectively. In a 16-year follow-up of children in a headache-free control group, 11% had developed migraine [28]. However, we found no extended follow-up studies using the same criterion for frequent headaches as used in the present study, in which 7.4% of participants had developed frequent headaches over the 14-year period. Importantly, we found a strong gender difference: females had a higher risk than males (11.3 and 1.5%, respectively) for developing frequent headaches in adulthood. A previous epidemiological survey conducted in the same health region [38] reported a similar gender difference in prevalence rates of frequent headaches (at least six episodes per month) among 20–29-years olds: 11.6 and 4.4% for females and males, respectively.

The predictors of outcomes have been examined further in long-term follow-up studies. For example, a 6-year follow-up of school children into adolescence in Turkey studies the predictors of incident cases and persistence of headache [29]. In that study, having a sibling with headache and a working mother increased the risk for developing headaches in adolescence for headache-free children, whereas having a mother with headache and female gender were associated with persistence of headaches. In the 15-year follow-up by the Turku, Finland, research group, headaches at school entry also predicted headache and migraine in early adulthood [32]. In the longer 26-year follow-up of children starting school in the UK, frequent headaches predicted headaches, multiple physical symptoms, and mental morbidity in adulthood [8].

In their extensive review of the potential risk factors that may differentiate between various headache disorders in cross-sectional clinical and school-based samples, Karwautz and collaborators [35] reported that parental divorce, low number of friends, and school absence were important discriminators between headache disorders such as migraine and tension-type headaches compared with headache-free controls. A previous study of adolescents in a community sample also found a strong relation between pubertal development and an increase in headaches and depressive symptoms in girls, which suggested a possible link to hormonal changes during puberty in girls [39].

Whether these potential indicators found in cross-sectional studies also predict short- and long-term outcomes in prospective outcome studies of children and adolescents with recurrent headaches in community-based studies is an important issue. We evaluated the importance of these short-term predictors and others in our previous 1-year follow-up study of early adolescents in the original sample [20]. In that study, unspecified frequent headaches at the baseline, gender (worse prognosis for girls), impairment of leisure-time activities and seeing friends, and high levels of depressive symptoms contributed significantly to the outcome. Of particular note is that the same set of baseline factors also predicted the frequency of headaches in the present 14-year follow-up evaluation of some of the original sample. This established model shows that the frequency of headaches, presence of comorbid depressive symptoms, and social impairment are important predictors of the short- and long-term prognosis for frequent headaches in early adolescents in unselected community samples.

The reasons for these variables having such a significant effect both in short term and long-term perspectives on frequent headaches are likely to be linked to relationships between vulnerability and resilience factors in adolescence. Increasing demands both developmentally, socially and academically might produce a stress pattern influencing the development and persistence of frequent headaches in youth. They may also lead to depressive symptoms, and their poor regulation often co-occuring with poor social skills and having few friends and avoidance of social activities, contribute to a negative and accumulative spiral into adulthood.

We note that many of these young people with such headaches do not seek or receive clinical treatment but rather learn to endure their headaches without complaint. One important factor increasing the likelihood that adolescents with frequent headaches also seek clinical treatment is degree of social disability as reflected by levels on a standardized measure such as the PedMIDAS [40] developed to assess social functioning among children and adolescents with migraine in a tertiary clinical sample. Here frequency of headaches was positively correlated to levels of disability, but less so for duration. While substantially lower disability levels have been observed in community samples of children and adolescents with frequent headaches [41, 42], those with a chronic migraine disorder have reported significantly higher disability levels.

Study limitations and strengths

Our study has some limitations. First, although the response rates at the long-term follow-up did not differ between adolescents with frequent headaches and those who were headache free at the baseline, the response rate after 14 years was fairly low (51.9%). Because of our assessment procedures and the use of self-report in the questionnaires and electronic responses, no formal headache diagnoses were established. Our definition of headache and other pain included "troublesome" complaints, which may have lowered the prevalence estimates in the present study. The reported data in the present study were part of an extensive long-term follow-up evaluation of adolescents and did not specifically focus on headache aspects only. Although our findings suggest a strong rate of persistence across the long-term follow-up period, we cannot rule out natural and spontaneous fluctuations in the rate of frequent headaches during the extended follow-up from adolescence into adulthood. Noteworthy here is that our predictive model at the 1-year follow-up was almost identical to the one obtained for our present long-term follow-up; however, our findings are likely to be restricted to the outcome for adolescents with frequent headaches in community samples. Whether it is also valid for adolescents with more complicated and frequent headaches in clinical samples should be confirmed.

Major strengths of the present study are the large sample, the long-term follow-up, and the inclusion of adolescents from various geographic (urban and rural) areas in the baseline sample. The assessment of headache was also based on the participants' current experience without the need for recall, which therefore minimized the potential for memory bias. The same predictive multivariate model of frequent headaches as obtained at the 1-year follow-up was reestablished in our long-term follow-up evaluation, which strengthens the validity of the present findings.

Conclusions

We found that a sizable proportion of adults aged 26–28 years reported frequent headaches to the same extent as they did in early adolescence. This and other findings of short- and long-term follow-up studies of community samples of children and adolescents suggest that there is strong risk for continuation of frequent headaches commonly associated with higher levels of emotional problems and impairment in social activities. In the long-term perspective, they are likely to have developed into chronic tension-type or migraine headaches or a combination. Although the prevalence of headaches improves in a substantial proportion of adolescents as they move into adulthood, the persistence of frequent headaches, particularly among girls, along with higher levels of depressive symptoms and impairment, emphasizes the need to provide effective psychological and pharmacological treatments to reduce frequent headache complaints and their associated social burden.

In future longitudinal research, more frequent and repeated assessment over time will reveal whether changes in persistence, improvement rates, and relapses occur in adolescents with recurrent headaches. This information will improve the identification of individuals experiencing persistent frequent headaches over extended periods. More importantly, for these people, the potential influence of gender, presence of depressive symptoms, and extent of impairment should be tested in the context of controlled treatment trials to examine whether these factors also contribute to changing the outcome.

Abbreviations

B: Unstandardized B coefficient; $CI_{95\%}$: Confidence interval; OR: Odds ratio; SE: Standard error; T1-T3: Time points

Acknowledgements

We thank all participants in the study.

Funding

This study has been financially supported by the Norwegian Research Council, National Council for Mental Health-Norway, Norwegian Extra Foundation for Health and Rehabilitation through EXTRA funds and the Liaison Committee between the Central Norway Regional Health Authority (RHA) and the Norwegian University of Science and Technology (NTNU).

Authors' contributions

BL design of the orginal study and the 1-year follow-up, statistical analysis and writing up the draft of the paper. AMS design of the study and supervisor of JFS who performed the long-term follow-up phase. All authors read and approved the final version of the manuscript.

Competing interests

The authors declare that they have no competing interests.

References

1. Scheidt P, Overpeck M, Wyatt W, Aszmann A (2000) Adolescent's general health and wellbeing. In: Health and health behaviour among young people. WHO policy series: health policy for children and adolescents. International report, vol 1. WHO series, Copenhagen, pp 24–38
2. van Geelen SM, Rydelius PA, Hagquist C (2015) Somatic symptoms and psychological concerns in a general adolescent population: exploring the relevance of DSM-5 somatic symptom disorder. J Psychosom Res 79(4):251–258
3. Perquin CW, Hazebroek-Kampschreur AAJM, Hunfeld JAM et al (2000) Pain in children and adolescents: a common experience. Pain 87:51–58
4. Wöber-Bingöl C (2013) Epidemiology of migraine and headache in children and adolescents. Curr Pain Headache Rep 17:341
5. Abu-Arafeh I, Razak S, Sivaraman B, Graham C (2010) Prevalence of headache and migraine in children and adolescents: a systematic review of population-based studies. Dev Med Child Neurol 52(12):1088–1097
6. Sillanpää M (1983) Changes in the prevalence of migraine and other headaches during the first seven school years. Headache 23:15–19
7. Sillanpää M. Classification of migraine. In: Guidetti V, Russell G, Sillanpää M, Winners P (eds) Headache and migraine in childhood and adolescence. London: Martin Dunitz Ltd;2002,134
8. Fearon P, Hotopf M (2001) Relation between headache in childhood and physical and psychiatric symptoms in adulthood: national birth cohort study. BMJ 322:1–5
9. Kernick D, Reinhold D, Campbell JL (2009) Impact of headache on young people in a school population. Br J Gen Pract 59(566):678–681
10. Balottin U, Poli PF, Termine C, Molteni S, Galli F (2012) Psychopathological symptoms in child and adolescent migraine and tension-type headache: a meta-analysis. Cephalalgia 33(2):112–122
11. Powers SW, Gilman DK, Hershey AD (2006) Headache and psychological functioning in children and adolescents. Headache 46(9):1404–1415
12. Strine TW, Okoro CA, McGuire LC, Balluz LS (2006) The associations among childhood headaches, emotional and behavioral difficulties, and health care use. Pediatrics 117(5):1728–1735
13. Kröner-Herwig B, Morris L, Heinrich M (2008) Biopsychosocial correlates of headache: what predicts pediatric headache occurrence? Headache 48(4):529–544
14. Larsson B (2002) The prognosis of recurrent headaches in childhood and adolescence. In: Guidetti V, Russell G, Sillanpää M, Winners P (eds) Headache and migraine in childhood and adolescence. Martin Dunitz Ltd, London, pp 203–214
15. Brna P, Dooley J, Gordon K, Dewan T (2005) The prognosis of childhood headache: a 20-year follow-up. Arch Pediatr Adolesc Med 159:1157–1160
16. Guidetti V, Galli F, Fabrizi P et al (1998) Headache and psychiatric comorbidity: clinical aspects and outcome in an 8-year follow-up study. Cephalalgia 18:455–462
17. Antonaci F, Voiticovschi-Iosob C, Di Stefano AL, Galli F, Ozge A, Balottin U (2014) The evolution of headache from childhood to adulthood: a review of the literature. J Headache Pain 15:15 Review
18. Metsähonkala L, Sillanpää M, Tuominen J (1996) Use of health care services in childhood migraine. Headache 36(7):423–428
19. Gassmann J, Morris L, Heinrich M, Kröner-Herwig B (2008) One-year course of paediatric headache in children and adolescents aged 8–15 years. Cephalalgia 28(11):1154–1162
20. Larsson B, Sund AM (2005) One-year incidence, course and outcome predictors of frequent headaches among early adolescents. Headache 45:684–691
21. Virtanen R, Aromaa M, Rautava P et al (2002) Changes in headache prevalence between pre-school and pre-pubertal ages. Cephalalgia 22:179–185
22. Laurell K, Larsson B, Mattsson P, Eeg-Olofsson O (2006) A 3-year follow-up of headache diagnoses and symptoms in Swedish schoolchildren. Cephalalgia 26:809–815
23. Wänman A, Agerberg G (1987) Recurrent headaches and craniomandibular disorders in adolescents: a longitudinal study. J Craniomandib Disord 1:229–236
24. Metsähonkala L, Sillanpää M, Tuominen J (1997) Outcome of early school-age migraine. Cephalalgia 17:662–665
25. Brattberg G (1993) Back pain and headache in Swedish schoolchildren: a longitudinal study. Pain Clin 6:153–162
26. Bille B (1962) Migraine in school children—a study of the incidence and short-term prognosis, and a clinical, psychological and electroencephalographic comparison between children with migraine and matched controls. Acta Paediatr Scand 51(Suppl. 136):1–151
27. Bille B (1981) Migraine in childhood and its prognosis. Cephalalgia 1:71–75
28. Bille B (1997) A 40-year follow-up of school children with migraine. Cephalalgia 17:487–491
29. Özge A, Sasmaz T, Cakmak SE, Kaleagasi H, Siva A (2010) Epidemiological-based childhood headache natural history study: after an interval of six years. Cephalalgia 30(6):703–712
30. Schmidt MH, Blanz B, Esser G (1992) Häufigkeit und Bedeutung des Kopfschmerzes im Kindes- und Jugendalter (Prevalence and importance of headaches in childhood and adolescence). Kindheit und Entwicklung 1:31–35
31. Brattberg G (2004) Do pain problems in young school children persist into early adulthood? A 13-year follow-up. Eur J Pain 8(3):187–199
32. Aromaa M, Sillanpää M, Aro H (2000) A population-based follow-up study of headache from age 7 to 22 years. J Headache Pain 1:11–15
33. Anttila P, Metsähonkala L, Sillanpää M (2006) Long-term trends in the incidence of headache in Finnish schoolchildren. Pediatrics 117(6):e1197–e1201
34. Sund AM, Larsson B, Wichström L (2001) Depressive symptoms among young Norwegian adolescents as measured by the Mood and feelings Questionnaire (MFQ). Eur Child Adolesc Psychiatry 10:222–229
35. Karwautz A, Wöber C, Böck A, Wagner-Ennsgraber C, Kienbacher C, Wöber-Bingöl C (1999) Psychosocial factors in children and adolescents with migraine and tension-type headache: a controlled study and review of the literature. Cephalalgia 19:32–43
36. Achenbach TM (1991) Manual for the Youth Self-Report and 1991 profile. University of Vermont. Department of Psychiatry, Burlington
37. Angold A (1989) Structured assessment of psychopathology in children and adolescents. In: Thompson C (ed) The instruments of psychiatric research. John Wiley, Chichester, pp 271–304
38. Hagen K, Zwart JA, Vatten L, Stovner LJ, Bovim G (2000) Prevalence of migraine and non-migrainous headache—head-HUNT, a large population-based study. Cephalalgia 20(10):900–906
39. LeResche L, Mancl LA, Drangsholt MT, Saunders K, Von Korff M (2005) Relationship of pain and symptoms to pubertal development in adolescents. Pain 118(1–2):201–209
40. Hershey A, Powers S, Vockell AL et al (2001) PedMIDAS. Development of a questionnaire to assess disability of migraines in children. Neurology 57:2034–2039
41. Krogh AB, Larsson B, Linde M (2015) Prevalence and disability of headache among Norwegian adolescents: A cross-sectional school-based study. Cephalalgia 35(13):1181–1191
42. Kröner-Herwig B, Heinrich M, Vath N (2010) The assessment of disability in children and adolescents with headache: adopting PedMIDAS in an epidemiological study. Eur J Pain 14:951–958

9

Vascular wall imaging in reversible cerebral vasoconstriction syndrome – a 3-T contrast-enhanced MRI study

Chun-Yu Chen[1,2], Shih-Pin Chen[1,2,3,4*], Jong-Ling Fuh[1,2], Jiing-Feng Lirng[2,5], Feng-Chi Chang[2,5], Yen-Feng Wang[1,2] and Shuu-Jiun Wang[1,2,6]

Abstract

Background: Limited histopathology studies have suggested that reversible cerebral vasoconstriction syndromes (RCVS) does not present with vascular wall inflammation. Previous vascular imaging studies have had inconsistent vascular wall enhancement findings in RCVS patients. The aim of this study was to determine whether absence of arterial wall pathology on imaging is a universal finding in patients with RCVS.

Methods: We recruited patients with RCVS from Taipei Veterans General Hospital prospectively from 2010 to 2012, with follow-up until 2017 ($n = 48$). We analyzed the characteristics of vascular wall enhancement in these patients without comparisons to a control group. All participants received vascular wall imaging by contrasted T1 fluid-attenuated inversion recovery with a 3-T magnetic resonance machine. The vascular wall enhancement was rated as marked, mild or absent.

Results: Of 48 patients with RCVS, 22 (45.8%) had vascular wall enhancement (5 marked and 17 mild). Demographics, clinical profiles, and cerebral artery flow velocities were similar across patients with versus without vascular wall enhancement, except that patients with vascular wall enhancement had fewer headache attacks than those without ($p = 0.04$). Follow-up imaging completed in 14 patients (median interval, 7 months) showed reduced enhancement in 9 patients, but persistent enhancement in 5.

Conclusion: Almost half of our RCVS patients exhibited imaging enhancement of diseased vessels, and it was persistent for approximately a third of those patients with follow-up imaging. Both acute and persistent vascular wall enhancement may be unhelpful for differentiating RCVS from central nervous system vasculitis or subclinical atherosclerosis.

Keywords: Reversible cerebral vasoconstriction syndromes, Thunderclap headache, Vascular wall imaging, Contrast enhancement

Background

Reversible cerebral vasoconstriction syndrome (RCVS) is a unifying term for a variety of clinical-radiological syndromes characterized by recurrent thunderclap headaches and reversible multifocal cerebral vasoconstrictions [1–4]. RCVS is not uncommon and potentially devastating because it is associated with a high risk of complications, such as posterior reversible encephalopathy syndrome, ischemic stroke, intracerebral hemorrhage and cortical subarachnoid hemorrhage (SAH) [3, 5–10]. The diagnosis is based primarily on angiography demonstrating cerebral vasoconstrictions and their reversibility, but its differentiation from central nervous system (CNS) vasculitis can be challenging [11, 12].

Conventional arterial imaging, such as computed tomography or magnetic resonance angiography (MRA), can be used to evaluate vascular stenosis in RCVS. However, the specificity of such imaging is limited by similar luminal defects being the result of other pathologies [13].

* Correspondence: chensp1977@gmail.com
[1]Department of Neurology, Neurological Institute, Taipei Veterans General Hospital, Taipei 112, Taiwan
[2]Faculty of Medicine, National Yang-Ming University School of Medicine, Taipei, Taiwan
Full list of author information is available at the end of the article

The small caliber and tortuosity of intracranial vessels hamper visualization of vascular walls by conventional imaging techniques [13]. After being used initially to characterize the luminal stenosis in carotid atherosclerotic disease [14], black-blood imaging techniques have been applied to intracranial vascular wall visualization and characterization of vascular wall pathologies, including intracranial atherosclerosis [15], vasculitis [16], arterial dissection [17], aneurysm [18] and RCVS [19, 20].

It is not known whether there are pathological vascular wall changes underlying RCVS vasoconstrictions. Generally, the limited histopathological data available do not support the presence of arterial wall inflammation in patients with RCVS [12, 21, 22]. However, in one case report, marked vascular wall enhancement was noted in a patient with cocaine vasculitis [23], and cocaine use has been considered to be an important etiology of RCVS [9, 12, 24]. In a recent case series, 3 patients with RCVS showed no apparent vascular wall enhancement on contrasted T1 fluid-attenuated inversion recovery (FLAIR) imaging, whereas marked vascular wall enhancement was found in 3 patients with CNS vasculitis and 1 patient with cocaine vasculopathy [19]. In another case series, 4 of 13 patients with RCVS had mild enhancement on T1-weighted sequences with fat suppression and a saturation band [20]; the remaining 9 patients had no enhancement. No congruous conclusions can be drawn from these studies. Therefore, we aimed to determine whether absence of arterial wall pathology on imaging is a universal finding in patients with RCVS or could be characteristic of a subgroup of RCVS patients, as well as to further refine these clinical-pathological syndromes into more specific disease entities.

Methods

Study subjects

We recruited 62 patients presenting with acute severe headaches prospectively from the headache clinic and emergency department at Taipei Veterans General Hospital from March 2010 to September 2012. Each subject completed a detailed headache intake form and provided comprehensive medical and headache histories before undergoing clinical and neurological examinations. Brain magnetic resonance imaging (MRI), MR venography and MRA were performed to exclude intracranial lesions attributable to the patients' headache. Spinal tap with cerebrospinal fluid analysis was performed to support diagnosis if patients agreed. Subjects were hospitalized to expedite completion of these diagnostic investigations if conditions allowed.

Diagnosis of RCVS required fulfillment of the following criteria: (1) at least two acute-onset severe headaches (thunderclap headaches), with or without focal neurological deficits; (2) vasoconstrictions demonstrated on MRA; and (3) reversibility of vasoconstrictions demonstrated by at least one follow-up MRA within 3 months. The diagnostic criteria were based on the definition of "benign (or reversible) angiopathy of the central nervous system" proposed by the International Classification of Headache Disorders, second edition (ICHD-2) (Code 6. 7.3) [25] and the essential diagnostic elements of RCVS proposed by Calabrese et al. [1]. The criteria were also in concordance with the newly proposed criteria for "headaches attributed to RCVS" in the ICHD-3 beta version (code 6.7.3) [26]. The exclusion criteria included: RCVS due to secondary causes, SAH or other intracranial disorders (but cortical SAH was allowed), and subjects with a poor vascular wall imaging quality, due to either a failure to focus on the large proximal vessels or difficulty with interpretation due to obscuration by motion artifacts.

Vascular wall imaging

All subjects underwent sequential brain MRI examinations with adequate sequences to exclude intracranial lesions, using a previously reported procedure [6, 7] except that a 3-T MR machine was used (MR750®, GE Medical Systems, Milwaukee, WI). Sequential MRAs were performed in all subjects until their vasoconstrictions normalized or until 3 months after disease onset.

We employed a vascular wall imaging protocol adapted from that proposed by Swartz et al. [15]. In brief, the protocol consisted of T1-weighted black blood vessel wall sequence (single inversion recovery-prepared two-dimensional fast spin echo acquisition with a 22 × 22 cm^2 field of view, 512 × 512 acquired matrix, 1.5 mm slice thickness, total slab thickness of 2–3 cm, and repetition/inversion/echo times of 2263/860/13 ms) before and after intravenous gadolinium administration (with constant scan parameters). All sequences were monitored for quality to ensure appropriate orientation to capture affected arteries at sites of stenosis. The acquisitions were targeted to ensure sampling of the middle cerebral arteries (MCAs).

Imaging analysis was performed on a radiology information system-picture archiving and communication system. Visual analysis was conducted to evaluate any focal wall thickening and postcontrast enhancement. Postcontrast enhancement was categorized as absent (none or minimal) or present by comparing pre- and post-gadolinium vessel wall imaging; enhancement was considered unequivocal if found in at least two imaging planes. The enhancement was characterized as mild if the arterial wall hyperintensity was mild or patchy (Fig. 1a), and as marked (Fig. 1b) if the arterial wall hyperintensity was strong and diffuse (involving the entire circumference of an arterial segment) in at least two imaging planes. The pattern of enhancement was characterized

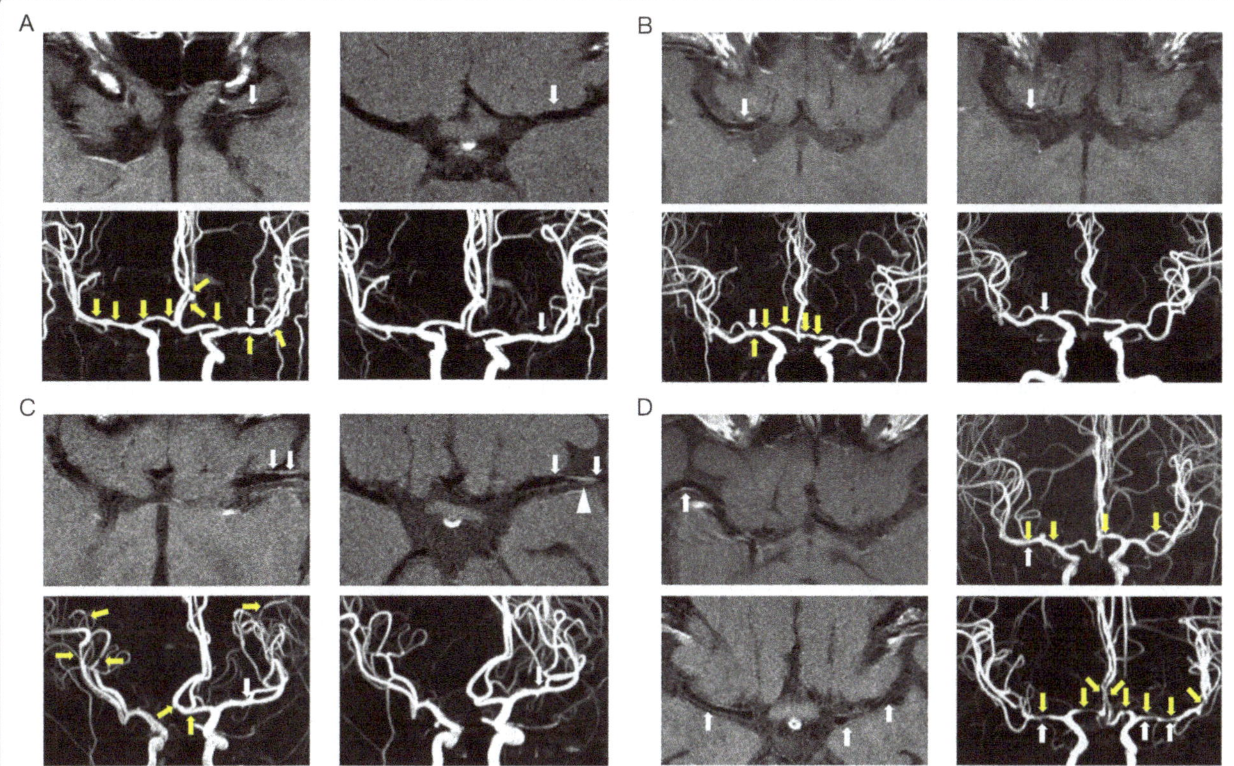

Fig. 1 Vascular wall enhancement in patients with RCVS. **a**, initially mild concentric enhancement, vascular imaging obtained 10 days after disease onset in a 48-year-old female; the enhancement was completely resolved at 7 years of follow-up; **b**, initially mild concentric enhancement, vascular imaging obtained 9 days after disease onset in a 52-year-old female; the enhancement was partially resolved 96 days later; **c**, initially marked concentric enhancement, vascular imaging obtained 10 days after disease onset in a 60-year-old female; the enhancement was partially resolved at 4.5 years of follow-up. The white arrowhead in **c** indicates partial volume of vein. Note that the enhanced vascular wall did not concordantly present at the site of vasoconstriction; **d**, upper, initially mild eccentric enhancement, vascular imaging obtained 25 days after disease onset in a 49-year-old female; lower, initially mild concentric enhancement, vascular imaging obtained 15 days after disease onset in a 48-year-old female. White arrows locate vascular wall enhancement. Yellow arrows locate vasoconstriction

as concentric if it was uniform and circumferential, and eccentric if nonuniform and noncircumferential [20]. If the patient had mild or marked vascular wall enhancement on the initial scan, they were invited to receive follow-up contrasted T1-FLAIR imaging, independent of their regular MRA follow-up. Any such targeted image findings were independently interpreted by two experienced neuroradiologists (J.F.L. and F.C.C.) who were blinded to the clinical data. The differences in grading were resolved by consensus.

Transcranial color-coded sonographic studies

Each patients' transcranial color-coded Doppler sonography was performed on the same day as the corresponding MRA. Mean flow velocities of major cerebral arteries, including the anterior cerebral arteries (ACAs), MCAs, posterior cerebral arteries, and basilar artery were recorded [6]. For bilateral vessels, the averaged velocity of both sides was taken as the mean velocity and maximal velocity was obtained from the side with a greater velocity.

Clinical follow-up

All eligible patients were followed up until their headaches subsided or the MRA follow-up endpoint. Patients with enhanced vessel walls were invited for an optional follow-up exploratory MRA study. As a result, the follow-up duration was quite variable across patients, but the information obtained may be useful for future follow-up study. The last follow-up was completed in 2017.

Statistical analysis

Descriptive statistics are presented as means ± standard deviations or percentages. Comparisons between two or more sets of normally distributed data were carried out with the t-tests (independent or paired) or one-way analyses of variance (ANOVAs). If normality was not assumed, the differences between two sets of data were tested with the Mann-Whitney U test, and the differences between three sets of data with the Kruskal Wallis test. For correlations between two continuous variables, we calculated the Pearson correlation coefficient, r. Predictors of vascular wall enhancement were identified by multiple logistic regression analyses. Statistical significance was set at $p < 0.05$. All analyses were performed with the IBM SPSS Statistics software package, version 18.0.

Results

Demographic profile

After excluding patients with poor vascular wall imaging quality or initial brain imaging beyond 30 days, 48 of 62 recruited RCVS patients remained in the final analysis. They were mostly women (42/48; 87.5%) with a mean age of 50.5 ± 9.4 years (range, 27–66 years). Triggers of their thunderclap headaches included defecation (37.5%), bathing (27.1%), intense emotions (20.8%), sex (18.8%), exertion (10.4%), and coughing (6.3%). A total of 12 patients received a spinal tap. All their CSF was clear and colorless, and pressure, cell count and metabolic analyses were within normal limit.

Ictal-stage vascular wall imaging

The mean latency from presentation to initial vessel wall imaging was 11.9 ± 7.1 days (range 1–30 days). The characteristics of the enhancement are presented in Table 1. A total of 22 patients (45.8%) had enhancement on contrasted vascular wall imaging, including 5 (22.7%) with marked and 17 (77.3%) with mild enhancement. The enhancement was concentric in 16 (72.7%, Fig. 1d, lower) and eccentric in 6 (27.3%, Fig. 1d, upper). The eccentric pattern was present only in vessels with mild enhancement (35.3%). The enhancement was not always co-localized with vasoconstriction. For example, the enhancement was colocalized with vasoconstriction in Fig. 1a, b and d, but incongruous with vasoconstriction in Fig. 1c. The enhancement involved the proximal M1 in 3 (13.6%), distal M1 in 6 (27.3%), and whole M1 in 13 (59.1%). Maximal flow velocity for the MCA and ACA did not differ significantly between patients with vascular wall enhancement (MCA, 114.5 ± 62.7 cm/s; and ACA, 75.1 ± 21.9 cm/s) and those without vascular wall enhancement (MCA, 97.2 ± 29.2 cm/s, $p = 0.25$, independent t test; and ACA, 69.7 ± 18.7 cm/s, $p = 0.42$, independent t test). There was no graded difference when the enhancement was characterized into mild and marked levels (Table 2). The demographics and headache profiles did not significantly differ between the patients with and without vascular wall enhancement (Table 3), except that patients with vascular wall enhancement had less frequent headache attacks (0.6 ± 0.3 per day) and fewer total headache attacks (4.7 ± 4.4) than those without vascular wall enhancement (0.9 ± 1.0 per day, $p = 0.07$, Mann-Whitney U test; 8.4 ± 8.4, $p = 0.04$, Mann-Whitney U test).

Table 1 Characteristics of vascular wall enhancement in patients with RCVS

Characteristics of vascular wall enhancement (*n* = 22)	
Segmental location, n (%)	22
Proximal M1	3 (13.6%)
Distal M1	6 (27.3%)
Whole M1 segment	13 (59.1%)
Degree of enhancement, n (%)	22
Mild	17 (77.3%)
Mark	5 (22.7%)
Reversibility, n (%)	14
Complete resolution	5 (35.7%)
Partial resolution	4 (28.6%)
No change	5 (35.7%)
Pattern, n (%)	22
Concentric	16 (72.7%)
Eccentric	6 (27.3%)

Follow-up vascular imaging

Follow-up vascular wall imaging was performed for 12 of the 17 patients with mild enhancement of the vascular wall and 4 of the 5 patients with marked enhancement with a median follow-up interval of 7 months (range, 17 days to 7 years). Analyzable images were obtained in 14 patients, of which 5 (35.7%) showed persistence of the initial enhancement and 9 (64.3%) showed partial or complete resolution of the initial enhancement (Fig. 1). Among 3 patients who received analyzable follow-up vascular wall imaging within 3 months, 1 patient (33%) showed persistence of the initial enhancement and 2 patients (67%) showed a reduction. Among 8 patients who received analyzable follow-up imaging within 3 years, 5 patients (62.5%) had persistent enhancement and 3 patients (37.5%) had a reduction. In patients with initially mild enhancement, the follow-up imaging showed no change in enhancement degree in 4 patients (with 35-, 96-, 168- and 641-day intervals), complete resolution in 4 patients, and partial improvement in 2 patients. Among patients with marked enhancement initially, follow-up vascular imaging showed complete regression in 1 patient after 46 days and residual mild enhancement in 2 patients. One patient had persistently marked enhancement, but the follow-up interval was short (17 days).

Discussion

In the present study, almost half of the RCVS patients showed some degree of enhancement in contrasted T1-FLAIR vascular imaging. In three fourths of the cases, the vascular wall enhancement was mild, and in the remaining fourth the enhancement was marked. The intensity of enhancement was not associated with MCA or ACA flow velocity. The enhancement of the vascular

Table 2 Cerebral blood flow velocity in RCVS patients with different degrees of vascular wall enhancement

	Extent of vessel wall enhancement			
	Absent (*n* = 23)	Mild (*n* = 12)	Marked (*n* = 5)	p
Maximal MCA (cm/s), mean ± SD	97.2 ± 29.2	115.3 ± 69.4	112.4 ± 49.4	0.52
Mean MCA (cm/s), mean ± SD	89.1 ± 23.0	102.6 ± 58.2	103.9 ± 53.3	0.56
Maximal ACA (cm/s), mean ± SD	69.7 ± 18.7	76.0 ± 20.7	73.2 ± 27.2	0.71
Mean ACA (cm/s), mean ± SD	66.2 ± 16.4	68.8 ± 17.8	66.6 ± 21.4	0.92

ACA anterior cerebral artery, *MCA* middle cerebral artery, *SEM* standard error of means

walls persisted at follow-up in a third of these patients, with a median follow-up duration of 7 months. The proportion of RCVS patients with vascular wall enhancement observed in this cohort was higher than that reported in previous studies [19, 20] and was persistent in some cases, suggesting that vascular wall enhancement may not be a reliable imaging sign as previously thought for clinical differentiation of RCVS from vasculopathy with an inflammatory component.

Differentiation from CNS vasculitis precludes unnecessary invasive brain biopsy, cerebral angiography, and lifelong immunosuppression in RCVS patients [12]. Previous studies with small numbers of patients found that arterial wall enhancement was mild (if present) in a minority of RCVS patients [20], as opposed to the strong wall enhancement frequently observed in vasculitis patients. In our present study, most of the vascular wall enhancement was also mild in the RCVS patients. However, the proportion of patients in which vascular wall enhancement was found was much higher than previously reported (47% vs. 31%) [20], and a fourth of the patients had strong vascular wall enhancement. Notwithstanding, the clinical hallmarks of recurrent thunderclap headaches and the reversibility of vasoconstriction without immunosuppressants in our patients support their being diagnosed with RCVS over CNS vasculitis.

Arterial wall enhancement in contrasted vascular imaging may reveal an inflammatory component of RCVS pathology. Although inflammation is not considered to

Table 3 Characteristics of the RCVS patients

	Vascular wall enhancement		p
	Absence (*n* = 26)	Presence (*n* = 22)	
Sex (female), n (%)	23 (88.5%)	19 (86.4%)	1.00
Age (years), man ± SD	49.7 ± 11.1	52.3 ± 7.5	0.53
Time to MRI from onset (days), mean ± SD	11.8 ± 6.9	12.0 ± 7.6	0.93
Vascular risk factors, n (%)			
Hypertension	2 (7.7%)	2 (9.1%)	0.86
Diabetes	1 (3.8%)	2 (9.1%)	0.59
CAD	0 (0.0%)	0 (0.0%)	NA
Headache attacks, n (%)			
Number of total attacks	8.4 ± 8.4	4.7 ± 4.4	0.04
Duration of whole course (d)	10.5 ± 6.3	8.8 ± 5.1	0.32
Frequency (number/duration)	0.9 ± 1.0	0.6 ± 0.3	0.07
Triggers, n (%)			
Bathing	8 (30.8%)	5 (22.7%)	0.53
Exertion	2 (7.7%)	3 (13.6%)	0.65
Cough	2 (7.7%)	1 (4.5%)	1.00
Defecation	7 (26.9%)	11 (50.0%)	0.10
Emotion	6 (23.1%)	4 (18.2%)	0.68
Sex	5 (19.2%)	4 (18.2%)	1.00
Mean number of triggers per patient	1.4 ± 0.9	1.6 ± 1.2	0.65
Mean total WMH volume (ml)	1.1 ± 1.2	1.3 ± 1.8	0.71

CAD coronary artery disease, *MRI* magnetic resonance imaging, *SEM* standard error of mean, *WHM* white matter hyperintensity

play a key role in the pathogenesis of RCVS, prolonged vasoconstriction per se has been proposed to be associated with an inflammatory process [23, 27]. Of note, an inflammatory cascade has been reported in cerebral vasospasm in SAH [28]. Although the pathologies of RCVS and SAH would be expected to differ from each other, they might share some pathomechanisms. For example, oxidative stress and endothelial dysfunction, which contribute to the vascular wall inflammation, have also been noted in patients with RCVS [29, 30]. Additionally, a postulated mechanism of cocaine-induced vasculitis includes cerebrovascular smooth muscle cells apoptosis and promotion of leukocyte migration across cerebral vascular walls [23, 31, 32], producing vessel wall inflammation. Because cocaine-induced vasculitis is considered a spectral disorder of RCVS [9, 12, 24], it is reasonable to deduce that vascular wall inflammation exists in at least some patients with secondary RCVS. Prolonged vasoconstriction has been hypothesized to contribute to the development of secondary angiitis [27]; similar mechanisms might also contribute to prolonged vascular wall enhancement. However, these were purely speculative; the nature of the persistent/residual vascular wall enhancement remains to be elucidated.

The enhancement of diseased vessels in RCVS was suggested to be reversible in a study completed in the USA [20]. In that study, 8 out of 9 RCVS patients showed complete resolution of their initial vascular wall imaging findings, with only 1 having minimal residual wall thickening after a median follow-up period of 3.5 months [20]. In contrast, one third of our patients with follow-up vascular imaging had persistent mild enhancement after a median period of 3 months (longest period, 21 months). Even among the 10 patients with some level of reduced enhancement on follow-up imaging (follow-up range, 55–95 months), four had residual enhancement. Slower resolution or greater persistence of the enhancement has been observed in atherosclerosis of the intracranial vessels [33], particularly if the enhancement is eccentric and heterogeneous with mild to moderate intensity [13]. Although atherosclerosis risk factors were not commonly present in our patients with persistent or residual enhancement (one patient had hypertension, and one patient had hypertension and diabetes), we could not completely exclude the possibility of subclinical atherosclerosis in our patients. Particularly, it has been found that subclinical atherosclerosis can be present in as high as 50% of patients with low cardiovascular risk [34] and about 60% of asymptomatic patients [34, 35], and that intracranial atherosclerosis is more prevalent in Asians [36]. Compared with the study by Mossa-Basha et al. [37], we focused more on the reversibility of vascular wall enhancement in RCVS, finding that the vascular wall enhancement was not always reversible in patients with RCVS, probably due to etiological heterogeneity. Hence, although vascular wall imaging is a powerful and reliable tool for evaluating diseases involving intracranial vessels, the use of it as an ancillary diagnostic tool for RCVS required deliberation. The persistence of vascular wall enhancement in RCVS did not depreciate the value of vessel wall imaging for differentiation of nonocclusive intracranial vasculopathies, but instead reminded the clinicians not making the diagnosis solely based on reversibility of the enhancement.

The headache characteristics of RCVS [38] are distinct from the primary headaches such as migraine [39] or cluster headache [40]. Although 20% of the patients with RCVS have pre-existing migraine [38], the cardiovascular or neurological comorbidities known to be associated with migraine [41–43] have not been well explored in patients with RCVS. Because both migraine [44] and RCVS [45] are associated increased risks of white matter hyperintensities, there could be some shared mechanisms between these two disorders. A higher headache frequency and long-term migraine may worsen the cardio-metabolic profile in migraineurs [44], which might partially be mediated by circulating microRNAs associated with vascular function [46, 47]. Whether similar mechanisms could contribute to RCVS pathogenesis or the imaging findings disclosed in this study deserve further investigation.

The present study had several limitations. First, we did not include a control group because doing so would involve unnecessary exposure of subjects to the potential risks of gadolinium deposition in the brain [48]. Second, because we did not recruit patients with secondary causes of RCVS, one should be cautious to extrapolate the findings to the general pathogenesis of RCVS. Given that secondary causes of RCVS are far less common than idiopathic ones in Asian patients [38, 49], elucidating the pathogenesis of the latter was our major concern. Third, although follow-up MRA evaluations for confirming vasoconstriction reversibility were obtained for all of our patients, the retention rate for vascular imaging was 70.8%, mainly due to the undesirable requirement of contrast injection. Fourth, the magnitudes of vascular wall enhancement observed in the present study do not correspond precisely with severity levels defined in the previous reports. However, vascular wall enhancement level differences across studies may reflect the particular machines, settings, and protocols used. In our study, we focused more on the presence of vascular wall enhancement, and the temporal change of the enhancement, both may have little to do with the degrees of the initial vascular wall enhancement. Fifth, these patients received the same treatment (nimodipine) but the resolution of enhancement was heterogeneous, so we cannot be sure if that enhancement of vascular wall imaging is altered by medical treatment. Sixth, the reluctance of patients to undergo spinal tap in Taiwanese society precluded CSF studies in many patients; therefore, the differential diagnosis of RCVS in our practice heavily relied on the presence of the clinical hallmark of RCVS (i.e. recurrent thunderclap headaches) and imaging findings (to demonstrate the reversibility of vasoconstrictions and to exclude SAH or other secondary causes of thunderclap headaches by susceptibility weighted imaging or other MR sequences [38, 45]. Nevertheless, the characteristics of the patients who received spinal tap were not different from those who did not receive spinal tap. Finally, our study could not confirm how long the persistent or residual enhancement could last. Studies with a longer follow-up period are needed.

Conclusion

Demographics, clinical profiles, and cerebral artery flow velocities were similar across patients with versus without vascular wall enhancement. Half of the RCVS patients had enhancement of diseased vessels and it was persistent for one third of them, so vascular wall enhancement may not be a reliable imaging marker for differentiating RCVS from central nervous system vasculitis or subclinical atherosclerosis. The clinical implication of our findings is that the differentiation of RCVS from other intracranial vasculopathy should not be made solely based on vascular wall imaging.

Abbreviations

ACA: Anterior cerebral artery; ANOVA: Analyses of variance; CNS: Central nervous system; FLAIR: Fluid-attenuated inversion recovery; ICHD-2: International Classification of Headache Disorders, second edition; MCA: Middle cerebral artery; MRA: Magnetic resonance angiogram; MRI: Magnetic resonance imaging; RCVS: Reversible cerebral vasoconstriction syndrome; SAH: Subarachnoid hemorrhage

Funding

This work was supported by the Brain Research Center, National Yang-Ming University from The Featured Areas Research Center Program within the framework of the Higher Education Sprout Project by the Ministry of Education (MOE) in Taiwan (to SJW); Taipei Veterans General Hospital [V100E6-001, V106C-117] (to SWJ & SPC); Ministry of Science and Technology of Taiwan [MOST 104-2314-B-010-015-MY2, MOST 104-2314-B-075 -006 -MY3, and MOST 103-2321-B-010-017-] (to SWJ & SPC); Ministry of Science and Technology support for the Center for Dynamical Biomarkers and Translational Medicine, National Central University, Taiwan [MOST 103-2911-I-008-001] (to SWJ); and Ministry of Health and Welfare, Taiwan [MOHW 103-TDU-B-211-113-003, MOHW 104-TDU-B-211-113-003, MOHW 105-TDU-B-211-113-003] (to SJW). The funders had no role in study design, data collection and analysis, decision to publish, or preparation of the manuscript.

Authors' contributions

CYC analyzed and interpreted the patient data and was a major contributor in writing the manuscript. SPC was responsible for study concept and design, acquisition of data, supervision of analysis and interpretation, and critical revision of the manuscript for important intellectual content. FCC and JFL analyzed the imaging data and contributed to manuscript writing. YFW, FJL, and SJW were responsible for patient recruitment, supervision of data acquisition and analysis, and critical revision of the manuscript for important intellectual content. All authors read and approved the final manuscript.

Competing interests

The authors declare that they have no competing interests.

Author details

[1]Department of Neurology, Neurological Institute, Taipei Veterans General Hospital, Taipei 112, Taiwan. [2]Faculty of Medicine, National Yang-Ming University School of Medicine, Taipei, Taiwan. [3]Institute of Clinical Medicine, National Yang-Ming University, Taipei, Taiwan. [4]Division of Translational Research, Department of Medical Research, Taipei Veterans General Hospital, Taipei, Taiwan. [5]Department of Radiology, Taipei Veterans General Hospital, Taipei, Taiwan. [6]Brain Research Center, National Yang-Ming University, Taipei, Taiwan.

References

1. Calabrese LH, Dodick DW, Schwedt TJ et al (2007) Narrative review: reversible cerebral vasoconstriction syndromes. Ann Intern Med 146:34–44
2. Chen SP, Fuh JL, Lirng JF et al (2006) Is vasospasm requisite for posterior leukoencephalopathy in patients with primary thunderclap headaches? Cephalalgia 26:530–536
3. Ducros A, Boukobza M, Porcher R et al (2007) The clinical and radiological spectrum of reversible cerebral vasoconstriction syndrome. A prospective series of 67 patients. Brain 130:3091–3101
4. Singhal AB, Caviness VS, Begleiter AF et al (2002) Cerebral vasoconstriction and stroke after use of serotonergic drugs. Neurology 58:130–133
5. Chen SP, Fuh JL, Lirng JF et al (2006) Recurrent primary thunderclap headache and benign CNS angiopathy: spectra of the same disorder? Neurology 67:2164–2169
6. Chen SP, Fuh JL, Chang FC et al (2008) Transcranial color doppler study for reversible cerebral vasoconstriction syndromes. Ann Neurol 63:751–757
7. Chen SP, Fuh JL, Wang SJ et al (2010) Magnetic resonance angiography in reversible cerebral vasoconstriction syndromes. Ann Neurol 67:648–656
8. Ducros A, Fiedler U, Porcher R et al (2010) Hemorrhagic manifestations of reversible cerebral vasoconstriction syndrome: frequency, features, and risk factors. Stroke 41:2505–2511
9. Singhal AB, Hajj-Ali RA, Topcuoglu MA et al (2011) Reversible cerebral vasoconstriction syndromes: analysis of 139 cases. Arch Neurol 68:1005–1012
10. Lee MJ, Cha J, Choi HA et al (2017) Blood-brain barrier breakdown in reversible cerebral vasoconstriction syndrome: implications for pathophysiology and diagnosis. Ann Neurol 81:454–466
11. Chen SP, Fuh JL, Wang SJ (2011) Reversible cerebral vasoconstriction syndrome: current and future perspectives. Expert Rev Neurother 11:1265–1276
12. Singhal AB, Topcuoglu MA, Fok JW et al (2016) Reversible cerebral vasoconstriction syndromes and primary angiitis of the central nervous system: clinical, imaging, and angiographic comparison. Ann Neurol 79: 882–894
13. Mossa-Basha M, Alexander M, Gaddikeri S et al (2016) Vessel wall imaging for intracranial vascular disease evaluation. J Neurointerv Surg 8:1154–1159
14. Edelman RR, Mattle HP, Wallner B et al (1990) Extracranial carotid arteries: evaluation with "black blood" MR angiography. Radiology 177:45–50
15. Swartz RH, Bhuta SS, Farb RI et al (2009) Intracranial arterial wall imaging using high-resolution 3-tesla contrast-enhanced MRI. Neurology 72:627–634
16. Kuker W, Gaertner S, Nagele T et al (2008) Vessel wall contrast enhancement: a diagnostic sign of cerebral vasculitis. Cerebrovasc Dis 26:23–29
17. Takano K, Yamashita S, Takemoto K et al (2013) MRI of intracranial vertebral artery dissection: evaluation of intramural haematoma using a black blood, variable-flip-angle 3D turbo spin-echo sequence. Neuroradiology 55:845–851
18. Horie N, Morikawa M, Fukuda S et al (2011) Detection of blood blister-like aneurysm and intramural hematoma with high-resolution magnetic resonance imaging. J Neurosurg 115:1206–1209

19. Mandell DM, Matouk CC, Farb RI et al (2012) Vessel wall MRI to differentiate between reversible cerebral vasoconstriction syndrome and central nervous system vasculitis: preliminary results. Stroke 43:860–862
20. Obusez EC, Hui F, Hajj-Ali RA et al (2014) High-resolution MRI vessel wall imaging: spatial and temporal patterns of reversible cerebral vasoconstriction syndrome and central nervous system vasculitis. AJNR Am J Neuroradiol 35: 1527–1532
21. Serdaru M, Chiras J, Cujas M et al (1984) Isolated benign cerebral vasculitis or migrainous vasospasm? J Neurol Neurosurg Psychiatry 47:73–76
22. Hajj-Ali RA, Furlan A, Abou-Chebel A et al (2002) Benign angiopathy of the central nervous system: cohort of 16 patients with clinical course and long-term followup. Arthritis Rheum 47:662–669
23. Han JS, Mandell DM, Poublanc J et al (2008) BOLD-MRI cerebrovascular reactivity findings in cocaine-induced cerebral vasculitis. Nat Clin Pract Neurol 4:628–632
24. Ducros A (2012) Reversible cerebral vasoconstriction syndrome. Lancet Neurol 11:906–917
25. (2004) The International Classification of Headache Disorders: 2nd edition. Cephalalgia 24 Suppl 1:9–160
26. (2013) The international classification of headache disorders, 3rd edition (beta version). Cephalalgia 33:629–808
27. Calabrese LH, Duna GF (1995) Evaluation and treatment of central nervous system vasculitis. Curr Opin Rheumatol 7:37–44
28. Carr KR, Zuckerman SL, Mocco J (2013) Inflammation, cerebral vasospasm, and evolving theories of delayed cerebral ischemia. Neurol Res Int 2013: 506584
29. Chen SP, Wang YF, Huang PH et al (2014) Reduced circulating endothelial progenitor cells in reversible cerebral vasoconstriction syndrome. J Headache Pain 15:82
30. Chen SP, Chung YT, Liu TY et al (2013) Oxidative stress and increased formation of vasoconstricting F2-isoprostanes in patients with reversible cerebral vasoconstriction syndrome. Free Radic Biol Med 61:243–248
31. Gan X, Zhang L, Berger O et al (1999) Cocaine enhances brain endothelial adhesion molecules and leukocyte migration. Clin Immunol 91:68–76
32. Su J, Li J, Li W et al (2003) Cocaine induces apoptosis in cerebral vascular muscle cells: potential roles in strokes and brain damage. Eur J Pharmacol 482:61–66
33. Skarpathiotakis M, Mandell DM, Swartz RH et al (2013) Intracranial atherosclerotic plaque enhancement in patients with ischemic stroke. AJNR Am J Neuroradiol 34:299–304
34. Baber U, Mehran R, Sartori S et al (2015) Prevalence, impact, and predictive value of detecting subclinical coronary and carotid atherosclerosis in asymptomatic adults: the BioImage study. J Am Coll Cardiol 65:1065–1074
35. Fernandez-Friera L, Penalvo JL, Fernandez-Ortiz A et al (2015) Prevalence, vascular distribution, and multiterritorial extent of subclinical atherosclerosis in a middle-aged cohort: the PESA (progression of early subclinical atherosclerosis) study. Circulation 131:2104–2113
36. Arenillas JF (2011) Intracranial atherosclerosis: current concepts. Stroke 42: S20–S23
37. Mossa-Basha M, Shibata DK, Hallam DK et al (2017) Added value of Vessel Wall magnetic resonance imaging for differentiation of nonocclusive intracranial Vasculopathies. Stroke 48:3026–3033
38. Chen SP, Fuh JL, Lirng JF et al (2015) Recurrence of reversible cerebral vasoconstriction syndrome: a long-term follow-up study. Neurology 84: 1552–1558
39. Charles A (2018) The pathophysiology of migraine: implications for clinical management. Lancet Neurol 17:174–182
40. Snoer A, Lund N, Beske R et al (2018) Cluster headache beyond the pain phase: a prospective study of 500 attacks. Neurology. https://doi.org/10.1212/01.wnl.0000542491.92981.03
41. Tana C, Santilli F, Martelletti P et al (2015) Correlation between migraine severity and cholesterol levels. Pain Pract 15:662–670
42. Giamberardino MA, Affaitati G, Martelletti P et al (2015) Impact of migraine on fibromyalgia symptoms. J Headache Pain 17:28
43. Lopez-de-Andres A, Luis Del Barrio J, Hernandez-Barrera V et al (2018) Migraine in adults with diabetes; is there an association? Results of a population-based study. Diabetes Metab Syndr Obes 11:367–374
44. Tana C, Tafuri E, Tana M et al (2013) New insights into the cardiovascular risk of migraine and the role of white matter hyperintensities: is gold all that glitters? J Headache Pain 14:9
45. Chen SP, Chou KH, Fuh JL et al (2018) Dynamic changes in white matter Hyperintensities in reversible cerebral vasoconstriction syndrome. JAMA Neurol. https://doi.org/10.1001/jamaneurol.2018.1321
46. Tana C, Giamberardino MA, Cipollone F (2017) microRNA profiling in atherosclerosis, diabetes, and migraine. Ann Med 49:93–105
47. Cheng CY, Chen SP, Liao YC et al (2018) Elevated circulating endothelial-specific microRNAs in migraine patients: a pilot study. Cephalalgia 38:1585–1591
48. Lenkinski RE (2017) Gadolinium retention and deposition revisited: how the chemical properties of gadolinium-based contrast agents and the use of animal models inform us about the behavior of these agents in the human brain. Radiology 285:721–724
49. Choi HA, Lee MJ, Choi H et al (2018) Characteristics and demographics of reversible cerebral vasoconstriction syndrome: a large prospective series of Korean patients. Cephalalgia 38:765–75

10

Feasibility of serum CGRP measurement as a biomarker of chronic migraine: a critical reappraisal

Mi Ji Lee[1], Sook-Yeon Lee[2], Soohyun Cho[1], Eun-Suk Kang[2] and Chin-Sang Chung[1,3*]

Abstract

Background: Calcitonin gene-related peptide (CGRP) has been reported as elevated in chronic migraine. We aimed to validate the role of interictal serum CGRP concentration in peripheral blood samples as a biomarker of chronic migraine.

Methods: We prospectively recruited patients with episodic and chronic migraine and normal controls (NCs) in the Samsung Medical Center between August 2015 and May 2016. Blood samples were collected interictally from antecubital veins per prespecified protocol. Serum CGRP measurement was performed in the central laboratory by a single experienced technician blinded to clinical information. Migraine subtype, headache days in the previous month, and the presence and characteristics of headache at ±2 days of measurement were evaluated at every visit.

Results: A total of 156 migraineurs (106 episodic and 50 chronic) and 27 NCs were recruited in this study. Compared to NCs (75.7 ± 20.07 pg/mL) and patients with episodic migraine (67.0 ± 20.70 pg/mL), patients with chronic migraine did not show an interictal elevation of serum CGRP levels (64.9 ± 15.32 pg/mL). Serum CGRP concentration was not associated with headache status (ictal vs. interictal), migraine subtype (migraine with vs. without aura), use of preventive or acute medications, and comorbid medication overuse. Higher serum CGRP concentration did not predict treatment response in patients with chronic migraine.

Conclusions: Serum CGRP concentration may not be a feasible biomarker for chronic migraine. Further validation is necessary before CGRP can be used in the clinical practice.

Keywords: Migraine, Biomarker, CGRP, Immunoassay

Background

Migraine is a common and disabling neurological disorder characterized by episodic attacks of headache and associated symptoms. When the migraine progresses to a chronic form (chronic migraine), the frequency of migraine attack increases, and head pain can persist even between attacks. The strategy of treatment differs between episodic migraine (EM) and chronic migraine (CM).

To date, the diagnosis of migraine is based on the patients' description of symptoms. Although the International Headache Society offers well-structured diagnostic criteria for migraine and its subtypes [1], it is often challenged in the clinic by the language barrier (e.g. deafness or cognitively impaired patient), recall bias, and instability of patient-reported headache frequency. Therefore, researchers have been seeking a biomarker which can aid the diagnosis and follow-up of migraine. Calcitonin gene-related peptide (CGRP) is one of the most promising candidates, since interictal serum CGRP concentration was reported as a possible biomarker of CM [2]. However, the diagnostic role of CGRP has not been validated yet. In this study, we aimed to reproduce the previous study results and validate with clinical data from normal subjects, patients with EM, and those with CM.

* Correspondence: cspaul@naver.com
[1]Department of Neurology, Samsung Medical Center, Sungkyunkwan University School of Medicine, 81 Irwon-Ro, Gangnam-Gu, Seoul 06351, South Korea
[3]Neuroscience Center, Samsung Medical Center, Seoul, South Korea
Full list of author information is available at the end of the article

Methods

Subjects

We prospectively recruited 156 adult patients with migraine (106 episodic and 50 chronic migraine) in the

Samsung Medical Center headache clinic from August 2015 to May 2016. The diagnosis of migraine was based on the International Classification of Headache Disorders 3rd edition beta version (ICHD-3 beta). The distinction between episodic migraine (EM) and chronic migraine (CM) was also based on the ICHD-3 beta. We included patients of > 1 year after migraine onset. Twenty-seven normal controls (NCs) were also recruited for this study. Subjects were considered as NC when they had no subjective headache, then investigators confirm that they did not have migraine, any headache of moderate or severe intensity, or any acute or chronic pain disorder and did not take any regular medications. This study was approved by the institutional review board of Samsung Medical Center. All the participants gave written consent.

Evaluation

All patients completed a structured questionnaire regarding headache characteristics, frequency, past medical history, and the use of acute and preventive medications. From the questionnaire, the presence of unilateral autonomic symptoms (UAS) and headache unilaterality were identified as clinical markers of trigeminal activation [3, 4]. Two headache neurologists (M.J.L. and C.-S.C.) interviewed all patients. We used Allodynia Symptom Checklist-12 (ASC-12) to estimate allodynia during migraine attack. CGRP was followed up after 3 months in patients with CM who underwent Botulinum toxin treatment. Selected patients with EM also underwent the follow-up measurement.

Blood collection

Blood sampling was conducted in our central laboratory between 8 and 10 a.m. after overnight fasting. A serum separator tube was used for sampling. After clotting at room temperature for 30 min, samples were centrifuged for 15 min at approximately 2000×*g*. Aliquots were stored immediately at − 80 °C. At the day of sampling, all patients and NCs were asked about the presence of headache since the past two days. When present, we collected information about the presence and characteristics of headache at the day (day 0) and the day before (day − 1) the sampling. It was considered interictal if patients did not have moderate or severe headache at both day − 1 and day 0 for EM patients and at day 0 for CM patients. Patients who took acute abortive medication at day − 1 or day 0 were excluded from the study, regardless of the severity of headache.

Serum CGRP measurement

All serum CGRP concentration was measured by an experienced laboratory technician who was blinded to clinical information or group assignment, using a commercially available ELISA kit (Wuhan USCN Business Co., Ltd., Hubei, China) based on the manufacturer's instructions. The principle of assay kit is the competitive inhibition enzyme immunoassay. The biotin labeled CGRP was added to reaction well with unlabeled CGRP from patient's serum, incubated and measured by binding of avidin conjugated to horseradish peroxidase. Five-point standard curve was generated with serially diluted standards and the concentration of CGRP in the sample was derived from it, which was reverse proportional to the intensity of final reaction. In-house prepared quality control sample was included at every batch of test. Analyses of between-run precision of control 1 and control 2 showed coefficients of variation of 13.1% and 11.2%, respectively. The detection range of kit was 12.35–1000 pg/mL.

Statistical analysis

Data are presented as mean (SD) or number (%) unless otherwise specified. The student t-test or Mann-Whitney test was used depending on the distribution of continuous variables. The Chi-Square test or Fisher's exact test was performed to compare categorical variables. The relationship between CGRP concentration and clinical characteristics including the presence of UAS and headache unilaterality was tested by using the linear regression analysis. All data analyses were performed using Stata (version 14). *P* values less than 0.05 were considered significant.

Results

Subjects

Among 156 patients recruited, 13 patients (7 with EM and 6 with CM) were excluded because they took an acute abortive medication at day − 1 or day 0. Finally, 143 (99 EM and 44 CM) patients and 27 NCs were included in the analysis. Interictal sampling was successful in 96 patients with EM and 34 with CM. Characteristics of patients and NCs are summarized in Table 1.

Serum CGRP concentration

Group comparison

Results on interictal serum CGRP concentrations are summarized in Fig. 1. The mean serum CGRP concentration in patients with CM (64.9 pg/mL, SD 15.32) was not different from that of compared to NCs (mean 75.7 (SD 20.07) pg/mL; $p = 0.104$). Patients with EM showed a wider distribution of CGRP concentrations (Fig. 1). The mean CGRP concentration was 67.0 (SD 20.70) pg/mL in patients with EM, which was not different from that in CM patients ($p > 0.999$) or NCs ($p = 0.133$). Group difference remained non-significant when adjusted for age, sex, and the presence of aura.

Table 1 Characteristics of study subjects

	Normal control ($n = 27$)	Episodic migraine ($n = 99$)	Chronic migraine ($n = 44$)	*P*-value
Age	34 (27–42)	44 (31–49)	39.5 (31–54)	0.016
Female sex	25 (92.6%)	78 (78.8%)	36 (81.8%)	0.258
Migraine with aura	NA	18 (18.2%)	8 (18.2%)	> 0.999
Headache days/month	NA	5 (2–10)	27 (15–30)	< 0.001
Hypertension	0 (0%)	6 (6.06%)	5 (11.36%)	0.162
Diabetes	0 (0%)	0 (0%)	1 (2.27%)	0.237
Dyslipidemia	0 (0%)	6 (6.06%)	5 (11.36%)	0.162
Stroke	0 (0%)	1 (1.01%)	1 (2.27%)	0.670
Cardiac disease	0 (0%)	2 (2.02%)	2 (4.55%)	0.445
Current smoking	0 (0%)	6 (6.06%)	5 (11.36%)	0.162
Fibromyalgia	0 (0%)	1 (1.01%)	2 (4.55%)	0.250
Depression	0 (0%)	4 (4.04%)	12 (27.27%)	< 0.001
Anxiety disorder	0 (0%)	1 (1.01%)	8 (18.18%)	< 0.001
Panic disorder	0 (0%)	2 (2.02%)	3 (6.82%)	0.180
Preventive medication	0 (0%)	19 (19.19%)	22 (50%)	< 0.001
TCA	0 (0%)	13 (13.13%)	18 (40.91%)	< 0.001
Beta-blocker	0 (0%)	15 (15.15%)	15 (34.09%)	0.001
CCB	0 (0%)	12 (12.12%)	13 (29.55%)	0.002
Antiepileptic drugs	0 (0%)	3 (3.03%)	11 (25%)	< 0.001
ARB	0 (0%)	2 (2.02%)	1 (2.27%)	0.745

NA = not assessed; *TCA* = tricyclic antidepressant; *CCB* = calcium-channel blocker; *ARB* = angiotensin-II receptor blocker

Clinical correlation

Interictal serum CGRP concentration was not correlated with monthly headache days (Spearman's rho = 0.087, $p = 0.324$; Fig. 2). It was also independent of reported severity of allodynia during migraine attacks (Spearman's rho = – 0.023, $p = 0.815$). The use of preventive medication was not associated with serum CGRP concentration ($p = 0.466$ and 0.673 for EM and CM, respectively). None of age, sex, migraine subtype (MA vs. MO), vascular risk factors, and fibromyalgia was significant for CGRP (Additional file 1: Table S1). In the CM group, serum CGRP concentrations did not differ by the presence of

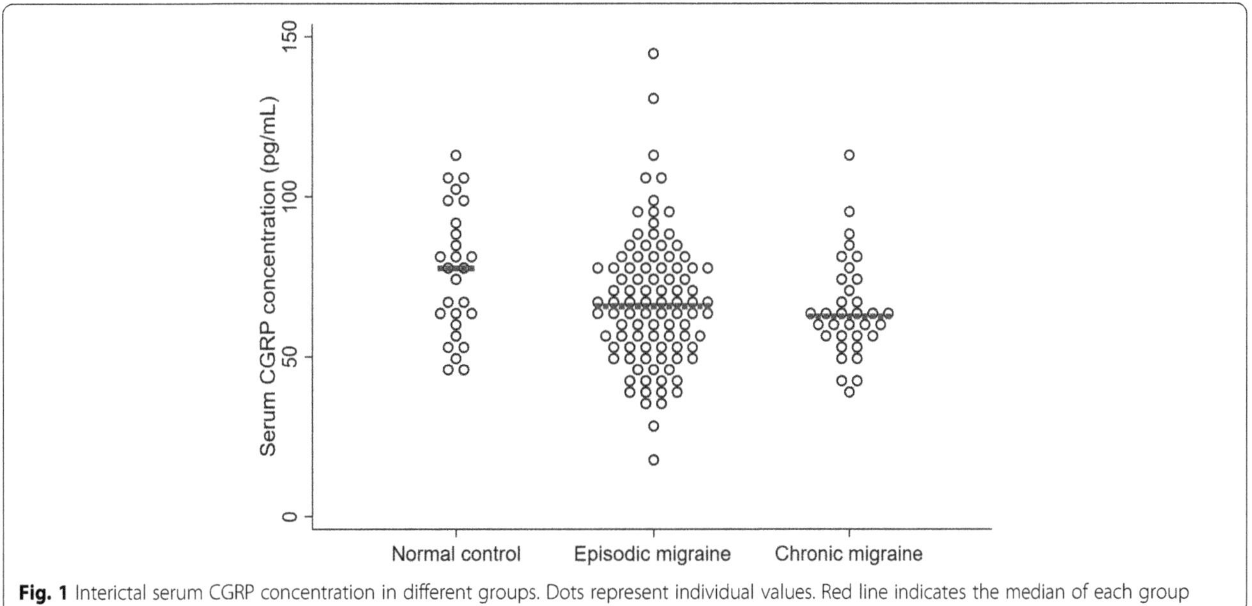

Fig. 1 Interictal serum CGRP concentration in different groups. Dots represent individual values. Red line indicates the median of each group

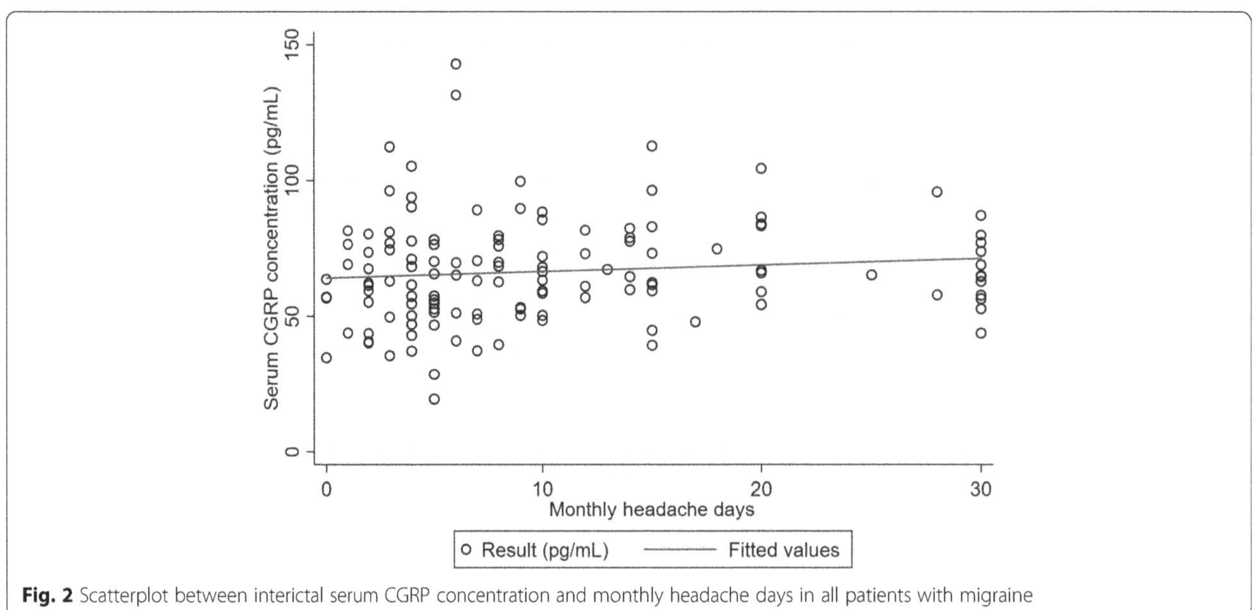

Fig. 2 Scatterplot between interictal serum CGRP concentration and monthly headache days in all patients with migraine

medication overuse (65.3 ± 4.70 pg/mL in 15 patients with CM without MOH vs. 64.6 ± 3.30 pg/mL in 19 patients with CM and MOH, $p = 0.902$).

Data on clinical markers of trigeminal activation were available in all but one patients (96 EM and 33 CM) who underwent the interictal CGRP testing. A total of 17 (17.7%) EM patients and 10 (30.3%) CM patients had at least one UAS. Unilateral headaches were reported by 36 (37.5%) EM and 11 (33.3%) CM patients. Either the presence of UAS or headache unilaterality showed no association with the interictal serum CGRP concentrations (Table 2).

Ictal vs interictal CGRP concentrations

When ictal and interictal samples were compared, serum CGRP concentration was not affected by the presence of moderate-severe headache on the day of measurement ($p = 0.307$ and 0.460 for EM and CM, respectively; Fig. 3).

Longitudinal changes in serum CGRP concentration

Among 16 patients with EM who were followed up with serum CGRP concentration, all showed a change in their serum CGRP concentration after 3 months. All EM patients did not use preventive medications during the follow-up. However, CGRP concentration was not an indicator of a > 50% reduction of headache frequency and did not correlate with changes in monthly headache frequency (Figs. 4 and 5).

Eleven patients with CM underwent follow-up sampling at 3 months after Botulinum toxin treatment. Baseline serum CGRP concentration of responders ($n = 4$) was not higher than those of non-responders ($n = 7$; median 60.1 [IQR 59.0–64.9] vs median 72.9 [IQR 62.9–79.8] pg/mL for responders and non-responders, respectively, $p = 0.130$). After treatment, all the non-responders showed a reduction in their serum CGRP concentrations, while responders showed a variable change (Fig. 4).

Discussion

In this study, we found no increase in serum CGRP concentration in patients with CM. It was not associated with headache days, allodynia severity, or the presence of headache on the day of measurement.

Table 2 Linear regression analysis results of clinical markers of trigeminal activation

	Beta	95% CI	*P*-value
Unilateral autonomic symptoms	2.07	−7.53 - 11.68	0.670
Conjunctival injection and/or lacrimation	−4.27	−21.90 - 13.37	0.633
Nasal congestion and/or rhinorrhea	−8.69	−36.22 - 18.85	0.534
Eyelid edema	−14.57	−34.06 - 4.92	0.141
Ptosis	−1.39	−9.76 - 6.98	0.743
Any	−2.87	−9.93 - 4.19	0.422
Headache unilaterality	2.07	−7.53 - 11.68	0.670

The dependent variable was the interictal serum CGRP concentrations

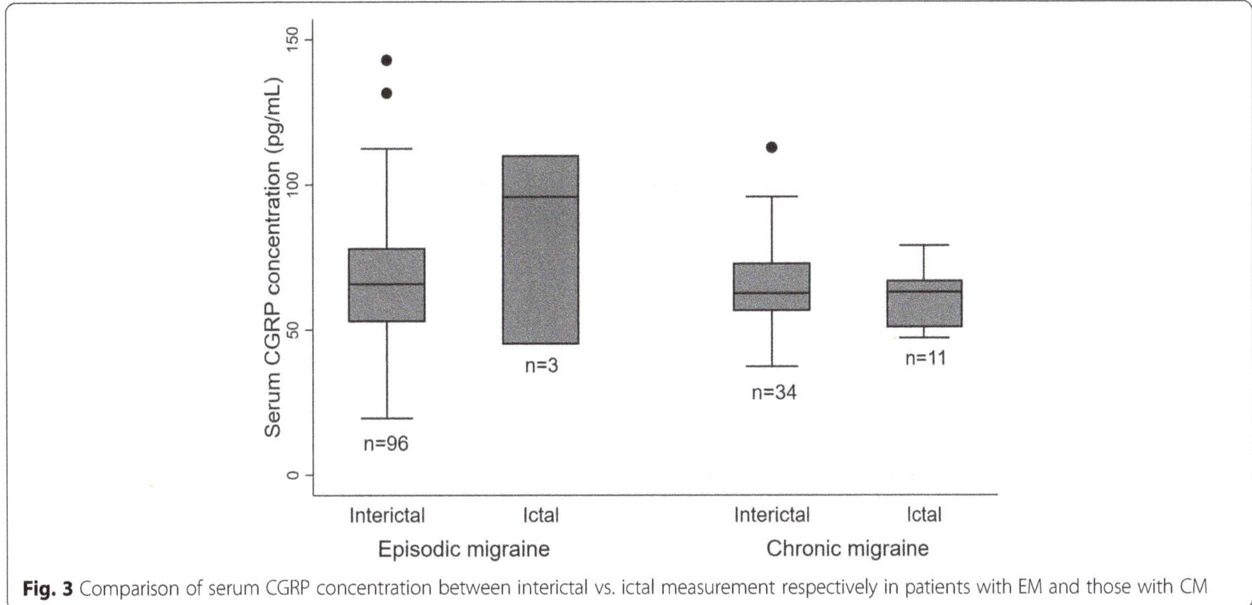

Fig. 3 Comparison of serum CGRP concentration between interictal vs. ictal measurement respectively in patients with EM and those with CM

A biomarker is defined as an indicator of normal biological processes, pathogenic processes or pharmacological responses to a therapeutic intervention [5]. Clinically, a good biomarker should aid the diagnosis of the disease, correlate with disease severity, or predict outcomes [6]. It also should be easy to measure with acceptable inter-rater and intra-subject reliability. Finally, a good biomarker is linked to pathophysiological explanation [5, 6].

To search for a biomarker of migraine, several candidates have been tested [6, 7]. Based on an early finding that jugular venous CGRP level is elevated during acute migraine attack [8], CGRP has been regarded as a key neuropeptide of migraine pathophysiology [9, 10]. Indeed, increasing evidences on the role of CGRP in migraine headache exist. CGRP-containing neurons are most frequently found in the human trigeminal ganglion [11]. CGRP antagonists and monoclonal antibodies to CGRP or its receptor have shown a good efficacy to prevent migraine attacks [12–14]. Based on these results, serum CGRP concentration is one of the most attractive candidates of biomarkers of migraine. Recently, a possible role of interictal serum CGRP measurement in the diagnosis of CM and prediction of treatment outcome has been suggested by researchers [2, 15, 16].

Our study results, however, do not support CGRP as a biomarker of CM. Serum CGRP concentration was not

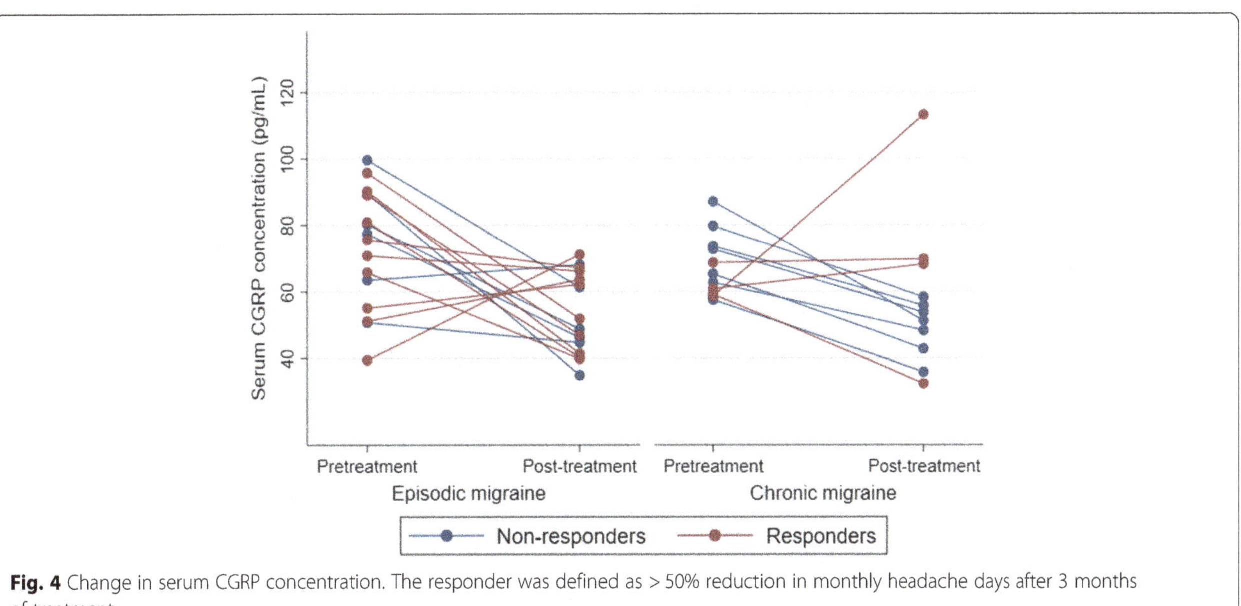

Fig. 4 Change in serum CGRP concentration. The responder was defined as > 50% reduction in monthly headache days after 3 months of treatment

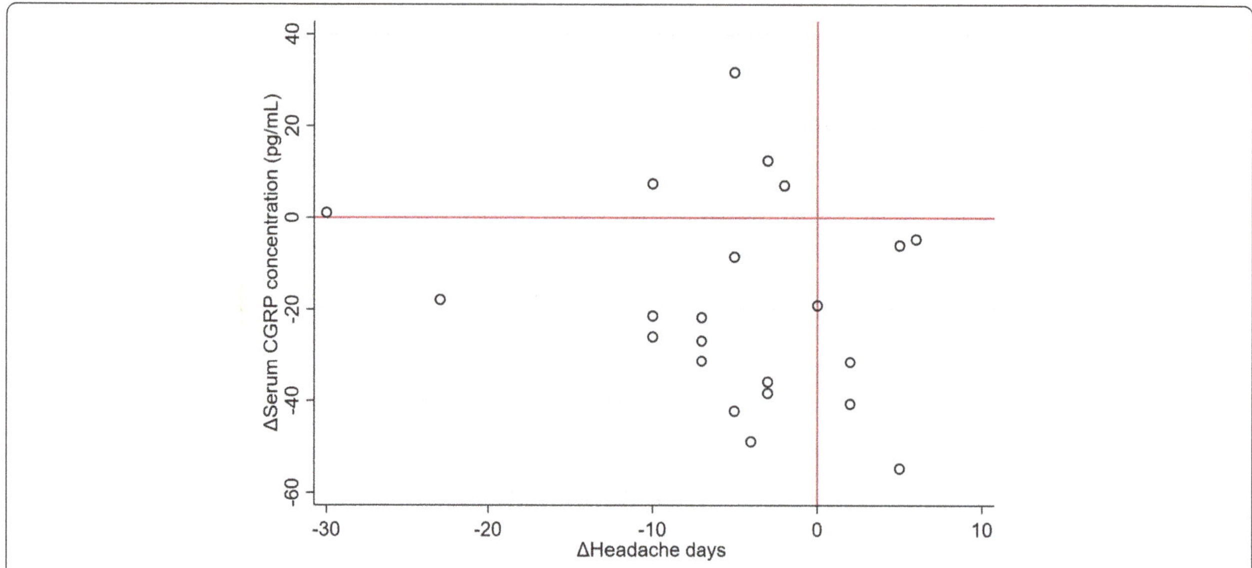

Fig. 5 Correlation between changes in monthly headache days and serum CGRP concentrations before and after 3 months. The right upper and left lower sections indicate positive correlation

diagnostic for CM, did not correlate with disease severity (headache frequency or allodynia), and did not predict the treatment outcome. CGRP concentrations did not differ according to migraine subtype (migraine with vs. without aura) or comorbidities such as fibromyalgia and medication overuse. Clinical markers of trigeminovascular activation were not associated with increased CGRP concentration. CGRP changed significantly over time, but it did not correlate with disease course. Based on our study results, CGRP might be neither a static biomarker in determining disease condition, nor dynamic biomarker which can reflect the disease severity. In addition, serum CGRP concentration may be prone to inter-subject fluctuations, without regard to treatment response.

Biomarker studies using CGRP has been challenged because of its short half-life in venous blood. In earlier studies using plasma samples, investigators made a supreme effort to reduce the time from sampling to freezing [8, 17]. However, Cernuda-Morollón et al. reported a promising result using serum samples which require a relatively long time to clot at room temperature [2]. We followed their methods and the same manufacturer's instruction with theirs. Our analysis of between-run precision showed acceptable variations to exclude batch effects. Role of CGRP as a biomarker of chronic migraine should be re-appraised after a critical review of detection methods.

Technical factors might have attributed to the discrepancy between our study results and the previous study results. In the study by Cernuda-Morollón et al. [2], CGRP concentrations were low in the NC and EM groups, while subjects with a high (> 100 pg/mL) CGRP level were present only in the CM group. In contrast, such a high CGRP concentration was detected in all NC, EM, and CM groups in our study. Technically, a batch effect should be considered if different batches were used for different groups. Different lots of ELISA kits, environments of experiments, or personnel who performed the experiment can affect the result. For example, when a researcher collects and analyzes blood samples of patients prior to the recruitment of matched control subjects, the between-group difference may be affected by the order of experiment because the two experiments can be different at least theoretically in terms of lot numbers of kits, time delay from the sampling and experiment, timing of experiments, or even temperature or humidity in the laboratory. In our study, we analyzed blood samples from two or more groups in each batch and repeated experiment using some samples of previous batch when we started a new batch.

Differences in demographics and characteristics should be also considered. Our CM patients have less fibromyalgia and more medication overuse than patients included in the study of Cernuda-Morollón et al., but these two comorbidities were not associated with serum CGRP levels in both studies [2]. According to Cernuda-Morollón et al. [2], migraine with aura was associated with higher serum CGRP concentration in women with CM. While nearly half of CM patients had aura in their study, the prevalence of migraine with aura was less than one fifth in our CM patients. This is not surprising because Asians have less prevalence of migraine with aura, although the prevalence of migraine is overall similar across countries [18–20]. This might explain the inconsistency in part between our and their study results. However, the association of migraine with aura and CGRP concentration was not reproduced in our study. Further validation studies are still warranted to further reproduce the association between migraine diagnosis, migraine subtype, and interictal CGRP concentrations before it can be implemented as a diagnostic procedure in clinics.

Taken together, our data raise questions regarding the validity of serum CGRP testing for the diagnosis of CM. In addition to clinical feasibility, fundamental questions also remain unanswered: whether the trigeminovascular system is persistently activated between attacks in CM, whether CGRP measured in peripheral blood can reflect the trigeminovascular activation, and what is the optimal method to detect and measure CGRP concentrations in human. In the future studies, it may be worthwhile to investigate if CM with a high level of interictal CGRP concentration is a clinically distinct subtype.

The strengths of our study are following. We conducted the CGRP measurement in our central laboratory which have been maintained under a strict quality control. Clinical information was completely blinded to the technician who performed the experiment. Also, several clinical features of migraine were tested. Our study also has limitations. Our NCs were not matched to patients in terms of age, sex, and comorbidities. However, we intended to determine the normal value in healthy young individuals. In addition, our study subjects were recruited from a single university hospital with a single ethnicity. Our study results might not be generalized to the whole migraine population until external validation is made.

Conclusion

Serum CGRP concentration may not be a feasible biomarker for CM. Technical, clinical, and pathophysiological factors should be addressed using more subjects in different laboratories before the interictal testing of CGRP can be used in the clinical practice.

Abbreviations

CGRP: Calcitonin gene-related peptide; CM: chronic migraine; EM: episodic migraine

Acknowledgements

We thank Ms. Miran Jung and Sujin Moon for their help in data management.

Funding

SK chemical and DongA ST supported the data management in part.

Authors' contributions

MJL conceived and designed the study, collected and analyzed data, and drafted the manuscript. SYL performed the ELISA experiment. SC drafted the manuscript. ESK designed and supervised the experiment and critically revised the manuscript. C-SC conceived of the study, collected the data, and critically revised the manuscript. All authors read and approved the final manuscript.

Competing interests

The authors declare that they have no competing interests.

Author details

[1]Department of Neurology, Samsung Medical Center, Sungkyunkwan University School of Medicine, 81 Irwon-Ro, Gangnam-Gu, Seoul 06351, South Korea. [2]Department of Laboratory Medicine and Genetics, Samsung Medical Center, Sungkyunkwan University School of Medicine, Seoul, South Korea. [3]Neuroscience Center, Samsung Medical Center, Seoul, South Korea.

References

1. Headache Classification Committee of the International Headache Society (IHS) (2018) The international classification of headache disorders, 3rd edition. Cephalalgia 38:1–211
2. Cernuda-Morollon E, Larrosa D, Ramon C, Vega J, Martinez-Camblor P, Pascual J (2013) Interictal increase of CGRP levels in peripheral blood as a biomarker for chronic migraine. Neurology 81:1191–1196
3. Sarchielli P, Pini LA, Zanchin G, Alberti A, Maggioni F, Rossi C et al (2006) Clinical-biochemical correlates of migraine attacks in rizatriptan responders and non-responders. Cephalalgia 26:257–265
4. Barbanti P, Aurilia C, Dall'Armi V, Egeo G, Fofi L, Bonassi S (2016) The phenotype of migraine with unilateral cranial autonomic symptoms documents increased peripheral and central trigeminal sensitization. A case series of 757 patients. Cephalalgia 36:1334–1340
5. Puntmann VO (2009) How-to guide on biomarkers: biomarker definitions, validation and applications with examples from cardiovascular disease. Postgrad Med J 85:538–545
6. Durham P, Papapetropoulos S (2013) Biomarkers associated with migraine and their potential role in migraine management. Headache 53:1262–1277
7. Nagata E, Hattori H, Kato M, Ogasawara S, Suzuki S, Shibata M et al (2009) Identification of biomarkers associated with migraine with aura. Neurosci Res 64:104–110
8. Goadsby PJ, Edvinsson L, Ekman R (1990) Vasoactive peptide release in the extracerebral circulation of humans during migraine headache. Ann Neurol 28:183–187
9. Edvinsson L, Warfvinge K (2017) Recognizing the role of CGRP and CGRP receptors in migraine and its treatment. Cephalalgia .https://doi.org/10.1177/0333102417736900.
10. Edvinsson L (2017) The Trigeminovascular pathway: role of CGRP and CGRP receptors in migraine. Headache 57(Suppl 2):47–55
11. Tajti J, Uddman R, Moller S, Sundler F, Edvinsson L (1999) Messenger molecules and receptor mRNA in the human trigeminal ganglion. J Auton Nerv Syst 76:176–183
12. Silberstein SD, Dodick DW, Bigal ME, Yeung PP, Goadsby PJ, Blankenbiller T et al (2017) Fremanezumab for the preventive treatment of chronic migraine. N Engl J Med 377:2113–2122
13. Tepper S, Ashina M, Reuter U, Brandes JL, Dolezil D, Silberstein S et al (2017) Safety and efficacy of erenumab for preventive treatment of chronic migraine: a randomised, double-blind, placebo-controlled phase 2 trial. Lancet Neurol 16:425–434
14. Ho TW, Connor KM, Zhang Y, Pearlman E, Koppenhaver J, Fan X et al (2014) Randomized controlled trial of the CGRP receptor antagonist telcagepant for migraine prevention. Neurology 83:958–966
15. Dominguez C, Vieites-Prado A, Perez-Mato M, Sobrino T, Rodriguez-Osorio X, Lopez A et al (2018) CGRP and PTX3 as predictors of efficacy of Onabotulinumtoxin type a in chronic migraine: an observational study. Headache 58:78–87
16. Cernuda-Morollon E, Martinez-Camblor P, Ramon C, Larrosa D, Serrano-Pertierra E, Pascual J (2014) CGRP and VIP levels as predictors of efficacy of Onabotulinumtoxin type a in chronic migraine. Headache 54:987–995

Poor sleep quality in migraine and probable migraine: a population study

Tae-Jin Song[1], Soo-Jin Cho[2], Won-Joo Kim[3], Kwang Ik Yang[4], Chang-Ho Yun[5] and Min Kyung Chu[6*]

Abstract

Background: Probable migraine (PM) is a subtype of migraine that is prevalent in the general population. Previous studies have shown that poor sleep quality is common among migraineurs and is associated with an exacerbation of migraine symptoms. However, information on the prevalence and clinical implication of poor sleep quality among individuals with PM is scarce. Thus, the aim of this study was to assess the prevalence and clinical impact of poor sleep quality in individuals with PM in comparison with those with migraine.

Methods: Two-stage cluster random sampling was used to perform the survey for sleep and headache in Korean general population. Participants with Pittsburgh Sleep Quality Index > 5 were considered as having poor sleep quality.

Results: Of 2695 participants, 379 (14.1%) had PM and 715 (26.5%) had poor sleep quality. Prevalence of poor sleep quality was 35.4% in the PM group, which was lower than that in the migraine group (47.6%, $p = 0.011$), but higher than that in the non-headache group (21.4%, $p < 0.001$). The PM participants with poor sleep quality showed increased headache frequency (median [interquartile range]: 2.0 [0.3–4.0] vs. 1.0 [0.2–2.0]; $p = 0.001$) and headache intensity (visual analogue scale, 6.0 [4.0–7.0] vs. 5.0 [3.5–6.0]; $p = 0.003$) compared to PM participants who had no poor sleep quality.

Conclusions: Poor sleep quality was prevalent among participants with PM. It was associated with an exacerbation of PM symptoms. Our findings suggest that proper evaluation and treatment for poor sleep quality are needed in the management of PM.

Keywords: Headache, Migraine, Pittsburgh sleep quality index, Sleep, Sleep quality

Background

Probable migraine (PM) is classified when one of diagnostic criteria of migraine in the third edition of the international classification of headache disorders (ICHD-3) is not applicable [1]. Probable migraine affects approximately 5–10% of the general population. It causes significant amount of disability owing to its symptoms such as migraine [2–4]. Although previous studies have demonstrated that patients with PM have relatively milder headache symptoms compared to individuals with migraine [3, 5], many patients with PM experience poor quality of life related to health with considerable disability [4].

Previous researches have revealed that sleep disturbances are frequent among migraineurs. Accompanying insomnia is more frequently noted in migraineurs than that in non-migraineurs [6]. Additionally, excessive daytime sleepiness is more prevalent among migraineurs. It is associated with worsening migraine symptoms [7]. Habitual snoring and bruxism are known to be risk factors of chronic migraine, a chronic form of migraine showing more severe symptoms and more frequent comorbidities compared to episodic migraine [8, 9]. Restless legs syndrome is also significantly associated with migraine [10].

Both sleep quantity and quality are important not only for health, but also for well-being [11]. Sleep studies have demonstrated that duration of sleep does not differ between non-migraineurs and migraineurs [12, 13]. Therefore, difference in sleep quality may explain the

* Correspondence: chumk@yonsei.ac.kr
[6]Department of Neurology, Yonsei University College of Medicine, 50-1 Yonsei-ro, Seodaemoon-gu, Seoul 03722, South Korea
Full list of author information is available at the end of the article

higher sleep disturbance in migraineurs. Several studies have shown that poor sleep quality in migraineurs is more frequently noted compared to that in non-migraine individuals with headache [14, 15]. Moreover, migraineurs who had poor sleep quality showed more frequent headache as well as symptoms of depression and anxiety [16].

Although PM is a common headache disorder, information about prevalence and clinical impact of poor sleep quality in individuals with PM is limited. We hypothesized that poor sleep quality would be prevalent in participants with PM and that it would be associated with an aggravation of clinical presentation of PM, as in the case with migraine. The Korean Headache-Sleep Study (KHSS) is a nationwide, general population-based survey about headache and sleep. The KHSS may give us a chance to investigate the relationship of PM with poor sleep quality. Thus, the aim of this study was to evaluate the prevalence and impact of poor sleep quality among participants with PM and those with migraine using data of the KHSS. Factors associated with poor sleep quality in participants with PM were also assessed.

Methods

Survey

KHSS is a nation-wide and cross-sectional study regarding headache and sleep characteristics among adult (19–69 years old) across Korean general population. Detailed protocol and methods of KHSS were described elsewhere [17]. Briefly, KHSS used two-stage random sampling methods. The study population of KHSS was based on the distribution of Korean population except Jeju-island [17]. To prevent interest bias, we informed all participants that our survey theme was a social health issue than neurological disorders such as headache and sleep problems. The survey was conducted by door-to-door visits and face-to-face interviews, using a structured questionnaire. The questionnaire covered information regarding characteristics of headache, sleep, anxiety, and depression. All interviewers were not medical related workers. They were members of Gallup Korea. The KHSS was approved by the Institutional Review Board of Hallym University Sacred Heart Hospital (approval No. 2011-I077). We received written consent from all participants before the survey interview. The survey was performed from November 2011 to January 2012.

Diagnosis of migraine and PM

Migraine and PM were diagnosed based on ICHD-2 diagnostic criteria which was valid at that time [18]. Migraine was defined based on code 1.1 migraine without aura of ICHD-2 [18]. If a participant satisfied A, B, C, and D criteria of 1.1 migraine without aura, she/he was classified as having migraine. If one of criteria for migraine was not satisfied, the participant was classified as having PM. It is difficult to define code 1.2.1 migraine with aura or code 1.6.2 PM with aura in epidemiological study using questionnaire survey methods [19]. Therefore, our study did not estimate the presence of aura. Our study's migraine included both code 1.1 migraine without aura and code 1.2 migraine with aura [18] while PM included both code 1.6.1 PM without aura and code 1.6.2 PM with aura [18]. Our study questionnaire exhibited a sensitivity of 75.0% and a specificity of 88.2% in migraine diagnosis compared to doctor's diagnosis via telephone interview and result in the survey [20]. Frequency of headache per month, visual analogue scale (VAS) for headache intensity, and Headache Impact Test-6 (HIT-6) for impact of headache was investigated. Non-headache participants were defined as those who reported no headache during the previous year.

Poor sleep quality, anxiety, and depression

Pittsburgh Sleep Quality Index (PSQI) was applied to assess sleep quality. Participants with total PSQI score > 5 were defined as having poor sleep quality [21]. We also investigated each component score of PSQI such as subjective quality of sleep, latency of sleep, duration of sleep, habitual sleep insufficiency, disturbance of sleep, use of hypnotics, and dysfunction at daytime [21]. Goldberg Anxiety Scale was used for the diagnosis of anxiety. The Goldberg Anxiety Scale includes four screening items and five supplementary items [22, 23]. Participants who presented positive answers with more than two of screening items or with more than five of all scale items were classified as persons with anxiety. The Korean version of Goldberg Anxiety Scale was validated in previous studies, with a sensitivity of 82.0% and a specificity of 94.4% [23, 24]. Patient Health Questionnaire-9 (PHQ-9) was applied to investigate the presence of depression [25]. In this scoring system, presence of depression was defined as 10 points or more. The Korean version of PHQ-9 was also validated with a sensitivity of 81.1% and a specificity of 89.9% [26].

Statistical analyses

All statistical analyses were performed using SPSS 22.0 (IBM, Armonk, NY, USA). Kolmogorov-Smirnov test was used to check normal distribution for continuous variables. If variables showed normal distribution, independent t-test or one-way analysis of variance was used. If variables did not show normal distribution, Mann-Whitney U-test or Kruskal-Wallis test was performed. Categorical variables were analysed using Chi-square test or Fisher's exact test. We used Mann–Whitney *U*-test to compare headache frequency per month, VAS score for headache intensity, and HIT-6 score between participants had PM with and without poor sleep quality.

For assessing factors contributing to poor sleep quality among participants with PM, we performed multivariable linear regression analyses after adjusting sociodemographic variables (age, sex, residential area size, and level of education), GAS score for anxiety, PHQ-9 score for depression, frequency of headache (per month), and intensity of headache (VAS score). Statistical significance was considered when p value (two-tailed) was less than 0.05.

Results

Survey

We interviewed 7430 people and 3114 people who agreed to participate in our study (58.1% of rejection rate). Of these, 419 people withdraw participation during the interview. Finally, 2695 people completed our survey (36.3% of cooperation rate, Fig. 1). Distribution of sex, age, residence size, or education level of our sample was not significantly different from that in the general population in Korea (Table 1).

Prevalence of migraine and PM

Of 2695 subjects included in our study, 1273 (47.2%) had at least one headache over the past year, including 143 (5.3%) migraineurs and 379 (14.1%) who had PM. Seven hundred and fifteen (26.5%) participants had poor sleep quality (Table 1). The prevalence of PM was the highest (16.8%) in 30–39 and 40–49 age groups. Of 379 PM participants, 339 (89.5%), 29 (7.7%), and 11 (2.8%) missed criterion B (typical duration of headache), criterion C (typical headache characteristics), and criterion D (typical accompanying symptoms) of code 1.1 migraine diagnostic criteria, respectively.

Prevalence of poor sleep quality and comparison of PSQI score according to headache diagnosis

The prevalence of poor sleep quality was significantly higher in participants with PM (35.4%) than that in participants with non-headache (21.0%, $p < 0.001$), but lower than that in participants with migraine (47.6%, $p = 0.011$). Regarding PSQI, component scores for latency of sleep (mean ± standard deviation) (1.1 ± 1.0 vs. 0.8 ± 0.9, $p = 0.001$), sleep duration (0.6 ± 0.8 vs. 0.4 ± 0.8, $p = 0.001$), sleep disturbance (0.9 ± 0.6 vs. 0.8 ± 0.5, $p = 0.001$), use of sleeping medication (0.1 ± 0.4 vs. 0.0 ± 0.2, $p = 0.001$), daytime dysfunction (0.8 ± 0.7 vs. 0.5 ± 0.6, $p = 0.001$), and total score (5.2 ± 2.4 vs. 4.2 ± 1.9, $p = 0.001$) were higher in PM participants than those in non-headache participants. However, PSQI component scores for subjective sleep quality (1.7 ± 0.7 vs. 1.7 ± 0.8, $p = 0.879$) and habitual sleep efficacy (0.0 ± 0.3 vs. 0.0 ± 1.5, $p = 0.119$) did not significantly differ between PM and non-headache participants. When comparing PM participants with migraineurs, PSQI component scores for sleep latency and sleep disturbance as well as total PSQI score were higher in participants with migraine than those in participants with PM (Table 2).

Clinical presentations of PM according to presence of poor sleep quality

Participants with PM combined with poor sleep quality had higher proportion of anxiety ($p < 0.001$), depression ($p < 0.001$), and frequency of headache attack (median [interquartile range]: 2.0 [0.3–4.0] vs. 1.0 [0.2–2.0], $p =$

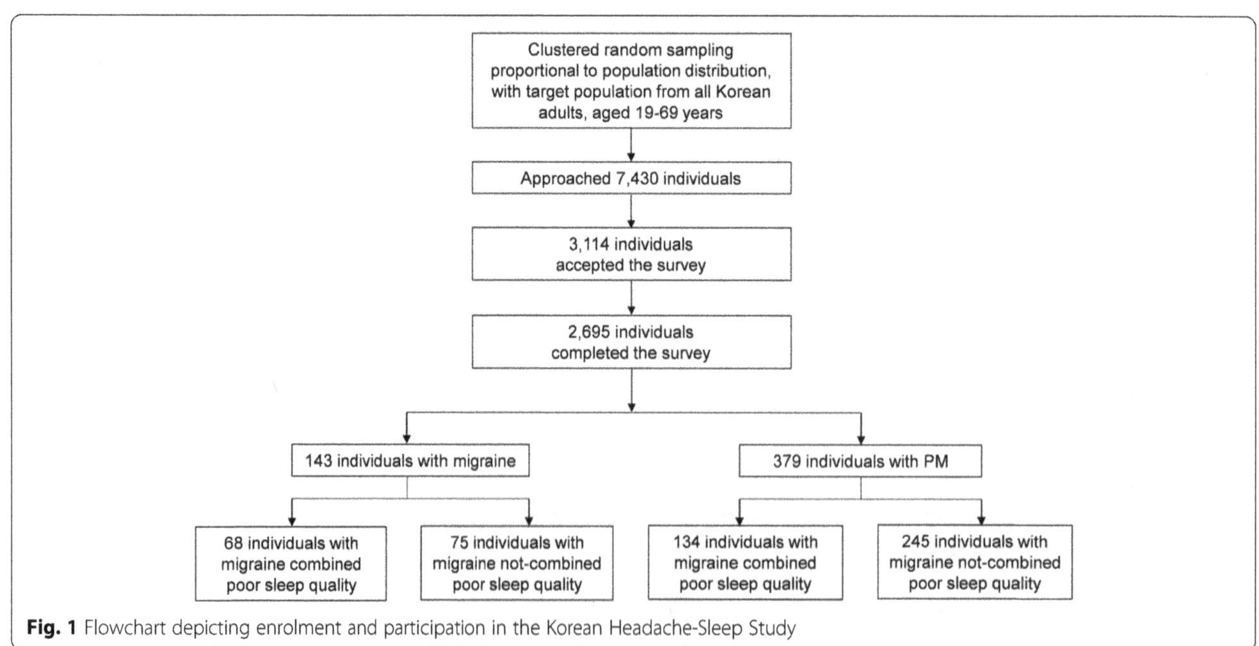

Fig. 1 Flowchart depicting enrolment and participation in the Korean Headache-Sleep Study

Table 1 Sociodemographic characteristics of survey participants, the total Korean population, and cases identified as having migraine, probable migraine, and poor sleep quality

Characteristic	Survey participants *N* (%)	Total population *N* (%)	*p*	Migraine *N*, % (95% CI)	Probable migraine *N*, % (95% CI)	Poor sleep quality *N*, % (95% CI) (PSQI > 5)
Sex						
Male	1345 (49.3)	17,584,365 (50.6)	0.854[a]	36, 2.7 (1.8–3.5)	136, 10.1 (8.5–11.8)	334, 24.8 (22.5–27.1)
Female	1350 (50.7)	17,198,350 (49.4)		107, 7.9 (6.5–9.4)	243, 17.9 (15.8–19.9)	381, 28.2 (25.8–30.6
Age, years						
19–29	542 (20.5)	7,717,947 (22.2)	0.917[a]	25, 4.5 (2.7–6.2)	69, 12.6 (9.8–15.4)	153, 28.3 (24.4–32.0)
30–39	604 (21.9)	8,349,487 (24.0)		42, 7.0 (4.9–9.1)	102, 16.8 (13.7–19.8)	136, 22.5 (19.2–25.9)
40–49	611 (23.1)	8,613,110 (24.8)		39, 6.5 (4.5–8.4)	102, 16.8 (13.9–19.8)	167, 27.3 (23.8–30.1)
50–59	529 (18.9)	6,167,505 (17.7)		22, 4.1 (2.4–5.9)	62, 11.6 (8.8–14.4)	160, 30.2 (26.3–34.2)
60–69	409 (15.6)	3,934,666 (11.3)		15, 3.9 (2.0–5.7)	44, 11.2 (8.1–14.2)	99, 24.2 (20.0–28.4)
Size of the residential area						
Large city	1248 (46.3)	16,776,771 (48.2)	0.921[a]	76, 6.1 (4.8–7.5)	180, 14.4 (12.4–16.3)	338, 27.1 (24.6–30.0)
Medium-to-small city	1186 (44.0)	15,164,345 (43.6)		48, 4.0 (2.9–5.2)	174, 14.7 (12.7–16.7)	303, 25.5 (23.1–28.0)
Rural area	261 (9.7)	2,841,599 (8.2)		19, 7.4 (4.2–10.6)	25, 9.7 (6.1–13.3)	74, 28.4 (22.8–33.9)
Education level						
Middle school or less	393 (14.9)	6,608,716 (19.0)	0.752[a]	22, 5.5 (4.2–7.7)	44, 11.5 (8.4–14.7)	110, 28.0 (23.5–32.4)
High school	1208 (44.5)	15,234,829 (43.8)		60, 5.0 (3.8–6.3)	178, 14.7 (12.7–16.7)	317, 26.2 (24.0–28.7)
College or more	1068 (39.6)	12,939,170 (37.2)		60, 5.6 (4.3–7.0)	155, 14.4 (12.3–16.5)	281, 26.3 (23.7–29.0)
Did not respond	26 (9.6)			1, 3.8 (0.0–11.8)	2, 7.7 (0.0–18.7)	7, 26.9 (8.7–45.2)
Total	2695 (100.0)	34,782,715 (100.0)		143, 5.3 (4.5–6.2)	379, 14.1 (12.7–15.4)	715, 26.5 (24.8–28.2)

N number, *CI* confidence interval, *PSQI* Pittsburgh Sleep Quality Index
[a]Compared with corresponding value reported in the general population of Korea

0.001) as well as higher headache intensity (VAS score, 6.0 [4.0–7.0] vs. 5.0 [3.5–6.0], $p = 0.003$) and higher HIT-6 score (50.0 [44.0–58.0] vs. 44.0 [40.0–50.0], $p = 0.001$) compared to participants with PM not combined with poor sleep quality (Table 3). Participants with migraine who combined with poor sleep quality had higher proportion of anxiety, depression, frequency of headache attack and higher HIT-6 score compared to participants with migraine who not combined with poor sleep quality (Table 3).

Table 2 Total and subcomponent PSQI scores among participants with no headache, probable migraine, and migraine

Component	Non-headache $N = 1422$	Probable migraine $N = 379$	Migraine $N = 143$	*p* value
Subjective sleep quality	1.7 ± 0.8	1.7 ± 0.7	1.7 ± 0.7	0.609
Sleep latency	0.8 ± 0.9	1.0 ± 1.0*	1.3 ± 1.1†‡	< 0.001
Sleep duration	0.4 ± 0.8	0.6 ± 0.8*	0.5 ± 0.8†‡	0.001
Habitual sleep efficacy	0.0 ± 1.5	0.0 ± 0.3	0.0 ± 0.0	0.116
Sleep disturbance	0.8 ± 0.6	0.9 ± 0.6*	1.1 ± 0.6†‡	< 0.001
Use of sleeping medication	0.0 ± 0.3	0.1 ± 0.4*	0.1 ± 0.5†	0.001
Daytime functioning	0.5 ± 0.7	0.8 ± 0.7*	0.9 ± 0.9†‡	< 0.001
Total	4.2 ± 1.9	5.2 ± 2.4*	5.6 ± 2.6†‡	< 0.001

PSQI Pittsburgh Sleep Quality Index
Data are presented as mean ± standard deviation
Each PSQI component score has a range of 0–3 points. Higher PSQI score indicates more severe disability
*$p < 0.05$ for non-headache vs. probable migraine, by Tukey's post-hoc analysis
†$p < 0.05$ for non-headache vs. migraine, by Tukey's post-hoc analysis
‡$p < 0.05$ for probable migraine vs. migraine, by Tukey's post-hoc analysis

Table 3 Demographics and clinical presentations of participants with migraine and probable migraine stratified according to the presence of poor sleep quality

Characteristic	Migraine with poor sleep quality *N* = 68 (47.5%)	Migraine without poor sleep quality *N* = 75 (52.5%)	*p* value	PM with poor sleep quality *N* = 134 (35.3%)	PM without poor sleep quality *N* = 245 (64.7%)	*p* value
Demographics						
Age, years	41.9 ± 13.0	40.6 ± 11.9	0.546	40.8 ± 13.0	42.5 ± 12.4	0.217
Female	51 (75.0)	56 (74.7)	0.963	86 (64.2)	157 (64.1)	0.985
Headache characteristics						
Bilateral pain	36 (52.9)	45 (60.0)	0.395	73 (54.5)	148 (60.4)	0.263
Non-pulsating quality	46 (67.6)	62 (82.7)	0.037	110 (82.1)	200 (81.6)	0.912
Mild-to-moderate severity	58 (85.3)	57 (76.0)	0.162	12 (9.0)	8 (3.3)	0.018
Not aggravated by movement	48 (70.6)	52 (69.3)	0.870	85 (63.4)	151 (61.6)	0.730
Accompanying symptoms						
Nausea	59 (86.8)	66 (88.0)	0.824	117 (87.3)	20.7 (84.5)	0.456
Vomiting	27 (39.7)	28 (37.3)	0.771	47 (35.1)	68 (27.8)	0.138
Photophobia	41 (60.3)	43 (57.3)	0.719	70 (52.2)	110 (44.9)	0.171
Phonophobia	50 (73.5)	51 (68.0)	0.468	101 (75.4)	167 (68.2)	0.140
Osmophobia	35 (51.5)	33 (44.0)	0.372	71 (53.0)	108 (44.1)	0.097
Accompanying psychiatric problems						
Anxiety (GAS score ≥ 5)	33 (48.5)	10 (13.3)	< 0.001	43 (32.1)	24 (9.8)	< 0.001
Depression (PHQ-9 score ≥ 10)	19 (27.9)	5 (6.7)	0.001	28 (20.9)	5 (2.0)	< 0.001
Headache frequency	2.0 (1.0–7.0)	1.0 (1.0–5.0)	0.009	2.0 (0.3–4.0)	1.00 (0.3–2.0)	0.001
VAS score for headache intensity	7.0 (4.0–10.0)	6.0 (4.0–8.0)	0.247	6.0 (4.0–7.0)	5.00 (3.5–6.0)	0.003
HIT-6 score	57.5 (50.0–65.0)	50.0 (43.0–57.0)	< 0.001	50.0 (44.0–58.0)	44.0 (40.0–50.0)	< 0.001

Data are presented as mean ± standard deviation, number (percent), or median (interquartile range)
PM probable migraine, *GAS* Goldberg Anxiety Scale, *PHQ* Patient Health Questionnaire, *VAS* visual analogue scale, *HIT* Headache Impact Test

Table 4 Analysis[a] of contributing factors related to the total PSQI score in participants with probable migraine

Factor	Unstandardized coefficients		Standardized coefficients	T	*p* value	Tolerance	VIF
	B	SE	β				
Age	−0.086	0.085	−0.046	−1.019	0.309	0.810	1.235
Sex	−0.177	0.202	−0.036	−0.877	0.381	0.969	1.032
Size of residential area	−0.086	0.157	−0.022	− 0.548	0.584	0.988	1.012
Educational level	−0.082	0.131	−0.028	−0.629	0.529	0.792	1.262
Anxiety (GAS score ≥ 5)	0.231	0.052	0.230	4.438	< 0.001	0.602	1.660
Depression (PHQ-9 score ≥ 10)	0.230	0.027	0.426	8.471	< 0.001	0.640	1.563
Headache frequency per month	0.039	0.018	0.090	2.166	0.031	0.928	1.077
VAS score for headache intensity	0.088	0.056	0.065	1.556	0.121	0.923	1.083

PSQI Pittsburgh Sleep Quality Index, *SE* standard error, *VIF* variation inflation factor, *GAS* Goldberg Anxiety Scale, *PHQ* Patient Health Questionnaire, *VAS* visual analogue scale
Independent variables included sociodemographic variables (age, sex, size of residential areas, and education level), anxiety (GAS score ≥ 5), depression (PHQ-9 score ≥ 10), headache frequency per month, and VAS score for headache intensity, whereas total PSQI score was included as the dependent variable
[a]multivariate linear regression: $R^2 = 0.194$, adjusted $R^2 = 0.139$

Factors associated with PSQI score among PM participants

In multivariable linear regression analysis, anxiety ($\beta = 0.230$, $p < 0.001$), depression ($\beta = 0.426$, $p < 0.001$), and headache frequency per month ($\beta = 0.090$, $p = 0.031$) were significant independent factors associated with total PSQI score in participants with PM (Table 4).

Discussion

The main findings of our research were as follows. First, prevalence of migraine, PM, and poor sleep quality in Korean general population were 5.3%, 14.1%, and 26.5%, respectively. Second, 35.3% of participants with PM had poor sleep quality, which was lower than the prevalence noted in participants with migraine, but higher than that in participants with non-headache. Third, among PM participants, those with poor sleep quality showed increased headache frequency, intensity, and impact.

Among migraineurs, poor sleep quality is not an uncommon problem. A clinic-based study in India has reported that 66.7% of migraineurs without aura show poor sleep quality. This proportion is higher than that in non-migraine participants [14]. A Chinese study investigating 1023 nurses has demonstrated that, compared to tension-type headache or non-headache participants, migraineurs have reported significantly higher frequency of poor sleep quality [27]. In our study, the first to assess the prevalence of poor sleep quality among individuals with PM in a population-based setting, approximately half of migraineurs and one-third of individuals with PM experienced poor sleep quality. This confirms that poor sleep quality is a common comorbidity not only in migraineurs, but also in individuals with PM.

Among PSQI components, latency of sleep, duration of sleep, sleep disturbance, hypnotics use, and daytime dysfunction scores were significantly higher in participants with PM than those in non-headache participants. This suggests that various aspects of sleep quality are impaired in individuals with PM. One interesting finding is the impairment of daytime functioning among participants with PM. Indeed, individuals with migraine or PM often report disability even during interictal period [28]. Migraineurs are less physically active with reduced vigour. They show higher levels of sleepiness and more anxiety and avoidance [28]. Our findings are in line with results of previous observation [28], additionally indicating that daytime dysfunction in PM patients might be associated with poor sleep quality.

Our study demonstrated that anxiety, depression, and headache frequency were associated with poor sleep quality. This is in agreement with previous observations showing that anxiety and depression are independently related factors for PSQI score [29, 30] and that headache frequency is positively associated with PSQI score among migraineurs [31]. Our results confirmed that anxiety, depression, and headache frequency were significant factors for PSQI score among individuals with PM.

Insomnia is a prevalent sleep disorder. Individuals with insomnia may have difficulty falling asleep, staying asleep or early awakening even if enough time is given [32]. Poor sleep quality can occur as a result of insomnia [33]. Nevertheless, it can be caused by other conditions such as sleep apnea, shift working, use of medications, environmental factors et al. [34–37]. Therefore, the poor sleep quality is related to insomnia but measures border sleep difficulties. We already investigated the association of poor sleep quality and migraine in a population-based sample [38]. Here, we firstly report the relationship of poor sleep quality and PM, another common and disabling headache disorder.

Based on findings of the present study, we propose the following strategies to improve sleep quality in participants with PM. Since anxiety, depression, and headache frequency are independent factors associated with poor sleep quality in individuals with PM, they could be successfully managed by pharmacological and non-pharmacological treatments. Anxiolytic drugs and antidepressants are effective in reducing anxiety and depression symptoms [39]. Non-pharmacological cognitive behaviour therapy (CBT) can be used to treat anxiety and depression [40]. Headache frequency can be reduced by preventive pharmacological treatment and non-pharmacological treatments such as relaxation techniques, CBT, education, and mindfulness [41]. Therefore, pharmacological and non-pharmacological treatments of anxiety, depression, and headache frequency might be able to improve sleep quality of individuals with PM. Such strategies may improve symptoms of PM by improving sleep quality.

In the present study, PM participants with poor sleep quality had more headache frequency and more severe headaches than PM participants without poor sleep quality. Considering that headache frequency and intensity are closely associated with headache-related disability and health-related quality of life, poor sleep quality may be an important factor for such aspects in individuals with PM [42]. Sleep quality may be improved using pharmacological and non-pharmacological treatments [43]. Our present findings suggest that, among individuals with PM, proper assessment and treatment of poor sleep quality may be needed to reduce headache-related disability and improve quality of life besides improving headache symptoms.

Our research has some limitations. First, although questionnaire was utilized to the diagnosis of PM and migraine, this questionnaire was only validated in migraine, but not validated in PM. According to ICHD-2, the diagnosis of PM is diagnosed only when one of the criteria of migraine is not satisfied. Thus, validation for PM itself is not necessarily required. Second, we evaluated sleep quality using a questionnaire without performing actigraphy or polysomnography to confirm the sleep quality objectively. Nevertheless, we found it not only practical, but also appropriate to use PSQI because this tool was validated for assessing sleep quality, showing good agreement with polysomnography and actigraphy measurements [44]. Therefore, it has been widely adopted in clinical and epidemiological studies. Third, although our study was population-based with low sampling error, its statistical power was limited because our study could not preform subgroup analysis due to limited sample size. Lastly, we did not included medications for migraine and PM treatment in analyses. Although a significant proportion of migraineurs did not receive medical treatment, some medications for acute and preventive treatments may influence on sleep quality. Caffeine, a common ingredient of acute migraine treatment, may impair sleep quality [45]. Topiramate is a widely used medication for preventive migraine treatment and may induce dysphoria or unmask latent mood disorder [46]. Further studies are needed the effect of migraine medications on sleep quality among individuals of migraine and PM.

On the other hand, the present study has several strengths. First, our study used a questionnaire whose Korean version was specifically validated for assessing migraine, anxiety, depression, and sleep quality. Second, we applied clustered random sampling proportional to the distribution in the Korean general population with low sampling error which allowed us to accurately assess the prevalence of migraine, PM, and poor sleep quality. Third, we investigated PSQI component scores in addition to total scores. PSQI comprises seven components including subjective sleep quality, latency of sleep, duration of sleep, habitual sleep efficacy, sleep disturbance, use of hypnotics, and dysfunction at daytime. By investigating these various aspects of sleep quality separately, we were able to determine that some components were impaired in participants with PM.

Conclusion

Although the prevalence of poor sleep quality was lower in participants with PM than that in migraineurs, prevalence remained high in those with PM. It was associated with worse symptoms of PM. Our results suggest that appropriate diagnostic approach and management of poor sleep quality are necessary to manage PM appropriately.

Abbreviations

HIT-6: Headache impact test-6; ICHD: International classification of headache disorders; KHSS: Korean headache-sleep study; PHQ-9: Patient health questionnaire-9; PM: Probable migraine; PSQI: Pittsburgh sleep quality index; VAS: Visual analogue scale

Acknowledgements

The authors would like to thank Gallup Korea for providing technical support for the Korean Headache-Sleep Study.

Funding

This Study was supported by a 2011-Grant from Korean Academy of Medical Sciences. This research was also supported by a grant (2018R1D1A1B07040959) of the Basic Science Research Program through the National Research Foundation (NRF) funded by the Ministry of Education, Republic of Korea.

Authors' contributions

T-JS, S-JC, W-JK, KIY, C-HY, and MKC contributed to the design of the analysis and interpretation of the data. T-JS and MKC drafted the paper with contributions from all authors. All authors approved the final version of the manuscript.

Competing interests

Tae-Jin Song has no potential conflicts of interest.
Soo-Jin Cho was a site investigator of multicenter trial sponsored by Otsuka Korea, Eli Lilly and Company, Korea BMS, and Parexel Korea Co., Ltd.. Soo-Jin Cho also worked as an advisory member for Teva. Soo-Jin Cho received research support from Hallym University Research Fund 2016 and Academic award of Myung In Pharm. Co. Ltd. Soo-Jin Cho also received lecture honoraria from Yuyu Pharmaceutical Company and Allergan Korea.
Won-Joo Kim has no potential conflicts of interest.
Kwang Ik Yang has no potential conflicts of interest.
Chang-Ho Yun has no potential conflicts of interest.
Min Kyung Chu was a site investigator for a multi-center trial sponsored by Eli Lilly and company; worked an advisory member for Teva, and received lecture honoraria from Allergan Korea and Yuyu Pharmaceutical Company in the past 24 months. The authors declare that they have no competing interest.

Author details

[1]Department of Neurology, College of Medicine, Ewha Womans University, Seoul, South Korea. [2]Department of Neurology, Dongtan Sacred Heart Hospital, Hallym University College of Medicine, Hwaseong, South Korea. [3]Department of Neurology, Gangnam Severance Hospital, Yonsei University, College of Medicine, Seoul, South Korea. [4]Department of Neurology, Soonchunhyang University College of Medicine, Cheonan Hospital, Cheonan, South Korea. [5]Department of Neurology, Clinical Neuroscience Center, Seoul National University Bundang Hospital, Seongnam, South Korea. [6]Department of Neurology, Yonsei University College of Medicine, 50-1 Yonsei-ro, Seodaemoon-gu, Seoul 03722, South Korea.

References

1. Headache Classification Committee of the International Headache Society (IHS) The International Classification of Headache Disorders, 3rd edition (2018). Cephalalgia 38 (1):1–211. http://journals.sagepub.com/toc/cepa/38/1
2. Bigal M, Kolodner K, Lafata J, Leotta C, Lipton R (2006) Patterns of medical diagnosis and treatment of migraine and probable migraine in a health plan. Cephalalgia 26(1):43–49
3. Lantéri-Minet M, Valade D, Geraud G, Chautard M, Lucas C (2005) Migraine and probable migraine–results of FRAMIG 3, a French nationwide survey carried out according to the 2004 IHS classification. Cephalalgia 25(12):1146–1158
4. Patel N, Bigal M, Kolodner K, Leotta C, Lafata JE, Lipton R (2004) Prevalence and impact of migraine and probable migraine in a health plan. Neurology 63(8):1432–1438

5. Kim BK, Chung YK, Kim JM, Lee KS, Chu MK (2013) Prevalence, clinical characteristics and disability of migraine and probable migraine: a nationwide population-based survey in Korea. Cephalalgia 33(13):1106–1116
6. Uhlig BL, Engstrom M, Odegard SS, Hagen KK, Sand T (2014) Headache and insomnia in population-based epidemiological studies. Cephalalgia 34(10):745–751
7. Kim J, Cho SJ, Kim WJ, Yang KI, Yun CH, Chu MK (2016) Excessive daytime sleepiness is associated with an exacerbation of migraine: a population-based study. J Headache Pain 17(1):62
8. Scher AI, Lipton RB, Stewart WF (2003) Habitual snoring as a risk factor for chronic daily headache. Neurology 60(8):1366–1368
9. Fernandes G, Franco AL, Goncalves DA, Speciali JG, Bigal ME, Camparis CM (2013) Temporomandibular disorders, sleep bruxism, and primary headaches are mutually associated. J Orofac Pain 27(1):14–20
10. Schurks M, Winter A, Berger K, Kurth T (2014) Migraine and restless legs syndrome: a systematic review. Cephalalgia 34(10):777–794
11. Pilcher JJ, Ginter DR, Sadowsky B (1997) Sleep quality versus sleep quantity: relationships between sleep and measures of health, well-being and sleepiness in college students. J Psychosom Res 42(6):583–596
12. Bruni O, Russo PM, Violani C, Guidetti V (2004) Sleep and migraine: an actigraphic study. Cephalalgia 24(2):134–139
13. Nayak C, Sinha S, Nagappa M, Nagaraj K, Kulkarni GB, Thennarasu K, Taly AB (2016) Study of sleep microstructure in patients of migraine without aura. Sleep Breath 20(1):263–269
14. Karthik N, Kulkarni GB, Taly AB, Rao S, Sinha S (2012) Sleep disturbances in 'migraine without aura'–a questionnaire based study. J Neurol Sci 321(1–2):73–76
15. Seidel S, Hartl T, Weber M, Matterey S, Paul A, Riederer F, Gharabaghi M, Wober-Bingol C, Wober C, Group PS (2009) Quality of sleep, fatigue and daytime sleepiness in migraine - a controlled study. Cephalalgia 29(6):662–669
16. Zhu Z, Fan X, Li X, Tan G, Chen L, Zhou J (2013) Prevalence and predictive factors for poor sleep quality among migraineurs in a tertiary hospital headache clinic. Acta Neurol Belg 113(3):229–235
17. Oh K, Cho SJ, Chung YK, Kim JM, Chu MK (2014) Combination of anxiety and depression is associated with an increased headache frequency in migraineurs: a population-based study. BMC Neurol 14:238
18. Headache Classification Subcommittee of the International Headache Society (2004) The International Classification of Headache Disorders: 2nd edition. Cephalalgia 24(1):9–160
19. Stang PE, Osterhaus JT (1993) Impact of migraine in the United States: data from the National Health Interview Survey. Headache 33(1):29–35
20. Kim BK, Chu MK, Lee TG, Kim JM, Chung CS, Lee KS (2012) Prevalence and impact of migraine and tension-type headache in Korea. J Clin Neurol 8(3): 204–211
21. Buysse DJ, Reynolds CF 3rd, Monk TH, Berman SR, Kupfer DJ (1989) The Pittsburgh sleep quality index: a new instrument for psychiatric practice and research. Psychiatry Res 28(2):193–213
22. Goldberg D, Bridges K, Duncan-Jones P, Grayson D (1988) Detecting anxiety and depression in general medical settings. BMJ 297(6653):897–899
23. Lim JY, Lee SH, Cha YS, Park HS, Sunwoo S (2001) Reliability and validity of anxiety screening scale. J Korean Acad Fam Med 22(8):1224–1232
24. Kim JS, Kim SY, Lee GY, Park TJ, Lee YH, Kong BK (1997) The standardization of Korean-translated Goldberg's shart screening scale for anxiety and depression. Korean J Fam Med 18:1452–1460
25. Pignone MP, Gaynes BN, Rushton JL, Burchell CM, Orleans CT, Mulrow CD, Lohr KN (2002) Screening for depression in adults: a summary of the evidence for the US preventive services task force. Ann Intern Med 136(10):765–776
26. Choi HS, Choi JH, Park KH, Joo KJ, Ga H, Ko HJ, Kim SR (2007) Standardization of the Korean version of patient health Questionnaire-9 as a screening instrument for major depressive disorder. J Korean Acad Fam Med 28(2):114–119
27. Wang Y, Xie J, Yang F, Wu S, Wang H, Zhang X, Liu H, Deng X, Xie W, Yu S (2015) Comorbidity of poor sleep and primary headaches among nursing staff in North China. J Headache Pain 16:88
28. Lampl C, Thomas H, Stovner LJ, Tassorelli C, Katsarava Z, Lainez JM, Lanteri-Minet M, Rastenyte D, Ruiz de la Torre E, Andree C, Steiner TJ (2016) Interictal burden attributable to episodic headache: findings from the Eurolight project. J Headache Pain 17:9
29. Feng Q, Zhang QL, Du Y, Ye YL, He QQ (2014) Associations of physical activity, screen time with depression, anxiety and sleep quality among Chinese college freshmen. PLoS One 9(6):e100914
30. Shim J, Kang SW (2017) Behavioral factors related to sleep quality and duration in adults. J Lifestyle Med 7(1):18–26
31. Lin YK, Lin GY, Lee JT, Lee MS, Tsai CK, Hsu YW, Lin YZ, Tsai YC, Yang FC (2016) Associations between sleep quality and migraine frequency: a cross-sectional case-control study. Medicine (Baltimore) 95(17):e3554
32. Roth T (2007) Insomnia: definition, prevalence, etiology, and consequences. J Clin Sleep Med 3(5 Suppl):S7–S10
33. Morin CM, Belleville G, Belanger L, Ivers H (2011) The insomnia severity index: psychometric indicators to detect insomnia cases and evaluate treatment response. Sleep 34(5):601–608
34. Macey PM, Woo MA, Kumar R, Cross RL, Harper RM (2010) Relationship between obstructive sleep apnea severity and sleep, depression and anxiety symptoms in newly-diagnosed patients. PLoS One 5(4):e10211
35. Agargun MY, Tekeoglu I, Gunes A, Adak B, Kara H, Ercan M (1999) Sleep quality and pain threshold in patients with fibromyalgia. Compr Psychiatry 40(3):226–228
36. Elliott JL, Lal S (2016) Blood pressure, sleep quality and fatigue in shift working police officers: effects of a twelve hour roster system on cardiovascular and sleep health. Int J Environ Res Public Health 13(2):172
37. Genderson MR, Rana BK, Panizzon MS, Grant MD, Toomey R, Jacobson KC, Xian H, Cronin-Golomb A, Franz CE, Kremen WS, Lyons MJ (2013) Genetic and environmental influences on sleep quality in middle-aged men: a twin study. J Sleep Res 22(5):519–526
38. Song TJ, Yun CH, Cho SJ, Kim WJ, Yang KI, Chu MK (2018) Short sleep duration and poor sleep quality among migraineurs: a population-based study. Cephalalgia 38(5):855–864
39. Farach FJ, Pruitt LD, Jun JJ, Jerud AB, Zoellner LA, Roy-Byrne PP (2012) Pharmacological treatment of anxiety disorders: current treatments and future directions. J Anxiety Disord 26(8):833–843
40. Hofmann SG, Asnaani A, Vonk IJ, Sawyer AT, Fang A (2012) The efficacy of cognitive behavioral therapy: a review of meta-analyses. Cognit Ther Res 36(5):427–440
41. Probyn K, Bowers H, Mistry D, Caldwell F, Underwood M, Patel S, Sandhu HK, Matharu M, Pincus T (2017) Non-pharmacological self-management for people living with migraine or tension-type headache: a systematic review including analysis of intervention components. BMJ Open 7(8):e016670
42. Bagley CL, Rendas-Baum R, Maglinte GA, Yang M, Varon SF, Lee J, Kosinski M (2012) Validating migraine-specific quality of life questionnaire v2.1 in episodic and chronic migraine. Headache 52(3):409–421
43. Khawaja IS, Dieperink ME, Thuras P, Kunisaki KM, Schumacher MM, Germain A, Amborn B, Hurwitz TD (2013) Effect of sleep skills education on sleep quality in patients attending a psychiatry partial hospitalization program. Prim Care Companion CNS Disord 15(1)
44. Landry GJ, Best JR, Liu-Ambrose T (2015) Measuring sleep quality in older adults: a comparison using subjective and objective methods. Front Aging Neurosci 7:166
45. Lohsoonthorn V, Khidir H, Casillas G, Lertmaharit S, Tadesse MG, Pensuksan WC, Rattananupong T, Gelaye B, Williams MA (2013) Sleep quality and sleep patterns in relation to consumption of energy drinks, caffeinated beverages, and other stimulants among Thai college students. Sleep Breath 17(3):1017–1028
46. Janowsky DS, Kraus JE, Barnhill J, Elamir B, Davis JM (2003) Effects of topiramate on aggressive, self-injurious, and disruptive/destructive behaviors in the intellectually disabled: an open-label retrospective study. J Clin Psychopharmacol 23(5):500–504

12

PACAP38 and PAC_1 receptor blockade: a new target for headache?

Eloisa Rubio-Beltrán[1*], Edvige Correnti[2], Marie Deen[3], Katharina Kamm[4], Tim Kelderman[5], Laura Papetti[6], Simone Vigneri[7], Antoinette MaassenVanDenBrink[1], Lars Edvinsson[8] and On behalf of the European Headache Federation School of Advanced Studies (EHF-SAS)

Abstract

Pituitary adenylate cyclase activating polypeptide-38 (PACAP38) is a widely distributed neuropeptide involved in neuroprotection, neurodevelopment, nociception and inflammation. Moreover, PACAP38 is a potent inducer of migraine-like attacks, but the mechanism behind this has not been fully elucidated.

Migraine is a neurovascular disorder, recognized as the second most disabling disease. Nevertheless, the antibodies targeting calcitonin gene-related peptide (CGRP) or its receptor are the only prophylactic treatment developed specifically for migraine. These antibodies have displayed positive results in clinical trials, but are not effective for all patients; therefore, new pharmacological targets need to be identified.

Due to the ability of PACAP38 to induce migraine-like attacks, its location in structures previously associated with migraine pathophysiology and the 100-fold selectivity for the PAC_1 receptor when compared to VIP, new attention has been drawn to this pathway and its potential role as a novel target for migraine treatment. In accordance with this, antibodies against PACAP38 (ALD 1910) and PAC_1 receptor (AMG 301) are being developed, with AMG 301 already in Phase II clinical trials. No results have been published so far, but in preclinical studies, AMG 301 has shown responses comparable to those observed with triptans. If these antibodies prove to be effective for the treatment of migraine, several considerations should be addressed, for instance, the potential side effects of long-term blockade of the PACAP (receptor) pathway. Moreover, it is important to investigate whether these antibodies will indeed represent a therapeutic advantage for the patients that do not respond the CGRP (receptor)-antibodies.

In conclusion, the data presented in this review indicate that PACAP38 and PAC_1 receptor blockade are promising antimigraine therapies, but results from clinical trials are needed in order to confirm their efficacy and side effect profile.

Keywords: PACAP, PAC_1 receptor, Migraine, Prophylactic treatment

Review

Discovery of PACAP

The description of the pituitary adenylate cyclase activating polypeptide-38 (PACAP38) was made by Arimura and his team in 1989, following the extraction of the peptide from more than 4000 samples of ovine hypothalamus. After the isolation, its characterization showed that it was formed by 38 amino acids, with a 68% homology with vasoactive intestinal peptide (VIP), described almost twenty years earlier [1]. Subsequently, the peptide was synthesized and shown to activate adenylyl cyclase (AC) in cultures of rat pituitary cells, thereby obtaining its name as pituitary adenylate cyclase activating polypeptide. A year later, a fragment of PACAP38 with similar AC activation profile was isolated. This was formed by 27 amino acids and thus named PACAP27 [2]. That same year, cloning of cDNA from ovine PACAP38 revealed that the amino acid sequence of the mature human PACAP38 was identical to that of the ovine. In addition, later studies showed that it was identical in all mammals [3], suggesting that it has been conserved during evolution.

This review will give an overview of PACAP, its complex signaling pathway, the role PACAP and its receptors have in physiological conditions and their involvement in some disorders, with special focus on

* Correspondence: a.rubiobeltran@erasmusmc.nl
[1]Division of Vascular Medicine and Pharmacology, Department of Internal Medicine, Erasmus University Medical Center, Rotterdam, The Netherlands
Full list of author information is available at the end of the article

migraine. Moreover, the preclinical results of PACAP (receptor) blockade in migraine models, the side effects that could be expected in clinical trials, and the considerations that must be taken if PACAP (receptor)-antibodies are effective for migraine treatment will be discussed.

Pharmacology

PACAP belongs to a wider group of peptides called the VIP/glucagon/growth hormone releasing factor/secretin superfamily. The ADCYAP1gene, located on chromosome 18, encodes PACAP; initially, a proprotein is expressed, and later processed to form a 38 amino acid peptide (PACAP38) with a cleavage-amidation site that can generate a 27-residue-amidated fragment (PACAP27). In mammals, the most prevalent form is PACAP38 [4], therefore, in this review PACAP38 will be referred as PACAP unless stated otherwise.

Three PACAP receptors have been described: $VPAC_1$, $VPAC_2$ and PAC_1, all coupled to G-proteins (Fig. 1). $VPAC_1$ and $VPAC_2$ receptors present equal affinity for PACAP and VIP and their activation stimulates AC. On the other hand, PAC_1 receptor is 100 times more selective for PACAP and presents a complex signaling pathway [4].

Alternative splicing of the PAC_1 receptor gene results in several isoforms. These receptor variants are characterized by shorter extracellular domains (PAC_1*short*, PAC_1*veryshort*), different inserts in an intracellular loop important for G-protein interaction (PAC_1*null*, PAC_1*hip*, PAC_1*hop1*, PAC_1*hop2*, PAC_1*hiphop1*, PAC_1*hiphop2*) and/or discrete sequences located in transmembrane domains II and IV (PAC_1*TM4*) [5–8]. Of relevance, in humans, twelve homologues have been reported [7, 9–11], which have been reviewed elsewhere [12, 13]. For each splice variant, PACAP38 and PACAP27 present similar affinity and potency for AC and phospholipase C (PLC) stimulation, but different efficacy (i.e. maximal effect) of PLC responses [14, 15]. Although in several processes the activation of AC or PLC can result in similar "stimulatory" responses, in smooth muscle cells (e.g. blood vessels), activation of AC leads to vasodilation, whereas PLC activation results in vasoconstriction. This plays an important role in disorders such as migraine, where expression of a PAC_1 receptor isoform with a lower PLC efficacy could favor AC stimulation, thus facilitating vasodilatory responses in cranial blood vessels [16, 17].

To study PAC_1 receptor-mediated responses, selective agonists and antagonists are used. Currently, one selective agonist has been described, maxadilan [18, 19] and three antagonists M65, Max.d.4 and PACAP6–38 [20]. However, no study has investigated whether such compounds are selective for one PAC_1 receptor variant, or whether they bind to all isoforms. Moreover, PACAP6–38 also binds to the $VPAC_2$ receptor, and, together with M65, has been shown to behave as agonist of the PAC_1 receptor in certain tissues [21, 22]. Hence, novel selective pharmacological tools are needed to characterize PAC_1 receptor-mediated responses. Indeed, an antibody against the PAC_1 receptor, such as AMG 301, could be useful for characterization; however, it is yet not clear

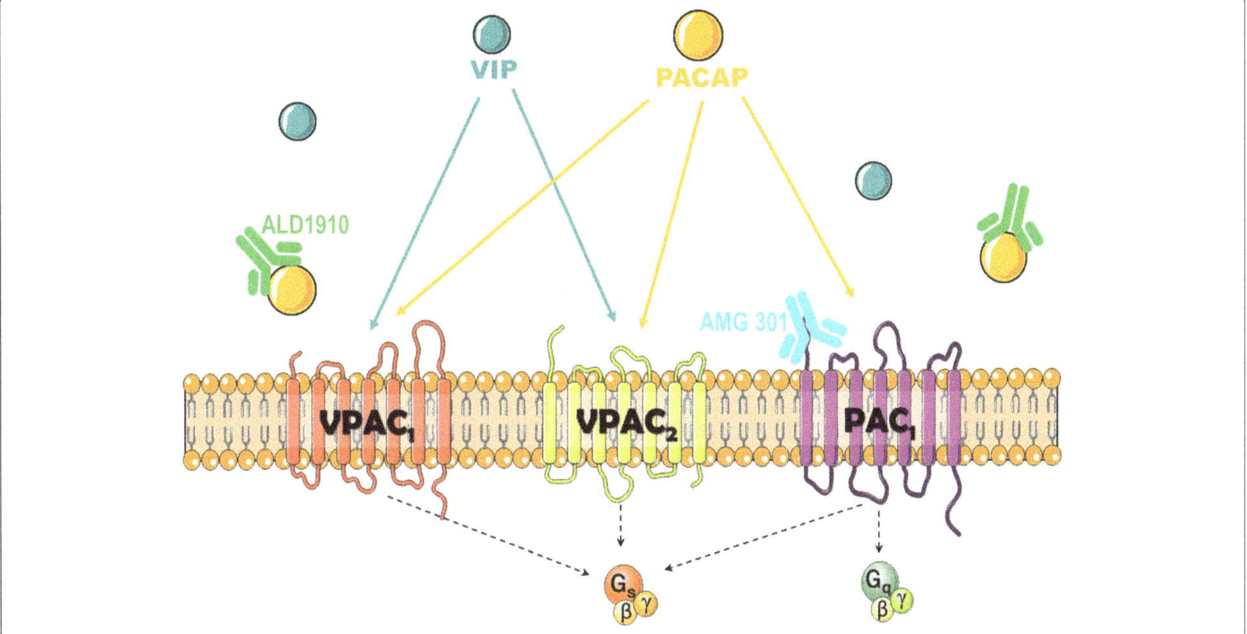

Fig. 1 PACAP receptors. Three receptors to PACAP have been described: $VPAC_1$, $VPAC_2$ and PAC_1. VIP and PACAP show similar affinity for $VPAC_1$ and $VPAC_2$, whereas PACAP is 100-fold more selective for PAC_1 receptor. The antibodies developed for prophylactic antimigraine treatment bind either to PACAP (PACAP38, ALD1910) or to the PAC_1 receptor (AMG 301)

wheter this antibody is selective for one specific variant. If the antibody would be selective for one of the splice variants, this may affect its therapeutic potential, in particular if there are different splice variants expressed in different human populations. On the other hand, different splice variants might hypothetically offer the possibility of designing a drug that would selectively affect the PAC_1 receptor in the trigeminovascular system, while not affecting PAC_1 receptors at other sites in the body, thus reducing its potential side effects.

Physiological roles of PACAP and the PAC_1 receptor

Preclinical studies have shown that PACAP and PAC_1 receptors are widely distributed, both centrally and peripherally. It is therefore not surprising that PACAP is described as a (neuro)hormone, neurotransmitter, neuromodulator, neurotrophic factor and immunomodulator [13]. As the PAC_1 receptor is currently under investigation for migraine treatment, only the distribution of this receptor will be reviewed, while the distribution of $VPAC_{1/2}$ receptors has been reviewed extensively elsewhere [13, 23, 24].

PACAP/PAC_1 receptor in the central nervous system

PACAP fibers and PAC_1 receptors are widely expressed throughout the central nervous system (CNS) with the highest density of both in the hypothalamus and supraoptic nucleus [25–31]. In accordance with this, PAC_1 receptor activation has been associated with release of vasopressin and regulation of drinking behavior [32, 33], decrease of food intake [34–36], modulation of the sleep/wake cycle [37, 38], clock gene expression [38], melatonin synthesis stimulation [39], sexual maturation [40, 41], stress and sexual behavior [41, 42], learning [43], pain processing [44] and psychomotor responsiveness [45] .

Of special interest for migraine, both PACAP fibers and the PAC_1 receptor are present in the paraventricular nucleus of the hypothalamus, the ventrolateral periaqueductal gray, the locus coeruleus, the solitary nucleus, the trigeminal nucleus caudalis (TNC) and the trigeminal ganglion (TG). These structures have all been associated with nociception and/or migraine pathophysiology [23, 46–49].

PACAP/PAC_1 receptor in the periphery

Peripherally, PACAP fibers and/or cell bodies have been described in acrosome caps of primary spermatocytes, mature spermatids, in the testis, epithelial cells from epididymal tubules, the ovaries, mammary glands, in stromal stem cells and terminal placental villi, where the amount of PACAP mRNA increases with the progression of pregnancy [50–52]. Similarly, PAC_1 receptors have been described in spermatids, the penile corpus cavernosum, the ovaries, the chorionic vessels and in stromal and decidual cells of the placenta [51, 53–55]. Considering the presence of PACAP and PAC_1 receptors also in hypothalamus and pituitary, an important role in modulation of the hypothalamo-pituitary-gonadal axis is suggested.

PACAP fibers and cell bodies are also found in the adrenal gland, pancreas, epithelium and smooth muscle cells of the urinary tract, the bladder, urethra, larynx, lungs, gastrointestinal smooth muscle cells, duodenal mucosa, thymus, spleen and innervating vascular smooth muscle cells [23, 26, 56–67]. PAC_1 receptors have been described in the adrenal medulla, pancreas, liver, lungs, enterochromaffin-like cells, thymus and vascular smooth muscle cells [47, 56, 62, 67–70].

Due to their vast distribution peripherally, PACAP and the PAC_1 receptor are involved in a variety of physiological processes, such as regulation of adrenaline release [71], stimulation of adipocyte thermogenesis [72], lipid metabolism [73], metabolic stress adaptation [74], glucose and energy homeostasis [75], renin production [76, 77] and inflammatory responses [78]. Furthermore, PACAP and the PAC_1 receptor have a crucial role in the long-term maintenance of neurogenic vasodilation in the periphery and in the homeostatic responses to cerebral, retinal, cardiac, hepatic, intestinal and renal ischemic events [79–88]. This topic has been extensively reviewed elsewhere [89].

PACAP and PAC_1 receptor in pathophysiological conditions

Besides being involved in several physiological processes, PACAP is thought to contribute to the pathophysiology of several conditions.

PACAP has been associated with regulation of inflammatory processes. In an arthritis model, $PACAP^{-/-}$ mice showed absence of arthritic hyperalgesia and reduction of joint swelling, vascular leakage and inflammatory cell accumulation. In the late phase of the disease, immune cell function and bone neoformation were increased [90]. In rheumatoid arthritis, the vasodilatory effects of PACAP through activation of the PAC_1 receptor facilitated plasma leakage, edema formation, and leukocyte migration [91, 92]. Furthermore, $PACAP^{-/-}$ mice developed more severe inflammation and tumors in a model of colitis [78]. In preclinical models, upregulation of PACAP and its receptors in micturition pathways contributed to the development of urinary bladder dysfunction, including symptoms of increased voiding frequency and pelvic pain [58], suggesting a role in low urinary tract dysfunction. In the nervous system, studies demonstrated anxiogenic actions of PACAP and the possibility of blocking anxiety-related behaviors with PAC_1 receptor antagonists [93–95]. In patients with post-traumatic stress disorder (PTSD), blood levels of PACAP correlated with severity of stress-related symptoms [96], and in females, a single nucleotide polymorphism in the estrogen response element of the PAC_1 receptor gene is predictive of PTSD diagnosis [97].

Furthermore, PACAP plays a complex role in pain transmission. At the peripheral sensory nerve terminals, pro- and anti-nociceptive effects are observed; while in CNS, central sensitization, increase of neuronal excitation and induction of chronic pain have been described [98]. In an acute somatic and visceral inflammatory model, PACAP decreased pain transmission; however, after application in the spinal cord, a transient induction of analgesia was followed by long-lasting algesia [99]. Moreover, injection of PACAP into the paraventricular nucleus of hypothalamus increased the activity of the TNC, an effect which was inhibited by the PAC_1 receptor antagonist [48]. Although it has been shown that PACAP is actively transported through the blood-brain barrier (BBB), it is rapidly degraded or returned by efflux pumps [100]. Thus, a direct central action of peripheral PACAP is unlikely.

Although the role of PACAP in pain processing remains elusive, clinical data strongly suggest the involvement of PACAP in the pathophysiology of migraine and cluster headache (CH) (see also [101, 102]). Recent evidence of a correlation between a genetic variant of the PAC_1 receptor gene (ADCYAP1R1) and susceptibility to CH was demonstrated [103]. Another study identified a relationship between altered PACAP levels in peripheral blood and different types of headache [104]. Further, two studies reported low interictal plasma levels of PACAP in migraine and CH when compared to controls [105, 106]. Particularly, a detailed analysis of PACAP mRNA expression in peripheral blood mononuclear cells detected a significantly lower level of PACAP in migraine patients compared to healthy controls, with no significant differences revealed between the control group and tension-type headache, CH or medication overuse headache groups. Interestingly, PACAP increased ictally in jugular or cubital blood of migraine [105, 107, 108] and CH patients [93, 106], and levels decreased as headache ameliorated after sumatriptan administration [108]. Finally, when administered to migraine patients, PACAP induced an instant headache in 90% of patients, which was later followed by a delayed headache similar to a migraine-like attack in two thirds of the subjects [109]. This has led to study the role of PACAP in migraine pathophysiology as will be discussed in the next section.

PACAP in migraine pathophysiology

The use and development of experimental animal and human models of headache, migraine in particular, have provided invaluable insight into the pathophysiological mechanisms underlying headache disorders [110, 111]. To investigate the molecular mechanisms behind the headache-inducing effects of PACAP, a number of animal studies have been conducted. Additionally, several human studies have been performed, some of these in combination with imaging techniques. In the following sections, both human and animal studies investigating the headache-related effects of PACAP will be reviewed.

Human studies

The headache-inducing effect of PACAP was first reported in a study on cerebral blood flow in healthy volunteers, where 10 out of 12 participants reported mild to moderate headache after PACAP infusion [112]. A double-blind, randomized, placebo-controlled, crossover study later showed that 12 out of 12 healthy subjects and 11 out of 12 migraine patients reported headache after intravenous infusion of PACAP, compared to two and three, respectively, after placebo [109]. Further, two healthy subjects and one migraine patient reported a migraine-like attack within 1 h after infusion, whereas six migraine patients reported a migraine-like attack after a mean of 6 h (range 2–11 h) after infusion. This study also found dilation of middle cerebral artery (MCA) and the superficial temporal artery after PACAP infusion.

The role of vasodilation in PACAP-induced headache was further explored in a magnetic resonance angiography (MRA) study in healthy volunteers [113]. Eight out of nine participants reported an immediate headache and 100% reported a delayed headache after PACAP infusion. Further, over a 5 h period PACAP induced a sustained dilation of the *extracranial* middle meningeal artery (MMA) but no change in intracerebral MCA. Collectively, these studies support the notion that PACAP induces headache via sustained vasodilation. In another MRA study, PACAP infusion induced headache in 91% of included migraine patients, and 73% reported migraine-like attacks compared to 82% and 18%, respectively, after VIP administration. Further, PACAP induced a long-lasting (> 2 h) dilation of extracranial arteries, whereas the dilation caused by VIP normalized after 2 h. In both cases, dilation of intracranial arteries was not observed. This further underlines prolonged extracranial vasodilation as the migraine inducing mechanism of PACAP [114]. Interestingly, in an in vitro study neither PACAP nor VIP were potent in inducing vasodilation of the intracranial portion of the human MMA [115].

In a resting-state magnetic resonance study, infusion of PACAP affected connectivity in the salience, the default mode and the sensorimotor network during migraine attacks. VIP had no effect on these networks [116]. Another study in migraine patients reproduced the induction of migraine-like attacks in 72% of patients and showed that PACAP induced premonitory symptoms in 48% of patients compared to 9% after CGRP [117], suggesting an effect on central PAC_1 receptors.

However, as described above, PACAP is rapidly degraded or transported back after actively crossing the BBB [100]; therefore, the premonitory symptoms could be mediated via activation of a central structure that is not protected by the BBB.

Two studies in migraine patients have further analysed plasma levels of markers of peptide release from parasympathetic (VIP) and sensory (CGRP) perivascular nerve fibres; mast cell degranulation (tumour necrosis factor alpha and tryptase); neuronal damage, glial cell activation or leakage of the BBB (S100 calcium binding protein B and neuron-specific enolase); and hypothalamic activation (prolactin, thyroid-stimulating hormone, follicle-stimulating hormone, luteinizing hormone and adrenocorticotropic hormone) after PACAP infusion [114, 118]. Only levels of VIP, S100 calcium binding protein B, prolactin and the thyroid-stimulating hormone were modified and did not differ between patients who developed migraine-like attacks and those who did not. However, it is important to consider that samples were obtained from the antecubital vein and it is not known yet if peripheral plasma changes reliably reflect cranial release of mediators.

The human studies point out PACAP as a key player in migraine pathophysiology [102]. As VIP does not induce migraine-like attacks, it is assumed that PACAP's actions are mediated by PAC_1 receptor activation. Nevertheless, it is still too early to rule out $VPAC_{1/2}$ receptors as additional potential antimigraine targets, since no studies in humans have been performed with antagonists. Further, the short plasma half-life of VIP, two minutes (as compared to 6–10 min of PACAP [119]), could be the cause of its lack of migraine-inducing effects.

Animal studies

To characterize the exact receptor involved in PACAP-mediated actions, the vasodilatory effect of PACAP was elucidated in animal studies, showing that VIP, PACAP38 and PACAP27 induce vasodilation of the rat MMA in vivo [120, 121]. Interestingly, this effect was blocked by $VPAC_1$ antagonists in the former [120] and $VPAC_2$ antagonists in the latter [121]. Both studies found no effect of PAC_1 antagonists on vasodilation. Similarly, in an in vitro study, PACAP induced vasodilation of the *human* middle meningeal and distal coronary arteries, and this effect was not modified by PACAP6–38 [115]. In contrast, an ex vivo study found that PAC_1 antagonists reversed the PACAP-induced vasodilation in the rat MMA [17]. As mentioned previously, PAC_1 receptor antagonists have shown agonistic behavior and affinity for $VPAC_2$ receptors. This could explain the contradictory results observed in the MMA vasodilation studies. Therefore, different methods must be used to elucidate the receptors involved in migraine pathophysiology. For example, in a in vivo model of chronic migraine, induced by recurrent chemical dural stimulation, PAC_1 receptor mRNA was shown to be increased in the TG, but not in the TNC, and no significant differences were found in the expression of the $VPAC_1$ and $VPAC_2$ receptors [122]. Moreover, in an in vivo rat model, intravenous administration of AMG 301, the PAC_1 receptor antibody, inhibited evoked nociceptive activity in the trigemino-cervical complex, and the results were comparable to the inhibition observed with sumatriptan [123].

In addition to sustained vasodilation, mast cell degranulation has also been suggested as one of the headache-inducing mechanisms of PACAP. This hypothesis is based on findings from animal studies showing that PACAP degranulates mast cells from the rat dura mater [124]. Further, PACAP-induced delayed vasodilation of the rat MMA is attenuated in mast cell depleted rats [125]. Interestingly administration of VIP did not result in mast cell release of histamine from the dura [126]. However, as mentioned previously, no changes in peripheral blood markers of mast cell degranulation have been observed in migraine patients [114, 118].

Collectively, the animal studies confirm that PACAP induces vasodilation and suggest that this effect might be mediated through degranulation of mast cells. Also, recent results show that these effects are most likely exerted through activation of the PAC_1 receptor. Due to the contradictory results, further studies are warranted to confirm this.

PACAP (receptor) blockade as a therapeutic target

As shown above, PACAP seems to play an important role in migraine pathophysiology. Although the exact receptor involved has not yet been elucidated, some studies indicate that the PAC_1 receptor is the most important [17, 48, 113, 117, 122, 123]. Therefore, both PACAP and PAC_1 receptor have been suggested as novel targets for migraine treatment and possibly a new therapeutic option for patients who do not respond to CGRP (receptor) blocking drugs. Although both neuropeptides co-localize in the trigeminal ganglion [49], and could share some biological cascades, the PACAP-induced migraine attacks indicate an independent role of PACAP in the genesis of migraine.

In this light, the interest from pharmaceutical companies for blocking the PACAP/PAC_1 receptor pathway has increased. There are two therapeutic approaches to inhibit PACAP: (i) PAC_1 receptor antagonists or antibodies directed against this receptor; or (ii) antibodies directed against the peptide PACAP [102]. Since PAC_1 receptor antagonists have been reported to act as agonists depending on the tissue (see Pharmacology), the antibodies seem a better option for blocking this receptor.

Currently, a phase 2a, randomized, double blind, placebo-controlled study is underway to evaluate the efficacy and safety of a PAC_1 receptor antibody (AMG 301) in subjects with chronic or episodic migraine (Clinical trials identifier: NCT03238781, [127]). Unfortunately, no preliminary results have been published so far. Preclinical studies are also evaluating a monoclonal antibody (ALD1910) targeting PACAP38 for its potential in the treatment of migraine patients who have an inadequate response to therapeutics directed at CGRP or its receptor [128].

Potential side effects of PACAP/PAC$_1$ receptor blockade

Indeed, the possibility of a new therapeutic target for prophylactic migraine treatment is exciting; however, it is important to consider that PACAP and PAC_1 receptor participate in numerous physiological processes (see Fig. 2). As antibodies are not likely to cross the BBB, only the possible side effects regarding peripheral blockade of PACAP and PAC_1 receptor will be discussed.

As PACAP and PAC_1 receptor are expressed throughout the components of the hypothalamo-pituitary-gonadal axis [50–52], and the pituitary gland is not protected by the BBB, a dysregulation of the functions of this axis could be a concern. Also, the immune system has been described to be regulated by activation of PAC_1 receptor [61]. This, together with its participation in the modulation of inflammatory processes, could result in alterations in the immune response and increased production of pro-inflammatory cytokines [78, 129]. In accordance with this, in a mouse model of colitis, PACAP-deficient mice developed a more severe disease [78].

Blocking PACAP might also alter the response to metabolic stress. Studies with PACAP-deficient mice have shown a more profound and longer lasting insulin-induced hypoglycemia and a reduction in glucose-stimulated insulin secretion [74, 75]. Moreover, PACAP-deficient mice had hepatic microvesicular steatosis, intracellular fat accumulation in muscle and skeletal muscle and depletion of subcutaneous white fat [73].

Furthermore, PACAP and the PAC_1 receptor participate in vasodilatory responses, renin release and regulation of cardiovascular function [77, 115, 125]. Although the density of $VPAC_{1/2}$ and PAC_1 receptors in coronary artery is less than that in cranial MMA [115], arguing for a limited role in cardiac ischemia, a protective role in ischemic events has been described. Thus, considering the increased cardiovascular risk that migraine patients present [130–133], careful monitoring of patients with preexisting cardiovascular risk factors is advised. However, similar concerns have been raised with the CGRP (receptor)-antibodies [134, 135], with no cardiovascular adverse events reported in the clinical trials [136].

Further considerations

If the antibodies against the PAC_1 receptor prove to be effective for the prophylactic treatment of migraine, some concerns should be addressed. Firstly, as previously discussed, it is important to consider the possible side effects of long-term blockade of PACAP/PAC_1

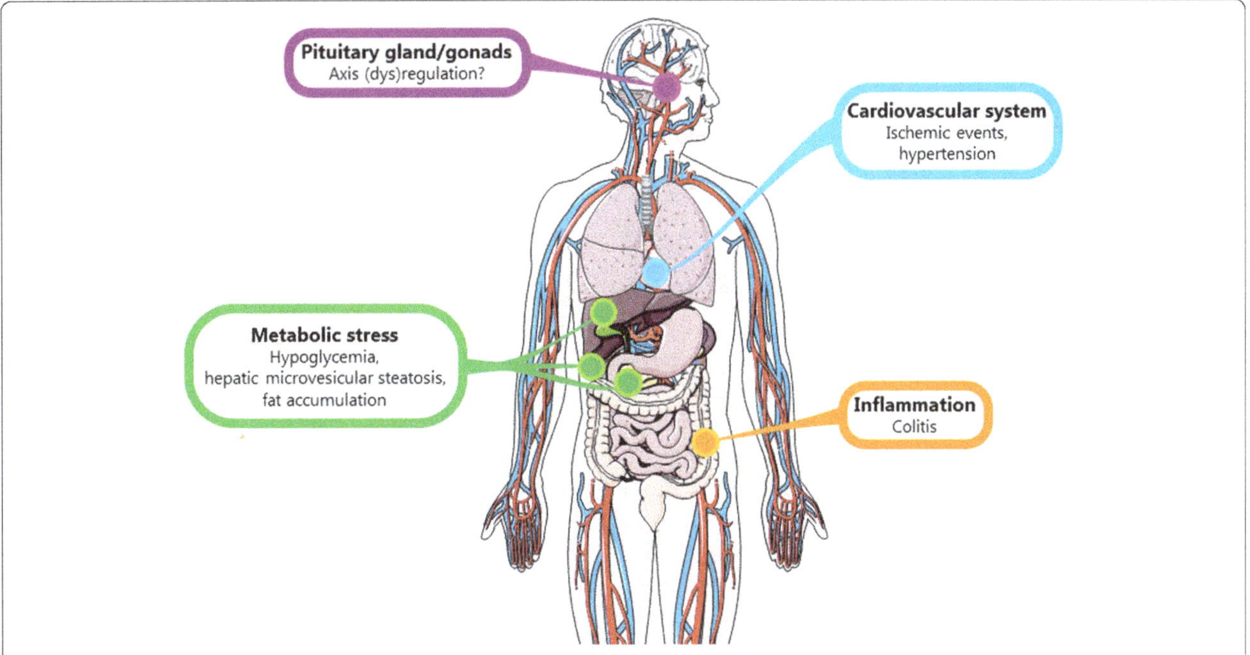

Fig. 2 Possible side effects after long-term exposure to PACAP (receptor)-antibodies. An overview of the organ systems where PACAP and PAC_1 receptor are present and the possible side effects that could be observed

receptor, with emphasis on the cardiovascular system, as migraine patients present a higher cardiovascular risk. Therefore, safety studies in patients with cardiovascular disease are needed. Moreover, the administration route of the antibody against the PAC_1 receptor is subcutaneous, thus erythema, pruritus and mild pain in the injection site could be expected, as it has been observed with the CGRP (receptor) – antibodies [136]. Nevertheless, the monthly administration represents an advantage for treatment adherence.

It will also be important to define whether PAC_1 receptor antibodies will really represent a therapeutic advantage for the patients that are not responding to the CGRP (receptor)-antibodies. Since studies have shown that PACAP and CGRP co-localize in structures relevant for migraine pathophysiology (e.g. trigeminal ganglion) [49], PACAP blockade may only be effective for the same patients to whom CGRP blockade is already effective. If a distinction can be made between patient groups this would also shed light on the pathophysiology of migraine, as it could distinguish between CGRP-associated or PACAP-associated migraine patients. Moreover, the PAC_1 receptor sequence that is recognized by the antibody has not been disclosed, thus, the variants of the receptor to which the antibody binds are not known. If revealed, it would be interesting to study whether certain receptor isoforms predispose patients to present migraine, or whether the treatment will only be effective in patients with those isoforms.

Finally, as mentioned previously, it is still too early to rule out $VPAC_{1/2}$ receptors as therapeutic targets for migraine treatment. Therefore, ALD1910, the antibody against PACAP38, currently undergoing preclinical studies [128], broadens the therapeutic options for migraine treatment. However, further safety studies should be addressed, as blocking PACAP38 would inhibit the actions of three different receptors, increasing the possibilities of adverse side effects.

Conclusion

The possible role of PACAP/PAC_1 receptor blockade as migraine treatment has been reviewed. All three PACAP receptors have been described in TG, TNC and (dural) arteries, structures previously related to migraine pathophysiology [47, 49]. Indeed, infusion of PACAP is able to induce migraine-like attacks [109]. Moreover, interictally, low plasma levels of PACAP have been described [105], while during a migraine attack, PACAP increases in jugular and cubital blood [105, 108] and decreases as headache ameliorates after sumatriptan administration [108].

Clinical studies have shown that infusion of VIP does not induce migraine-like headaches [114], therefore, it is considered that the possible receptor involved in PACAP actions is PAC_1 receptor, as VIP has affinity for $VPAC_1$ and $VPAC_2$ receptors; although this could be attributed to pharmacokinetic (i.e. half-life), rather than pharmacodynamic aspects. Pharmacological characterization in preclinical studies has provided contradictory results, indicating a complex pharmacology of the PAC_1 receptor [21, 22]. However, a recent in vivo study showed that intravenous infusion of PAC_1 receptor antibody, inhibited evoked nociceptive activity in the trigemino-cervical complex in rats, and these results were comparable to the inhibition observed with sumatriptan [123]. These results have led to the development of antibodies against PACAP (ALD1910) and PAC_1 receptor (AMG 301) for migraine treatment.

In conclusion, the data presented in this review indicate that PACAP and PAC_1 receptor blockade are promising migraine therapies but results from clinical trials are needed in order to confirm their efficacy and their side effects profile.

Abbreviations

AC: Adenylyl cyclase; BBB: Blood-brain barrier; CGRP: Calcitonin gene-related peptide; CH: Cluster headache; CNS: Central nervous system; MCA: Middle cerebral artery; MMA: Middle meningeal artery; MRA: Magnetic resonance angiography; PACAP38: Pituitary adenylate cyclase activating polypeptide-38; PLC: Phospholipase C; PTSD: Post-traumatic stress disorder; TG: Trigeminal ganglion; TNC: Trigeminal nucleus caudalis; VIP: Vasoactive intestinal peptide

Acknowledgements

The European Headache Federation and the Department of Clinical and Molecular Medicine, Sapienza University of Rome, are gratefully acknowledged for supporting this work. Figs. 1 and 2 were modified from Servier Medical Art, licensed under a Creative Common Attribution 3.0 Generic License, https://smart.servier.com/.

Funding

This work was supported by the European Headache Federation.

Authors' contributions

AMvdB and LE conceived the review. All authors designed the review, drafted the manuscript and revised it for intellectual content. All authors read and approved the final manuscript.

Competing interests

AMvdB received research grants and/or consultation fees from Amgen/Novartis, Lilly/CoLucid, Teva and ATI. LE has given talks and received grant for preclinical studies sponsored by Novartis and TEVA. All other authors declare no conflicts of interest.

Author details

[1]Division of Vascular Medicine and Pharmacology, Department of Internal Medicine, Erasmus University Medical Center, Rotterdam, The Netherlands. [2]Department of Child Neuropsychiatry, University of Palermo, Palermo, Italy. [3]Danish Headache Center, Department of Neurology, Rigshospitalet Glostrup, Glostrup, Denmark. [4]Department of Neurology, University Hospital, LMU

Munich, Munich, Germany. [5]Department of Neurology, Ghent University Hospital, Ghent, Belgium. [6]Headache Center, Bambino Gesù Children's Hospital, IRCCS, Rome, Italy. [7]Department of Experimental Biomedicine and Clinical Neurosciences, University of Palermo; Pain Medicine Unit, Santa Maria Maddalena Hospital, Occhiobello, Italy. [8]Department of Internal Medicine, Institute of Clinical Sciences, Lund University, Lund, Sweden.

References

1. Miyata A, Arimura A, Dahl RR, Minamino N, Uehara A, Jiang L, Culler MD, Coy DH (1989) Isolation of a novel 38 residue-hypothalamic polypeptide which stimulates adenylate cyclase in pituitary cells. Biochem Biophys Res Commun 164(1):567–574 https://doi.org/10.1016/0006-291X(89)91757-9
2. Miyata A, Jiang L, Dahl RD, Kitada C, Kubo K, Fujino M, Minamino N, Arimura A (1990) Isolation of a neuropeptide corresponding to the N-terminal 27 residues of the pituitary adenylate cyclase activating polypeptide with 38 residues (PACAP38). Biochem Biophys Res Commun 170(2):643–648 https://doi.org/10.1016/0006-291X(90)92140-U
3. Kimura C, Ohkubo S, Ogi K, Hosoya M, Itoh Y, Onda H, Miyata A, Jiang L, Dahl RR, Stibbs HH, Arimura A, Fujino M (1990) A novel peptide which stimulates adenylate cyclase: molecular cloning and characterization of the ovine and human cDNAs. Biochem Biophys Res Commun 166(1):81–89 https://doi.org/10.1016/0006-291X(90)91914-E
4. Harmar AJ, Fahrenkrug J, Gozes I, Laburthe M, May V, Pisegna JR, Vaudry D, Vaudry H, Waschek JA, Said SI (2012) Pharmacology and functions of receptors for vasoactive intestinal peptide and pituitary adenylate cyclase-activating polypeptide: IUPHAR review 1. Br J Pharmacol 166(1):4–17. https://doi.org/10.1111/j.1476-5381.2012.01871.x
5. Shinohara K, Funabashi T, Nakamura TJ, Mitsushima D, Kimura F (2002) Differential regulation of pituitary adenylate cyclase-activating peptide receptor variants in the rat suprachiasmatic nucleus. Neuroscience 110(2): 301–308 https://doi.org/10.1016/S0306-4522(01)00479-1
6. Joumot L, Waeber C, Pantaloni C, Holsboer F, Seeburg PH, Bockaert J, Spengler D (1995) Differential signal transduction by six splice variants of the pituitary adenylate cyclase-activating peptide (PACAP) receptor. Biochem Soc Trans 23(1):133–137. https://doi.org/10.1042/bst0230133
7. Pantaloni C, Brabet P, Bilanges B, Dumuis A, Houssami S, Spengler D, Bockaert J, Journot L (1996) Alternative splicing in the N-terminal extracellular domain of the pituitary adenylate cyclase-activating polypeptide (PACAP) receptor modulates receptor selectivity and relative potencies of PACAP-27 and PACAP-38 in phospholipase C activation. J Biol Chem 271(36):22146–22151. https://doi.org/10.1074/jbc.271.36.22146
8. Chatterjee TK, Sharma RV, Fisher RA (1996) Molecular cloning of a novel variant of the pituitary adenylate cyclase-activating polypeptide (PACAP) receptor that stimulates calcium influx by activation of L-type calcium channels. J Biol Chem 271(50):32226–32232. https://doi.org/10.1074/jbc.271.50.32226
9. Lutz EM, Ronaldson E, Shaw P, Johnson MS, Holland PJ, Mitchell R (2006) Characterization of novel splice variants of the PAC_1 receptor in human neuroblastoma cells: consequences for signaling by VIP and PACAP. Mol Cell Neurosci 31(2):193–209 https://doi.org/10.1016/j.mcn.2005.09.008
10. Dautzenberg FM, Mevenkamp G, Wille S, Hauger RL (1999) N-terminal splice variants of the type I PACAP receptor: isolation, characterization and ligand binding/selectivity determinants. J Neuroendocrinol 11(12):941–949. https://doi.org/10.1046/j.1365-2826.1999.00411.x
11. Pisegna JR, Wank SA (1996) Cloning and characterization of the signal transduction of four splice variants of the human pituitary adenylate cyclase activating polypeptide receptor: evidence for dual coupling to adenylate cyclase and phospholipase C. J Biol Chem 271(29):17267–17274. https://doi.org/10.1074/jbc.271.29.17267
12. Blechman J, Levkowitz G (2013) Alternative splicing of the pituitary adenylate cyclase-activating polypeptide receptor PAC_1: mechanisms of fine tuning of brain activity. Front Endocrinol 4(55):1–19
13. Dickson L, Finlayson K (2009) VPAC and PAC receptors: from ligands to function. Pharmacol Ther 121(3):294–316 https://doi.org/10.1016/j.pharmthera.2008.11.006
14. Spengler D, Waeber C, Pantaloni C, Holsboer F, Bockaert J, Seeburgt PH, Journot L (1993) Differential signal transduction by five splice variants of the PACAP receptor. Nature 365:170. https://doi.org/10.1038/365170a0
15. Braas KM, May V (1999) Pituitary adenylate cyclase-activating polypeptides directly stimulate sympathetic neuron neuropeptide Y release through PAC_1 receptor isoform activation of specific intracellular signaling pathways. J Biol Chem 274(39):27702–27710. https://doi.org/10.1074/jbc.274.39.27702
16. Erdling A, Sheykhzade M, Maddahi A, Bari F, Edvinsson L (2013) VIP/PACAP receptors in cerebral arteries of rat: characterization, localization and relation to intracellular calcium. Neuropeptides 47(2):85–92. https://doi.org/10.1016/j.npep.2012.12.005
17. Syed AU, Koide M, Braas KM, May V, Wellman GC (2012) Pituitary adenylate cyclase-activating polypeptide (PACAP) potently dilates middle meningeal arteries: implications for migraine. J Mol Neurosci 48(3):574–583. https://doi.org/10.1007/s12031-012-9851-0
18. Moro O, Lerner EA (1997) Maxadilan, the vasodilator from sand flies, is a specific pituitary adenylate cyclase activating peptide type I receptor agonist. J Biol Chem 272(2):966–970. https://doi.org/10.1074/jbc.272.2.966
19. Tatsuno I, Uchida D, Tanaka T, Saeki N, Hirai A, Saito Y, Moro O, Tajima M (2001) Maxadilan specifically interacts with PAC1 receptor, which is a dominant form of PACAP/VIP family receptors in cultured rat cortical neurons. Brain Res 889(1):138–148 https://doi.org/10.1016/S0006-8993(00)03126-7
20. Uchida D, Tatsuno I, Tanaka T, Hirai A, Saito Y, Moro O, Tajima M (1998) Maxadilan is a specific agonist and its deleted peptide (M65) is a specific antagonist for PACAP type 1 receptor. Ann N Y Acad Sci 865(1):253–258. https://doi.org/10.1111/j.1749-6632.1998.tb11185.x
21. Sághy É, Payrits M, Helyes Z, Reglődi D, Bánki E, Tóth G, Couvineau A, Szőke É (2015) Stimulatory effect of pituitary adenylate cyclase-activating polypeptide 6-38, M65 and vasoactive intestinal polypeptide 6-28 on trigeminal sensory neurons. Neuroscience 308:144–156 https://doi.org/10.1016/j.neuroscience.2015.08.043
22. Reglodi D, Borzsei R, Bagoly T, Boronkai A, Racz B, Tamas A, Kiss P, Horvath G, Brubel R, Nemeth J, Toth G, Helyes Z (2008) Agonistic behavior of PACAP6-38 on sensory nerve terminals and Cytotrophoblast cells. J Mol Neurosci 36(1):270–278. https://doi.org/10.1007/s12031-008-9089-z
23. Vaudry D, Falluel-Morel A, Bourgault S, Basille M, Burel D, Wurtz O, Fournier A, Chow BKC, Hashimoto H, Galas L, Vaudry H (2009) Pituitary adenylate cyclase-activating polypeptide and its receptors: 20 years after the discovery. Pharmacol Rev 61(3):283–357. https://doi.org/10.1124/pr.109.001370
24. Sherwood NM, Krueckl SL, McRory JE (2000) The origin and function of the pituitary adenylate cyclase-activating polypeptide (PACAP)/glucagon superfamily*. Endocr Rev 21(6):619–670
25. Köves K, Arimura A, Görcs TG, Somogyvári-Vigh A (1991) Comparative distribution of Immunoreactive pituitary adenylate cyclase activating polypeptide and vasoactive intestinal polypeptide in rat forebrain. Neuroendocrinology 54(2):159–169
26. Kóves K, Arimura A, Somogyvári-Vigh A, Vigh S, Miller JIM (1990) Immunohistochemical demonstration of a novel hypothalamic peptide, pituitary adenylate cyclase-activating polypeptide, in the ovine hypothalamus*. Endocrinology 127(1):264–271
27. Hannibal J (2002) Pituitary adenylate cyclase-activating peptide in the rat central nervous system: an immunohistochemical and in situ hybridization study. J Comp Neurol 453(4):389–417. https://doi.org/10.1002/cne.10418
28. Kivipelto L, Absood A, Arimura A, Sundler F, Håkanson R, Panula P (1992) The distribution of pituitary adenylate cyclase-activating polypeptide-like immunoreactivity is distinct from helodermin- and helospectin-like immunoreactivities in the rat brain. J Chem Neuroanat 5(1):85–94 https://doi.org/10.1016/0891-0618(92)90036-P
29. Joo KM, Chung YH, Kim MK, Nam RH, Lee BL, Lee KH, Cha CI (2004) Distribution of vasoactive intestinal peptide and pituitary adenylate cyclase-activating polypeptide receptors ($VPAC_1$, $VPAC_2$, and PAC_1 receptor) in the rat brain. J Comp Neurol 476(4):388–413. https://doi.org/10.1002/cne.20231
30. Mikkelsen JD, Hannibal J, Larsen PJ, Fahrenkrug J (1994) Pituitary adenylate cyclase activating peptide (PACAP) mRNA in the rat neocortex. Neurosci Lett 171(1):121–124 https://doi.org/10.1016/0304-3940(94)90620-3
31. Suda K, Smith DM, Ghatei MA, Murphy JK, Bloom SR (1991) Investigation and characterization of receptors for pituitary adenylate cyclase-activating polypeptide in human brain by Radioligand binding and chemical cross-linking. J Clin Endocrinol Metabol 72(5):958–964
32. Kageyama K, Hanada K, Iwasaki Y, Sakihara S, Nigawara T, Kasckow J, Suda T (2007) Pituitary adenylate cyclase-activating polypeptide stimulates corticotropin-releasing factor, vasopressin and interleukin-6 gene

transcription in hypothalamic 4B cells. J Endocrinol 195(2):199–211. https://doi.org/10.1677/joe-07-0125
33. Nomura M, Ueta Y, Larsen PJ, Hannibal J, Serino R, Kabashima N, Shibuya I, Yamashita H (1997) Water deprivation increases the expression of pituitary adenylate cyclase-activating polypeptide gene in the rat Subfornical organ*. Endocrinology 138(10):4096–4100
34. Mizuno Y, Kondo K, Terashima Y, Arima H, Murase T, Oiso Y (1998) Anorectic effect of pituitary adenylate cyclase activating polypeptide (PACAP) in rats: lack of evidence for involvement of hypothalamic neuropeptide gene expression. J Neuroendocrinol 10(8):611–616. https://doi.org/10.1046/j.1365-2826.1998.00244.x
35. Mounien L, Bizet P, Boutelet I, Gourcerol G, Fournier A, Vaudry H, Jégou S (2006) Pituitary adenylate cyclase-activating polypeptide directly modulates the activity of proopiomelanocortin neurons in the rat arcuate nucleus. Neuroscience 143(1): 155–163 https://doi.org/10.1016/j.neuroscience.2006.07.022
36. Mounien L, Do Rego J-C, Bizet P, Boutelet I, Gourcerol G, Fournier A, Brabet P, Costentin J, Vaudry H, Jégou S (2008) Pituitary adenylate cyclase-activating polypeptide inhibits food intake in mice through activation of the hypothalamic Melanocortin system. Neuropsychopharmacology 34:424. https://doi.org/10.1038/npp.2008.73
37. Kawaguchi C, Tanaka K, Isojima Y, Shintani N, Hashimoto H, Baba A, Nagai K (2003) Changes in light-induced phase shift of circadian rhythm in mice lacking PACAP. Biochem Biophys Res Commun 310(1):169–175 https://doi.org/10.1016/j.bbrc.2003.09.004
38. Hannibal J, Fahrenkrug J (2004) Target areas innervated by PACAP-immunoreactive retinal ganglion cells. Cell Tissue Res 316(1):99–113. https://doi.org/10.1007/s00441-004-0858-x
39. Hannibal J, Jamen F, Nielsen HS, Journot L, Brabet P, Fahrenkrug J (2001) Dissociation between light-induced phase shift of the circadian rhythm and clock gene expression in mice lacking the pituitary adenylate cyclase activating polypeptide type 1 receptor. J Neurosci 21(13):4883–4890
40. Apostolakis EM, Riherd DN, O'Malley BW (2005) PAC_1 receptors mediate pituitary adenylate cyclase-activating polypeptide- and progesterone-facilitated receptivity in female rats. Mol Endocrinol 19(11):2798–2811
41. Shintani N, Mori W, Hashimoto H, Imai M, Tanaka K, Tomimoto S, Hirose M, Kawaguchi C, Baba A (2002) Defects in reproductive functions in PACAP-deficient female mice. Regul Pept 109(1):45–48 https://doi.org/10.1016/S0167-0115(02)00169-6
42. Amir-Zilberstein L, Blechman J, Sztainberg Y, Norton William HJ, Reuveny A, Borodovsky N, Tahor M, Bonkowsky Joshua L, Bally-Cuif L, Chen A, Levkowitz G (2012) Homeodomain protein Otp and activity-dependent splicing modulate neuronal adaptation to stress. Neuron 73(2):279–291 https://doi.org/10.1016/j.neuron.2011.11.019
43. Otto C, Kovalchuk Y, Wolfer DP, Gass P, Martin M, Zuschratter W, Gröne HJ, Kellendonk C, Tronche F, Maldonado R, Lipp H-P, Konnerth A, Schütz G (2001) Impairment of mossy Fiber long-term potentiation and associative learning in pituitary adenylate cyclase activating polypeptide type I receptor-deficient mice. J Neurosci 21(15):5520–5527. https://doi.org/10.1523/jneurosci.21-15-05520.2001
44. Ohnou T, Yokai M, Kurihara T, Hasegawa-Moriyama M, Shimizu T, Inoue K, Kambe Y, Kanmura Y, Miyata A (2016) Pituitary adenylate cyclase-activating polypeptide type 1 receptor signaling evokes long-lasting nociceptive behaviors through the activation of spinal astrocytes in mice. J Pharmacol Sci 130(4):194–203 https://doi.org/10.1016/j.jphs.2016.01.008
45. Hashimoto H, Shintani N, Tanaka K, Mori W, Hirose M, Matsuda T, Sakaue M, J-i M, Niwa H, Tashiro F, Yamamoto K, Koga K, Tomimoto S, Kunugi A, Suetake S, Baba A (2001) Altered psychomotor behaviors in mice lacking pituitary adenylate cyclase-activating polypeptide (PACAP). Proc Natl Acad Sci 98(23):13355–13360. https://doi.org/10.1073/pnas.231094498
46. Tajti J, Uddman R, Edvinsson L (2001) Neuropeptide localization in the 'migraine generator' region of the human brainstem. Cephalalgia 21(2):96–101. https://doi.org/10.1046/j.1468-2982.2001.00140.x
47. Knutsson M, Edvinsson L (2002) Distribution of mRNA for VIP and PACAP receptors in human cerebral arteries and cranial ganglia. NeuroReport 13(4): 507–509
48. Robert C, Bourgeais L, Arreto CD, Condes-Lara M, Noseda R, Jay T, Villanueva L (2013) Paraventricular hypothalamic regulation of trigeminovascular mechanisms involved in headaches. J Neurosci 33(20):8827–8840. https://doi.org/10.1523/JNEUROSCI.0439-13.2013
49. Eftekhari S, Salvatore CA, Johansson S, Chen TB, Zeng Z, Edvinsson L (2015) Localization of CGRP, CGRP receptor, PACAP and glutamate in trigeminal ganglion. Relation to the blood-brain barrier. Brain Res 1600:93–109. https://doi.org/10.1016/j.brainres.2014.11.031
50. Koh P-O, Won C-K, Noh H-S, Cho G-J, Choi W-S (2005) Expression of pituitary adenylate cyclase activating polypeptide and its type I receptor mRNAs in human placenta. J Vet Sci 6(1):1–5
51. Scaldaferri ML, Modesti A, Palumbo C, Ulisse S, Fabbri A, Piccione E, Frajese G, Moretti C (2000) Pituitary adenylate cyclase-activating polypeptide (PACAP) and PACAP-receptor type 1 expression in rat and human placenta*. Endocrinology 141(3):1158–1167. https://doi.org/10.1210/endo.141.3.7346
52. Vaccari S, Latini S, Barberi M, Teti A, Stefanini M, Canipari R (2006) Characterization and expression of different pituitary adenylate cyclase-activating polypeptide/vasoactive intestinal polypeptide receptors in rat ovarian follicles. J Endocrinol 191(1):287–299. https://doi.org/10.1677/joe.1.06470
53. Koh PO, Kwak SD, Kim HJ, Roh G, Kim JH, Kang SS, Choi WS, Cho GJ (2003) Expression patterns of pituitary adenylate cyclase activating polypeptide and its type I receptor mRNAs in the rat placenta. Mol Reprod Dev 64(1):27–31. https://doi.org/10.1002/mrd.10221
54. Guidone G, Müller D, Vogt K, Mukhopadhyay AK (2002) Characterization of VIP and PACAP receptors in cultured rat penis corpus cavernosum smooth muscle cells and their interaction with guanylate cyclase-B receptors. Regul Pept 108(2):63–72 https://doi.org/10.1016/S0167-0115(02)00107-6
55. Li M, Funahashi H, Mbikay M, Shioda S, Arimura A (2004) Pituitary adenylate cyclase activating polypeptide-mediated intracrine signaling in the testicular germ cells. Endocrine 23(1):59–75. https://doi.org/10.1385/endo:23:1:59
56. Mazzocchi G, Malendowicz LK, Rebuffat P, Gottardo L, Nussdorfer GG (2002) Expression and function of vasoactive intestinal peptide, pituitary adenylate cyclase-activating polypeptide, and their receptors in the human adrenal gland. J Clin Endocrinol Metabol 87(6):2575–2580
57. Portela-Gomes GM, Lukinius A, Ljungberg O, Efendic S, Ahrén B, Abdel-Halim SM (2003) PACAP is expressed in secretory granules of insulin and glucagon cells in human and rodent pancreas: evidence for generation of cAMP compartments uncoupled from hormone release in diabetic islets. Regul Pept 113(1):31–39 https://doi.org/10.1016/S0167-0115(02)00295-1
58. Girard BM, Tooke K, Vizzard MA (2017) PACAP/receptor system in urinary bladder dysfunction and pelvic pain following urinary bladder inflammation or stress. Front Syst Neurosci 11(90):1–23
59. Luts A, Uddman R, Alm R, Basterra J, Sundler F (1993) Peptide-containing nerve fibers in human airways: distribution and coexistence pattern. Int Arch Allergy Immunol 101(1):52–60
60. Sundler F, Ekblad E, Absood A, Håkanson R, Köves K, Arimura A (1992) Pituitary adenylate cyclase activating peptide: a novel vasoactive intestinal peptide-like neuropeptide in the gut. Neuroscience 46(2):439–454 https://doi.org/10.1016/0306-4522(92)90064-9
61. Abad C, Martinez C, Leceta J, Juarranz MG, Delgado M, Gomariz RP (2002) Pituitary adenylate-cyclase-activating polypeptide expression in the immune system. Neuroimmunomodulation 10(3):177–186
62. Tokuda N, Arudchelvan Y, Sawada T, Adachi Y, Fukumoto T, Yasuda M, Sumida H, Shioda S, Fukuda T, Arima A, Kubota S (2006) PACAP receptor (PAC1-R) expression in rat and rhesus monkey Thymus. Ann N Y Acad Sci 1070(1):581–585. https://doi.org/10.1196/annals.1317.085
63. Ny L, Larsson B, Alm P, Ekström P, Fahrenkrug J, Hannibal J, Andersson KE (1995) Distribution and effects of pituitary adenylate cyclase activating peptide in cat and human lower oesophageal sphincter. Br J Pharmacol 116(7):2873–2880
64. Cardell Lars O, Hjert O, Uddman R (1997) The induction of nitric oxide-mediated relaxation of human isolated pulmonary arteries by PACAP. Br J Pharmacol 120(6):1096–1100. https://doi.org/10.1038/sj.bjp.0700992
65. Martin F, Baeres M, Møller M (2004) Origin of PACAP-immunoreactive nerve fibers innervating the Subarachnoidal blood vessels of the rat brain. J Cereb Blood Flow Metab 24(6):628–635. https://doi.org/10.1097/01.wcb.0000121234.42748.f6
66. Filipsson K, Tornøe K, Holst J, Ahrén B (1997) Pituitary adenylate cyclase-activating polypeptide stimulates insulin and glucagon secretion in humans*. J Clin Endocrinol Metab 82(9):3093–3098
67. Borboni P, Porzio O, Pierucci D, Cicconi S, Magnaterra R, Federici M, Sesti G, Lauro D, D Agata V, Cavallaro S, LNJL M (1999) Molecular and functional characterization of pituitary adenylate cyclase-activating polypeptide (PACAP-38)/vasoactive intestinal polypeptide receptors in pancreatic β-cells and effects of PACAP-38 on components of the insulin secretory System1. Endocrinology 140(12):5530–5537
68. Gottschall PE, Tatsuno I, Miyata A, Arimura A (1990) Characterization and distribution of binding sites for the hypothalamic peptide, pituitary adenylate cyclase-activating polypeptide*. Endocrinology 127(1):272–277

69. Busto R, Prieto JC, Bodega G, Zapatero J, Carrero I (2000) Immunohistochemical localization and distribution of VIP/PACAP receptors in human lung. Peptides 21(2):265–269 https://doi.org/10.1016/S0196-9781(99)00202-8
70. Zeng N, Kang TAO, Lyu RM, Wong H, Wen YI, Walsh John H, Sachs G, Pisegna Joseph R (1998) The pituitary adenylate cyclase activating polypeptide type 1 receptor (PAC1-R) is expressed on gastric ECL cells: evidence by immunocytochemistry and RT-PCR. Ann N Y Acad Sci 865(1): 147–156. https://doi.org/10.1111/j.1749-6632.1998.tb11173.x
71. Fukushima Y, Hikichi H, Mizukami K, Nagayama T, Yoshida M, Suzuki-Kusaba M, Hisa H, Kimura T, Satoh S (2001) Role of endogenous PACAP in catecholamine secretion from the rat adrenal gland. Am J Phys Regul Integr Comp Phys 281(5):R1562–R1567. https://doi.org/10.1152/ajpregu.2001.281.5.R1562
72. Diané A, Nikolic N, Rudecki AP, King SM, Bowie DJ, Gray SL (2014) PACAP is essential for the adaptive thermogenic response of brown adipose tissue to cold exposure. J Endocrinol 222(3):327–339. https://doi.org/10.1530/joe-14-0316
73. Gray SL, Cummings KJ, Jirik FR, Sherwood NM (2001) Targeted disruption of the pituitary adenylate cyclase-activating polypeptide gene results in early postnatal death associated with dysfunction of lipid and carbohydrate metabolism. Mol Endocrinol 15(10):1739–1747
74. Hamelink C, Tjurmina O, Damadzic R, Young WS, Weihe E, Lee H-W, Eiden LE (2002) Pituitary adenylate cyclase-activating polypeptide is a sympathoadrenal neurotransmitter involved in catecholamine regulation and glucohomeostasis. Proc Natl Acad Sci 99(1):461–466. https://doi.org/10.1073/pnas.012608999
75. Jamen F, Persson K, Bertrand G, Rodriguez-Henche N, Puech R, Bockaert J, Ahrén B, Brabet P (2000) PAC_1 receptor–deficient mice display impaired insulinotropic response to glucose and reduced glucose tolerance. J Clin Investig 105(9):1307–1315
76. Lutz-Bucher B, Monnier D, Koch B (1996) Evidence for the presence of receptors for pituitary adenylate cyclase-activating polypeptide in the neurohypophysis that are positively coupled to cyclic AMP formation and Neurohypophyseal hormone secretion. Neuroendocrinology 64(2):153–161
77. Hautmann M, Friis UG, Desch M, Todorov V, Castrop H, Segerer F, Otto C, Schütz G, Schweda F (2007) Pituitary adenylate cyclase–activating polypeptide stimulates renin secretion via activation of PAC1 receptors. J Am Soc Nephrol 18(4):1150–1156. https://doi.org/10.1681/asn.2006060633
78. Nemetz N, Abad C, Lawson G, Nobuta H, Chhith S, Duong L, Tse G, Braun J, Waschek JA (2008) Induction of colitis and rapid development of colorectal tumors in mice deficient in the neuropeptide PACAP. Int J Cancer 122(8): 1803–1809. https://doi.org/10.1002/ijc.23308
79. Babai N, Atlasz T, Tamás A, Reglodi D, Tóth G, Kiss P, Gábriel R (2005) Degree of damage compensation by various pacap treatments in monosodium glutamate-induced retinal degeneration. Neurotox Res 8(3): 227–233. https://doi.org/10.1007/bf03033976
80. Chen Y, Samal B, Hamelink CR, Xiang CC, Chen Y, Chen M, Vaudry D, Brownstein MJ, Hallenbeck JM, Eiden LE (2006) Neuroprotection by endogenous and exogenous PACAP following stroke. Regul Pept 137(1):4–19 https://doi.org/10.1016/j.regpep.2006.06.016
81. Dejda A, Seaborn T, Bourgault S, Touzani O, Fournier A, Vaudry H, Vaudry D (2011) PACAP and a novel stable analog protect rat brain from ischemia: insight into the mechanisms of action. Peptides 32(6):1207–1216 https://doi.org/10.1016/j.peptides.2011.04.003
82. László E, Kiss P, Horváth G, Szakály P, Tamás A, Reglödi D (2014) The effects of pituitary adenylate cyclase activating polypeptide in renal ischemia/reperfusion. Acta Biol Hung 65(4):369–378. https://doi.org/10.1556/ABiol.65.2014.4.1
83. Lazarovici P, Cohen G, Arien-Zakay H, Chen J, Zhang C, Chopp M, Jiang H (2012) Multimodal neuroprotection induced by PACAP38 in oxygen–glucose deprivation and middle cerebral artery occlusion stroke models. J Mol Neurosci 48(3):526–540. https://doi.org/10.1007/s12031-012-9818-1
84. Muzzi M, Buonvicino D, De Cesaris F, Chiarugi A (2017) Acute and chronic triptan exposure neither alters rodent cerebral blood flow nor worsens ischemic brain injury. Neuroscience 340:1–7. https://doi.org/10.1016/j.neuroscience.2016.10.046
85. Ohtaki H, Nakamachi T, Dohi K, Aizawa Y, Takaki A, Hodoyama K, Yofu S, Hashimoto H, Shintani N, Baba A, Kopf M, Iwakura Y, Matsuda K, Arimura A, Shioda S (2006) Pituitary adenylate cyclase-activating polypeptide (PACAP) decreases ischemic neuronal cell death in association with IL-6. Proc Natl Acad Sci 103(19):7488–7493. https://doi.org/10.1073/pnas.0600375103
86. Reglodi D, Somogyvari-Vigh A, Vigh S, Kozicz T, Arimura A (2000) Delayed systemic administration of PACAP38 is neuroprotective in transient middle cerebral artery occlusion in the rat. Stroke 31(6):1411–1417. https://doi.org/10.1161/01.str.31.6.1411
87. Reglodi D, Tamás A, Somogyvári-Vigh A, Szántó Z, Kertes E, Lénárd L, Arimura A, Lengvári I (2002) Effects of pretreatment with PACAP on the infarct size and functional outcome in rat permanent focal cerebral ischemia. Peptides 23(12): 2227–2234 https://doi.org/10.1016/S0196-9781(02)00262-0
88. Vaczy A, Reglodi D, Somoskeoy T, Kovacs K, Lokos E, Szabo E, Tamas A, Atlasz T (2016) The protective role of PAC1-receptor agonist Maxadilan in BCCAO-induced retinal degeneration. J Mol Neurosci 60(2):186–194. https://doi.org/10.1007/s12031-016-0818-4
89. Reglodi D, Vaczy A, Rubio-Beltran E, MaassenVanDenBrink A (2018) Protective effects of PACAP in ischemia. J Headache Pain 19(1):19. https://doi.org/10.1186/s10194-018-0845-3
90. Botz B, Bölcskei K, Kereskai L, Kovács M, Németh T, Szigeti K, Horváth I, Máthé D, Kovács N, Hashimoto H, Reglődi D, Szolcsányi J, Pintér E, Mócsai A, Helyes Z (2014) Differential regulatory role of pituitary adenylate cyclase–activating polypeptide in the serum-transfer arthritis model. Arthritis Rheumatol 66(10):2739–2750. https://doi.org/10.1002/art.38772
91. Warren JB, Larkin SW, Coughlan M, Kajekar R, Williams TJ (1992) Pituitary adenylate cyclase activating polypeptide is a potent vasodilator and oedema potentiator in rabbit skin in vivo. Br J Pharmacol 106(2):331–334. https://doi.org/10.1111/j.1476-5381.1992.tb14336.x
92. Svensjö E, Saraiva EM, Amendola RS, Barja-Fidalgo C, Bozza MT, Lerner EA, Teixeira MM, Scharfstein J (2012) Maxadilan, the Lutzomyia longipalpis vasodilator, drives plasma leakage via PAC1–CXCR1/2-pathway. Microvasc Res 83(2):185–193 https://doi.org/10.1016/j.mvr.2011.10.003
93. Watanabe J, Nakamachi T, Matsuno R, Hayashi D, Nakamura M, Kikuyama S, Nakajo S, Shioda S (2007) Localization, characterization and function of pituitary adenylate cyclase-activating polypeptide during brain development. Peptides 28(9):1713–1719 https://doi.org/10.1016/j.peptides.2007.06.029
94. Ghzili H, Grumolato L, Thouënnon E, Tanguy Y, Turquier V, Vaudry H, Anouar Y (2008) Role of PACAP in the physiology and pathology of the sympathoadrenal system. Front Neuroendocrinol 29(1):128–141 https://doi.org/10.1016/j.yfrne.2007.10.001
95. Lezak KR, Roelke E, Harris OM, Choi I, Edwards S, Gick N, Cocchiaro G, Missig G, Roman CW, Braas KM, Toufexis DJ, May V, Hammack SE (2014) Pituitary adenylate cyclase-activating polypeptide (PACAP) in the bed nucleus of the stria terminalis (BNST) increases corticosterone in male and female rats. Psychoneuroendocrinology 45:11–20 https://doi.org/10.1016/j.psyneuen.2014.03.007
96. King SB, Toufexis DJ, Hammack SE (2017) Pituitary adenylate cyclase activating polypeptide (PACAP), stress, and sex hormones. Stress 20(5):465–475. https://doi.org/10.1080/10253890.2017.1336535
97. Ressler KJ, Mercer KB, Bradley B, Jovanovic T, Mahan A, Kerley K, Norrholm SD, Kilaru V, Smith AK, Myers AJ, Ramirez M, Engel A, Hammack SE, Toufexis D, Braas KM, Binder EB, May V (2011) Post-traumatic stress disorder is associated with PACAP and the PAC1 receptor. Nature 470:492. https://doi.org/10.1038/nature09856
98. Tajti J, Tuka B, Botz B, Helyes Z, Vecsei L (2015) Role of pituitary adenylate cyclase-activating polypeptide in nociception and migraine. CNS Neurol Disord Drug Targets 14(4):540–553 https://doi.org/10.2174/1871527314666150429114234
99. Sándor K, Bölcskei K, McDougall JJ, Schuelert N, Reglodi D, Elekes K, Petho G, Pintér E, Szolcsányi J, Helyes Z (2009) Divergent peripheral effects of pituitary adenylate cyclase-activating polypeptide-38 on nociception in rats and mice. Pain 141(1):143–150. https://doi.org/10.1016/j.pain.2008.10.028
100. Amin FM, Schytz HW (2018) Transport of the pituitary adenylate cyclase-activating polypeptide across the blood-brain barrier: implications for migraine. J Headache Pain 19(1):35. https://doi.org/10.1186/s10194-018-0861-3
101. Edvinsson L, Tajti J, Szalárdy L, Vécsei L (2018) PACAP and its role in primary headaches. J Headache Pain 19(1):21. https://doi.org/10.1186/s10194-018-0852-4
102. Vollesen ALH, Ashina M (2017) PACAP38: emerging drug target in migraine and cluster headache. Headache: J Head Face Pain 57(S2):56–63. https://doi.org/10.1111/head.13076
103. Bacchelli E, Cainazzo MM, Cameli C, Guerzoni S, Martinelli A, Zoli M, Maestrini E, Pini LA (2016) A genome-wide analysis in cluster headache points to neprilysin and PACAP receptor gene variants. J Headache Pain 17(1):114. https://doi.org/10.1186/s10194-016-0705-y
104. Guo S, Petersen AS, Schytz HW, Barløse M, Caparso A, Fahrenkrug J, Jensen RH, Ashina M (2017) Cranial parasympathetic activation induces autonomic symptoms but no cluster headache attacks. Cephalalgia 38 (8):1418-1428

105. Tuka B, Helyes Z, Markovics A, Bagoly T, Szolcsányi J, Szabó N, Tóth E, Kincses ZT, Vécsei L, Tajti J (2013) Alterations in PACAP-38-like immunoreactivity in the plasma during ictal and interictal periods of migraine patients. Cephalalgia 33(13):1085–1095. https://doi.org/10.1177/0333102413483931
106. Tuka B, Szabó N, Tóth E, Kincses ZT, Párdutz Á, Szok D, Körtési T, Bagoly T, Helyes Z, Edvinsson L, Vécsei L, Tajti J (2016) Release of PACAP-38 in episodic cluster headache patients – an exploratory study. J Headache Pain 17(1):69. https://doi.org/10.1186/s10194-016-0660-7
107. Hou L, Wan D, Dong Z, Tang W, Han X, Li L, Yang F, Yu S (2016) Pituitary adenylate cyclase-activating polypeptide expression in peripheral blood mononuclear cells of migraineurs. Cell Biosci 6:40. https://doi.org/10.1186/s13578-016-0106-6
108. Zagami AS, Edvinsson L, Goadsby PJ (2014) Pituitary adenylate cyclase activating polypeptide and migraine. Ann Clin Transl Neurol 1(12):1036–1040. https://doi.org/10.1002/acn3.113
109. Schytz HW, Birk S, Wienecke T, Kruuse C, Olesen J, Ashina M (2009) PACAP38 induces migraine-like attacks in patients with migraine without aura. Brain 132(1):16–25. https://doi.org/10.1093/brain/awn307
110. Ashina M, Hansen JM, á Dunga BO, Olesen J (2017) Human models of migraine — short-term pain for long-term gain. Nat Rev Neurol 13:713. https://doi.org/10.1038/nrneurol.2017.137
111. Bergerot A, Holland PR, Akerman S, Bartsch T, Ahn AH, MaassenVanDenBrink A, Reuter U, Tassorelli C, Schoenen J, Mitsikostas DD, VanDenMaagdenberg AMJM, Goadsby PJ (2006) Animal models of migraine: looking at the component parts of a complex disorder. Eur J Neurosci 24(6):1517–1534. https://doi.org/10.1111/j.1460-9568.2006.05036.x
112. Birk S, Sitarz JT, Petersen KA, Oturai PS, Kruuse C, Fahrenkrug J, Olesen J (2007) The effect of intravenous PACAP38 on cerebral hemodynamics in healthy volunteers. Regul Pept 140(3):185–191 https://doi.org/10.1016/j.regpep.2006.12.010
113. Amin FM, Asghar MS, Guo S, Hougaard A, Hansen AE, Schytz HW, RJvd G, de PJH K, HBW L, Olesen J, Ashina M (2012) Headache and prolonged dilatation of the middle meningeal artery by PACAP38 in healthy volunteers. Cephalalgia 32(2):140–149. https://doi.org/10.1177/0333102411431333
114. Amin FM, Hougaard A, Schytz HW, Asghar MS, Lundholm E, Parvaiz AI, de Koning PJH, Andersen MR, Larsson HBW, Fahrenkrug J, Olesen J, Ashina M (2014) Investigation of the pathophysiological mechanisms of migraine attacks induced by pituitary adenylate cyclase-activating polypeptide-38. Brain 137(3):779–794. https://doi.org/10.1093/brain/awt369
115. Chan KY, Baun M, de Vries R, van den Bogaerdt AJ, Dirven CM, Danser AH, Jansen-Olesen I, Olesen J, Villalon CM, MaassenVanDenBrink A, Gupta S (2011) Pharmacological characterization of VIP and PACAP receptors in the human meningeal and coronary artery. Cephalalgia 31(2):181–189. https://doi.org/10.1177/0333102410375624
116. Amin FM, Hougaard A, Magon S, Asghar MS, Ahmad NN, Rostrup E, Sprenger T, Ashina M (2016) Change in brain network connectivity during PACAP38-induced migraine attacks A resting-state functional MRI study. Neurology 86(2):180–187. https://doi.org/10.1212/wnl.0000000000002261
117. Guo S, Vollesen ALH, Olesen J, Ashina M (2016) Premonitory and nonheadache symptoms induced by CGRP and PACAP38 in patients with migraine. Pain 157(12):2773–2781. https://doi.org/10.1097/j.pain.0000000000000702
118. Guo S, Vollesen ALH, Hansen YBL, Frandsen E, Andersen MR, Amin FM, Fahrenkrug J, Olesen J, Ashina M (2017) Part II: biochemical changes after pituitary adenylate cyclase-activating polypeptide-38 infusion in migraine patients. Cephalalgia 37(2):136–147. https://doi.org/10.1177/0333102416639517
119. Hassan M, Refai E, Andersson M, Schnell P-O, Jacobsson H (1994) In vivo dynamical distribution of ^{131}I-VIP in the rat studied by gamma-camera. Nucl Med Biol 21(6):865–872. https://doi.org/10.1016/0969-8051(94)90166-X
120. Boni LJ, Ploug KB, Olesen I, Jansen-Olesen I, Gupta S (2009) The in vivo effect of VIP, PACAP-38 and PACAP-27 and mRNA expression of their receptors in rat middle meningeal artery. Cephalalgia 29(8):837–847. https://doi.org/10.1111/j.1468-2982.2008.01807.x
121. Akerman S, Goadsby PJ (2015) Neuronal PAC_1 receptors mediate delayed activation and sensitization of trigeminocervical neurons: relevance to migraine. Sci Transl Med 7(308):308ra157. https://doi.org/10.1126/scitranslmed.aaa7557
122. Han X, Ran Y, Su M, Liu Y, Tang W, Dong Z, Yu S (2017) Chronic changes in pituitary adenylate cyclase-activating polypeptide and related receptors in response to repeated chemical dural stimulation in rats. Mol Pain 13:1–10
123. Hoffmann J, Martins-Oliveira M, Akerman S, Supronsinchai W, Xu C, Goadsby PJ (2016) PAC-1 receptor antibody modulates nociceptive trigeminal activity in rat. Cephalalgia 36(1S):141–141
124. Baun M, Pedersen MHF, Olesen J, Jansen-Olesen I (2012) Dural mast cell degranulation is a putative mechanism for headache induced by PACAP-38. Cephalalgia 32(4):337–345. https://doi.org/10.1177/0333102412439354
125. Bhatt DK, Gupta S, Olesen J, Jansen-Olesen I (2014) PACAP-38 infusion causes sustained vasodilation of the middle meningeal artery in the rat: possible involvement of mast cells. Cephalalgia 34(11):877–886. https://doi.org/10.1177/0333102414523846
126. Ottosson A, Edvinsson L (1997) Release of histamine from Dural mast cells by substance P and calcitonin gene-related peptide. Cephalalgia 17(3):166–174. https://doi.org/10.1046/j.1468-2982.1997.1703166.x
127. Study to Evaluate the Efficacy and Safety of AMG 301 in Migraine Prevention. https://clinicaltrials.gov/ct2/show/NCT03238781. Accessed 02 May 2018.
128. ALD1910 – migraine prevention. alderbio.com. https://www.alderbio.com/pipeline/ald1910/. Accessed 19 May 2018.
129. Martínez C, Juarranz Y, Abad C, Arranz A, Miguel BG, Rosignoli F, Leceta J, Gomariz RP (2005) Analysis of the role of the PAC_1 receptor in neutrophil recruitment, acute-phase response, and nitric oxide production in septic shock. J Leukoc Biol 77(5):729–738. https://doi.org/10.1189/jlb.0704432
130. Chang CL, Donaghy M, Poulter N (1999) Migraine and stroke in young women: case-control study. BMJ : Br Med J 318(7175):13–18. https://doi.org/10.1136/bmj.318.7175.13
131. Etminan M, Takkouche B, Isorna FC, Samii A (2005) Risk of ischaemic stroke in people with migraine: systematic review and meta-analysis of observational studies. BMJ : Br Med J 330(7482):63–63. https://doi.org/10.1136/bmj.38302.504063.8F
132. Schurks M, Rist PM, Bigal ME, Buring JE, Lipton RB, Kurth T (2009) Migraine and cardiovascular disease: systematic review and meta-analysis. BMJ: Br Med J 339:b3914
133. Spector JT, Kahn SR, Jones MR, Jayakumar M, Dalal D, Nazarian S (2010) Migraine headache and ischemic stroke risk: an updated meta-analysis. Am J Med 123(7):612–624. https://doi.org/10.1016/j.amjmed.2009.12.021
134. Deen M, Correnti E, Kamm K, Kelderman T, Papetti L, Rubio-Beltran E, Vigneri S, Edvinsson L, Maassen Van Den Brink A, European Headache Federation School of Advanced S (2017) Blocking CGRP in migraine patients - a review of pros and cons. J Headache Pain 18(1):96. https://doi.org/10.1186/s10194-017-0807-1
135. MaassenVanDenBrink A, Meijer J, Villalón CM, Ferrari MD (2016) Wiping out CGRP: potential cardiovascular risks. Trends Pharmacol Sci 37(9):779–788. https://doi.org/10.1016/j.tips.2016.06.002
136. Mitsikostas DD, Reuter U (2017) Calcitonin gene-related peptide monoclonal antibodies for migraine prevention: comparisons across randomized controlled studies. Curr Opin Neurol 30(3):272–280. https://doi.org/10.1097/wco.0000000000000438

13

Migraine and greater pain symptoms at 10-year follow-up among patients with major depressive disorder

Ching-I Hung[1], Chia-Yih Liu[1], Ching-Hui Yang[2] and Shuu-Jiun Wang[3,4*]

Abstract

Background: No study has investigated the associations of migraine with pain symptoms over a ten-year period among outpatients with major depressive disorder (MDD). This study aimed to investigate this issue.

Methods: At baseline, the study enrolled 290 outpatients with MDD and followed-up the patients at six-month, two-year, and ten-year time points. MDD and anxiety comorbidities were diagnosed using the Structured Clinical Interview for DSM-IV-text revision. Migraine was diagnosed based on the International Classification of Headache Disorders. The bodily pain subscale of the Short Form 36 (SF-BP) and the pain subscale (PS) of the Depression and Somatic Symptoms scale were also used. Generalized Estimating Equation models were employed to investigate the longitudinal impacts of migraine on pain symptoms.

Results: MDD patients with migraine had lower SF-BP and higher PS scores than those without. Depression, anxiety, and headache indices were significantly correlated with SF-BP and PS scores. The higher the frequency of migraine, the more often patients suffered from pain symptoms. Patients with migraine at all investigated time points suffered from pain symptoms most of the time (ranging from 60.0% to 73.7%) over the 10 years. After controlling for depression and anxiety, migraine was independently associated with a decreased SF-BP score (by 8.93 points) and an increased PS score (by 1.33 points).

Conclusion: Migraine was an important comorbidity associated with greater severities of pain symptoms during long-term follow-up. Migraine treatment should be integrated into the treatment of depression to improve pain symptoms and quality of life in the pain dimension.

Keywords: Depression, Headache, Pain, Somatization, Quality of life

Background

Painful physical symptoms and depression interact with each other [1, 2]. Major depressive disorder (MDD) and pain symptoms may have a shared neurobiological mechanism and may be genetically correlated [3, 4]. Among patients with MDD, pain symptoms are common, and are associated with a greater severity of depression, a poorer treatment response, inability to achieve full remission, impaired function, a poorer quality of life, and an increased suicidal risk [3, 5–9].

MDD, migraine, anxiety, and pain symptoms mutually affect each other [10–12]. For example, strong bidirectional associations have been suggested to exist between psychiatric disorders, migraine, and suicide [13]. Among patients with chronic migraine, a higher affective dysregulated temperament score was found to be associated with a greater feeling of hopelessness and a higher suicidal risk [13]. Shared underlying genetic mechanisms have been reported for MDD and migraine [14]. In addition, migraine is also associated with increased risks of other diseases, such as cardiovascular diseases, cerebrovascular diseases, and fibromyalgia [15–19].

Nearly half of patients with MDD have comorbid migraine [20, 21]. MDD patients with migraine have greater severities of depression, anxiety, and pain symptoms than

* Correspondence: sjwang@vghtpe.gov.tw
[3]Faculty of Medicine and Brain Research Center, National Yang-Ming University and Neurological Institute, Taipei Veterans General Hospital, Taipei, Taiwan
[4]Department of Neurology, Taipei Veterans General Hospital, No. 201 Shi-Pai Road, Section 2, Taipei 112, Taiwan
Full list of author information is available at the end of the article

those without migraine [21, 22]. Migraine also has negative impacts on the recovery of health-related quality of life (HRQoL) and some pain symptoms after acute treatment [22, 23]. However, most of these studies were cross-sectional or acute treatment studies, and few studies have investigated the impacts of migraine on MDD during a long-term follow-up period. In a two-year follow-up study, migraine at baseline was an independent factor associated with upper and lower limb muscle soreness at the two-year follow-up point [24]. Another study found that migraine with active headache at follow-up was associated with greater severities of anxiety and somatic symptoms [25].

Several studies have investigated the associations of migraine with pain symptoms [22–24]. However, to our knowledge, no study has investigated the associations of migraine with the pain dimension of the HRQoL and pain symptoms among patients with MDD during a ten-year period. This issue is important for the following reasons: 1) pain symptoms are common, and are associated with a poorer prognosis of MDD [3, 7]; 2) migraine is a common comorbidity of MDD [20, 21], and the associations of migraine with pain symptoms should be clarified; and 3) in some patients with MDD, depression and pain symptoms are chronic and fluctuating. Several factors have been identified to be associated with chronic depression, such as a younger age at onset, a longer duration of depressive episode, a family history of mood disorders, and psychiatric comorbidities, including anxiety disorders, personality disorders, and substance abuse [26]. Factors associated with persisting pain symptoms post-three-month treatment among patients with MDD include a greater depressive severity, age < 40 years, more than one comorbidity, and previous MDD episodes [8]. In addition, persisting pain symptoms post-treatment were found to be associated with a poorer remission rate of depression [8]. Therefore, the outcomes of depression and pain symptoms interact and are correlated. Long-term follow-up studies are mandatory. Therefore, this study aimed to investigate the associations of migraine with the pain dimension of the HRQoL and pain symptoms among patients with MDD during a ten-year period. We hypothesized that migraine was associated with more severe pain symptoms and a poorer score in the pain dimension of the HRQoL among patients with MDD during a ten-year period, because migraine does not only encompass headache, but is also associated with other pain symptoms.

Methods

Subjects

This study was performed in the psychiatric outpatient clinics of the Chang Gung Memorial Hospital at Linkou, a medical center in northern Taiwan. At baseline (January 2004 to August 2007), consecutive outpatients who fulfilled the following three criteria were considered eligible subjects: 1) 18–65 years of age; 2) no antidepressants or other psychotropic drugs administered within the previous four weeks; and 3) met the DSM-IV-TR criteria for MDD and were experiencing a current major depressive episode (MDE) [27]. MDD and anxiety disorders were diagnosed according to the Structured Clinical Interview for DSM-IV-TR Axis I Disorders [28]. Moreover, three exclusion criteria were established to prevent confounding of somatic and pain symptoms, including 1) catatonic features, psychotic symptoms or severe psychomotor retardation with obvious difficulty in being interviewed; 2) a history of substance abuse or dependence without full remission in the previous month; and 3) chronic medical diseases such as hypertension, diabetes mellitus, and other medical diseases, except for headache.

At baseline, 290 subjects were enrolled. These patients were followed-up at the six-month, two-year, and ten-year points. The ten-year follow-ups were performed from August 2014 to December 2016. The study was approved by the Institutional Review Board of the Chang Gung Memorial Hospital. Based on the guidelines regulated in the Declaration of Helsinki, written informed consent was obtained from all subjects.

Assessment of headache

At baseline, all subjects completed a structured headache intake form, which reported headache patterns over the past year and included headache intensity, frequency, location, duration, aggravation by physical activities, phonophobia, photophobia, nausea, vomiting, precipitating factors, painkiller use, and aura. Then, an experienced headache specialist, who was blind to other results, interviewed all subjects and made headache diagnoses. This procedure was also performed at the two-year and ten-year follow-up points. At the six-month follow-up, diagnosis of migraine was taken as the baseline diagnosis.

At baseline and the two-year follow-up point, headache was diagnosed based on the International Classification of Headache Disorders, 2nd edition (ICHD-2) [29]. At the ten-year follow-up point, headache was diagnosed based on the ICHD-3 beta, and headache diagnoses at baseline and the two-year follow-up point were also updated to ICHD-3 beta diagnoses [30].

At each time point, subjects who fulfilled the criteria of migraine without aura (MO) and/or migraine with aura (MA) were classified as the "migraine" group, while the other subjects were categorized as the "non-migraine" group. The intensity and frequency of headaches were assessed at baseline and the three follow-up points. We used the visual analog scale (VAS) to evaluate the average headache intensity in the past week, rated from 0 (no pain) to 10 (pain as severe as I can imagine), and recorded the frequency of headache days.

Assessment of anxiety comorbidities

One psychiatrist, who was blind to other psychiatric data and headache diagnoses, used the Structured Clinical Interview for DSM-IV-TR Axis I Disorders to diagnose the following anxiety comorbidities: panic disorder, agoraphobia, specific phobia, social phobia, post-traumatic stress disorder, obsessive–compulsive disorder, and generalized anxiety disorder [28]. Subjects with any one of the seven anxiety disorders were classified as the "with any anxiety disorder" group, while the others were classified as the "without any anxiety disorder" group.

Instruments for the evaluation of pain, depression, and anxiety

The bodily pain subscale of the Short Form-36 (SF-BP) and the pain subscale (PS) of the Depression and Somatic Symptoms Scale (DSSS) were used to evaluate the pain dimension of HRQoL and pain severities, respectively [31–35]. The acute version of the Short Form-36 was used. SF-BP scores ranged from 0 to 100, a higher score indicating a better HRQoL [32, 33]. The PS of the DSSS evaluated the severities of five pain symptoms (headache, back pain, chest pain, neck and/or shoulder pain, and general muscle pain) in the past week. The total score of the PS ranged from 0 to 15, a higher score indicating a greater severity of pain symptoms.

To understand the longitudinal course of pain symptoms in the past 10 years, subjects were requested to report the percentages of time during which they had suffered the following pain symptoms in the past 10 years: headache, back pain, shoulder and/or neck pain, and general muscle pain.

The Hamilton Depression Rating Scale (HAMD) and the anxiety subscale of the Hospital Anxiety and Depression Scale (HADS-A) were used to evaluate depression and anxiety, respectively [35–37]. The scores ranged from 0 to 52 and 0–21 for the HAMD and HADS-A, respectively, and higher scores indicated a greater severity of symptoms.

The native language of our subjects was Chinese. The reliability and validity of the Chinese versions of the three administered scales (SF-36, HADS, and DSSS) have been established [31, 33–35].

Procedures

Subjects were followed-up at the time points of 6 months, 2 years, and 10 years after baseline enrollment. The SF-BP, PS, and HADS-A were administered at the three follow-up points, and the HAMD was evaluated by the same psychiatrist.

During the ten-year period, subjects might have quit pharmacotherapy or accepted pharmacotherapy intermittently. Pharmacotherapy was not controlled at the three follow-up points. At the index month of the follow-up point, patients who were not receiving pharmacotherapy were classified into the "without pharmacotherapy (in the index month)" group, whereas patients who were receiving pharmacotherapy were classified as the "with pharmacotherapy (in the index month)" group. This classification was used to avoid the confounding effects of pharmacotherapy in statistical analysis.

Statistical methods

All statistical analyses were performed using SPSS for Windows 20.0. The independent *t* test, Mann-Whitney U test, Kruskal-Wallis H test, Pearson's correlation, Spearman's correlation, and Chi-square test were used in appropriate situations.

Generalized Estimating Equation (GEE) models with robust error estimation and an unstructured covariance matrix were used to estimate the differences in SF-BP and PS scores between patients with and without migraine. The dependent variables were the SF-BP and PS scores. Initially, 10 variables were placed into the GEE model as independent variables, including six variables at baseline (age, gender, marital status, educational years, employment, with any anxiety disorders or not) and four variables at each follow-up point (with migraine or not, with pharmacotherapy or not, HAMD score, HADS-A score). Then, insignificant factors were removed from the GEE model one by one until all independent factors were significant.

A two-tailed P value of < 0.05 was taken to indicate statistical significance, and Bonferroni correction was used in appropriate situations.

Results

Subjects

For clarity, the labels "(B)", "(6 M)", "(2Y)" and "(10Y)" are used to represent data collected at baseline, and at the six-month, two-year, and ten-year follow-up points, respectively. At baseline, 290 subjects were enrolled. Table 1 shows the demographic variables, percentages of subjects with comorbidities, pain indices, and psychometric scores. There were no significant differences between patients who were and were not followed-up at the three follow-up points in terms of the five demographic variables, with the exception of the variable of age at the ten-year follow-up point (with vs. without follow-up: 41.3 ± 8.1 vs. 39.3 ± 8.2 years, $p = 0.04$). At the six-month and two-year time points, the percentage of subjects who attended follow-up was over 80%. At the ten-year follow-up point, approximately half of the subjects attended follow-up appointments. Of the subjects who did not complete the ten-year follow-up assessment ($n = 153$), 34.1% ($n = 99$) were unable to be contacted by phone or mail; 16.9% ($n = 49$) refused to participate in the follow-up; 1.0% ($n = 3$) had expired due to medical diseases; and 0.7% ($n = 2$) had their psychiatric diagnosis shifted to schizophrenia.

Table 1 Demographic variables, pain indices, and psychometric scores at different time points among patients with major depressive disorder

Time point	Baseline	Six-month follow-up	Two-year follow-up	Ten-year follow-up
Case number	290	254	237	137
Percentage of loss follow-up	–	12.4	18.3	52.8
Age (years)	30.2 ± 8.2	30.6 ± 8.2	32.5 ± 8.4	41.0 ± 8.1
Educational years	13.2 ± 2.4	13.3 ± 2.4	13.3 ± 2.4	13.3 ± 2.5
Female (%)	71.4	70.9	69.2	69.3
In employment (%)	57.2	56.7	55.7	57.7
Married (%)	42.1	42.1	43.0	44.5
With migraine (%)	46.9	46.5	22.8	38.0
With any anxiety disorders (%)	51.4	50.4	54.4	49.6
With pharmacotherapy (%)	0	47.6	27.4	27.7
BMI	21.4 ± 4.0	–	–	23.8 ± 4.3
SF-BP scores	48.3 ± 22.9	65.5 ± 23.6	68.4 ± 21.8	65.3 ± 20.5
PS scores	7.6 ± 3.8	4.1 ± 3.6	4.2 ± 3.3	4.7 ± 3.0
HAMD scores	23.4 ± 4.2	10.6 ± 7.8	10.4 ± 7.4	9.4 ± 6.4
HADS-A scores	15.0 ± 3.3	8.6 ± 4.8	9.0 ± 4.5	8.4 ± 4.7

BMI: body mass index; HAMD: Hamilton Depression Rating scale; HADS-A: anxiety subscale of the Hospital Anxiety and Depression scale; SF-BP: the bodily pain subscale of the Short Form 36; PS: pain subscale of the Depression and Somatic Symptoms scale

Headache and psychiatric diagnoses

Table 1 shows the percentages of patients with migraine at the different time points. At baseline, 136 subjects (46.9%) had migraine, including 116 MO (headache code 1.1) and 20 MO and MA (headache code 1.2). At the two-year follow-up point, 54 subjects (22.8%) had migraine, including 37 MO and 17 MO and MA. At the ten-year follow-up point, 52 subjects (38.0%) had migraine, including 42 MO and 10 MO and MA.

At baseline, 51.4% ($n = 149$) of the subjects had at least one anxiety disorder, including 12.1% ($n = 35$) with panic disorder, 11.7% ($n = 34$) with agoraphobia, 22.1% ($n = 64$) with specific phobia, 27.6% ($n = 80$) with social phobia, 10.7% ($n = 31$) with post-traumatic stress disorder, 9.3% ($n = 27$) with obsessive-compulsive disorder, and 5.5% ($n = 16$) with generalized anxiety disorder. Compared with the subjects without anxiety disorders, a higher percentage of the subjects with anxiety disorders had comorbid migraine (63.1% vs. 29.8%, $p < 0.001$).

Patients with migraine at the two-year and 10-year follow-up points had a longer total duration of pharmacotherapy (11.3 ± 8.1 vs. 7.8 ± 7.0 months, $p = 0.002$ at the two-year point; 28.3 ± 37.5 vs. 27.0 ± 35.8 months, $p = 0.84$ at the 10-year point) as compared with those without.

Differences in pain indices between groups

Table 2 shows the differences in the SF-BP and PS scores between groups at the four time points. Patients with migraine had a lower SF-BP score and a higher PS score than patients without migraine at all four time points after Bonferroni correction, with the exception of the PS score $_{(2Y)}$ in patients with pharmacotherapy.

Differences in the severities of depression, anxiety and headache indices between groups

Patients with migraine had a higher headache intensity and frequency than patients without migraine after Bonferroni correction (Table 3). Patients with migraine also had greater severities of depression and anxiety after Bonferroni correction, with the exception of the severities of depression $_{(6M)}$ and anxiety $_{(6M \text{ and } 10Y)}$ in patients without pharmacotherapy, and the severity of depression $_{(10Y)}$ in patients with pharmacotherapy.

Correlations of pain indices with depression, anxiety, and headache indices at the same time points

The SF-BP and PS scores were significantly (all $p < 0.001$) correlated with the severities of depression and anxiety, as well as the headache indices, at all four time points. The correlations of the SF-BP score with depression (correlation coefficient (r) ranged from − 070 to − 0.41), anxiety (r = − 0.59 to − 0.24), and headache intensity (r = − 0.59 to − 0.41) and frequency (r = − 0.54 to − 0.33) were negative. The correlations of the PS score with depression (r = 0.67 to 0.37), anxiety (r = 0.57 to 0.27), and headache intensity (r = 0.63 to 0.49) and frequency (r = 0.60 to 0.43) were positive.

Self-reported percentages of time with pain symptoms in the past ten years

The mean (± SD) percentages of time spent suffering pain in the head, neck and/or shoulder, back, and general

Table 2 The differences of the pain indices at four time points between patients with and without migraine

	Migraine	N	Without pharmacotherapy SF-BP	Without pharmacotherapy PS	N	With pharmacotherapy SF-BP	With pharmacotherapy PS
Baseline	Yes	136	37.7 ± 19.3**	9.6 ± 3.4**	–	–	–
Baseline	No	154	57.6 ± 21.8	5.9 ± 3.2	–	–	–
Six month	Yes	58	56.1 ± 26.9**	5.6 ± 4.1**	60	60.9 ± 21.8**	4.5 ± 3.9**
Six month	No	75	68.9 ± 22.6	3.8 ± 3.2	61	74.9 ± 18.9	2.5 ± 2.8
Two year	Yes	34	53.1 ± 22.2**	7.1 ± 4.3**	20	52.6 ± 18.7**	6.0 ± 2.7*
Two year	No	138	74.5 ± 19.9	3.1 ± 2.6	45	68.4 ± 19.8	4.4 ± 2.8
Ten year	Yes	38	59.0 ± 18.3**	5.9 ± 2.6**	14	47.3 ± 17.2**	7.3 ± 3.4**
Ten year	No	61	73.4 ± 19.5	3.6 ± 2.7	24	64.9 ± 19.0	4.1 ± 2.8

SF-BP the bodily pain subscale of the Short Form 36, *PS* the pain subscale of the Depression and Somatic Symptoms scale
*$P < 0.05$; ** Significance after Bonferroni correction with $P < 0.025$

muscles in the past 10 years were 30.2 ± 28.0, 47.0 ± 31.5, 32.6 ± 30.5, and 29.8 ± 30.8, respectively. The self-reported percentages of time spent with pain in the head (r ranged from − 0.27 to − 0.50 for the SF-BP; 0.35 to 0.55 for the PS), neck and/or shoulder (r = − 0.29 to − 0.60 for the SF-BP; 0.28 to 0.68 for the PS), back (r = − 0.23 to − 0.56 for the SF-BP; 0.35 to 0.67 for the PS), and general muscles (r = − 0.28 to − 0.59 for the SF-BP; 0.35 to 0.79 for the PS) were significantly (all $p < 0.01$) correlated with the SF-BP and PS scores at the four time points.

Figure 1 presents the differences in the self-reported percentages of time spent with pains in the different groups. Patients with migraine at the three time points $_{(B, 2Y, 10Y)}$ (group III) spent the highest percentage of time with the four pain symptoms (ranging from 60.0% to 73.7%), followed by patients with migraine at any two of the three points (group II). In contrast, patients without migraine at the three time points (group 0) had the lowest percentage of time spent with pain. In the post hoc analysis, significant differences between groups were noted for headache (group 0 vs. group I, II, and III; group I vs. group III), neck/shoulder pain (group 0 vs. group I, II, and III), back pain (group 0 vs. group II and III) and general muscle pain (group III vs. group 0, I, and II).

Factors independently associated with pain indices

Migraine was a significant factor associated with the SF-BP and PS scores after controlling for demographic variables, anxiety disorders at baseline, the severities of depression and anxiety at the same time points, and pharmacotherapy (Table 4). Compared with patients without migraine, in patients with migraine, the SF-BP score was lower by 8.93 points and the PS score was higher by 1.33 points after controlling for other factors.

Discussion

Migraine was a significant factor associated with the two pain indices after controlling for depression, anxiety, pharmacotherapy, and other factors (Table 4). Compared with MDD patients without migraine, MDD patients with migraine had a poorer HRQoL in the pain dimension and a higher pain severity at the four time points (Table 2). Moreover, patients with migraine also had greater severities of depression and anxiety (Table 3). Table 4 shows

Table 3 The difference of psychometric scores and headache indices at four time points between patients with and without migraine[a]

	Migraine	N	Without pharmacotherapy HAMD	Without pharmacotherapy HADS-A	Without pharmacotherapy HI	Without pharmacotherapy HF	N	With pharmacotherapy HAMD	With pharmacotherapy HADS-A	With pharmacotherapy HI	With pharmacotherapy HF
Baseline	Yes	136	24.8 ± 4.3**	15.7 ± 3.2**	6.4 ± 3.0**	4.3 ± 2.4**	–	–	–	–	–
Baseline	No	154	22.2 ± 3.8	14.3 ± 3.3	3.2 ± 2.7	2.3 ± 2.2	–	–	–	–	–
Six month	Yes	58	14.2 ± 9.1*	10.0 ± 5.0	3.7 ± 3.0**	2.8 ± 2.5**	60	10.5 ± 6.7**	9.1 ± 4.5**	2.9 ± 2.8**	2.2 ± 2.0***
Six month	No	75	11.0 ± 7.8	9.2 ± 4.7	1.5 ± 1.8	1.5 ± 2.2	61	6.7 ± 5.8	6.1 ± 4.1	1.4 ± 2.0	0.9 ± 1.4
Two year	Yes	34	16.3 ± 7.3**	12.0 ± 4.4**	5.2 ± 3.0**	2.6 ± 2.2**	20	15.7 ± 6.4**	11.9 ± 3.7**	4.8 ± 2.9**	2.6 ± 2.0**
Two year	No	138	8.4 ± 6.6	7.9 ± 4.1	1.5 ± 2.0	1.0 ± 1.5	45	9.6 ± 6.8	8.7 ± 4.3	2.3 ± 2.3	1.6 ± 1.8
Ten year	Yes	38	10.4 ± 5.5**	8.7 ± 4.8*	3.9 ± 3.0**	1.6 ± 1.5**	14	16.0 ± 6.8*	13.4 ± 4.5**	4.5 ± 3.5**	3.2 ± 2.7**
Ten year	No	61	6.4 ± 5.3	6.6 ± 4.1	1.3 ± 2.1	1.0 ± 1.5	24	11.3 ± 6.2	9.6 ± 3.7	1.3 ± 2.0	1.2 ± 1.7

HAMD hamilton depression rating scale, *HADS-A* anxiety subscale of the Hospital Anxiety and Depression scale, *HI* headache intensity, *HF* headache frequency
*$P < 0.05$; ** Significance after Bonferroni correction with $P < 0.0125$
[a]Headache intensity and frequency were measured using a 0–10 visual analog scale and the pain days of the past week, respectively

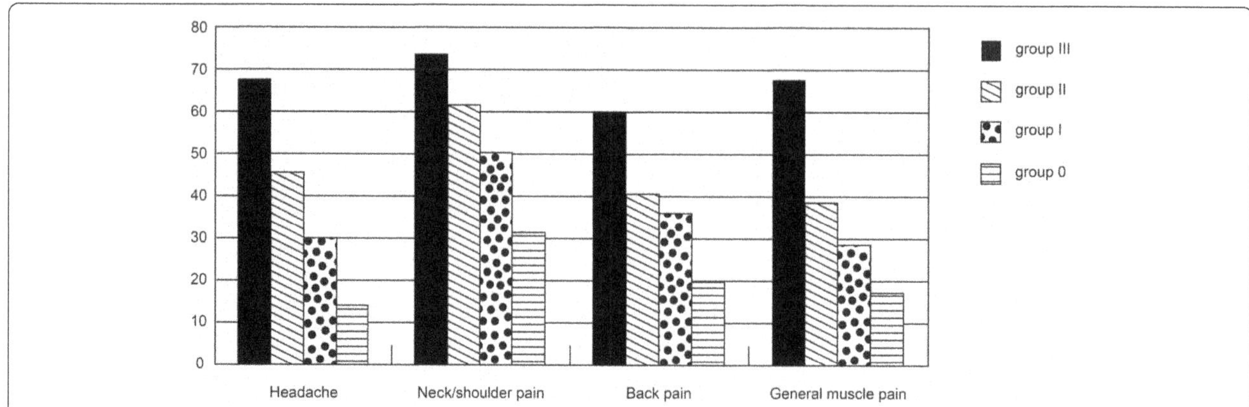

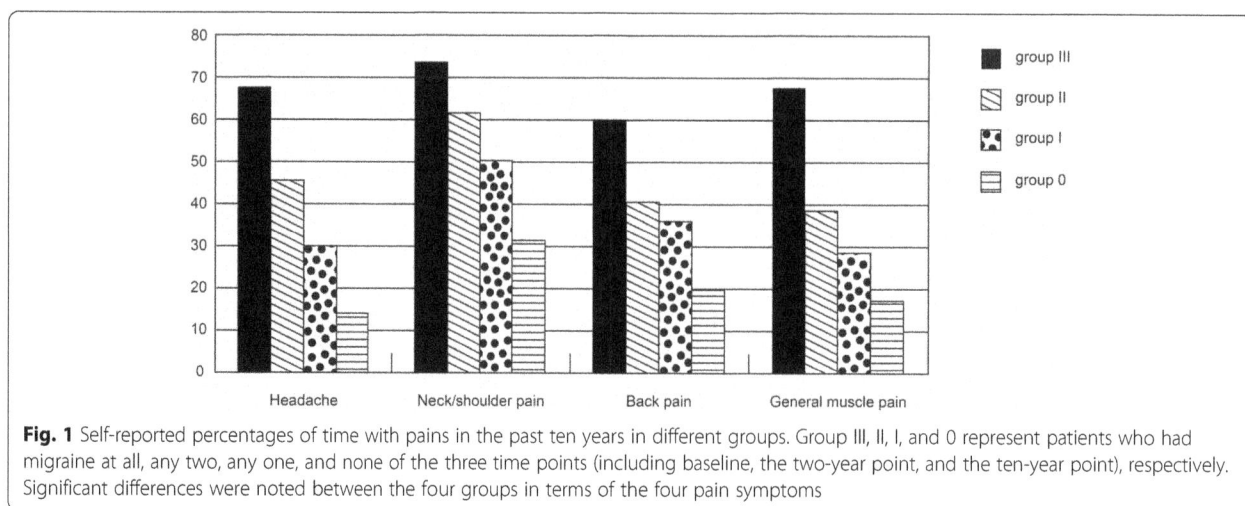

Fig. 1 Self-reported percentages of time with pains in the past ten years in different groups. Group III, II, I, and 0 represent patients who had migraine at all, any two, any one, and none of the three time points (including baseline, the two-year point, and the ten-year point), respectively. Significant differences were noted between the four groups in terms of the four pain symptoms

that migraine, HAMD score, and HADS-A score were independent factors associated with the PS and SF-BP. Therefore, the severities of depression and anxiety could only explain part of the pain symptoms in MDD patients. Migraine is an important but relatively neglected factor associated with pain symptoms, and was found to be independent of the effects of depression and anxiety. In fact, a previous study reported that migraine affects pain symptoms among psychiatric outpatients to a greater degree than MDE [20]. As discussed above, migraine was an important factor associated with pain symptoms in this study (Table 4). Pharmacotherapy for MDD that focuses on depression and anxiety only and neglects the role of migraine in pain symptoms might fail to fully resolve pain symptoms and lead to residual symptoms. This might be one of reasons why pain symptoms often become residual symptoms [38]. Our results implied that depression and migraine should be treated simultaneously. Migraine prevention is important, because migraine is not only associated with pain, but also with cardiovascular diseases, cerebrovascular diseases, and fibromyalgia [15–19]. In an animal study, decreases in pain symptoms were associated with improvement of depressive-like behaviors [39]. Depression and pain symptoms interact. There is a possibility that improving pain symptoms might decrease depressive symptoms among patients with depression; however, more research and evidence are indicated to support this hypothesis. Nonsteroidal anti-inflammatory drugs are commonly-used medications for headache [40]. Patients with MDD who use nonsteroidal anti-inflammatory drugs for headache should be monitored for medication overuse, because depression and anxiety are associated with a higher risk of medication-overuse headache [41, 42]. In fact, some therapeutic strategies for depression are also effective in treating migraine, including antidepressants (such as serotonin-norepinephrine re-uptake inhibitors and amitriptyline), cognitive behavioral therapy, and relaxation techniques [43]. Cognitive behavioral therapy might

Table 4 Independent variables associated with pain indices[a]

Dependent variable	Independent variable	Estimate	Standard error	95% CI	*P*
SF-BP	Migraine (yes vs. no)	−8.93	1.40	−6.20 to −11.67	< 0.001
	HAMD (one-point increment)	−1.20	0.10	−1.00 to − 1.40	< 0.001
	HADS-A (one-point increment)	−0.59	0.19	−0.22 to −0.96	< 0.01
	Educational years (one-year increment)	0.90	0.29	1.47 to 0.32	< 0.01
PS	Migraine (yes vs. no)	1.33	0.23	1.78 to 0.89	< 0.001
	HAMD (one-point increment)	0.19	0.02	0.22 to 0.16	< 0.001
	HADS-A (one-point increment)	0.12	0.03	0.18 to 0.06	< 0.001
	Educational years (one-year increment)	−0.13	0.05	−0.03 to −0.23	0.01
	Married (yes vs. no)	0.53	0.21	0.95–0.12	0.01
	Age (one-year increment)	0.03	0.01	0.05 to 0.004	0.02
	Anxiety disorders (yes vs. no)	0.52	0.24	1.00 to 0.05	0.03

HAMD hamilton depression rating scale, *HADS-A* anxiety subscale of the Hospital Anxiety and Depression scale, *SF-BP* the bodily pain subscale of the Short Form 36, *PS* pain subscale of the Depression and Somatic Symptoms scale
[a]Generalized Estimating Equations models were used in this Table

improve patients' self-management of diseases and promote adaptive behaviors and skills for coping with stress [43]. Physicians might use multi-model therapeutic strategies based on patient preference, disease severity, possible adverse side effects, and prior adherence history.

Two points are worth noting: 1) The patients in group III had the highest percentage of time spent with pain in the past 10 years (Fig. 1). The higher the frequency of migraine, the more often the patient suffered from pain symptoms. In fact, the patients in group III suffered from pain most of the time during the 10 years (ranging from 60.0% to 73.7%). Therefore, migraine should be treated and prevented during treatment for MDD. 2) For a long time, pain symptoms were considered a part of MDD symptoms [3]. In this study, the severities of depression and anxiety were significantly correlated with the SF-BP and PS scores at the same time points. This demonstrated that pain symptoms were associated with the severities of depression and anxiety. Moreover, our results also showed that pain symptoms in MDD patients might be partially associated with the comorbidity of migraine. Among patients without migraine at all time points (group 0), the self-reported percentage of time with pain was significantly lower than that of the other groups. The causal relationships between depression, anxiety, migraine, and pain symptoms should be further studied.

Migraine resulted in a poorer HRQoL in the pain dimension and a higher pain severity at the long-term follow-up points. This may result from several reasons: 1) Migraine is associated with sensory hypersensitivity [44]. Patients with migraine exhibit generalized pressure pain hypersensitivity in the head as compared with healthy controls [45]. Sensory stimuli can trigger migraine attacks, and central sensitization, characterized by abnormal neuronal excitability, allodynia, and hyperalgesia, may occur when headache attacks are experienced repeatedly [10, 46]. Compared with healthy controls, patients with migraine demonstrated increased neural activity in response to negative emotional stimuli [47]. Therefore, MDD patients with migraine may be more susceptible to other pain symptoms. Central sensitization may be one of the possible mechanisms shared between migraine, pain symptoms, and somatization [48]. 2) The SF-BP and PS include a headache component. Based on the ICH-3 beta criteria, migraine attack is characterized by moderate to severe headache, and is accompanied with physical activity limitation and other somatic symptoms. These may cause functional impairment and significant negative impacts on HRQoL. In fact, migraine was ranked as the seventh leading cause of functional disability [49].

Some limitations or bias should be addressed. 1) Approximately half of the subjects did not attend the ten-year follow-up appointment. Patients who refused to continue to participate in the study or who were unable to be contacted might be associated with a greater severity of depression, which may have caused bias. 2) The interval between the two-year and ten-year follow-up points was long. Unequal follow-up intervals might have caused bias. Frequent follow-up is required in future studies. 3) Due to memory bias, the self-reported percentage of time spent suffering pain in the past 10 years might be not very accurate. Although the self-reported percentages of time with pain were gross estimations, the self-reported indices were significantly correlated with the SF-BP and PS scores at all time points. 4) Although pharmacotherapy was included in the GEE model, the kind and amount of medication were not controlled, because the study was of an observational design. 5) The study excluded MDD patients with other chronic medical diseases at baseline and did not monitor whether these medical diseases and factors related to cardiovascular risk had developed at the follow-up points. In future studies, medical comorbidities should be monitored at follow-up, because these comorbidities might influence the pain threshold [50].

Conclusion

After controlling for depression, anxiety and other factors, migraine was independently associated with a poorer HRQoL in the pain dimension and more severe pain symptoms among patients with MDD. During the ten-year study period, the higher the frequency of migraine, the more often patients with MDD suffered from pain symptoms. Migraine prevention should be integrated into the treatment of depression, because simultaneous treatment of depression and migraine might help to improve pain symptoms and the score in the pain dimension of the HRQoL. Physicians should employ therapeutic strategies, including pharmacotherapy, cognitive behavioral therapy, and relaxation techniques, for the simultaneous treatment of depression and migraine.

Abbreviations

DSSS: Depression and Somatic Symptoms Scale; GEE: Generalized Estimating Equations; HADS-A: anxiety subscale of the Hospital Anxiety and Depression Scale; HRQoL: health-related quality of life; ICHD-2: International Classification of Headache Disorders, 2nd edition; ICHD-3 beta: International Classification of Headache Disorders, 3rd edition (beta version); MA: migraine with aura; MDD: major depressive disorder; MDE: major depressive episode; MO: migraine without aura; PS: pain subscale of the Depression and Somatic Symptoms Scale; SF-BP: bodily pain subscale of the Short Form-36; VAS: visual analog scale

Acknowledgements

This study was supported in part by Chang Gung Memorial Hospital Research Programs (CMRPG 3E2141, CMRPG 3G0251, and CLRPG3D0043). The funding sources had no further role in study design; in the collection, analysis and interpretation of data; in the writing of the report; and in the decision to submit the paper for publication. We also would like to thank the Brain Research Center, National Yang-Ming University from the Featured Areas Research Center Program within the framework of the Higher Education Sprout Project by the Ministry of Education (MOE) in Taiwan.

Funding

This study was supported in part by Chang Gung Memorial Hospital Research Programs (CMRPG 3E2141, CMRPG 3G0251, and CLRPG3D0043).

Authors' contributions

SJW and CIH participated in the design of the study. CIH, CYL, and CHY managed data collection. All authors contributed to data analysis and interpretation. CIH wrote the first draft of the manuscript. All authors contributed to and have approved the final version.

Competing interests

All authors declare that they have no conflicts of interest.

Author details

[1]Department of Psychiatry, Chang-Gung Memorial Hospital at Linkou and Chang-Gung University College of Medicine, Tao-Yuan, Taiwan. [2]Department of Nursing, Chang Gung University of Science and Technology, Tao-Yuan, Taiwan. [3]Faculty of Medicine and Brain Research Center, National Yang-Ming University and Neurological Institute, Taipei Veterans General Hospital, Taipei, Taiwan. [4]Department of Neurology, Taipei Veterans General Hospital, No. 201 Shi-Pai Road, Section 2, Taipei 112, Taiwan.

References

1. Ligthart L, Gerrits MM, Boomsma DI, Penninx BW (2013) Anxiety and depression are associated with migraine and pain in general: an investigation of the interrelationships. J Pain 14:363–370
2. Hung CI, Liu CY, Fu TS (2015) Depression: an important factor associated with disability among patients with chronic low back pain. Int J Psychiatry Med 49:187–198
3. Jaracz J, Gattner K, Jaracz K, Górna K (2016) Unexplained painful physical symptoms in patients with major depressive disorder: prevalence, pathophysiology and management. CNS Drugs 30:293–304
4. Mcintosh AM, Hall LS, Zeng Y, Adams MJ, Gibson J, Wigmore E et al (2016) Genetic and environmental risk for chronic pain and the contribution of risk variants for major depressive disorder: a family-based mixed-model analysis. PLoS Med 13:e1002090
5. Harada E, Satoi Y, Kikuchi T, Watanabe K, Alev L, Mimura M (2016) Residual symptoms in patients with partial versus complete remission of a major depressive disorder episode: patterns of painful physical symptoms in depression. Neuropsychiatr Dis Treat 12:1599–1607
6. Jeon HJ, Woo JM, Kim HJ, Fava M, Mischoulon D, Cho SJ et al (2016) Gender differences in somatic symptoms and current suicidal risk in outpatients with major depressive disorder. Psychiatry Investig 13:609–615
7. Lin HS, Wang FC, Lin CH (2015) Pain affects clinical patterns and treatment outcomes for patients with major depressive disorder taking fluoxetine. J Clin Psychopharmacol 35:661–666
8. Novick D, Montgomery W, Aguado J, Peng X, Haro JM (2017) Factors associated with and impact of pain persistence in Asian patients with depression: a 3-month, prospective observational study. Int J Psychiatry Clin Pract 21:29–35
9. Novick D, Montgomery W, Moneta MV, Peng X, Brugnoli R, Haro JM (2015) Chinese patients with major depression: do concomitant pain symptoms affect quality of life independently of severity of depression? Int J Psychiatry Clin Pract 19:174–181
10. De Tommaso M, Sciruicchio V (2016) Migraine and central sensitization: clinical features, main comorbidities and therapeutic perspectives. Curr Rheumatol Rev 12:113–126
11. Dindo LN, Recober A, Haddad R, Calarge CA (2017) Comorbidity of migraine, major depressive disorder, and generalized anxiety disorder in adolescents and young adults. Int J Behav Med 24:528–534
12. Plesh O, Adams SH, Gansky SA (2012) Self-reported comorbid pains in severe headaches or migraines in a US national sample. Headache 52: 946–956
13. Serafini G, Pompili M, Innamorati M, Gentile G, Borro M, Lamis DA et al (2012) Gene variants with suicidal risk in a sample of subjects with chronic migraine and affective temperamental dysregulation. Eur Rev Med Pharmacol Sci 16(10):1389–1398
14. Yang Y, Ligthart L, Terwindt GM, Boomsma DI, Rodriguez-Acevedo AJ, Nyholt DR (2016) Genetic epidemiology of migraine and depression. Cephalalgia 36:679–691
15. Mahmoud AN, Mentias A, Elgendy AY, Qazi A, Barakat AF, Saad M et al (2018) Migraine and the risk of cardiovascular and cerebrovascular events: a meta-analysis of 16 cohort studies including 1152407subjects. BMJ Open 8(3):e020498
16. Tana C, Giamberardino MA, Cipollone F (2017) microRNA profiling in atherosclerosis, diabetes, and migraine. Ann Med 49(2):93–105
17. Giamberardino MA, Affaitati G, Martelletti P, Tana C, Negro A, Lapenna D et al (2015) Impact of migraine on fibromyalgia symptoms. J Headache Pain 17:28
18. Tana C, Tafuri E, Tana M, Martelletti P, Negro A, Affaitati G et al (2013) New insights into the cardiovascular risk of migraine and the role of white matter hyperintensities: is gold all that glitters? J Headache Pain 14:9
19. Tana C, Santilli F, Martelletti P, di Vincenzo A, Cipollone F, Davì G et al (2015) Correlation between migraine severity and cholesterol levels. Pain Pract 15(7):662–670
20. Hung CI, Liu CY, Wang SJ (2013) Migraine predicts physical and pain symptoms among psychiatric outpatients. J Headache Pain 14:19
21. Oedegaard KJ, Fasmer OB (2005) Is migraine in unipolar depressed patients a bipolar spectrum trait? J Affect Disord 84:233–242
22. Hung CI, Liu CY, Chen CY, Yang CH, Wang SJ (2014) The impacts of migraine and anxiety disorders on painful physical symptoms among patients with major depressive disorder. J Headache Pain 15:73
23. Hung CI, Liu CY, Yang CH, Wang SJ (2012) The negative impact of migraine on quality of life after four weeks of treatment in patients with major depressive disorder. Psychiatry Clin Neurosci 66:8–16
24. Hung CI, Liu CY, Yang CH, Wang SJ (2016) Headache: an important factor associated with muscle soreness/pain at the two-year follow-up point among patients with major depressive disorder. J Headache Pain 17:57
25. Hung CI, Liu CY, Yang CH, Wang SJ (2015) The impacts of migraine among outpatients with major depressive disorder at a two-year follow-up. PLoS One 10:e0128087
26. Hölzel L, Härter M, Reese C, Kriston L (2011) Risk factors for chronic depression–a systematic review. J Affect Disord 129:1–13
27. American Psychiatric Association (2000) Diagnostic and statistical manual of mental disorders, fourth edition text revision (DSM-IV-TR). American Psychiatric Association, Washington, DC
28. First MB, Spitzer RL, Gibbon M, Williams JBW (2002) Structured clinical interview for DSM-IV-TR Axis I disorders, research version, patient edition (SCID-I/P). Biometrics Research, New York State Psychiatric Institute, New York
29. Headache Classification Subcommittee of the International Headache Society (2004) The international classification of headache disorders, 2nd ed. Cephalalgia 24(Suppl 1):1–160
30. Headache Classification Subcommittee of the International Headache Society (2013) The international classification of headache disorders, 3rd edition (beta version). Cephalalgia 33:629–808
31. Hung CI, Weng LJ, Su YJ, Liu CY (2006) Depression and somatic symptoms scale: a new scale with both depression and somatic symptoms emphasized. Psychiatry Clin Neurosci 60:700–708
32. Ware JE, Sherboune CD (1992) The MOS 36-item short-form health survey (SF-36). I Conceptual framework and item selection. Med Care 30:473–483
33. Tseng HM, Lu JF, Tsai YJ (2003) Assessment of health-related quality of life, II: norming and validation of SF-36 Taiwan version. Taiwan J Public Health 22:512–518
34. Chou YH, Lee CP, Liu CY, Hung CI (2017) Construct validity of the depression and somatic symptoms scale: evaluated by Mokken scale analysis. Neuropsychiatr Dis Treat 13:205–211
35. Hung CI, Liu CY, Wang SJ, Yao YC, Yang CH (2012) The cut-off points of the depression and somatic symptoms scale and the hospital anxiety and depression scale in detecting non-full remission and a current major depressive episode. Int J Psychiatry Clin Pract 16:33–40

36. Hamilton M (1967) Development of a rating scale for primary depressive illness. Br J Soc Clin Psychol 6:278–296
37. Zigmond AS, Snaith RP (1983) The hospital anxiety and depression scale. Acta Psychiatr Scand 67:361–370
38. Hung CI, Liu CY, Wang SJ, Yang CH (2014) Residual symptoms related to physical and panic symptoms at baseline predict remission of depression at follow-up. Psychopathology 47:51–56
39. Zhao X, Wang C, Zhang JF, Liu L, Liu AM, Ma Q et al (2014) Chronic curcumin treatment normalizes depression-like behaviors in mice with mononeuropathy: involvement of supraspinal serotonergic system and GABAA receptor. Psychopharmacology 231(10):2171–2187
40. Affaitati G, Martelletti P, Lopopolo M, Tana C, Massimini F, Cipollone F et al (2017) Use of nonsteroidal anti-inflammatory drugs for symptomatic treatment of episodic headache. Pain Pract 17(3):392–401
41. Lampl C, Thomas H, Tassorelli C, Katsarava Z, Laínez JM, Lantéri-Minet M et al (2016) Headache, depression and anxiety: associations in the Eurolight project. J Headache Pain 17:59
42. Sarchielli P, Corbelli I, Messina P, Cupini LM, Bernardi G, Bono G et al (2016) Psychopathological comorbidities in medication-overuse headache: a multicentre clinical study. Eur J Neurol 23(1):85–91
43. Peck KR, Smitherman TA, Baskin SM (2015) Traditional and alternative treatments for depression: implications for migraine management. Headache 55:351–355
44. Demarquay G, Mauguiere F (2016) Central nervous system underpinnings of sensory hypersensitivity in migraine: insights from neuroimaging and electrophysiological studies. Headache 56:1418–1438
45. Baron J, Ruiz M, Palacios-Cena M, Madeleine P, Guerrero ÁL, Arendt-Nielsen L et al (2017) Differences in topographical pressure pain sensitivity maps of the scalp between patients with migraine and healthy controls. Headache 57:226–235
46. De Tommaso M, Sciruicchio V, Delussi M, Vecchio E, Goffredo M, Simeone M et al (2017) Symptoms of central sensitization and comorbidity for juvenile fibromyalgia in childhood migraine: an observational study in a tertiary headache center. J Headache Pain 18:59
47. Wilcox SL, Veggeberg R, Lemme J, Hodkinson DJ, Scrivani S, Burstein R et al (2016) Increased functional activation of limbic brain regions during negative emotional processing in migraine. Front Hum Neurosci 10:366
48. Grassini S, Nordin S (2017) Comorbidity in migraine with functional somatic syndromes, psychiatric disorders and inflammatory diseases: a matter of central sensitization? Behav Med 43:91–99
49. Steiner TJ, Stovner LJ, Birbeck GL (2013) Migraine: the seventh disabler. J Headache Pain 14:1
50. Costantini R, Affaitati G, Massimini F, Tana C, Innocenti P, Giamberardino MA (2016) Laparoscopic cholecystectomy for gallbladder calculosis in fibromyalgia patients: impact on musculoskeletal pain, somatic hyperalgesia and central sensitization. PLoS One 11(4):e0153408

14

Increased thalamic glutamate/glutamine levels in migraineurs

Adina Bathel[1,2], Lauren Schweizer[1], Philipp Stude[1], Benjamin Glaubitz[1], Niklas Wulms[3], Sibel Delice[1] and Tobias Schmidt-Wilcke[3,4*]

Abstract

Background: Increased cortical excitability has been hypothesized to play a critical role in various neurological disorders, such as restless legs syndrome, epilepsy and migraine. Particularly for migraine, local hyperexcitability has been reported. Levels of regional excitatory and inhibitory neurotransmitters are related to cortical excitability and hence may play a role in the origin of the disease. Consequently, a mismatch of the excitatory-inhibitory neurotransmitter network might contribute to local hyperexcitability and the onset of migraine attacks. In this study we sought to assess local levels of glutamate / glutamine (GLX) and gamma-aminobutyric acid (GABA) in the occipital cortex and right thalamus of migraineurs and healthy subjects.

Methods: We measured interictally local biochemical concentrations in the occipital lobe and the right thalamus in patients with migraine (without aura) and healthy controls (HCs) using proton magnetic resonance spectroscopy at 3 T. GLX levels were acquired using PRESS and GABA levels using the GABA-sensitive editing sequence MEGA-PRESS. Regional GLX and GABA levels were compared between groups.

Results: Statistical analyses revealed significantly increased GLX levels in both the primary occipital cortex and thalamus. However, we found no group differences in GABA levels for these two regions. Correlation analyses within the migraine group revealed no significant correlations between pain intensity and levels of GLX or GABA in either of the two brain regions.

Conclusions: Further research is needed to investigate the role of GABA/GLX ratios in greater depth and to measure changes in neurotransmitter levels over time, i.e. during migraine attacks and interictally.

Keywords: Migraine, Headache, Thalamus, Occipital cortex, GABA, Spectroscopy

Background

Migraine is one of the most common neurological disorders, thought to affect up to 6% of men and 18% of women in western industrialized countries [1]. Apart from severe headaches, migraine patients often experience additional symptoms such as nausea and phono- and photophobia, strongly suggesting a multisystem involvement of the disease. The underlying mechanisms of migraine attacks, however, are not fully understood and different pathophysiological mechanisms have been proposed, such as dysfunction of the nucleus coeruleus [2], sterile neurogenic inflammation of the meninges [3] and cortical spreading depression [4]. Genetic studies have exposed a potential involvement of both glutamatergic and GABAergic receptors [5–8]. Additionally, there has been evidence of interictal hyperexcitability, e.g. in the visual cortex [9–12], suggesting a mechanistic role of an excitatory-inhibitory dysbalance contributing to the pathophysiology of migraine. However, the specific roles of glutamate and glutamine (GLX) on the one hand and gamma-amino-butyric acid (GABA) on the other hand, the major excitatory and inhibitory neurotransmitters in the brain, respectively, remain to be fully elucidated.

In vivo measurement of neurometabolite concentrations in the brain remains challenging; standardized clinical techniques, such as lumbar puncture and cerebrospinal

* Correspondence: tobias-schmidt-wilcke@t-online.de
[3]Department of Neurology, St. Mauritius Therapieklinik, Meerbusch, Germany
[4]Institute of Clinical Neuroscience and Medical Psychology, Universitätsklinikum Düsseldorf, Düsseldorf, Germany
Full list of author information is available at the end of the article

fluid (CSF) analysis exclude the possibility to link abnormal metabolite levels to specific regions, but instead generalize the pathophysiology to the entire CNS. In vivo proton magnetic resonance spectroscopy (^{1}H-MRS), however, can be used to measure local concentrations of neurometabolites in the human brain non-invasively. Recent studies have investigated altered neurometabolite levels in migraine patients during interictal periods and have presented evidence of both, increased GLX levels in the occipital cortex [12, 13] as well as altered GABA levels in the occipital and posterior cingulate cortices [14, 15]. GABA levels in the occipital cortex were shown to be either reduced in migraine patients as compared to HCs [15] or unchanged, but with an association between GABA levels and disease severity, such that lower levels were related to higher disease severity [16]. Using a more GABA-sensitive editing sequence, Mescher-Garwood-Point Resolved Spectroscopy (MEGA-PRESS), Aguila and colleagues could show that migraine patients also displayed altered GABA in the posterior cingulate cortex, in this case increased levels [14].

Apart from the occipital and cingulate cortices there are several other brain regions that have implications in the pathophysiology of migraine, but also in pain in general. One of these regions is the thalamus, a subcortical brain structure that is tightly coupled in a bidirectional manner with the cortex. The thalamus is best known for its role in relaying almost all sensory modalities to the brain [17, 18]. The presence of multi-sensory symptoms during migraine attacks and the central role of thalamic indicate a potential involvement of the thalamus during the attacks themselves. Interestingly Noseda et al. could recently demonstrate the direct effect of GLX and GABA on the activity of thalamic trigeminovascular neurons [19]. However, to our knowledge, no studies have been performed that specifically looked at thalamic GLX and GABA levels in migraine patients.

Using ^{1}H-MRS, and specifically the MEGA-PRESS technique, we investigated migraine patients (without aura) and HCs to determine whether thalamic and occipital GLX and GABA levels are altered in migraine patients, and whether local transmitter concentrations relate to any pain features. Migraine patients were scanned interictally at least three days after their last attack and two days before the next. We hypothesized that migraine patients would show a shift towards an increased excitatory tone, either in terms of increased GLX or decreased GABA levels.

Methods

Subjects

Migraine patients were recruited consecutively from the headache-outpatient clinic of the Neurology Department of the University Hospital Bergmannsheil Bochum. Study participants provided informed written consent prior to study enrollment. The local ethics committee had approved of the study (No. 4823–13). Migraine was diagnosed by an experienced neurologist (PS) according to the revised criteria for migraine of the International Headache Society [20]. To participate in the study migraineurs had to report (prior to enrolment) a migraine frequency of at least two migraine attacks per month. Only patients with migraine without aura were included. Participants were therapy naïve, or paused a consisting migraine prophylaxis 14 days prior to the MR scan. Only patients who had been pain free for at least 72 h prior to scanning and 48 h thereafter were enrolled. Migraine patients were compared to HCs. HCs had no personal or family history of migraine. Participants were excluded if they were taking medication affecting CNS metabolism (e.g. anticonvulsant/antidepressant medications) or had a history of neurological or psychiatric diseases, e.g. multiple sclerosis, schizophrenia, or mood disorders. All subjects underwent a thorough neurological examination. Patients additionally rated pain intensity during the last two attacks and completed the Migraine Disability Assessment (MIDAS). Since depression frequently co-occurs with migraine, we also screened for depressive symptoms. Patients filled out the Beck depression inventory questionnaire (BDI). Only patients with BDI scores < 20 (where 20 or more indicate the presence of a moderate or severe depression) were included. For details see Table 1.

Spectroscopy

^{1}H-MRS was performed using a Philips 3.0 T Achieva X-series scanner with a 32-channel head coil. The MRI session consisted of a high resolution T1-weighted scan (MPRAGE, TR/TE: 8.5/3.9 ms, voxel size $(1\ \text{mm})^3$ isotropic, FOV $240 \times 240 \times 220$ mm) allowing an accurate voxel placement, as well as PRESS and MEGA-PRESS scans of the occipital cortex ($3 \times 3 \times 3\ \text{cm}^3$, centered around the midline projecting to the primary visual cortex), and the right thalamus ($3 \times 3 \times 2.5\ \text{cm}^3$). For the thalamic voxel the medial edge was aligned with the third ventricle, its anterior edge with the most anterior point of the thalamus. Of note, the thalamic voxel included to some degree the right globus pallidus and putamen in the average subject (for voxel placement and representative spectra see also Figs. 1 and 2).

PRESS sequences used here had the following parameters: TR/TE: 2000/30 ms, spectral bandwidth of 2 kHz, sampling rate of 2048 points, 90-degree flip angle, number of signals averaged = 32. The MEGA-PRESS sequence used a longer TE (TR/TE: 2000/68 ms) and contained a 14-ms sinc-gaussian ON editing pulse at

Table 1 Study cohort

Study#	Gender	Age	Maximum Pain Intensity	Average Pain Intensity	Number of Days with Headache (last 3 months)	MIDAS Grade	BDI Score
1	F	39	7	7	3	3	7
2	F	23	6	6	27	4	1
4	F	29	7	7	40	4	6
6	M	32	10	5	4	3	3
7	M	35	7	7	18	3	3
9	M	45	7	7	3	4	11
10	F	39	4	4	6	3	5
15	F	43	5	5	5	3	0
16	F	31	8	8	5	3	0
19	F	26	8	6	20	3	1
20	F	36	8	8	35	4	2
21	F	32	9	8	12	4	16
48	F	24	8	7	6	2	2
49	F	66	8	8	20	4	4
50	F	29	3	3	2	1	0

Clinical descriptors: *BDI* Beck depression inventory, *F* female, *M* male, *MIDAS* Migraine Disability Assessment

1.9 ppm and an OFF editing pulse at 7.46 ppm (spectral bandwidth of 2 kHz and a sampling rate of 2048 points). A total of 320 transients were acquired: 10 averages of 16 ON and 10 averages 16 OFF scans. For both Point-RESolved Spectroscopy (PRESS) and MEGA-PRESS sequences, a PB-auto second order shim was used to reduce field inhomogeneities and water suppression was accomplished using VAPOR (80 Hz window). Macromolecules were not suppressed; therefore, GABA in this study refers to GABA+ macromolecules (GABA+).

Glutamate/glutamine (GLX), N-acetylaspartate (NAA), and creatine (Cr) concentrations from the PRESS acquisition were quantified using LCModel's (version 6.3) standard basis set including water scaling. Of note, since there is no Cr in the CSF, the metabolite to Cr ratio serves the additional purpose of tissue correction, which is an alternative to referencing the metabolite in question to water with an additional correction for tissue volume (gray and white matter). As Cr and phosphocreatine (PCr) cannot be resolved reliably at 3 T, Cr_{total} here refers to Cr and PCr.

After metabolite quantification, we assessed spectral quality before performing statistical analyses, e.g. group comparison. First of all, spectra were inspected visually, in some cases no metabolite signal could be detected and data were excluded from further analyses. Additionally, LCModel allows for the estimation of signal to noise ratios (SNRs). SNR is defined as the ratio of the maximum in the spectrum minus the baseline (within the analysis window) to twice the root mean square of the

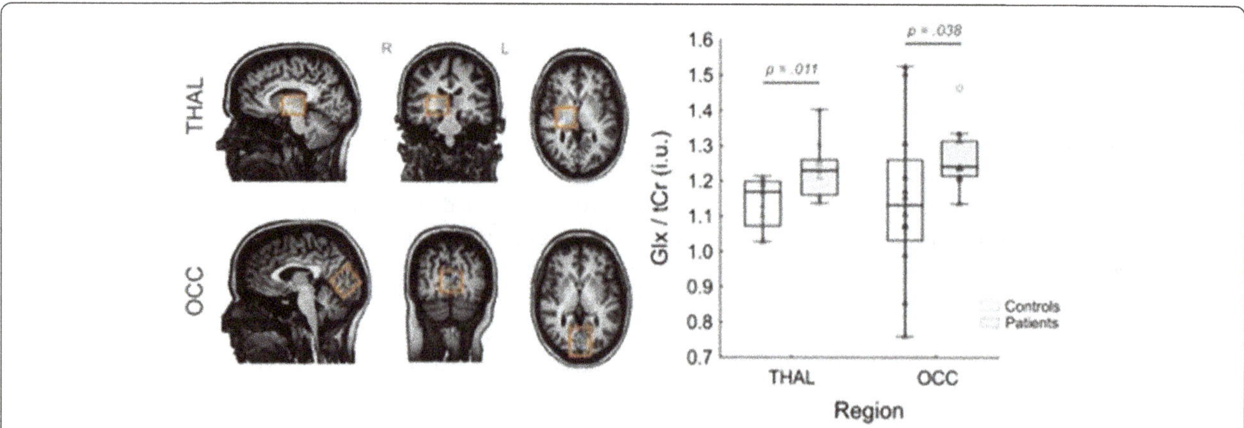

Fig. 1 Placement of spectroscopy voxels. Abbreviations: Cr = creatine, GLX = glutamate/glutamine, OCC = occipital cortex Thal = thalamus. Orange box depicts voxel placement in the thalamus and occipital cortex

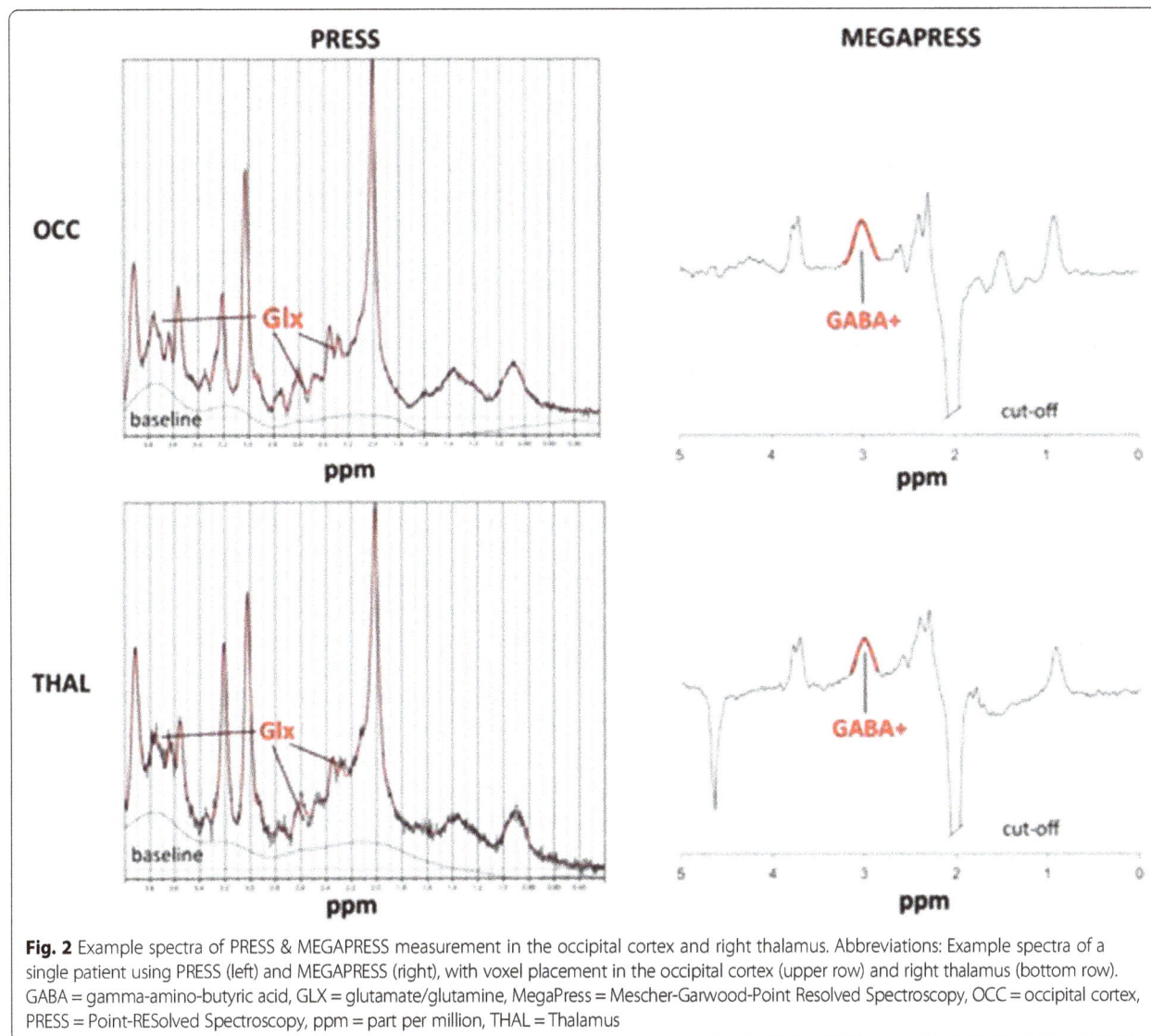

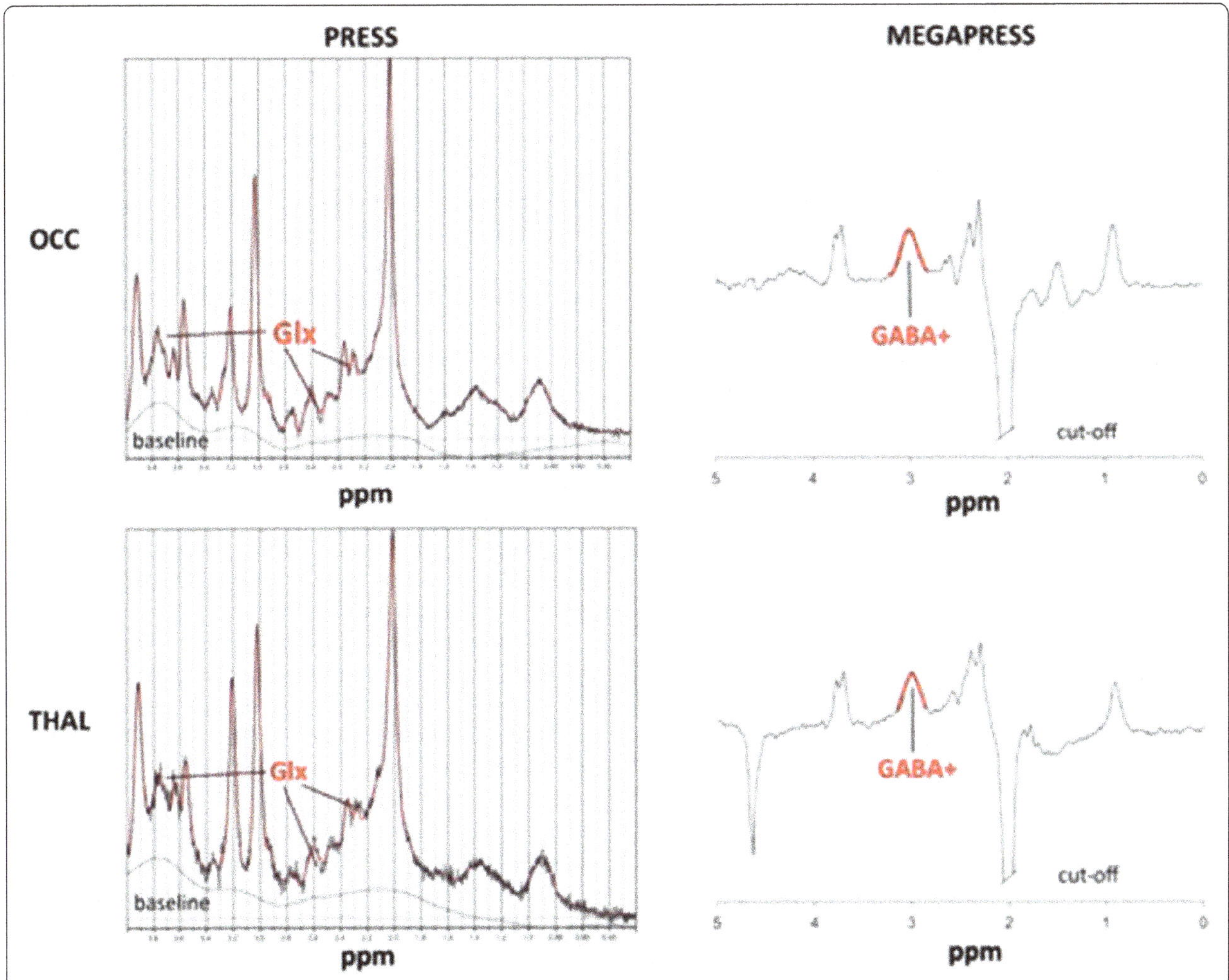

Fig. 2 Example spectra of PRESS & MEGAPRESS measurement in the occipital cortex and right thalamus. Abbreviations: Example spectra of a single patient using PRESS (left) and MEGAPRESS (right), with voxel placement in the occipital cortex (upper row) and right thalamus (bottom row). GABA = gamma-amino-butyric acid, GLX = glutamate/glutamine, MegaPress = Mescher-Garwood-Point Resolved Spectroscopy, OCC = occipital cortex, PRESS = Point-RESolved Spectroscopy, ppm = part per million, THAL = Thalamus

residuals. If spectra displayed a SNR > 20, resulting metabolites with a %SD < 15 were submitted to further statistical analyses.

GABA+ and Cr_{total} concentrations were acquired using MEGA-PRESS and quantified from the difference (ON – OFF) and OFF spectra, respectively, using GANNET version 2.0, a GABA Analysis Toolkit (http://www.gabamrs.com). After correcting for any frequency drifts using changes in peak Cr_{total} frequency as a reference, GANNET fits a Gaussian + baseline fit to the averaged ON-OFF difference spectra and uses the area under the curve to determine the GABA+ concentration (i.u.). Again, Cr_{total} served as an internal reference to control for interindividual differences in tissue volume; Cr_{total} was quantified using a Lorentz-Gaussian lineshape to fit the averaged OFF spectrum, where again the area under the curve quantifies the Cr concentration in the voxel, yielding GABA+/Cr_{total} ratios.

Statistical analysis

Mann-Whitney tests (MWU) were performed on each MRS measure [GABA+/Cr, GLX/Cr_{total}, Cr/H2O, (NAA + NAAG)/Cr] separately for each of the two MRS voxel regions (THAL and OCC) to detect differences between migraneurs and HCs. Relationships between local GABA and/or GLX concentrations and pain measures were determined using a Spearman correlation. Statistical significance was set at $p < .05$.

Results

Originally 19 migraineurs and 18 healthy controls were scanned using PRESS and MEGA-PRESS sequences. After careful examination 4 migraine patients were removed for the following reasons: One patient due to the presence of ninety headache days during the observation period making a chronic migraine or medication overuse headache the likely diagnosis, two patients due to a lack of any migraine attacks during the observation period, and one due to recurrent aura symptoms. Exclusion of four migraine patients did not affect the group statistic: Fifteen migraine patients (12 females, 3 males; age 35.2 ± 10.8 years) and fifteen control subjects (12 females, 3 males, age 33.4 ± 8.5 years, $p > 0.7$)) were included in the statistical analyses. Quality control of the MRS spectra excluded 4 patients and 3 HCs from the GABA thalamus, GLX thalamus and GLX occipital analyses, as well as 2 patients and 1 HC from the GABA occipital voxel.

Within the migraine group both average pain intensity and number of headache days were both positively correlated with the MIDAS score ($r = 0{,}54$, $p = 0{,}037$; and $r = 58$, $p = 0.024$ respectively). There were no significant correlations between pain measures and BDI scores ($p > .05$).

MWU tests revealed higher levels of Glx/Cr_{total} in both the THAL ($z = 2.54$, $p = .011$) and OCC ($z = 2.08$, $p = .038$) voxel locations (Table 2, Fig. 1). Levels of $GABA/Cr_{total}$, Cr/H20, and NAA/Cr_{total} were similar between patients and HCs. Correlation analyses within the migraine group revealed no significant correlations between GLX/Cr_{total} and/or $GABA+/Cr_{total}$ in either of the two brain regions with pain intensity or MIDAS scores ($p > .05$).

Discussion

The purpose of this study was to further elucidate the role of the neurotransmitters GLX and GABA in migraine. We specifically investigated local GLX and GABA concentrations in the occipital lobe including the primary visual cortex, and the right thalamus of migraine patients and HCs. Migraine patients had increased GLX levels in both the occipital cortex and the right thalamus, but showed no group differences in GABA in these two regions. Within the migraine group, no association between neurotransmitter concentrations and pain intensity or disability scores were found.

Our results support recent findings indicating that higher regional GLX levels are linked to the presence of migraine [13]. Zielmann et al. could demonstrate in a larger cohort (at a field strength of 7 T) that specifically glutamate levels were increased in the occipital cortex of patients with migraine [12]. Interestingly the effect was only observed in patients with migraine without aura, but not in patients with migraine with aura. Increased glutamatergic activity has been hypothesized to play an important role in the pathophysiology in migraine for a long time, specifically that increased glutamate levels lead to a cortical hyperexcitability within sensory cortices [21]. Of note, other studies applying spectroscopy in migraine could not confirm increased GLX levels, for example when looking at cerebellar GLX in patients with familiar hemiplegic migraine [22, 23]. Against this background one might argue that altered GLX levels are either region dependent or, from a statistical point of view, that the cohorts investigated so far are too small to consistently identify subtle differences.

The thalamus, our second region of interest, is known to play a crucial role in relaying not only nociception, but almost all sensory modalities [17, 18]. During migraine attacks most patients, apart from pain, additionally suffer from photo- and phonophobia. Given that hyperexcitability also plays a role in the genesis of multi-sensory symptoms during a migraine attack, this might either be a common phenomenon across different sensory cortices or one might postulate hyperexcitability within a structure with sensory input to the sensory cortices, i.e. the thalamus. Although at the current stage one can only speculate on the origin and spread of the pathophysiological processes leading to the clinical outbreak of a migraine attack, our data at least provide evidence for thalamic involvement in terms of an interictal increase of glutamatergic activity.

Interestingly, increased GLX levels have also been observed in other pain conditions [24]. Harris et al., for

Table 2 Metabolite concentrations

MWU - Test: Patients vs. Controls

Variable	Region	Rank Sum MIGA	Rank Sum Control	U	Z	*p*-value	Z adjusted	Valid N Patients	Valid N Control
GABA+/Cr	THAL	136	140	62	0,215	0,829	0,215	11	12
	OCC	180	198	89	−0,073	0,942	−0,073	13	14
Glx/Cr	THAL	177	99	21	2739	0,006	2739	11	12
	OCC	166	110	32	2062	0,039	2062	11	12
Cr/H2O	THAL	134	119	53	0,460	0,646	0,460	11	11
	OCC	167	184	76	-0,410	0,682	-0,410	13	13
(NAA + NAAG)/Cr	THAL	131	122	44	1022	0,307	1022	10	12
	OCC	133	143	65	0,031	0,975	0,031	11	12

GLX glutamate/glutamine, *GABA* gamma-amino-butyric acid, *NAA* N-actetyl-aspartate, *Cr* creatine

example, found elevated GLX levels in the insular cortex of fibromyalgia patients [25], while Fayed et al. described increased GLX level in the posterior cingulate cortex of patients with fibromyalgia and somatization disorder [26], suggesting that GLX plays a role in the pathogenesis of chronic pain. To date, only a few studies have looked at thalamic GLX in chronic pain conditions and the results are not yet conclusive [27, 28]. Our group has recently shown a link between GLX and pain sensitivity in healthy subjects where subjects more sensitive to pain stimuli had higher level of GLX in a network of brain regions known to play a role in pain perception, including the thalamus [29]. Against this background it is tempting to hypothesize, that there is a link between pain sensitivity and also the development of either chronic or recurrent pain conditions on the one hand and GLX levels in brain regions related to sensory and nociceptive processing on the other hand. However, this needs to be further elucidated; for now our results indicate increased interictal GLX levels in both the occipital cortex and the right thalamus in patients with migraine, supporting the notion of an extended network displaying cortical hyperexcitability.

With respect to GABA, several studies have investigated local GABA concentrations in migraine patients. Bigal et al. reported no significant differences in occipital GABA concentrations between migraine patients and HCs [16]. When pooling the migraine groups, patients with a higher disease burden had lower occipital GABA levels than patients with a lower disease burden. Using the MEGA-PRESS technique, Bridge et al. reported decreased GABA levels in the occipital cortex in migraine patients with aura [15], whereas Aguila et al. reported higher GABA levels in migraine patients in the posterior cingulate [14]. A later investigation of the same cohort could show that pain measures were negatively correlated with GABA concentrations. Our data are in line with the study of Bigal et al., indicating that migraine patients without aura display no altered GABA levels in the occipital cortex [16].

Taking all studies investigating local GABA concentrations in migraine patients into account, the results are not yet conclusive. The studies conducted so far looked at similar group sizes and age ranges, as well as cohorts with female predominance. Furthermore, all patients were investigated interictally. However, there were differences with respect to data acquisition, especially voxel placement, and migraine subtypes. As outlined above, our data do not support the notion of altered GABA levels in the occipital lobe of patients with migraine without aura and we speculate that altered GABA levels in that region might either be specific to migraine with aura or a characteristic of the migraine attack, but not of the interictal state.

Importantly, GABA has been found to be decreased in several other pain conditions such as fibromyalgia, diabetic neuropathic pain and trigeminal pain. Decreased GABA levels were found in the insular cortex of fibromyalgia patients [30] and patients with diabetic pain [24], while decreased thalamic GABA levels were found in patients with neuropathic pain after spinal trauma [31] and patients with neuropathic trigeminal pain [32]. As such it will be of interest to also look at GABA levels in other brain region related to nociceptive processing and multisensory integration, such as the insular cortex and cingulate cortex, in migraine patients.

Limitations

There are several limitations in our study that need to be pointed out. One drawback of this and other studies is the cross-sectional nature at a time point outside the actual migraine attack. As we measured GLX interictally, it cannot be derived from our data, if the elevated GLX level is a rebound phenomenon of a migraine attack, or if it is permanently elevated and facilitates nociceptive transmission. It will be of major importance to assess GLX and GABA levels during a migraine attack (or the day before), with the option to also account for laterality effects, or even longitudinally in- and outside a migraine attack to assess dynamic changes in neurotransmitters as they related to the pain event. Furthermore, with respect to headache frequency the group was rather heterogeneous, with number of headache days ranging from 2 to 40 (within 3 months). In future studies it will be important to investigate more homogeneous (and larger cohorts) to capture potential associations between neurotransmitter ratios and disease burden.

Another drawback from a methodological point of view is that GLX reflects both glutamate and glutamine levels. One might criticize that our interpretation of local hyperexcitability is based on the assumption that increased GLX levels are primarily caused by glutamate rather than glutamine, which is not necessarily the case. However, glutamate is one of the major components of the glutamic acid cycles taking place in both astrocytes and neurons, as such GLX is likely to also reflect the glutamate pool and/or turn around. Higher field strengths hold promise to separate both metabolites which will be helpful to further shed light onto the underlying pathophysiology [12].

Conclusion

We report increased GLX levels in the right thalamus and occipital cortex in migraineurs, but no changes in local GABA levels, supporting an extended network of cortical hyperexcitability.

We propose that thalamic GLX plays a role in the pathophysiology of migraine, but the full relevance of both neurotransmitters remains to be elucidated. Further research is needed to investigate the role of GLX-GABA-ratios in more depth, particularly over time and within larger cohorts, with migraineurs with and without aura and possibly other subgroups, since different pathomechanisms might play a role in migraine subtypes. It will also be interesting to relate thalamic metabolite levels during the migraine attack not only to headache intensity, but also to decreased pain thresholds, as well as phono- and photophobia, symptoms often present during migraine attacks, indicating altered multisensory perception.

Abbreviations

BDI: Beck depression inventory; Cr: Creatine; CSF: Cerebrospinal fluid; CSF: Cerebrospinal fluid; GABA: gamma-amino-butyric acid; GLX: Glutamate/glutamine; HC: Healthy control; H-MRS: Proton magnetic resonance spectroscopy; H-MRS: Proton magnetic resonance spectroscopy; MegaPress: Mescher-Garwood-Point Resolved Spectroscopy; MIDAS: Migraine Disability Assessment; MWU: Mann-Whitney-U; NAA: N-actetyl-aspartate; OCC: Occipital; PCr: Phosphocreatine; PRESS: Point-RESolved Spectroscopy; THAL: Thalamus

Acknowledgements

This work was supported by the Mercator research Center Ruhr (MERCUR, Pr-2014-0017). We appreciate the continuous support of Philips Germany. Tobias Schmidt-Wilcke is currently supported by a grant of the DFG (Deutsche Forschungsgemeinschaft, GZ: SCHM 2665/4-1).

Authors'contributions

AB wrote proposal, designed study, recruited healthy controls, involved in manuscript writing. LS performed data acquisition, involved in manuscript writing. PS designed study, recruited patients. BG performed data acquition and data analysis. NW performed data analysis, reviewed manuscript. SD recruited healthy controls, performed data acquisition, reviewed manuscript. TSW wrote proposal, designed study, performed data analysis, involved in manuscript writing, reviewed manuscript. All authors read and approved the final manuscript.

Competing interest

The authors declare that they have no competing interests.

Author details

[1]Department of Neurology, Berufsgenossenschaftliches Universitätsklinikum Bergmannsheil, Ruhr-University-Bochum, Bochum, Germany. [2]Department of Anesthesiology, Unfallkrankenhaus Berlin, Berlin, Germany. [3]Department of Neurology, St. Mauritius Therapieklinik, Meerbusch, Germany. [4]Institute of Clinical Neuroscience and Medical Psychology, Universitätsklinikum Düsseldorf, Düsseldorf, Germany.

References

1. Stovner LJ, Zwart JA, Hagen K, Terwindt GM, Pascual J (2006) Epidemiology of headache in Europe. Eur J Neurol. https://doi.org/10.1111/j.1468-1331.2006.01184.x
2. Weiller C, May A, Limmroth V et al (1995) Brain stem activation in spontaneous human migraine attacks. Nat Med. https://doi.org/10.1038/nm0795-658
3. Moskowitz MA (1990) Basic mechanisms in vascular headache. Neurol Clin 8(4):801–815.
4. Charles A (2009) Advances in the basic and clinical science of migraine. Ann Neurol. https://doi.org/10.1002/ana.21691
5. Quintas M, Neto JL, Pereira-Monteiro J et al (2013) Interaction between gamma-aminobutyric acid a receptor genes: new evidence in migraine susceptibility. PLoSOne. 2013;8(9):e74087. https://doi.org/10.1371/journal.pone.0074087
6. Chen T, Murrell M, Fowdar J, Roy B, Grealy R, Griffiths LR (2012) Investigation of the role of the GABRG2 gene variant in migraine. J Neurol Sci. https://doi.org/10.1016/j.jns.2012.03.014
7. Plummer PN, Colson NJ, Lewohl JM et al (2011) Significant differences in gene expression of GABA receptors in peripheral blood leukocytes of migraineurs. Gene doi:https://doi.org/10.1016/j.gene.2011.08.031; https://doi.org/10.1016/j.gene.2011.08.031
8. Fernandez F, Esposito T, Lea RA et al (2008) Investigation of gamma-aminobutyric acid (GABA) a receptors genes and migraine susceptibility. BMC Med Genet. https://doi.org/10.1186/1471-2350-9-109
9. Coppola G, Pierelli F, Schoenen J (2007) Is the cerebral cortex hyperexcitable or hyperresponsive in migraine? Cephalalgia. https://doi.org/10.1111/j.1468-2982.2007.01500.x
10. Khedr EM, Ahmed MA, Mohamed KA (2006) Motor and visual cortical excitability in migraineurs patients with or without aura: transcranial magnetic stimulation. Neurophysiol Clin. https://doi.org/10.1016/j.neucli.2006.01.007
11. Höffken O, Stude P, Lenz M, Bach M, Dinse HR, Tegenthoff M (2009) Visual paired-pulse stimulation reveals enhanced visual cortex excitability in migraineurs. Eur J Neurosci. https://doi.org/10.1111/j.1460-9568.2009.06859.x
12. Zielman R, Wijnen JP, Webb A et al (2017) Cortical glutamate in migraine. Brain 140(7):1859–1871. https://doi.org/10.1093/brain/awx130
13. Siniatchkin M, Sendacki M, Moeller F et al (2012) Abnormal changes of synaptic excitability in migraine with aura. Cereb Cortex 22(10):2207–2216. https://doi.org/10.1093/cercor/bhr248
14. Aguila MER, Lagopoulos J, Leaver AM et al (2015) Elevated levels of GABA+ in migraine detected using1H-MRS. NMR Biomed. https://doi.org/10.1002/nbm.3321
15. Bridge H, Stagg CJ, Near J, Lau CI, Zisner A, Zameel Cader M (2015) Altered neurochemical coupling in the occipital cortex in migraine with visual aura. Cephalalgia. https://doi.org/10.1177/0333102414566860
16. Bigal ME, Hetherington H, Pan J et al (2008) Occipital levels of GABA are related to severe headaches in migraine. Neurology. https://doi.org/10.1212/01.wnl.0000313376.07248.28
17. Magon S, May A, Stankewitz A et al (2015) Morphological abnormalities of thalamic subnuclei in migraine: a multicenter MRI study at 3 tesla. J Neurosci. https://doi.org/10.1523/JNEUROSCI.2154-15.2015
18. Messina R, Rocca MA, Colombo B et al (2015) White matter microstructure abnormalities in pediatric migraine patients. Cephalalgia. https://doi.org/10.1177/0333102415578428
19. Noseda R, Kainz V, Borsook D, Burstein R (2014) Neurochemical pathways that converge on thalamic trigeminovascular neurons: potential substrate for modulation of migraine by sleep, food intake, stress and anxiety. PLoS One. https://doi.org/10.1371/journal.pone.0103929
20. Olesen J, Marie-Germaine B (2004) The international classification of headache disorders 2nd edition ICHD-II. Headache. https://doi.org/10.1111/j.1526-4610.2008.01121.x
21. Ferrari MD, Odink J, Bos KD, Malessy MJ, Bruyn GW (1990) Neuroexcitatory plasma amino acids are elevated in migraine. Neurology. 1990;40(10):1582–6.
22. Dichgans M, Herzog J, Freilinger T, Wilke M, Auer DP (2005) 1H-MRS alterations in the cerebellum of patients with familial hemiplegic migraine type 1. Neurology. https://doi.org/10.1212/01.WNL.0000151855.98318.50
23. Zielman R, Teeuwisse WM, Bakels F et al (2014) Biochemical changes in the brain of hemiplegic migraine patients measured with 7 tesla 1H-MRS. Cephalalgia. https://doi.org/10.1177/0333102414527016
24. Petrou M, Pop-Busui R, Foerster BR et al (2012) Altered excitation-inhibition balance in the brain of patients with diabetic neuropathy. Acad Radiol. https://doi.org/10.1016/j.acra.2012.02.004
25. Harris RE, Sundgren PC, Craig AD et al (2009) Elevated insular glutamate in fibromyalgia is associated with experimental pain. Arthritis Rheum 60(10):3146–3152. https://doi.org/10.1002/art.24849
26. Fayed N, Andres E, Rojas G et al (2012) Brain dysfunction in fibromyalgia and somatization disorder using proton magnetic resonance spectroscopy: a controlled study. Acta Psychiatr Scand. https://doi.org/10.1111/j.1600-0447.2011.01820.x

27. Feraco P, Bacci a PF et al (2011) Metabolic abnormalities in pain-processing regions of patients with fibromyalgia: a 3T MR spectroscopy study. AJNR Am J Neuroradiol. https://doi.org/10.3174/ajnr.A2550
28. Widerström-Noga E, Cruz-Almeida Y, Felix ER, Pattany PM (2015) Somatosensory phenotype is associated with thalamic metabolites and pain intensity after spinal cord injury. Pain. https://doi.org/10.1016/j.pain.0000000000000019
29. Zunhammer M, Geis S, Busch V, Eichhammer P, Greenlee MW (2016) Pain modulation by intranasal oxytocin and emotional picture viewing-a randomized double-blind fMRI study. Sci Rep. https://doi.org/10.1038/srep31606
30. Foerster BR, Petrou M, Edden RA et al (2012) Reduced insular gamma-aminobutyric acid in fibromyalgia. Arthritis Rheum 64(2):579–583. https://doi.org/10.1002/art.33339
31. Gustin SM, Wrigley PJ, Youssef AM et al (2014) Thalamic activity and biochemical changes in individuals with neuropathic pain after spinal cord injury. Pain 155(5):1027–1036. https://doi.org/10.1016/j.pain.2014.02.008.
32. Henderson LA, Peck CC, Petersen ET et al (2013) Chronic pain: lost inhibition? J Neurosci 33(17):7574–7582. https://doi.org/10.1523/JNEUROSCI.0174-13.2013

15

Migraine induction with calcitonin gene-related peptide in patients from erenumab trials

Casper Emil Christensen[†], Samaira Younis[†], Marie Deen, Sabrina Khan, Hashmat Ghanizada and Messoud Ashina[*]

Abstract

Background: Migraine prevention with erenumab and migraine induction by calcitonin gene-related peptide (CGRP) both carry notable individual variance. We wanted to explore a possible association between individual efficacy of anti-CGRP treatment and susceptibility to migraine induction by CGRP.

Methods: Thirteen migraine patients, previously enrolled in erenumab anti-CGRP receptor monoclonal antibody trials, received CGRP in a double-blind, placebo-controlled, randomized cross-over design to investigate their susceptibility to migraine induction. A standardized questionnaire was used to assess the efficacy of previous antibody treatment. The patients were stratified into groups of high responders and poor responders. Primary outcomes were incidence of migraine-like attacks and area under the curve of headache intensity after infusion of CGRP and placebo. All interviews and experiments were performed in laboratories at the Danish Headache Center, Copenhagen, Denmark.

Results: Ten high responders and three poor responders were included. CGRP induced migraine-like attacks in ten (77%) patients, whereof two were poor responders, compared to none after placebo ($p = 0.002$). The area under the curve for headache intensity was greater after CGRP, compared to placebo, at 0–90 min ($p = 0.009$), and 2–12 h ($p = 0.014$). The median peak headache intensity score was 5 (5–9) after CGRP, compared to 2 (0–4) after placebo ($p = 0.004$).

Conclusions: Patients with an excellent effect of erenumab are highly susceptible to CGRP provocation. If an association is evident, CGRP provocation could prove a biomarker for predicting antibody treatment efficacy.

Trial registration: Retrospectively registered at clinicaltrials.gov with identifier: NCT03481400.

Keywords: Headache, CGRP, Biomarker, Monoclonal antibody

Background

Clinicians treating migraine have, until now, been limited to preventive drugs that were initially developed for cardiovascular, psychiatric or neurological diseases other than migraine. [1] Four anti calcitonin gene-related peptide (anti-CGRP) monoclonal antibodies (mAbs) are in late-phase development as the first class of preventive therapeutics targeting migraine-specific mechanisms. [2] Three mAbs (fremanezumab, eptinezumab and galcanezumab) are ligand specific, and bind to CGRP, while one (erenumab) binds to the receptor complex (Fig. 1). [3–6] Overall efficacy and tolerability between the four antibodies are quite similar, but individual efficacy is widespread. While some patients report excellent efficacy, 35% report less than 50% reduction in monthly migraine days when treated with erenumab. [7] The question is whether we can identify which patients to treat with the new therapeutics by predicting efficacy response and thereby introduce personalized treatment schemes.

Calcitonin gene-related peptide induces migraine-like attacks in an average of 62% of migraine patients across placebo-controlled and open-label provocation studies. [8–11] Individual differences in mAb efficacy and migraine induction suggest that CGRP involvement in migraine varies between patients, and susceptibility to provocation could be a possible biomarker for anti-CGRP treatment efficacy.

We sought to investigate a possible association between anti-CGRP treatment efficacy and susceptibility

* Correspondence: ashina@dadlnet.dk
[†]Casper Emil Christensen and Samaira Younis contributed equally to this work.
Danish Headache Center and Department of Neurology, Rigshospitalet Glostrup, Faculty of Health and Medical Sciences, University of Copenhagen, Copenhagen, Denmark

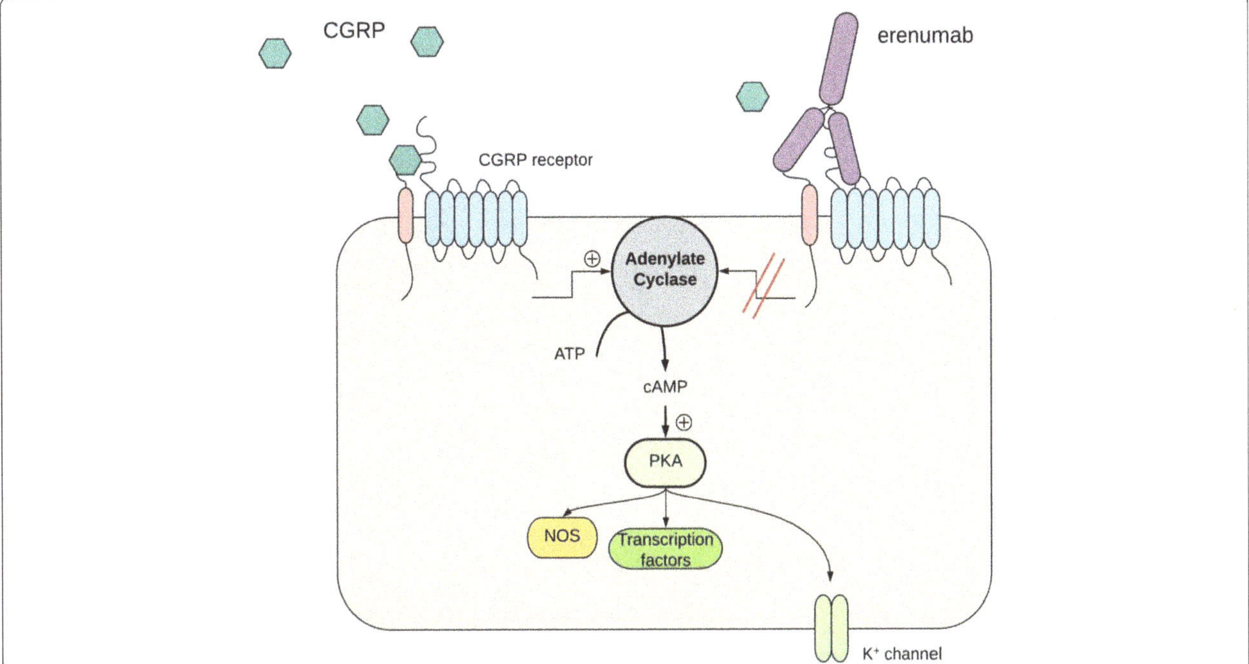

Fig. 1 Intracellular signaling pathways of calcitonin gene-related peptide receptor activation. One effect of CGRP receptor activation is adenylate cyclase-mediated cyclic adenosine monophosphate (cAMP) elevation, which leads to protein kinase A (PKA) activation, and activation of multiple targets depending on cell type. Nitric oxide synthesis may be the result of nitric oxide synthase (NOS) phosphorylation, gene transcription changes may be a result of cAMP response element binding protein (CREB) activation, and relaxation of vascular smooth muscle cells is partly a result of ATP-sensitive potassium channels (K+ channels) activation

to CGRP-induced migraine-like attacks. Our hypotheses were that CGRP would conduce to a small migraine-like attack rate in a group of patients with little to no effect of erenumab and a large attack rate in a group who experienced an excellent effect of erenumab.

Methods

Recruitment process

Patients, who had participated in the episodic and chronic erenumab trials (ClincalTrials.gov IDs: NCT02483585 and NCT02066415), were recruited from the Danish Headache Center. These patients were contacted and enrolled after completing their participation in the mAb trial. Patients, who were likely eligible for participation in up-coming anti-CGRP mAbs clinical trials, were recruited from the Danish Headache Center as well. The patients were enrolled from July 25 2016 to June 21 2017. Inclusion criteria: migraine with and/or without aura according to the International Classification of Headache Disorders (ICHD-3 beta) [12], age 18 to 65 years, and previous/probable participation in an anti-CGRP mAb trial. Exclusion criteria: use of pharmacological agents (except contraceptives and preventive migraine medication), cardiovascular disease and other serious somatic or psychiatric disorders.

Study design

Response to anti-CGRP mAb treatment was evaluated using a standardized questionnaire (Fig. 2). Patients rated treatment efficacy for reduction in: migraine days, headache days, days using rescue medication, and headache intensity. Treatment efficacy was assessed based on the patients' last month of receiving mAbs. Patients, who reported an excellent effect of treatment (efficacy score ≥ 50%) in at least two of the four outcome variables, were defined as high responders. The remaining patients were defined as poor responders.

Patients received 1.5 μg/min human α-CGRP (PolyPeptide, Strasbourg, France) and placebo isotonic saline as infusions over 20 min on two separate study days in a double-blind, placebo-controlled, randomized, cross-over design.

Experimental protocol

Patients reported to the clinic headache-free for at least 48 h. Coffee, tea, cocoa, cola, tobacco, and alcohol were not allowed for 12 h before study start. Patients were instructed to fast for four hours before study start. Fertile female participants underwent a pregnancy test upon arrival at the hospital.

Questionnaire:
Provoked migraine-like attacks using calcitonin gene-related peptide (CGRP) in migraine patients, who have previously received treatment with CGRP antibodies or CGRP receptor antibodies.

1. How would you rate the effect of the medication you have received through your participation in the clinical trial for migraine preventive treatment?
The assessment of the effect should be based on your last month of receiving the drug.

For each outcome (i-iv), please mark the score that best represents the efficacy of the drug.

	Efficacy score:	0 %	25 %	50 %	75 %	100 %
i.	Reduction in number of migraine days					
ii.	Reduction of the headache intensity					
iii.	Reduction in number of headache days					
iv.	Reduction in number of days, where you used rescue medication					

2. Global assessment of effect:
Based on the last month of receiving the drug, how satisfied were you with the effect of the drug you received through your participation in the clinical trial for migraine preventive treatment?

This evaluation should represent a global assessment based on both reduction of headache days as well as headache intensity.

	Effect score:	0 %	25 %	50 %	75 %	100 %
i.	Global assessment					

		Yes	No
3	Would you buy the drug, if it were available?		
4.	Would you recommend the drug to others?		

Fig. 2 Questionnaire used for monoclonal antibody response stratification. Patients who reported excellent effect of treatment (efficacy score ≥ 50%) in at least two of the four outcome variables (i-iv) were defined as high responders. The remaining patients were defined as poor responders

Patients underwent a medical examination on the first study day. A venous catheter was inserted into a cubital vein, followed by rest in supine position for 30 min, before initiating the infusion. Intensity and characteristics of headache, heart rate (HR), blood pressure, and adverse events were registered every 10 min from 10 min before to 90 min after infusion.

Headache intensity and characteristics

Headache intensity was rated based on a 0 to 10 numeric rating scale (NRS) where '0' denoted no headache, and '10' the worst possible headache.

Headache characteristics were recorded using a standardized questionnaire including headache intensity, location, quality, aggravation by physical activity, and accompanying symptoms.

Upon discharge from the hospital, patients were instructed to self-report headache intensity and characteristics in a standardized headache diary hourly from 2 to 12 h after infusion start. Patients were allowed to use their usual migraine medication after discharge.

Migraine-like attack criteria

Pharmacologically-induced migraine attacks are not spontaneous attacks, and cannot fulfill the ICHD-3 beta criteria. [12] Therefore, modified criteria for experimentally-induced attacks were developed based on the following considerations. [13, 14] Firstly, the majority of patients report that the induced attacks mimic their spontaneous attacks. [10, 15] Secondly, spontaneous migraine attacks mostly develop in a matter of hours, and in the beginning of the attack phenomenologically fulfill the criteria for tension-type headache. Only hereafter, the headache worsens, becomes unilateral and presents the associated symptoms required for a migraine diagnosis. Finally, most patients can predict an impending migraine attack in the early attack stage and cannot be denied treatment in an experimental setting. Thus, induced attacks are frequently treated before all migraine criteria are fulfilled. Accordingly, we used the following two criteria to define a pharmacologically-induced migraine-like attack [14]:

The headache fulfills criteria C and D of the ICHD-3 beta [12].

C: Headache has at least two of the following characteristics: Unilateral location, pulsating quality, moderate to severe intensity, or aggravation by physical activity.

D: At least one of the following accompanying symptoms: Nausea and/or vomiting, or photophobia and phonophobia.

or

Headache described as mimicking the patient's spontaneous attack and treated with acute migraine rescue medication.

Statistical analysis

Headache intensity scores are presented as median (range). Heart rate and mean arterial pressure (MAP) are presented as mean ± standard deviation under the assumption that they adhere to a normal distribution. Primary endpoints were incidence of migraine-like attacks from 0 to 12 h after infusion and area under the curve (AUC), using the trapezoidal rule [16], for headache intensity score at 0 to 90 min and 90 min to 12 h on the CGRP day, as compared to the placebo day for all patients. McNemar's test and Wilcoxon signed-rank test were used as appropriate. Secondary endpoints were HR and MAP, which were compared between the two study days using paired t-tests. Peak headache intensity score and time to peak headache were compared between the study days using Wilcoxon signed-rank test. Adverse events are reported as incidences on the CGRP and placebo day and compared between days using McNemar's test in explorative analysis. Predictive values, sensitivity and specificity were also calculated as post hoc analyses.

Separate meaningful inference statistics within each mAb response groups could not be performed due to small subgroup sample sizes. Data from patients without previous experience from the erenumab trials were excluded from the final analyses as this recruitment was limited by the competitive enrollment strategies of the anti-CGRP mAbs clinical trials. No statistical power calculation was conducted prior to the study as the sample size was based on the available data. R (Version 3.4.2) was used to conduct the statistical analyses. *P* values are reported as two-tailed with a 5% level of significance.

Results

Participants

Thirteen patients (12 women) completed the study (Fig. 3). Seven were enrolled from the episodic migraine erenumab trial (ClincalTrials.gov ID: NCT02483585), and six were enrolled from the chronic migraine erenumab trial (ClincalTrials.gov ID: NCT02066415). All 13 patients were enrolled after completing the safety follow-up visit 12 weeks after the last dose of erenumab. Mean age was 39 years (standard deviation ±11 and range 22 to 53).

Clinical characteristics, migraine incidence and intensity

Headache characteristics and accompanying symptoms are presented in Table 1. Ten of 13 patients (77%) developed migraine-like attacks after CGRP, compared to none after placebo ($p = 0.002$) (Fig. 4). Two of the 10 patients, who experienced migraine-like attacks, reported poor response to treatment (patients 5 and 12).

The three patients, who did not develop migraine-like attacks after CGRP, were chronic migraine patients (patients 9, 10 and 11). One of these patients (patient 11) was a poor responder with an efficacy score of zero for all four outcome variables. The other two patients were high responders (patients 9 and 10).

The AUC for headache intensity was greater after CGRP compared to placebo at both 0 to 90 min ($p = 0.009$) and 2 to 12 h ($p = 0.014$) (Fig. 5). The median peak headache intensity score was 5 (5 to 9) after CGRP, compared to 2 (0 to 4) after placebo ($p = 0.004$). Time to peak headache was 180 min (110 to 270) after CGRP and 330 min (72.5 to 660) after placebo ($p = 0.250$).

Vital signs and adverse events

The AUC for HR was higher ($p < 0.001$) and AUC for MAP was lower ($p < 0.001$) after CGRP compared to placebo. All patients reported warm sensations (13/13 (100%)) after CGRP compared to only one patient reporting warm sensation (1/13, (8%)) after placebo ($p < 0.001$). Flushing was observed after CGRP in all patients (13/13 (100%)) compared to none after placebo ($p < 0.001$). Five of 13 patients (63%) reported palpitations after CGRP, compared to two of 13 (15%) after placebo ($p = 0.014$).

Predictive values, sensitivity and specificity

Positive predictive value for CGRP-induced attacks in erenumab high responders was 0.80 (95% CI 0.49 to 0.96) and sensitivity was 0.80 (95% CI 0.66 to 0.89). Negative predictive value was 0.33 (95% CI 0.08 to 0.73) and specificity was 0.33 (95% CI 0.01 to 0.91).

Discussion

Our major finding was that patients with response to erenumab showed hypersensitivity to CGRP infusion in a placebo-controlled experiment. In addition to a high

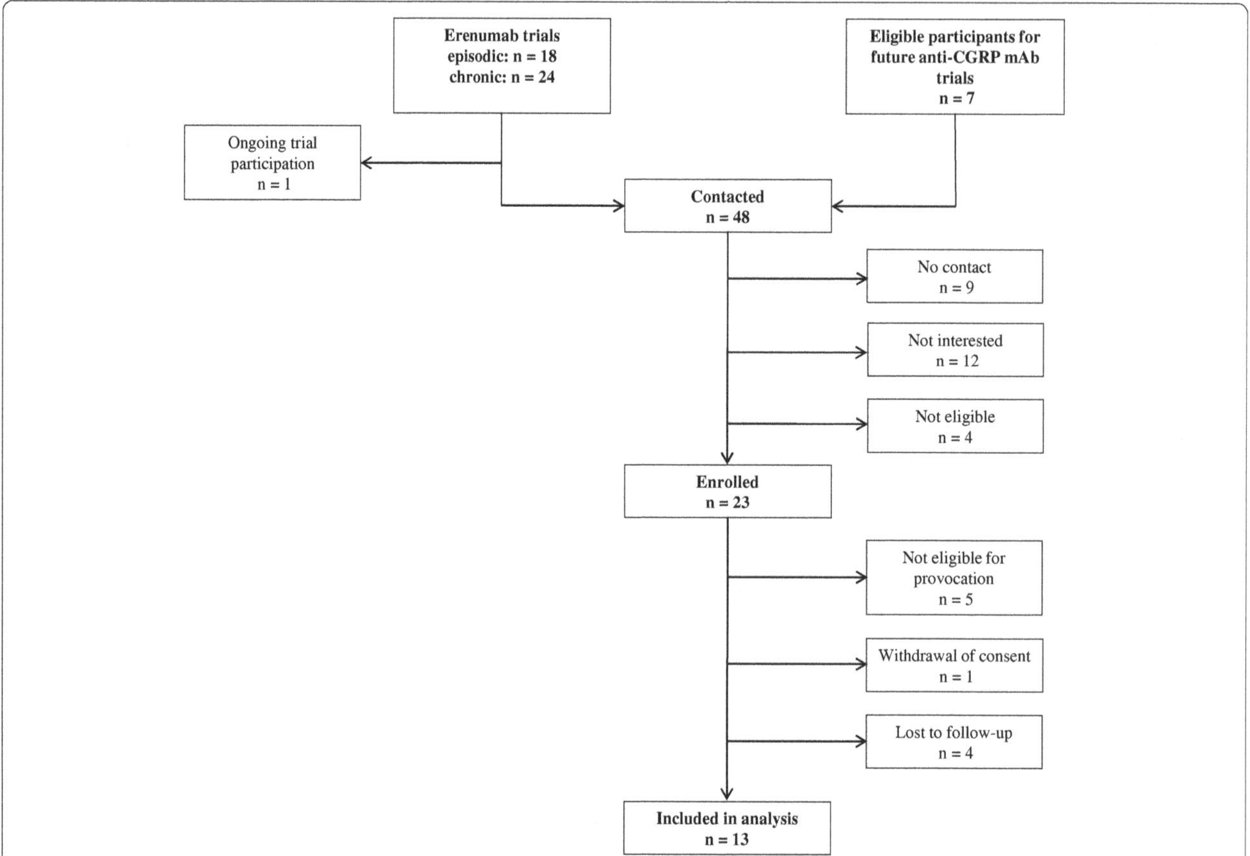

Fig. 3 Inclusion flowchart. Twenty-three patients were enrolled in the study. Ten of these were excluded subsequently. One patient was excluded due to a cardiac conduction disease and one due to diabetes mellitus (well-regulated), according to the conventional CGRP provocation protocol. Three patients were excluded from analysis as they did not participate in the erenumab trials. One patient withdrew consent before the experiments. Four patients were lost to follow-up and one of these had participated in the first study day. Data from these days were excluded from analyses. Of the ten patients, who were excluded, seven had received erenumab and six of these were high responders. Response status was not obtained from the last of the seven subjects

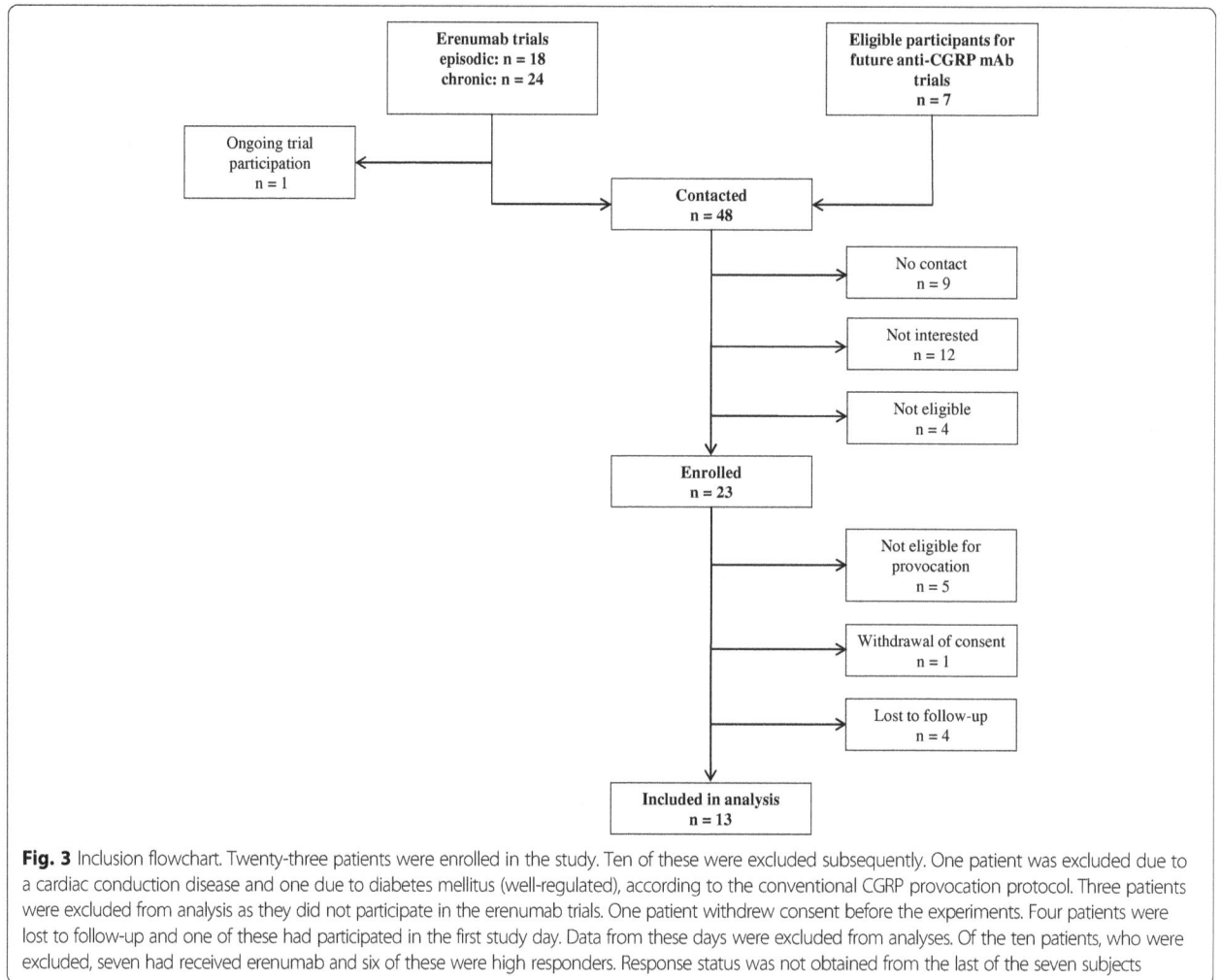

migraine induction rate (77%), compared to previous studies, participants also reported moderate to severe (median peak intensity of 5, range 5 to 9) and long-lasting headaches (Fig. 5), which further points toward high CGRP susceptibility. Previous studies reported median peak headache intensities ranging from 1 to 4. [9, 10]

Mechanisms of migraine initiation by CGRP and migraine prevention by anti-CGRP mAbs are unknown. Calcitonin gene-related peptide is expressed in the trigeminal C fibers [17], trigeminal ganglion [18] and trigeminal nucleus caudalis [19], and its receptors are expressed in vascular smooth muscle cells [20], A-delta fibers [17] and trigeminal ganglia. [18] Calcitonin gene-related peptide binds to its receptor and activates multiple intracellular signaling pathways of which the most well-known is activation of adenylate cyclase and formation of cyclic adenosine monophosphate (cAMP). [21] In arteries, this leads to dilation through an endothelial-dependent synthesis of nitric oxide or relaxation of vascular smooth muscle cells via opening of ATP-sensitive potassium channels (Fig. 1). [22, 23] In trigeminal ganglion cells, the cAMP increase may cause sensitization of nociceptive neurons through upregulation of gene transcription and algogenic receptors in the cell membranes. [21, 24] In healthy volunteers, CGRP modulates inputs from noxious heat stimulation of the trigeminal area in the brain stem and insula. [25] The phosphodiesterase-3 inhibitor, cilostazol, potentiates the accumulation of cAMP in a receptor independent manner, and induces migraine in 86% of patients [26, 27], supporting the notion that cAMP upregulation may induce migraine. To what extent erenumab interacts with these mechanisms and exerts its anti-migraine effect is not fully clarified. Interestingly, erenumab inhibits CGRP-driven increases in dermal blood flow after capsaicin injections suggesting peripheral effects of CGRP receptor blockage. [28]

Our study explored a possible association between self-reported erenumab efficacy and sensitivity to migraine induction by CGRP. Identifying a link between poor response to mAb treatment and not developing migraine when challenged with CGRP (a so-called *non-CGRP phenotype*) could provide a biomarker for treatment response. In an effort to provide test reliability

Table 1 Clinical characteristics of headache and associated symptoms after CGRP and placebo

Patient	Efficacy score (%)	Day	Time to peak headache (duration)	Headache characteristics	Associated symptoms	Mimics usual migraine	Migraine-like attack (onset)	Treatment (time)/ efficacy
1 CM	50/75/0/25	CGRP	3 h (4 h)	Bilat/10/Throb+Pres/+	+/+/+	Yes	Yes (20min)	Sumatriptan 100 mg (6 h) / No
		Placebo[a]	80 min (NA)	Bilat/6/Pres/M	+/+/–	No	No	NR
		Spon		Bilat/Throb/+	+/+/+			
2 EM	100/100/ 100/100	CGRP	2 h (NA)[b]	Bilat/10/Pres/+	–/+/–	Yes	Yes (20 min)	Sumatriptan 50 mg (2 h) / Yes
		Placebo	None					
		Spon		Right/Throb/+	+/+/–			
3 EM	100/0/0/100	CGRP	3 h (1 h)	Bilat/7/Throb/+	+/+/+	Yes	Yes (70 min)	Sumatriptan 50 mg (3 h) / Yes, Treo (9 h) / NR
		Placebo	30 min (1h)	Bilat/3/Pres/M	–/+/–	No	No	None
		Spon		Left/ Throb/+	+/+/+			
4 EM	100/50/0/100	CGRP[c]	6 h (1 h)	Bilat/7/Throb+Pres/NR	+/+/+	NR	Yes (5 h)	2 x KP (5 h) / No, Riza 10 mg (6 h) / NR[d], KP (10 h) / Yes
		Placebo	10 h (NA)	Left/5/Throb/+	–/–/+	Yes	No (NA)[e]	Riza + 2 x KP (10 h) / NR[f]
		Spon		Left/Throb/+	+/+/+			
5 EM	0/25/0/0	CGRP	3 h (1 h)	Bilat/5/Pres/+	–/+/+	Yes	Yes (20 min)	Sumatriptan 100 mg (3 h) / Yes
		Placebo	None					
		Spon		Bilat/Throb/+	–/+/+			
6 EM	75/50/50/75	CGRP	3 h (2 h)	Right/4/Pres/–	–/+/–	Yes	Yes (2 h)	Zolmitriptan 2.5 mg (3 h) / Yes, 2 x Treo (6 h) / Yes
		Placebo	9 h (2 h)	Right/3/NR/-	–/+/–	Yes	No (NA)	Treo (9 h) / NR
		Spon		Unilat[g]/Throb/+	+/+/+			
7 EM	75/75/0/75	CGRP	1 h (10 min)	Right/5/Throb/NR	–/+/–	Yes	Yes (20 min)	2 x Treo (3 h) / Yes, Sumatriptan 50 mg (4 h) / Yes
		Placebo	4 h (2 h)	Left/2/Pres/+	–/+/–	Yes	No (NA)	None
		Spon		Unilat[7]/Throb/+	+/+/+			
8 EM	100/50/75/75	CGRP	8 h (5 h)	Left/9/Pres/+	+/+/+	Yes	Yes (2 h)	None
		Placebo	50 min (10 min)	Bilat/2/Pres/M	–/+/–	No	No (NA)	None
		Spon		Left/Throb/+	+/+/+			
9 CM	75/0/75/75	CGRP	4 h (5 h)	Right/2/Throb/+	–/–/–	Yes	No (NA)[e]	None
		Placebo	None					
		Spon		Bilat+Unilat[h]/Throb/+	+/+/+			
10 CM	100/0/25/100	CGRP	None					
		Placebo	None					
		Spon		Right/Throb/+	+/+/+			
11 CM	0/0/0/0	CGRP	50 min (10 min)	Bilat/5/Throb/M	–/–/–	No	No (NA)	Panadol Extra + Ibuprofen 600 mg (2 h) / Yes
		Placebo	None					
		Spon		Left/Throb/+	+/+/+			
12 CM	50/25/0/25	CGRP	6 h (1 h)	Right/9/Throb/+	+/+/+	Yes	Yes (40 min)	2 x Treo + Paracetamol 1 g + Meto 10 mg (6 h) / Yes
		Placebo	None					
		Spon		Right/Throb/+	+/+/+			
13 CM	50/50/75/50	CGRP	80 min (20 min)	Right/5/Throb/+	–/+/+	Yes	Yes (60 min)	Sumatriptan 100 mg + Naproxen 500 mg (2 h) / Yes
		Placebo	7 h (1 h)	Bilat/2/Pres/+	–/–/–	No	No (NA)	None
		Spon		Right/Throb/+	+/+/+			

Efficacy score: Reduction in migraine days/reduction of the headache intensity/reduction in headache days/reduction in days of used rescue medication. Headache characteristics: Localization/intensity/quality/aggravation. Associated symptoms: Nausea/photophobia/phonophobia. The criteria for a migraine-like attack are described in 'Methods'. Treatment efficacy: ≥ 50% decrease of headache intensity within 2 h

Bilat Bilateral, *Throb* Throbbing, *Pres* Pressing, *M* Missing data, *NR* Not reported, *CM* Chronic migraine, *EM* Episodic migraine

KP Codeine 30.6 mg + Paracetamol 500 mg, *Panadol Extra* Paracetamol 500 mg + Caffeine 65 mg, *Treo* Aspirin 500 mg + Caffeine 50 mg, Meto: Metoclopramide 10 mg, Riza: Rizatriptan 10 mg

[a]2–12 h data not reported; [b] 3–4 h data not reported; [c] 2–12 h data not reported for aggravation and mimics usual migraine; [d] Sleep at 8–9 h, headache intensity score was 1 at 10 h; [e] Possible migraine-like attack; [f] 11–12 h data missing, but reported pain relief and sleep after medication intake; [g] Unilateral, no side preference; [h] Shifting between bilateral and unilateral (no side preference)

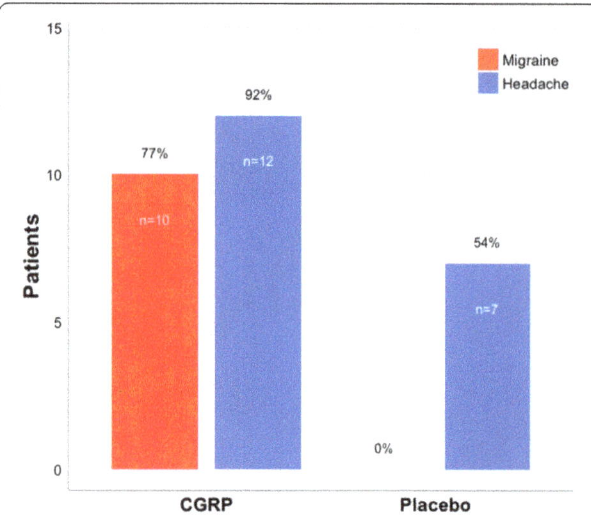

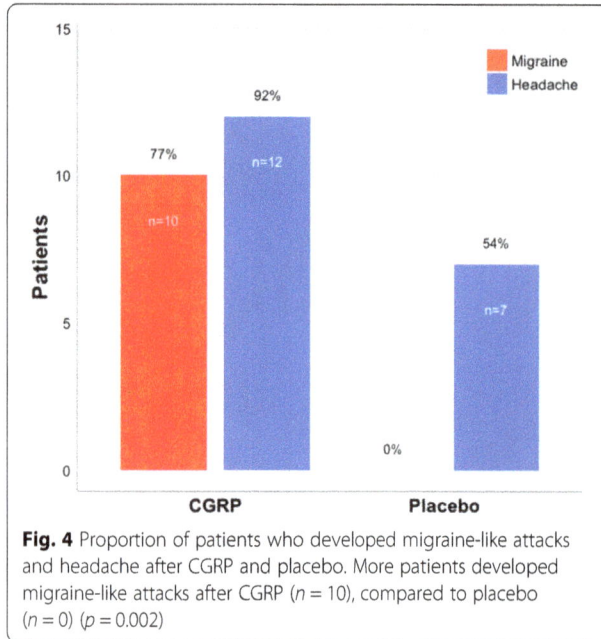

Fig. 4 Proportion of patients who developed migraine-like attacks and headache after CGRP and placebo. More patients developed migraine-like attacks after CGRP ($n = 10$), compared to placebo ($n = 0$) ($p = 0.002$)

measures, we calculated predictive values, sensitivity and specificity as post hoc analyses. Positive predictive value and sensitivity for CGRP-induced attacks in erenumab high responders were high. In contrast, negative predictive value and specificity were low, impaired by the small sample of erenumab poor responders. We evaluated erenumab treatment response using four variables: reduction in migraine days, reduction in headache intensity, reduction in headache days and reduction in days using rescue medication. Our predefined criteria for "poor response" identified three such participants (subjects 5, 11 and 12 in Table 1). One of these was a *non-responder* who scored zero in all four efficacy variables. This participant reported no migraine after CGRP infusion. The other two poor responders reported migraine-like attacks after CGRP. We obtained treatment efficacy from 19 patients (Fig. 3) and only the three above-mentioned patients reported "poor response". Therefore, we could not include enough poor responders to calculate a correlation to low migraine induction, which is a limitation. Furthermore, we cannot ignore the fact that having a poor response to erenumab in mAb trials might affect a patient's willingness to participate in our study,

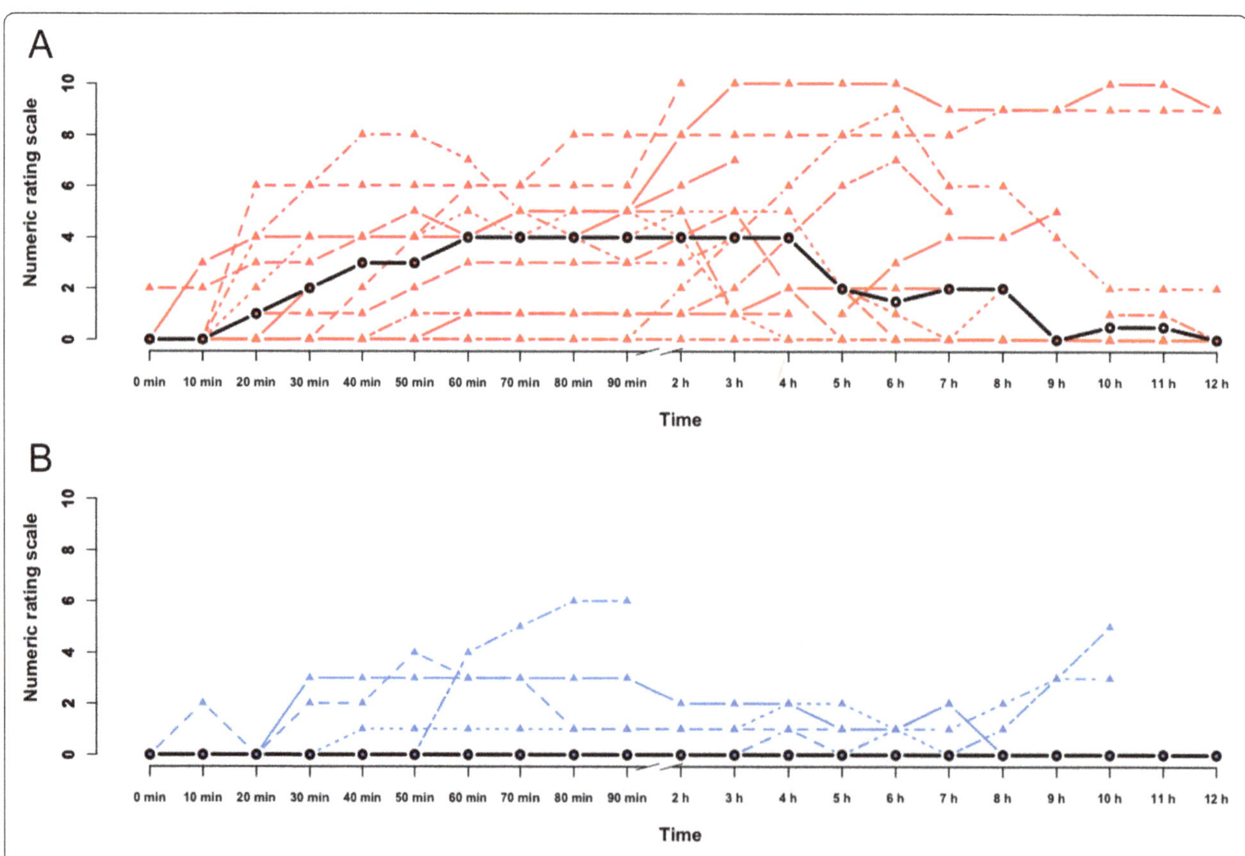

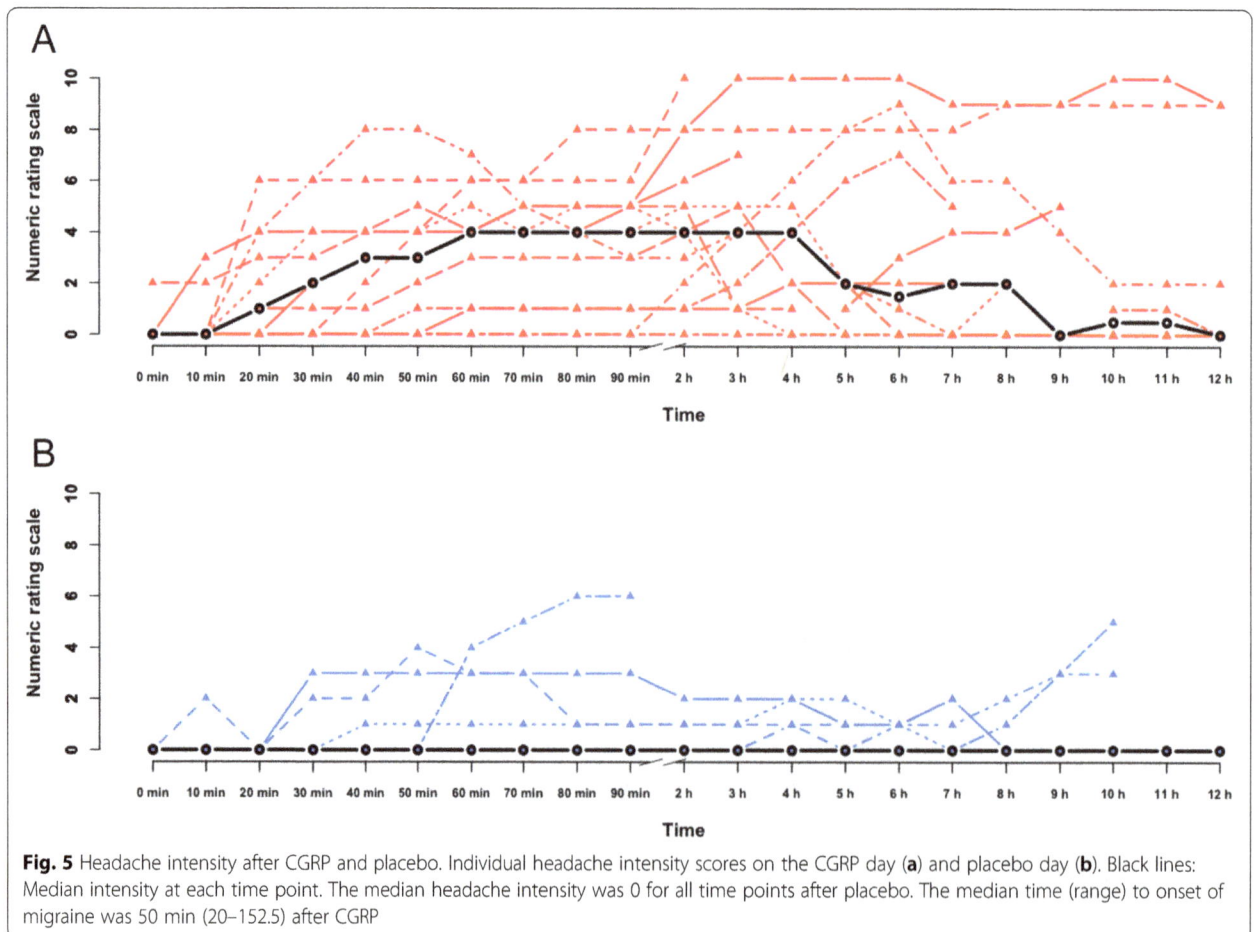

Fig. 5 Headache intensity after CGRP and placebo. Individual headache intensity scores on the CGRP day (**a**) and placebo day (**b**). Black lines: Median intensity at each time point. The median headache intensity was 0 for all time points after placebo. The median time (range) to onset of migraine was 50 min (20–152.5) after CGRP

subsequently leading to sampling bias. Our findings suggest that having a positive response to erenumab, based on our questionnaire variables, is associated with a high susceptibility to migraine induction by CGRP. The lack of a larger group of poor responders inhibits us from drawing conclusions on a possible association between those patients and a low susceptibility to CGRP. The question remains whether a CGRP provocation model can be used to predict efficacy of anti-CGRP mAb treatment when it becomes available. A large-scale prospective provocation study in patients, before they receive anti-CGRP treatment, would allow us to draw conclusions on poor responders i.e. patients with a possible *non-CGRP* migraine phenotype. When a sufficient number of *non-responders* have been provoked, we will be able to determine if the CGRP model of migraine is a biomarker for treatment response. Consequently, we will be able to provide biomarker reliability tests with sensitivity and specificity as outcome measures.

Conclusion

In this study we showed high migraine induction capabilities with CGRP in migraine patients who responded to erenumab treatment compared to data from previous CGRP provocation experiments. [8–11] If an association between poor migraine induction and poor treatment efficacy is also evident, the CGRP model of migraine could become the basis for a biomarker for mAb treatment response. Such a biomarker would be a powerful tool for clinicians choosing therapeutics for the prevention of migraine.

Abbreviations

AUC: Area under the curve; cAMP: Cyclic adenosine monophosphate; CGRP: Calcitonin gene-related peptide; HR: Heart rate; ICHD-3 beta: International classification of headache disorders version 3 beta; mAb: Monoclonal antibody; MAP: Mean arterial pressure; NRS: Numerical rating scale

Acknowledgments

The authors gratefully thank laboratory technicians Lene Elkjær and Winnie Grønning for their assistance with data extraction.

Funding

This study was supported by the Lundbeck Foundation (R155–2014-171 and R249–2017-1608) and the Research Foundation of Rigshospitalet (E-23327-02). The funding parties had no influence on study design, inclusion of participants, collection or interpretation of data.

Authors' contributions

CC: study concept and design, acquisition, analysis and interpretation of data, and drafting and revision of manuscript. SY: study concept and design, acquisition, analysis and interpretation of data, and drafting and revision of manuscript. MD, SK and HG: study concept and design, critical revision of manuscript for intellectual content. MA: study concept and design, interpretation of data, critical revision of manuscript, and study initiation and supervision. All authors read and approved the final manuscript.

Competing interests

MA is a consultant or scientific advisor for Allergan, Amgen, Alder, Eli Lilly, Novartis and Teva, principal investigator for: Amgen 20120178 (Phase 2), 20120295 (Phase 2), 20130255 (Open label extension), 20120297 (Phase 3), 20150308 (Phase 2), ElectroCore GM-11 gamma-Core-R, TEVA TV48125-CNS-30068 (Phase 3), Novartis CAMG334A2301 (Phase 3) and Alder PROMISE-2. MA has no ownership interest and does not hold stock in any pharmaceutical company. MA serves as associated editor of Cephalalgia and co-editor of the Journal of Headache and Pain. SK has acted as invited speaker for Novartis. The remaining authors report no competing interests.

References

1. Evers S, Áfra J, Frese A, Goadsby PJ, Linde M, May A et al (2009) EFNS guideline on the drug treatment of migraine - revised report of an EFNS task force. Eur J Neurol 16:968–981
2. Khan S, Olesen A, Ashina M. CGRP, a target for preventive therapy in migraine and cluster headache: systematic review of clinical data. Cephalalgia. 2017. https://doi.org/10.1177/0333102417741297
3. Bigal ME, Dodick DW, Rapoport AM, Silberstein SD, Ma Y, Yang R et al (2015) Safety, tolerability, and efficacy of TEV-48125 for preventive treatment of high-frequency episodic migraine: a multicentre, randomised, double-blind, placebo-controlled, phase 2b study. Lancet Neurol 14:1081–1090
4. Dodick DW, Goadsby PJ, Spierings ELH, Scherer JC, Sweeney SP, Grayzel DS (2014) Safety and efficacy of LY2951742, a monoclonal antibody to calcitonin gene-related peptide, for the prevention of migraine: a phase 2, randomised, double-blind, placebo-controlled study. Lancet Neurol 13:885–892
5. Dodick DW, Goadsby PJ, Silberstein SD, Lipton RB, Olesen J, Ashina M et al (2014) Safety and efficacy of ALD403, an antibody to calcitonin gene-related peptide, for the prevention of frequent episodic migraine: a randomised, double-blind, placebo-controlled, exploratory phase 2 trial. Lancet Neurol 13:1100–1107
6. Sun H, Dodick DW, Silberstein S, Goadsby PJ, Reuter U, Ashina M et al (2016) Safety and efficacy of AMG 334 for prevention of episodic migraine: a randomised, double-blind, placebo-controlled, phase 2 trial. Lancet Neurol 15:382–390
7. Ashina M, Dodick D, Goadsby PJ, Reuter U, Silberstein S, Zhang F et al (2017) Erenumab (AMG 334) in episodic migraine: interim analysis of an ongoing open-label study. Neurology 89:1237–1243
8. Guo S, Vollesen ALH, Olesen J, Ashina M (2016) Premonitory and nonheadache symptoms induced by CGRP and PACAP38 in patients with migraine. Pain 157:2773–2781
9. Hansen JM, Hauge AW, Olesen J, Ashina M (2010) Calcitonin gene-related peptide triggers migraine-like attacks in patients with migraine with aura. Cephalalgia 30:1179–1186
10. Lassen LH, Haderslev PA, Jacobsen VB, Iversen HK, Sperling B, Olesen J (2002) CGRP may play a causative role in migraine. Cephalalgia 22:54–61
11. Asghar MS, Hansen AE, Amin FM, van der Geest RJ, Koning P, Der V, HBW L et al (2011) Evidence for a vascular factor in migraine. Ann Neurol 69:635–645
12. Society HCC of the IH (2013) The international classification of headache disorders, 3rd edition (beta version). Cephalalgia 33:629–808
13. Guo S, Christensen AF, Liu ML, Janjooa BN, Olesen J, Ashina M (2017) Calcitonin gene-related peptide induced migraine attacks in patients with and without familial aggregation of migraine. Cephalalgia 37:114–124
14. Schytz HW, Birk S, Wienecke T, Kruuse C, Olesen J, Ashina M et al (2009) PACAP38 induces migraine-like attacks in patients with migraine without aura. Brain 132:16–25
15. Olesen J, Thomsen LL, Iversen H (1994) Nitric oxide is a key molecule in migraine and other vascular headaches. Trends Pharmacol Sci 15:149–153
16. Matthews JN, Altman DG, Campbell MJ, Royston P (1990) Analysis of serial measurements in medical research. BMJ 300:230–235
17. Eftekhari S, Warfvinge K, Blixt FW, Edvinsson L (2013) Differentiation of nerve fibers storing CGRP and CGRP receptors in the peripheral Trigeminovascular system. J Pain 14:1289–1303
18. Eftekhari S, Salvatore CA, Calamari A, Kane SA, Tajti J, Edvinsson L (2010) Differential distribution of calcitonin gene-related peptide and its receptor components in the human trigeminal ganglion. Neuroscience 169:683–696
19. Eftekhari S, Edvinsson L (2011) Calcitonin gene-related peptide (CGRP) and its receptor components in human and rat spinal trigeminal nucleus and spinal cord at C1-level. BMC Neurosci 12:112

20. Jansen-Olesen I, Jørgensen L, Engel U, Edvinsson L (2003) In-depth characterization of CGRP receptors in human intracranial arteries. Eur J Pharmacol 481:207–216
21. Russell FA, King R, Smillie S-J, Kodji X, Brain SD (2014) Calcitonin gene-related peptide: physiology and pathophysiology. Physiol Rev 94:1099–1142
22. Brain SD, Grant AD (2004) Vascular actions of calcitonin gene-related peptide and Adrenomedullin. Physiol Rev 84:903–934
23. Nelson MT, Huang Y, Brayden JE, Hescheler J, Standen NB (1990) Arterial dilations in response to calcitonin gene-related peptide involve activation of K+ channels. Nature 344:770–773
24. Fabbretti E, D'Arco M, Fabbro A, Simonetti M, Nistri A, Giniatullin R (2006) Delayed upregulation of ATP P2X3 receptors of trigeminal sensory neurons by calcitonin gene-related peptide. J Neurosci 26:6163–6171
25. Asghar MS, Becerra L, Larsson HBW, Borsook D, Ashina M (2016) Calcitonin gene-related peptide modulates heat nociception in the human brain - an fMRI study in healthy volunteers. PLoS One 11:1–20
26. Guo S, Olesen J, Ashina M (2014) Phosphodiesterase 3 inhibitor cilostazol induces migraine-like attacks via cyclic AMP increase. Brain 137:2951–2959
27. Khan S, Deen M, Hougaard A, Amin FM, Ashina M (2018) Reproducibility of migraine-like attacks induced by phosphodiesterase-3-inhibitor cilostazol. Cephalalgia 38:892–903
28. Vu T, Ma P, Chen JS, de Hoon J, Van Hecken A, Yan L et al (2017) Pharmacokinetic-Pharmacodynamic relationship of Erenumab (AMG 334) and capsaicin-induced dermal blood flow in healthy and migraine subjects. Pharm Res 34:1784–1795

16

Multigroup latent class model of musculoskeletal pain combinations in children/adolescents: identifying high-risk groups by gender and age

Iman Dianat[1], Arezou Alipour[1] and Mohammad Asghari Jafarabadi[2,3*]

Abstract

Background: To investigate the combinations of Musculoskeletal pain (MSP) (neck, shoulder, upper and low back pain) among a sample of Iranian school children.

Methods: The MSP combinations was modeled by latent class analysis (LCA) to find the clusters of high–risk individuals and multigroup LCA taking into account the gender and age (≤ 13 years and ≥ 14 years of age categories).

Results: The lowest and highest prevalence of MSP was 14.2% (shoulder pain in boys aged ≥14 years) and 40.4% (low back pain in boys aged ≤13 years), respectively. The likelihood of synchronized neck and low back pain (9.4–17.7%) was highest, while synchronized shoulder and upper back pain (4.5–9.4%) had the lowest probability. The probability of pain at three and four locations was significantly lower in boys aged ≥14 years than in other gender–age categories. The LCA divided the children into *minor*, *moderate*, and *major pain classes*. The likelihood of shoulder and upper back pain in the *major pain class* was higher in boys than in girls, while the likelihood of neck pain in the *moderate pain class* and low back pain in the *major pain class* were higher in children aged ≥14 years than those aged ≤13 years. Gender–age specific clustering indicated a higher likelihood of experiencing *major pain* in children aged ≤13 years.

Conclusions: The findings highlight the importance of gender– and age–specific data for a more detailed understanding of the MSP combinations in children and adolescents, and identifying high-risk clusters in this regard.

Keywords: Age–specific, Gender–specific, Pain combination, Schoolchildren, Widespread pain, Multigroup LCA

Background

Musculoskeletal pain (MSP) is an extremely common health problem in both genders and in all age groups all around the world [1, 2]. MSP is the most common cause of severe long-term pain and physical disability with significant cost to the individual and society [2, 3]. The current burden of MSP is substantial, and is predicted to increase in both the developed and developing countries [3, 4].

Recent evidence has shown that MSP is very common among school children and youth [5–7]. According to the literature, the reported incidence of neck, shoulder and spinal pain in school children and adolescents ranges from 7% to 74% [5, 6, 8–10]. There is evidence that MSP in childhood and adolescence is a contributory factor for experiencing such complaints in adulthood [11–13]. Therefore, improvement of the understanding of the characteristics of MSP among children and adolescents is necessary for designing appropriate interventions to prevent this phenomenon.

So far, most epidemiological studies on MSP in children and adolescents have evaluated one or at most two pain locations concurrently. As a result, there is limited knowledge with regard to the pain in multiple anatomic locations in this group. The need for studies on MSP combinations in children and adolescents is also well emphasized [14]. In an attempt to address this issue, the present study

* Correspondence: m.asghari862@gmail.com
[2]Road Traffic Injury Research Centre, Faculty of Health, Tabriz University of Medical Sciences, Tabriz, Iran
[3]Department of Statistics and Epidemiology, Faculty of Health, Tabriz University of Medical Sciences, Tabriz 14711, Iran
Full list of author information is available at the end of the article

was conducted to evaluate the MSP combinations in neck, shoulder, upper back and low back areas. Pain combinations can be best addressed by latent class analysis (LCA). However, it has been acknowledged that LCA has been little used in the field of medical research [15], and particularly for evaluation of MSP [14]. LCA provides assessment of whether associations between observed categorical variables (e.g. neck, shoulder, upper back and low back pain in this study) can be described by the presence of an unobserved categorical variable (risk group defined by MSP) (Fig. 1). To better understand the causal mechanisms of the MSP combinations, the LCA can be utilized to determine whether the risk group defined by the MSP adequately gives details on the neck, shoulder, upper back and low back pain combinations among children and adolescents. In addition, information on gender and age subgroups can provide a basis for better identifying high–risk groups (gender– and age–specific groups) and developing interventions as well as dealing with MSP in this population. Therefore, the objective of this study was to investigate the combinations of MSP and clusters of high risk individuals among school children and adolescents using LCA and multigroup gender– and age–specific LCA.

Methods

Study population and procedure

This cross-sectional analytical study was performed in the city of Tabriz, Iran. Tabriz is the capital of East Azerbaijan province in North-western Iran and the fourth major city in Iran with a population of about 1.58 million. School children aged 11–15 years and were in grades 6–8 were included in the study. A three-stage sampling method was utilized to acquire a representative sample of schoolchildren. In the first stage, five educational districts were chosen as strata. In the second stage, a total of 40 schools were selected randomly from these districts, which comprised four girl's schools and four boy's schools. Finally, within each school, the study participants were selected randomly by simple random sampling scheme. The sample size of the study was calculated to be approximately 1105 cases, based on the main outcome of the study, the prevalence of MSP (the minimum about 7% to reach maximum sample size), considering 95% confidence, a precision about 20% and using sample size formula on single proportion in the descriptive studies. Taking into account the design effect about 1.5, the sample size increased to 1611 cases. The samples were allocated to each district and school based on a proportion to size scheme.

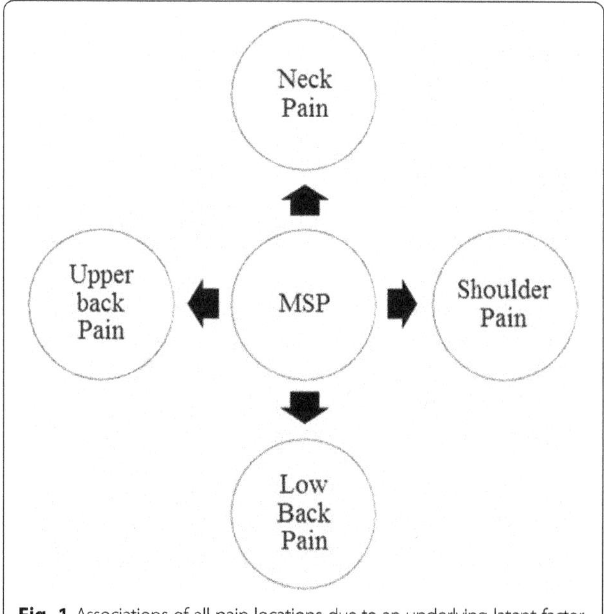

Fig. 1 Associations of all pain locations due to an underlying latent factor

Ethics approval and consent to participate

Before any participation, permission was taken from the education department of Tabriz as well as the school authorities involved. Additionally, the parental permission and informed consent for school children was also taken asking for them to contribute in the study. The study was approved by institutional review board of Tabriz university of medical sciences (code: IR.TBZMED.1394.1166). The research was conducted in accordance with the Declaration of the World Medical Association and the Helsinki Declaration on human subjects testing.

Data collection

The data were collected using a checklist consisting of demographic and MSP data after confirmation by ethics committee. The demographic variables included gender (girls: 1, boys: 2) and age (years). The data on MSP included neck, shoulder, upper back and low back complaints during the preceding month was evaluated using a pre-shaded manikin picture showing the pain location and the modified standardized Nordic Musculoskeletal Questionnaire (NMQ) [16]. The response alternatives were: "no" and "yes". The Farsi version of the NMQ with an established reliability and validity was used in the study [17].

Statistical analyses

Data were analysed using LCA utilizing SAS 9.4 PROC LCA software to find the clusters of individuals by similar pattern of reported MSP [18]. The reports of symptoms were dichotomized as neck pain (no = 0, yes = 1), shoulder pain (no = 0, yes = 1), low back pain (no = 0, yes = 1), and upper back pain (no = 0, yes = 1). Simple LCA was used to estimate the probability and class membership. The study participants were assigned to the latent class clusters with the highest posterior probability as calculated based on Bayes' theorem. A successful model fit was evaluated by a Chi-square Goodness of Fit (GOF) statistic $p > 0.05$.

The conditional independence assumption was intuitively fulfilled since the measures of symptoms in anatomical sites were independently assessed. Multigroup LCA was also used to assess various features of data taking into account the effect of gender (girls = 1 and boys = 2) and age (≤ 13 years = 1 and ≥ 14 years = 2) as well as gender–age combinations (girls ≤13 years = 1, girls ≥14 years = 2, boys ≤13 years = 1, and boys ≥14 years = 4) as the grouping variables. The multigroup models were fitted based on three number of classes obtained in the first step taking into account the effect of gender, age as well as gender–age as the grouping variables in the model. To achieve an appropriate number of classes, a sequence of models were fitted with two, three and four number of classes, and the optimal model was selected by Akaike's Information Criterion (AIC) [19] and Bayesian Information Criterion (BIC) [20]. A smaller AIC and BIC for a particular model proposes a preferable model. A 5% decrease in these measures was used to reach the conclusion. In addition, model interpretability was also considered (e.g. on the basis of the item-response probabilities, each class was distinguishable from others and no class was trivial in size) so that a meaningful label was assigned to each class. In multiple-group LCA, both the class memberships and item response probabilities can change across groups, and therefore measurement invariance can be empirically verified across groups. The parameters were estimated by the maximum likelihood procedure using the EM algorithm. The Newton-Raphson technique was used to estimate the parameters. The convergence index used was the maximum absolute deviation (MAD) to achieve the iteration limit. Missing data on the latent class and latent status indicators were permitted and treated under the assumption that data were missing at random (MAR). Any record with missing data on grouping variables specified in the model was eliminated from the analysis.

Results

Demographic data

A total of 1611 school children participated in the study, of which the percentage of gender–age combinations were 29.8%, 23.1%, 22.9% and 24.2% for girls ≤13 years, girls ≥14 years, boys ≤13 years and boys ≥14 years of age categories, respectively.

The mean weight of the participants were 49.7 (SD 11.36) kg; [girls ≤13 years: 48.1 (SD 10.5) kg, girls ≥14 years: 47.2 (SD 11.7) kg, boys ≤13 years: 51.1 (SD 10.1) kg and boys ≥14 years: 53.2 (SD 12.2) kg] and BMI, 19.9 (3.83) kg/m^2 [girls ≤13 years: 19.6 (SD 3.8) kg/m^2, girls ≥14 years: 20.0 (SD 4.2) kg/m^2, boys ≤13 years: 19.8 (SD 3.3) kg/m^2 and boys ≥14 years: 20.3 (SD 4.0) kg/m^2]. More details on characteristics of the physical leisure activity, use of schoolbags and psychological trait among the schoolchildren are presented in [5, 6].

Prevalence of symptoms

The prevalence of neck, shoulder, low back, and upper back symptoms were 27.9% (95% Confidence Interval (CI): 25.8–30.2%), 20.7% (95% CI: 18.8–22.8%), 34.3% (95% CI: 32.0–36.7%) and 19.0% (95% CI: 17.1–21.0%), respectively. Also 31.5% (95% CI: 29.3–33.9%) of participants reported pain in any of the four body regions.

Gender–age differences in prevalence of symptoms in different body regions

Table 1 shows that prevalence of MSP in gender–age categories in different body regions. The results for *pain at one location* showed a significantly lower prevalence of shoulder symptoms in boys aged ≥14 years and higher prevalence of low back symptoms in boys and girls aged ≤13 years ($p < 0.05$) than in other gender–age categories. The results for *pain at 2 locations* showed significantly lower prevalence of neck/shoulder and shoulder/upper back symptoms in boys aged ≥14 years as well as higher prevalence of shoulder/low back and low back/upper back symptoms in boys and girls aged ≤13 years ($p < 0.05$) than in other gender–age categories. The results for *pain at 3 locations* and *pain at all 4 locations* showed significantly lower prevalence of symptoms in boys ≥14 years of age category ($p < 0.05$) than in other groups.

Choosing the number of latent classes in LCA

A smaller AIC (32.36) and BIC (107.75) for a model by three classes support this model compared to the models with two and four number of classes. Additionally, each class was distinguishable from others on the basis of item-response probabilities, so that a meaningful label was assigned to each class. The first class included those participants (60.2%) with small/moderate value (around 0.3 or lower) of probability of pain in all anatomic locations which was assigned as *moderate pain class.* The second class consisted of participants (7.1%) with high value (> 0.65) of probability of pain in all anatomic locations, which was named as *major pain class.* A small probability of pain (around 0.1 or lower) was observed in the third class with 32.7% of participants as *minor pain class* (Table 2).

Gender-specific LCA modeling

The results of gender-specific LCA modeling are presented in Table 3. As can be seen from this table, the *minor pain class* consisted of 30.7% of girls and 34.5% of boys. With the same pattern of difference, the *moderate pain class* involved 57.9% and 61.6% of girls and boys, respectively. While the *major pain class* had a higher rate of pain in girls (11.4%) compared to boys (4.0%), the test of invariance across gender groups showed no significant difference between girls and boys in the pain clusters ($p > 0.05$). The findings indicated that the

Table 1 Prevalence of MSP (*n* (%)) in gender–age categories in different body regions

	Gender–age categories				*P*-value*
	Girls ≤13 years	Girls ≥14 years	Boys ≤13 years	Boys ≥14 years	
	n (%)	*n* (%)	*n* (%)	*n* (%)	
Pain at 1 location					
Neck pain	136 (28.9%)	99 (27.2%)	112 (31.0%)	90 (23.6%)	0.135
Shoulder pain	108 (23.0%)[a]	77 (21.2%)[a]	87 (24.1%)[a]	**54 (14.2%)[b]**	**0.003**
Upper back pain	84 (17.9%)	64 (17.6%)	83 (23.0%)	67 (17.6%)	0.164
Low back pain	**181 (38.5%)[a]**	111 (30.5%)[b]	**146 (40.4%)[a]**	105 (27.6%)[b]	**< 0.001**
Pain at 2 locations					
Neck/shoulder pain	190 (40.4%)[a]	145 (39.8%)[a]	155 (42.9%)[a]	**116 (30.4%)[b]**	**0.002**
Shoulder/upper back pain	166 (35.3%)[a]	121 (33.2%)[a,b]	136 (37.7%)[a]	**104 (27.3%)[b]**	**0.018**
Shoulder/low back pain	**222 (47.2%)[a,b]**	149 (40.9%)[b,c]	**191 (52.9%)[a]**	139 (36.5%)[c]	**< 0.001**
Low back/upper back pain	**171 (36.4%)[a]**	101 (27.7%)[b]	**131 (36.3%)[a]**	108 (28.3%)[b]	**0.006**
Neck/low back pain	161 (34.3%)	120 (33.0%)	130 (36.0%)	123 (32.3%)	0.722
Neck/upper back pain	150 (31.9%)	99 (27.2%)	101 (28.0%)	95 (24.9%)	0.145
Pain at 3 locations					
Neck/shoulder/low back pain	264 (56.2%)[a,b]	193 (53.0%)[b,c]	224 (62.0%)[a]	**178 (46.7%)[c]**	**< 0.001**
Neck/shoulder/upper back pain	227 (48.3%)[a]	170 (46.7%)[a]	179 (49.6%)[a]	**147 (38.6%)[b]**	**0.010**
Neck/low back/upper back pain	267 (56.8%)[a,b]	182 (50.0%)[b,c]	211 (58.4%)[a]	**180 (47.2%)[c]**	**0.004**
Shoulder/low back/upper back pain	251 (53.4%)[a,b]	172 (47.3%)[b,c]	215 (59.6%)[a]	**170 (44.6%)[c]**	**< 0.001**
Pain at all 4 locations					
Neck/shoulder/low back/upper back pain	286 (60.9%)[a,b]	206 (56.6%)[b,c]	236 (65.4%)[a]	**197 (51.7%)[c]**	**0.001**

**P*-value based on Chi-Squared test (using exact procedure)
In each row, each subscript letter denotes a subset of gender–age categories whose column proportions do not differ significantly from each other at the 0.05 level. Significant differences are shown in bold

likelihood of shoulder and upper back pain in the *major pain class* was considerably higher in boys than girls.

Age-specific LCA modeling

Table 4 shows the results of age-specific LCA modeling. Based on the test of invariance, there was significant difference across children ≤13 years and ≥ 14 years of age categories in membership probability ($p < 0.05$). The *minor pain class* involved a higher percentage of children aged ≥14 years (61.4%) compared to those aged ≤13 years (29.1%). In the *moderate pain class,* children aged ≤13 years (63.9%) were more probable to experience pain than those aged ≥14 years (33.3%). The *major pain class* consisted of 7.0% and 5.3% of children aged ≤13 years and ≥ 14 years, respectively. The results showed considerable differences in the neck and low back pain in the *moderate pain class* as well as neck pain in the *major pain class* across age categories.

Table 2 Membership and item response probabilities in general LCA modeling

Class name	minor pain class	moderate pain class	major pain class
Membership probabilities (%)	32.7%	60.2%	7.1%
MSP			
Neck pain	< 0.01[a]	0.36	0.88
Shoulder pain	0.04	0.24	0.70
Upper back pain	< 0.01	0.24	0.65
Low back pain	0.13	0.38	1.00

[a]Rho estimates (item response probabilities) were presented

Gender-age specific LCA

The results of gender and age (combined)-specific LCA modeling are presented in Table 5. The results indicated that boys (77.8%) and girls (59.7%) aged ≥14 years were the most probable groups for experiencing MSP in the *minor* and *moderate pain classes*, respectively. Girls (30.0%) and boys (34.7%) aged ≤13 years were the most probable groups to experience MSP in the *major pain class.* However, the test of invariance across gender–age categories showed no significant difference between gender–age categories in the pain clusters ($p > 0.05$). Nevertheless, the item response probabilities showed considerable differences across gender–age categories. In the *major pain class,* girls aged ≥14 years were more likely to experience pain in all four anatomical areas than other groups. In the

Table 3 Membership and item response probabilities in gender-specific LCA modeling

	Gender	Latent class		
		minor pain class	moderate pain class	major pain class
Class Membership Probabilities (%)	Girl	30.7%	57.9%	**11.4%**
	Boy	34.5%	61.6%	**4.0%**
MSP				
Neck pain	Girl	< 0.01 #	0.35	**0.84**
	Boy	< 0.01	0.35	**0.94**
Shoulder pain	Girl	0.02	0.27	**0.61**
	Boy	0.04	0.21	**0.79**
Upper back pain	Girl	< 0.01	0.25	**0.50**
	Boy	< 0.01	0.23	**0.95**
Low back pain	Girl	**0.18**	0.38	1.00
	Boy	**0.08**	0.36	1.00

#: Rho estimates (item response probabilities) were presented. Considerable differences between boys and girls are shown in bold (≥ 0.1). Test the invariance across gender groups (Chi^2_{dif} (12) = 16.76, *P*-value = 0.159)

moderate pain class, the likelihood of neck and shoulder complaints in boys aged ≥14 years and also low back pain in girls aged ≥14 were higher than in other categories.

Discussion

Although there are various studies on MSP, pain combinations in children and adolescents are poorly addressed in the literature [14]. The present study was therefore conducted to investigate the combinations of MSP among school children using LCA and multigroup gender– and age–specific LCA. One of the main findings of this study was that the MSP occurred frequently at multiple sites in the study population, which is in line with the findings of previous studies conducted in this regard [14, 21].

From a descriptive point of view, the lowest and highest levels of recorded MSP was 14.2% (shoulder pain in boys ≥14 years of age) and 40.4% (low back pain in boys ≤13 years of age), respectively. With regard to synchronized pain, the likelihood of experiencing synchronized neck and low back pain (prevalence rate was between 9.4% and 17.7%) was highest, while synchronized shoulder and upper back pain (prevalence rate was between 4.5% and 9.4%) had the lowest probability. This is similar to the findings for slightly older (16 and 18 year olds) children reported by Auvinen et al. (2009) [14]. The probability of pain at two locations was relatively the same for both genders as well as for both age categories. However, the probability of pain at three and four locations was significantly lower in boys aged ≥14 years than in other gender–age categories. This finding is relatively similar to the findings of Auvinen et al. (2009) [14], who found that MSP generally occurred more frequently in

Table 4 Membership and item response probabilities in age-specific LCA modeling

	Age (years)	Latent class		
		minor pain class	moderate pain class	major pain class
Class Membership probabilities (%)	≤ 13	29.1%	63.9%	7.0%
	≥ 14	61.4%	33.3%	5.3%
MSP				
Neck pain	≤ 13	0.07 #	**0.30**	**0.97**
	≥ 14	< 0.01	**0.71**	**0.70**
Shoulder pain	≤ 13	< 0.01	0.27	0.69
	≥ 14	0.09	0.29	0.71
Low back pain	≤ 13	0.02	0.21	**0.57**
	≥ 14	0.08	0.30	**1.00**
Upper back pain	≤ 13	**< 0.01**	0.44	1.00
	≥ 14	**0.24**	0.42	1.00

#: Rho estimates (item response probabilities) was presented. Considerable differences between age groups are shown in bold (≥0.1). Test the invariance across age groups ($Chi2_{dif}$ (12) =22.46, *P*-value = 0.033)

Table 5 Membership and item response probabilities in gender–age (combined) specific LCA modeling

	Gender-age categories	Latent class		
		minor pain class	moderate pain class	major pain class
Class Membership Probabilities (%)	Girls ≤13	38.8%	31.2%	**30.0%**
	Girls ≥14	35.5%	**59.7%**	4.8%
	Boys ≤13	28.6%	36.7%	**34.7%**
	Boys ≥14	**77.8%**	5.4%	16.8%
MSP				
Neck pain	Girls ≤13	< 0.01#	0.39	0.55
	Girls ≥14	0.10	0.32	**1.00**
	Boys ≤13	0.14	0.10	0.67
	Boys ≥14	0.13	**0.49**	0.66
Shoulder pain	Girls ≤13	< 0.01	0.28	0.48
	Girls ≥14	0.07	0.25	**0.75**
	Boys ≤13	< 0.01	0.19	0.49
	Boys ≥14	0.03	**1.00**	0.39
Low back pain	Girls ≤13	0.22	< 0.01	**1.00**
	Girls ≥14	< 0.01	**0.43**	**1.00**
	Boys ≤13	**0.63**	< 0.01	0.65
	Boys ≥14	0.22	< 0.01	0.65
Upper back pain	Girls ≤13	0.08	0.18	0.31
	Girls ≥14	< 0.01	0.23	**0.87**
	Boys ≤13	0.08	0.06	0.53
	Boys ≥14	0.09	< 0.01	0.63

#: Rho estimates (item response probabilities) was presented. Considerable differences between gender-age categories are shown in bold (≥ 0.1). Test the invariance across age groups ($Chi2_{dif}$ (36) = 44.78, *P*-value = 0.150)

girls than in boys of the same age. This is also, in part, similar to the findings of other studies, which have reported significant associations between age and pains at multiple locations in school children and adolescents [14, 21, 22]. Also, it should be noted that the probability of pain in multiple locations had a direct relationship with the number of locations, which is also similar to the findings of Auvinen et al. (2009) [14].

It is of interest to note that this study applied multi-group LCA for better understanding and a more detailed analysis of the MSP in school children and the results showed a three-class unobserved factor explaining associations among the musculoskeletal observed components. The associations between this factor and observed musculoskeletal components were fairly modeled totally and in gender and age subgroups, which is relatively new to the literature. In summary, the LCA showed promise in expanding the current understanding of the MSP. The results of modeling demonstrated that a three-class latent factor, which is *moderate pain, minor pain* and *major pain*, can best describes associations among observed features of the MSP among all age categories of both genders in the studied population. Based on the results of the LCA, similar pain profiles were observed for individuals belonging to a given class. The findings demonstrated that the percentage of children with moderate, minor and high probability of experiencing pain in all anatomical locations (representing three pain classes) were 60%, 33% and 7%, respectively. This is relatively similar to the findings of previous studies conducted among school children and adolescents [14, 22]. It is of interest to note that, in the line with our results, Auvinen et al. (2009) reported that belonging to a class with high probability of pain predicted pain at all anatomic sites [14], but with a slight difference, Adamson et al. (2007) did not find any class with a single main pain site and only showed the co-occurrence of neck and back pain among their study subjects [22]. With regard to gender–specific findings, both genders had a relatively similar pattern of pain, although the likelihood of shoulder and upper back pain in the *major pain class* was higher in boys than in girls. From an age–specific point of view, a similar pattern of pain was also observed for children ≤13 years and ≥ 14 years of age categories, although the likelihood of neck pain in the *moderate pain class* and low back pain in the *major pain class* were higher in children aged ≥14 years than those aged ≤13 years. With regard to gender–age specific clustering, the results of invariance test showed a same pattern of classes for boys and girls; although the likelihood of experiencing *major pain* was considerably higher in children aged ≤13 years than in those aged ≥14 years. These findings add to the significance of gender– and age–specific data, which is new to the literature, to develop guidelines and interventions in preventing MSP in school children and adolescents, particularly for those who are at greater risk of experiencing such complaints.

The strength of the present study can be considered by the LCA which identified high-risk clusters of school children and adolescents according to their MSP profile in a large sample. The definition of the widespread pain suggested by the American College of Rheumatology [23] or the definition offered by MacFarlane et al. (1996) (e.g. The Manchester definition) for screening fibromyalgia, require experiencing pain in at least 2 contralateral body quadrants (e.g. right or left and above or below the waist) and in the axial skeleton (e.g. spine or anterior chest) [24]. Such definitions, although they may be useful clinical tools to detect and diagnose fibromyalgia and other MSP, are too specific for describing widespread pain in epidemiological studies. It seems that assessing the MSP profile clustering by LCA, and particularly in subgroups by multigroup LCA, provide a compensation for this problem.

Individuals with MSP are typically referred to physiotherapists in primary health care and physiotherapy may relieve local pain and somehow multisite pain. In MSP, the treatment aims to support change processes that can attend to pain relief and should be time-limited, but this is not the case and was a great concern and limitation for physiotherapy. The results of Whal et al. (2018) showed the relation between being the long-term consumers of physiotherapy and self-management competency and they concluded that a treatment goal for people with MSP should include development of self-management capacity [25]. The findings of current study may provide a useful framework to taking into account the diversity of the children'/adolescents' MSP with regard to self-management capacity when referring to MSP therapy.

Furthermore, there are many comorbidities of MSP: in particular migraine [26, 27] and fibromyalgia [28]. Also, MSP may have potential interaction with other comorbidities which may affect the therapy outcome [29].

The large sample size in a general population and considering pain combinations form gender–and age–specific perspective are the major strengths of this study. Another advantage was that the data were collected by one of the authors interviewing the school children in order to decrease the likelihood of non-participation bias and to prevent observer error (e.g. as opposed to self-reporting or parental-assisted reporting). However, as in any epidemiological study, there may be possible limitation with regard to the accuracy and reliability of self-reported data on MSP as the outcome measure. However, as it has been acknowledged, this may be the only measure to understand whether and how the school children and adolescents feel any pain or discomfort, especially in large-scale populations [5, 14]. As another limitation, we performed the LCA in a cross-sectional study and have focused on gender- and age-specific MSP clusters in the population but we didn't taking into account the risk factors; to better find the relationship between the risk factors and MSP combinations in a LCA scheme, stronger epidemiological studies (case-control and cohort designs) are recommended. Additionally, in such a large epidemiological study, the etiologies cannot be considered. However, the results may be biased by mixing benign diseases with more serious clinical conditions. As another shortcoming, the interview concerned only the preceding month. Therefore there is the risk to include both chronic pain conditions, lasting more than 6 months, and minor episodic painful situations.

Conclusions

In conclusion, the findings of this study add to the understanding of the MSP combinations in school children and adolescents and help to identify high-risk clusters of this population according to their MSP profile. It was shown that the MSP was frequent at multiple sites among the study population. The LCA divided the studied children into three pain clusters including *moderate pain class*, *minor pain class* and *major pain class*. The LCA demonstrated that both genders had a relatively similar pattern of pain, although the likelihood of shoulder and upper back pain in the *major pain class* was higher in boys than in girls. A similar pattern of pain was also observed for the two age groups, although the likelihood of neck pain in the *moderate pain class* and low back pain in the *major pain class* were higher in children aged ≥14 years than those aged ≤13 years. The results of gender–age specific clustering indicated a same pattern of classes for boys and girls, although the likelihood of experiencing *major pain* was considerably higher in children aged ≤13 years. These findings highlight the importance of gender– and age–specific data for better understanding and a more detailed analysis of the MSP in school children and adolescents using the LCA, which can consequently lead to developing guidelines and interventions to prevent MSP in this population (particularly for those who are at greater risk of developing MSP). The findings have also implications for assessment of MSP in epidemiological studies.

Abbreviations

AIC: Akaike's Information Criterion; BIC: Bayesian Information Criterion; CI: Confidence Interval; GOF: Goodness of Fit; LCA: Latent class analysis; MAR: Missing at random; MSP: Musculoskeletal pain

Acknowledgements

The support of Research deputy of Tabriz University of Medical Sciences is appreciated.

Funding
This work was supported by the Research deputy of Tabriz University of Medical Sciences.

Authors' contributions
All authors read and approved the final manuscript. ID and AA conceived of the study and participated in the design and data collection. MAJ and ID participated in the data analyses, interpretation of the results and MS preparation.

Authors' information
ID is associate professor of Ergonomics and an instructor at Tabriz University of Medical Sciences, Tabriz, Iran, AA is MSc of Ergonomics and MAJ is associate professor of Biostatistics and an instructor at Tabriz University of Medical Sciences, Tabriz, Iran.

Competing interests
The authors declare that they have no competing interests.

Author details
[1]Department of Occupational Health and Ergonomics, Tabriz University of Medical Sciences, Tabriz, Iran. [2]Road Traffic Injury Research Centre, Faculty of Health, Tabriz University of Medical Sciences, Tabriz, Iran. [3]Department of Statistics and Epidemiology, Faculty of Health, Tabriz University of Medical Sciences, Tabriz 14711, Iran.

References
1. Henschke N, Harrison C, McKay D, Broderick C, Latimer J, Britt H, Maher CG (2014) Musculoskeletal conditions in children and adolescents managed in Australian primary care. BMC Musculoskelet Disord 15(1):164
2. Woolf AD, Erwin J, March L (2012) The need to address the burden of musculoskeletal conditions. Best Pract Res Clin Rheumatol 26(2):183–224
3. Brooks PM (2006) The burden of musculoskeletal disease—a global perspective. Clin Rheumatol 25(6):778–781
4. Hoy D, March L, Brooks P, Blyth F, Woolf A, Bain C, Williams G, Smith E, Vos T, Barendregt J (2014) The global burden of low back pain: estimates from the global burden of disease 2010 study. Ann Rheum Dis 73(6):968–974
5. Dianat I, Alipour A, Asgari Jafarabadi M (2018) Risk factors for neck and shoulder pain among schoolchildren and adolescents. J Paediatr Child Health 54(1):20–27
6. Dianat I, Alipour A, Jafarabadi MA (2017) Prevalence and risk factors of low back pain among school age children in Iran. Health promotion perspectives 7(4):223
7. MacDonald J, Stuart E, Rodenberg R (2017) Musculoskeletal low back pain in school-aged children: a review. JAMA Pediatr 171(3):280–287
8. Diepenmaat A, Van der Wal M, De Vet H, Hirasing R (2006) Neck/shoulder, low back, and arm pain in relation to computer use, physical activity, stress, and depression among Dutch adolescents. Pediatrics 117(2):412–416
9. Jeffries LJ, Milanese SF, Grimmer-Somers KA (2007) Epidemiology of adolescent spinal pain: a systematic overview of the research literature. Spine (Phila Pa 1976) 32(23):2630–2637
10. Murphy S, Buckle P, Stubbs D (2007) A cross-sectional study of self-reported back and neck pain among English schoolchildren and associated physical and psychological risk factors. Appl Ergon 38(6):797–804
11. Hakala P, Rimpelä A, Salminen JJ, Virtanen SM, Rimpelä M (2002) Back, neck, and shoulder pain in Finnish adolescents: national cross sectional surveys. BMJ 325(7367):743
12. Hestbaek L, Leboeuf-Yde C, Kyvik KO, Manniche C (2006) The course of low back pain from adolescence to adulthood: eight-year follow-up of 9600 twins. Spine (Phila Pa 1976) 31(4):468–472
13. Siivola SM, Levoska S, Latvala K, Hoskio E, Vanharanta H, Keinänen-Kiukaanniemi S (2004) Predictive factors for neck and shoulder pain: a longitudinal study in young adults. Spine (Phila Pa 1976) 29(15):1662–1669
14. Auvinen JP, Paananen MV, Tammelin TH, Taimela SP, Mutanen PO, Zitting PJ, Karppinen JI (2009) Musculoskeletal pain combinations in adolescents. Spine (Phila Pa 1976) 34(11):1192–1197
15. Boyko EJ, Doheny RA, McNeely MJ, Kahn SE, Leonetti DL, Fujimoto WY (2010) Latent class analysis of the metabolic syndrome. Diabetes Res Clin Pract 89(1):88–93
16. Kuorinka I, Jonsson B, Kilbom A, Vinterberg H, Biering-Sørensen F, Andersson G, Jørgensen K (1987) Standardised Nordic questionnaires for the analysis of musculoskeletal symptoms. Appl Ergon 18(3):233–237
17. Dianat I, Karimi MA (2014) Association of parental awareness of using schoolbags with musculoskeletal symptoms and carrying habits of schoolchildren. J Sch Nurs 30(6):440–447
18. Kaplan D. The sage handbook of quantitative methodology for the social sciences: sage; 2004
19. Akaike H (1974) A new look at the statistical model identification. IEEE Trans Autom Control 19(6):716–723
20. Schwarz G (1978) Estimating the dimension of a model. Ann Stat 6(2):461–464
21. Petersen S, Brulin C, Bergström E (2006) Recurrent pain symptoms in young schoolchildren are often multiple. Pain 121(1–2):145–150
22. Adamson G, Murphy S, Shevlin M, Buckle P, Stubbs D (2007) Profiling schoolchildren in pain and associated demographic and behavioural factors: a latent class approach. Pain 129(3):295–303. https://doi.org/10.1016/j.pain.2006.10.015
23. Wolfe F, Clauw DJ, Fitzcharles MA, Goldenberg DL, Katz RS, Mease P, Russell AS, Russell IJ, Winfield JB, Yunus MB (2010) The American College of Rheumatology preliminary diagnostic criteria for fibromyalgia and measurement of symptom severity. Arthritis Care Res (Hoboken) 62(5):600–610
24. Macfarlane G, Croft P, Schollum J, Silman A (1996) Widespread pain: is an improved classification possible? J Rheumatol 23(9):1628–1632
25. Wahl AK, Opseth G, Nolte S, Osborne RH, Bjørke G, Mengshoel AM (2018) Is regular use of physiotherapy treatment associated with health locus of control and self-management competency? A study of patients with musculoskeletal disorders undergoing physiotherapy in primary health care. Musculoskeletal Sci Pract 36:43–47. https://doi.org/10.1016/j.msksp.2018.04.008
26. Tana C, Giamberardino MA, Cipollone F (2017) microRNA profiling in atherosclerosis, diabetes, and migraine. Ann Med 49(2):93–105
27. Giamberardino MA, Affaitati G, Martelletti P, Tana C, Negro A, Lapenna D, Curto M, Schiavone C, Stellin L, Cipollone F (2016) Impact of migraine on fibromyalgia symptoms. J Headache and Pain 17(1):28
28. Costantini R, Affaitati G, Massimini F, Tana C, Innocenti P, Giamberardino MA (2016) Laparoscopic cholecystectomy for gallbladder Calculosis in fibromyalgia patients: impact on musculoskeletal pain, somatic hyperalgesia and central sensitization. PLoS One 11(4):e0153408. https://doi.org/10.1371/journal.pone.0153408
29. Giamberardino MA, Tana C, Costantini R (2014) Pain thresholds in women with chronic pelvic pain. Curr Opin Obstet Gynecol 26(4):253–259

17

Headache in transient ischemic attacks

Elena R. Lebedeva[1,2*], Natalia M. Gurary[3] and Jes Olesen[4]

Abstract

Background: Headache is a common feature in acute cerebrovascular disease but no studies have evaluated the prevalence of specific headache types in patients with transient ischemic attacks (TIA). The purpose of the present study was to analyze all headaches within the last year and the last week before TIA and at the time of TIA.

Methods: Eligible patients with TIA ($n = 120$, mean age 56.1, females 55%) had focal brain or retinal ischemia with resolution of symptoms within 24 h without presence of new infarction on MRI with DWI ($n = 112$) or CT ($n = 8$). All patients were evaluated within one day of admission by a single neurologist. As a control group we used patients ($n = 192$, mean age 58.7, females 64%) admitted with diagnoses "lumbago", "lumbar spine osteochondrosis" or "gastrointestinal ulcer".

Results: One-year prevalence of migraine without aura was significantly higher in TIA patients than in controls: 20.8% and 7.8% respectively ($p = 0.002$, OR 3.1, 95% CI 1.6–6.2). 22 patients (18.3%) had sentinel or warning headache within the last week before TIA. At the time of TIA a new type of headache was observed in 16 patients (13.3%). No controls had a new type of headache. 12 of these 16 patients had migraine-like headache, 8 patients had tension-type-like headache and one patient thunderclap headache. Posterior circulation TIA was associated with headaches within last week before TIA and at the time of TIA much more frequently than anterior circulation TIA.

Conclusions: The one year prevalence of migraine was significantly higher in TIA patients than in controls and so was the prevalence of headache within the last week before TIA and at the time of TIA. A previous headache that worsens and a new type of headache can be a warning of impending TIA.

Keywords: Transient ischemic attack, TIA, Secondary headache disorders, Migraine, Warning headache

Background

Several previous studies have shown that headache is a common feature in TIA, its frequency varies from 16% till 36% in different studies [1–10]. These studies have mostly included all kinds of CVD with a minority of transient ischemic attacks (TIA). No recent studies have specifically evaluated the prevalence of headache in patients with TIA and none have diagnosed previous headaches and headaches at the time of TIA according to internationally accepted diagnostic criteria [11].

For a detailed analysis of headaches in TIA it is necessary to characterize not only the headache occurring at the time of TIA but also previous headaches such as migraine and tension-type headache. Otherwise it is impossible to distinguish between an attack of usual headache and a new type of headache occurring at the time of TIA. In order to make this distinction, extensive semi-structured neurologically conducted interviews are necessary, and they should be done as soon as possible after TIA. To the best of our knowledge no such study has ever been performed.

Here we present a prospective study of 120 consecutive patients with TIA using a validated extensive semistructured professionally conducted interview done as soon as the TIA diagnosis including neuroimaging had been secured after admission. The aims of this study were to analyze all headaches within the last year before TIA, all headaches within the last week before TIA (sentinel headache) and all headaches occurring within 24 h after TIA. Our hypothesis was that TIA may cause headaches and that headache may be a warning sign of impending TIA.

* Correspondence: elenalebedeva1971@gmail.com
[1]Department of Neurology and Neurosurgery, The Ural State Medical University, Repina 3, Yekaterinburg 620028, Russia
[2]International Headache Center "Europe-Asia", Yekaterinburg, Russia
Full list of author information is available at the end of the article

Methods

Study populations

The period of recruitment of patients was from April 2014 till May 2016. The study population was admitted to the stroke unit of city hospital "New Hospital" in Yekaterinburg, Russia. Inclusion criteria were focal brain or retinal ischemia with resolution of symptoms within 24 h and without presence of new infarction on magnetic resonance imaging (MRI) with diffusion weighted imaging (DWI) or *computed tomography*(CT). Excluded were patients with previous cerebrovascular disease or other serious neurological disease and memory problems. All patients were evaluated within one day of admission, usually within a few hours by a neurologist. 62 patients had TIA < 6 h before admission to the hospital, 50 patients had TIA in interval from 6 to 12 h, 6 had TIA in interval from 13 to 24 h and two had TIA in interval from 24 to 36 h before admission.

A total of 131 patients were examined, 11 patients were excluded because most of them had difficulties to recall essential information and memory problems. 112 patients had MRI with DWI and 8 had CT. These examinations were done immediately after admission to the hospital. All TIA cases were subdivided into anterior and posterior circulation TIA.

As a control group we used patients who were admitted to the emergency room without acute neurological deficits or serious neurological or somatic disorders. We examined 225 controls.33 patients were excluded and 192 patients were included.

Evaluation

One neurologist (N.M.G.) collected patient data prospectively, using a standardized case-report form during face-to-face interviews during admission to the emergency room in controls. Information about patients, medical history and risk factors imaging and laboratory tests were recorded. We recorded history of headache during last year, during 1 week before TIA and at the time of TIA defined as within 24 h of TIA onset. We used extensive semi-structured interview forms that contained all necessary information to diagnose previous headaches.

Definitions and diagnostic criteria

TIA was defined as a transient episode of neurological dysfunction caused by focal brain, spinal cord, or retinal ischemia, without acute infarction [12].

The diagnoses of previous and present headaches were made according to the explicit diagnostic criteria of the International Headache Society, the International Classification of Headache Disorders ICHD-3 [11]. We recorded headache within the last year and last week before TIA and within 24 h after onset of TIA. We distinguished between previous headache without change of characteristics, headache with change of characteristics and new type of headache. We defined a new type of headache in TIA as a headache which arose for the first time in the week before or within 24 h after onset of TIA. Migraine or tension type headache with changes of characteristics within the last week before TIA or within 24 h after onset of TIA as well as migraine or tension type headache as a new type of headache were defined as migraine-like headache and tension- type-like headache respectively. We did not apply the diagnostic criteria for "headache attributed to TIA" of the ICHD-3 because the purpose of the present study was to compare all kinds of headaches in patients with TIA to a matched control group.

Ethical considerations

The Medical Ethics Committee of the Urals State Medical University approved this study. All respondents were informed of the purpose of the survey. Written informed consent was obtained from all participants.

Statistical analysis

Statistical analyses were performed with SPSS 17.0 software. Continuous variables were summarized as means, and categorical variables as numbers and percentages. We used chi-squared to compare distributions of categorical variables between groups. We set statistical significance at $P < 0.05$. We first used binary logistic regression to estimate odds ratios (OR) with 95% confidence intervals (CI) for consulting and laboratory data. Prevalence estimates and 95% CI for the prevalence estimates of migraine and other headache were determined using previously described methods [13, 14].

Results

Characteristics of patients with TIA and controls

Table 1 shows the distribution of patients with TIA and controls by age and sex. The mean age of patients with TIA and controls did not differ significantly: 56.1 and 58.7 respectively. Females prevailed in the control group (64%). Control patients were admitted to the emergency room with the following diagnoses: "lumbago" or "lumbar spine osteochondrosis" ($n = 99$), "pancreatitis" ($n= 62$), "gastrointestinal ulcer" ($n = 7$), tick bite ($n = 14$), irritable bowel syndrome ($n = 2$), paroxysmal benign positional vertigo ($n = 2$), arthritis ($n = 5$), allergic reaction ($n = 1$). Most patients (106 patients, 88%) had TIA in the anterior circulation system and only few (14 patients, 12%) in the posterior circulation system. Seven patients (5.8%) had two or more attacks of TIA. Table 2 shows clinical characteristics of patients with TIA and controls. The prevalence of the following factors was significantly higher in TIA patients than in controls: consumption of strong alcoholic beverages, arterial hypertension, atrial fibrillation, low physical

Table 1 Distribution of patients with TIA and controls by age and sex

Sex	Age interval							
	15–25	26–35	36–45	46–55	56–65	66–75	76–90	Mean age
Male TIA patinets ($n = 55$)	3 (5.5%)	4 (7.3%)	5 (9.1%)	7 (12.7%)	22 (40%)	10 (18.2%)	4 (7.3%)	56.5
Male controls ($n = 69$)	0 (0.0%)	2 (2.9%)	11 (15.9%)	24 (34.8%)	17 (24.6%)	9 (13.0%)	6 (8.7%)	56.5
Female TIA patients ($n = 65$)	5 (7.7%)	7 (10.8%)	7 (10.8%)	9 (13.8%)	16 (24.6%)	11 (16.9%)	10 (15.4%)	55.7
Female controls ($n = 123$)	0 (0.0%)	5 (4.1%)	11 (8.9%)	25 (20.3%)	41 (33.3%)	26 (21.1%)	15 (12.2%)	59.9
All TIA patients ($n = 120$)	8 (6.7%)	11 (9.2%)	12 (10.0%)	16 (13.3%)	38 (31.7%)	21 (17.5%)	14 (11.7%)	56,1
All control patients ($n = 192$)	0 (0.0%)	7 (3.6%)	22 (11.5%)	49 (25.5%)	58 (30.2%)	35 (18.2%)	21 (10.9%)	58.7

activity, family history of stroke in first degree relatives, hypercholesterolemia, angina pectoris.

The duration of TIA varied from 5 min to 24 h. 42 patients (35%) had resolution of all symptoms within 60 min. Among them 22 patients (18,3%) had duration of TIA from 2 till 15 min and 20 patients (16,7%) 16–60 min. 18 patients (15%) had duration of TIA from 1 h to 3 h and 60 patients (50%) had duration from 3 h to 24 h. 86 patients with TIA had sensory deficits, 68 patients had speech disturbances, 73 patients had unilateral motor weakness [14].

All patients with TIA underwent a stroke risk assessment according to the ABCD2 score. A low risk of stroke (0–3 points) was registered in 62 patients (51.6%), moderate risk (4–5 points) in 54 patients (45%), high risk (6–7 points) in 4 patients (3.3%).

Headache within last year (excepting last week) before TIA

The prevalence of all primary headache disorders in patients with TIA during the last year (excepting the last week) before TIA and in controls is presented in Table 3. Ninety patients (75%) had tension-type headache (TTH) and 27 patients (22.5%) had migraine during 1 year before TIA. Most patients with migraine also had TTH. 20 patients had no headache at all. The prevalence of chronic headaches was 4%. These patients all had TTH and/or migraine and were thus included in the above numbers. Only the one-year prevalence of migraine without aura was significantly higher in patients with TIA than in controls: 20.8% and 7.8% respectively ($p = 0.002$, OR 3.1, 95% CI 1.6–6.2). This was also true for females only: 33.8% and 11.4% respectively ($p < 0.001$, OR 4.0, 95% CI 1.9–8.5).

Headache within the last week before TIA

These headaches and headaches in controls are described in Table 4. 26 of 120 patients with TIA (21.6%) had headache within the last week before TIA versus 12 of 192 of controls (6.2%) ($p < 0.01$). All patients ($n = 14$, 100%)with posterior circulation TIA and 12 of 106 patients (11.3%) with anterior circulation TIA had headache in this period. Headache occurred most often within one day before TIA

Table 2 Clinical characteristics of patients with TIA and controls

Characteristics	Patients with TIA ($n = 120$)	Controls ($n = 192$)	*P* value
Mean age	56.1	58.7	0.1
Male, n (%)	55 (45.8%)	69 (35.9%)	0.1
Current smoker, n (%)	38 (31.7%)	45 (23.4%)	0.1
Consumption of light alcoholic beverages, n (%)	5 (4.2%)	11 (5.7%)	0.7
Consumption of strong alcoholic beverages, n (%)	23 (19.2%)	18 (9.4%)	0.02
Arterial hypertension, n (%)	94 (78.3%)	108 (56.3%)	< 0.001
Diabetes mellitus, n (%)	10 (8.3%)	14 (7.3%)	0.9
Hyperglycemia n (%)	23 (19.2%)	26 (13.5%)	0.2
Atrial fibrillation, n (%)	14 (11.6%)	7 (3.6%)	0.01
Body mass index > 25, n (%)	68 (56.7%)	118 (61.5%)	0.5
Low physical activity, n (%)	45 (37.5%)	28 (14.6%)	< 0.001
Family history of stroke in first degree relatives, n (%)	53 (44.2%)	48(25.0%)	0.001
Peripheral artery disease, n (%)	2 (1.7%)	1 (0.5%)	0.7
Hypercholesterolemia, n (%)	56 (46.7%)	55 (28.6%)	0.002
Angina pectoris, n (%)	32 (26.7%)	18 (9.4%)	< 0.001
Myocardial infarction, n (%)	11 (9.2%)	7 (3.6%)	0.07

Table 3 One-year prevalence[a] of primary headache disorders in patients with TIA ($n = 120$) and in controls ($n = 192$) according ICHD 3

Type of headaches	Males with TIA ($n = 55$)	Male controls ($n = 69$)	P, OR (95% CI)	Females with TIA ($n = 65$)	Female controls ($n = 123$)	P, OR (95% CI)	All patients with TIA ($n = 120$)	All controls ($n = 192$)	P, OR (95% CI)
Migraine without aura	3 (5.5%)[b]	1 (1.4%)	0.5	22 (33.8%)	14 (11.4%)	< 0.001, 4.0; 1.9–8.5	25 (20.8%)	15 (7.8%)	0.002, 3.1; 1.6–6.2
Migraine with aura	0	0	–	1 (1.5%)	1 (0.8%)	0.8	1 (0.8%)	1 (0.52%)	0.7
Chronic migraine	0	0	–	1 (1.5%)	1 (0.8%)	0.8	1 (0.8%)	1 (0.52%)	0.7
Episodic TTH[c]	40 (72.7%)	48 (69%)	0.9	46 (70.8%)	84 (68.3%)	0.9	86 (71.7%)	132 (68.7%)	0.6
Chronic TTH	0	0	–	4 (6.2%)	3 (2.4%)	0.4	4 (3.3%)	3 (1.6%)	0.5
Cluster headache	1 (1.8%)	0	0.9	0	1 (0.81%)	0.7	1 (0.8%)	1 (0.52%)	0.7
Medication overuse headache (analgesics)	0	0	–	2 (3.1%)	0	0.2	2 (1.7%)	0	0.3
Absence of headache	11 (20%)	20 (29%)	0.3	9 (13.8%)	14 (11.4%)	0.8	20 (16.6%)	34 (17.7%)	0.9

[a]Prevalence of primary headache disorders in patients with TIA were calculated during last year excepting the last week before TIA
[b]Percentages in this table were calculated using number of patients with TIA and controls (males, females, all) indicated in upper row of the table
[c]TTH – tension type of headache

Table 4 Headache in patients during 1 week before TIA ($n = 120$) and during last week before interview in controls ($n = 192$)

Type of headache	Previous headache without changes in patients with TIA	Previous headache without changes in controls	P, OR (95% CI)	Previous headache with changes in patients with TIA	Previous headache with changes in controls	P, OR (95% CI)	New type of headache in patients with TIA	New type of headache in controls	P, OR (95% CI)
Migraine without aura[a]	2(1.6%)	0 (0%)	0.07	4 (3.3%)	0	0.01	2 (1.6%)	0	0.07
Migraine with aura[a]	0	0	–	0	0	–	1 (0.8%)	0	0.2
TTH[a]	2 (1.6%)	10 (5.2%)	0.1	12 (10%)	2 (1.0%)	0.0002	2 (1.6%)	0	0.01
Cluster headache	0	0	–	0	0	–	0	0	–
Thunderclap headache	N/A[b]	N/A	–	N/A		–	1 (0.8%)	0	0.2
All headaches	4 (3.3%)	10 (5.2%)	0.4	16 (13.3%)	2 (1.0%)	0.00001	6 (5%)	0	0.0003

[a]Here and in the Table 5: migraine with and without aura with changes of characteristics and tension type headache with changes of characteristics as well as migraine with and without aura or tension type headache as a new type of headache were defined as migraine-like headache and tension type-like headache respectively in the text of the article because they were probably attributed to TIA

[b]Here and in the Table 5: N/A not applicable

(15 out of 26 patients, 57.6%), 11 out of 26 patients (42.3%) had headache 2–7 days before TIA.

Four patients (3.3%) had previous headache without changes of characteristics within a week of TIA and 10 controls (5.2%).Seven patients (5.8%) and no controls had migraine-like headaches within the last week before TIA. Patients with posterior circulation TIA had migraine-like headache more often (6 of 14, 42.8%) than patients with anterior circulation TIA (1 of 106, 0.9%). Four of 7 patients had a past history of migraine during the last year. Before TIA their migraine attacks became daily and stronger than usual. In three patients the migraine-like attacks appeared for the first time. All these seven patients could have sentinel or warning headache.

Fourteen patients (11.6%) had tension-type-like headache during the last week before TIA and 2 controls (1.0%). The percentage of patients with posterior circulation TIA with such headaches was much greater (57.1%) than the percentage with anterior circulation TIA (7.5%).12 of these patients had a past history of headache. They had increases in duration, frequency, and/or intensity of their previous headaches. The prevalence of TTH with changes of characteristics was significantly higher in TIA patients (10%) than in controls (1.0%). Two patients with TIA had a new tension-type- like headache and no controls. All these 14 patients with tension-type-like headache could have sentinel or warning headache.

Totally 22 patients (14 with tension-type-like headache, 7 with migraine-like headache and one with thunderclap headache) had sentinel or warning headache within the last week before TIA.

Headache at the time of TIA

A new type of headache was observed in 16 patients (13.3%) (Table 5). No controls had a new type of headache. 12 of the 16patients had migraine-like headache, 8 patients had tension-type-like headache and one patient thunderclap headache. Among the sixteen patients, 12 had posterior circulation TIA (86% of patients with posterior circulation TIA) and 4 had anterior circulation TIA (3.7% of patients with anterior circulation TIA). There was no relation between duration of TIA symptoms and occurrence of a new type of headache. 11 patients with a new type of headache (69%) were older than 45 years.

A previous headache with changed characteristics was found in 9 of 120 patients (7.5%) and no in controls. Four of these patients had migraine-like headache and 5 tension-type-like headache. Six patients had TIA in the posterior circulation (42.8%) and 3 in the anterior circulation (2.8%). Four patients had a past history of migraine without aura and 5 a history of TTH. They had increased intensity, frequency or altered localization or they became refractory to usual treatment Seven patients had headache at the same time as TIA and two after TIA. Six patients had duration of TIA more than 3 h and three patients had duration 10–15 min.

Eight of 120 patients (6.6%) and 9 controls (4.6%) had a usual headache without any changes. Four patients had TIA in the posterior circulation and the remaining four in the anterior circulation. Six patients had headache at the same time as TIA and two after TIA. Six patients had duration of TIA more than 3 h and two patients had duration 15–30 min.

We performed follow-up of 118 out of 120 patients with TIA, the average follow-up period was 30 months. Four patients reported repeated TIA. Ischemic strokes happened in 7 patients. We found only one case of migraine with aura which was missed during the first interview.

Table 5 Headaches at the time of TIA onset ($n = 120$) and at admission of controls ($n = 192$)

Type of headache	Headaches at the time of development of TIA								
	Previous headache without changes in patients with TIA	Previous headache without changes in controls	P, OR (95% CI)	Previous headache with changes in patients with TIA	Previous headache with changes in controls	P, OR (95% CI)	New type of headache in patients with TIA	New type of headache in patients with controls	P, OR (95% CI)
Migraine without aura	2 (1.6%)	5 (4.1%)	0.6	4 (3.3%)	0	0.01	11 (9.1%)	0	0.00001
Migraine with aura	0	0	–	0	0	–	1 (0.83%)	0	0.2
TTH	6 (5%)	4 (3.3%)	0.1	5 (4.1%)	0	0.004	3 (2.5%)	0	0.02
Cluster headache	0	0	–	0	0	–	0	0	0
Thunderclap headache	N/A	N/A	–	N/A	N/A	–	1 (0.83%)	0	0.2
All headaches	8 (6.6%)	9 (4.6%)	0.4	9 (7.5%)	0	0.0001	16 (13.3%)	0	0.00001

Discussion

The major findings of the present study were that TIA patients compared to controls more frequently had migraine within the previous year, more often had headache within one week before TIA and at the time of TIA.

Previous studies of headache in TIA

Only few studies have attempted to characterize headache in patients with TIA and no studies were performed in the past 10 years [1–10]. In most studies headaches were analyzed in TIA patients together with stroke patients [1, 2, 4, 9] but two studies analyzed TIA patients separately [5, 10]. Patients were asked in one study about the presence and localization of headache at symptom onset and to describe the quality of headache according to predefined categories: dull, pressing, stabbing, burning, pulsate, or circular [2]. In the other study patients were asked about the presence and nature (throbbing versus constant) of headache [4]. In three other studies patients were asked about onset, duration, location and quality of headache [1, 5, 9, 10]. Patients were asked about headache prior to TIA only in two studies [1, 5]. All previous studies used CT but not MRI with DWI for detection of infarct and many studies therefore may have included small infarcts. Besides no study could make a specific diagnosis of headache because of absence of classification that time or lack of information about necessary characteristics of the headache. The few studies with a big number of TIA patients did not use a detailed interview about previous and current headache [2, 3]. Therefore, it is difficult to compare our results with previous studies. The character of headaches at TIA onset was different in different studies: throbbing [1, 9] or diffuse [5] or generalized non-localized [10]. The overall prevalence of headache at the time of TIA varied from 16% to 36% and is thus in accordance with our results [1–10].

Methodological considerations

Several principles should be taken into account in studies of headache in TIA patients. First of all, it is impossible to know the exact diagnosis of headache without using the diagnostic criteria of the International classification of headache [11]. This requires a professional semi-structured interview about previous and current headache, preferably face to face, because some important characteristics of headache can otherwise be missed in acutely ill patients. It is also necessary to record the exact timing of headache and TIA and to use a generally accepted definition of transient ischemic attacks including MRI with DWI to exclude acute infarcts.

Headache can only manifest in a limited number of ways. Thus, most secondary headaches including headache in TIA patients have the characteristics of tension-type headache or migraine without aura. If there is a close temporal relation, it must, however, be classified as a secondary headache attributed to the causative disorder according to ICHD-3 [11]. Since most of the headaches encountered in the present study were new or had altered characteristics and occurred significantly more often than in the control group, we have chosen to call those occurring in the week before or at the time of TIA migraine–like headaches and tension-type-like headaches.

Significance of our findings

Our results have important clinical implications and also bespeak to some extent the possible mechanisms of headache and migraine.

Can headache be a warning sign of TIA?

From transcranial doppler monitoring it is well known that patients have many neurologically silent cerebral emboli [15]. Perhaps some of them cause headache. Our study showed beyond doubts that headache, more specifically migraine-like headache, is more common within the previous year before TIA than in controls. The difference was even more pronounced within one week of TIA and particularly within the last day before TIA. It seems overwhelmingly likely, therefore, that headache, especially headache of a new type or with altered characteristics can be a warning about impending TIA. But is headache a useful warning symptom? In other words, should such a headache lead to vascular work-up? In our opinion the answer is yes, under some circumstances. All middle aged to elderly patients who encounter a new type of headache should definitely have a vascular work-up. But also middle aged to elderly patients with a previously existing headache such as migraine or tension-type headache should be studied if the headache changes markedly in frequency or character despite the fact that the diagnosis is still the same. Special attention should be paid to patients with accelerating frequency of migraine that cannot otherwise be explained. Some may consider this a too aggressive attitude, but it must be remembered that diagnostic methods needed for prevention of cerebrovascular disorders are quite simple, pose no risk to the patient and that vascular episodes that can be prevented are often serious. Ultrasound examination of the neck vessels and blood tests may suffice, supplemented as necessary according to the degree of risk and other factors.

Anterior versus posterior circulation TIA

In agreement with previous studies in stroke and TIA [1–10], we confirm that headaches in TIA patients are more prevalent with posterior circulation TIA. In fact, all our patients with posterior circulation TIA had headache within the week before TIA and many at the time of TIA. The reason for this remains unclear but it is noteworthy that the interest in brain stem and hypothalamic mechanisms of migraine is increasing. During attack of migraine without aura, blood flow was increased in a small area of the ventro-medial medulla and this finding has later been confirmed [16, 17]. The vast majority of migraine auras are caused by blood flow changes thought to be caused by cortical spreading depression in the occipital cortex [18] and, finally, white matter abnormalities in migraine patients are primarily seen in the posterior fossa circulatory territory [15]. There are also reports of small pathologies in the brain stem associated with headache or migraine [17].

Strengths and weaknesses of the present study

To the best of our knowledge this is the first study that has examined headache in TIA patients using a professional, face to face, semistructured interview describing all relevant characteristics of headaches associated with TIA.

One limitation of this study is the quick disappearance of clinical symptoms in TIA patients before admission to the hospital. Some of them could not remember details which are important in the differential diagnosis of TIA and MA. For example, some patients could have missed gradual spread of symptoms or presence of succession of symptoms. Some patients could not describe the characteristics of headache during TIA very well. Therefore some cases of MA could have been missed. However, we performed follow-up of 118 out of 120 patients with TIA. The period of follow-up varied from 6 months till 4 years. We found only one case of migraine with aura which was missed during the first interview. This patient experienced three more similar attacks of migraine with aura during two following years.

The weakness of the present study was using only CT in 8 patients which is not an accurate method for detection of small infarcts, especially in the posterior territory. However we performed a follow-up of these 8 patients during 3 years and nobody from them had recurrent episodes and other neurological problems. Also, the inaccuracy of patient's recall of headache during the last year may have been a limiting factor.

Conclusions

The one year prevalence of migraine was significantly higher in TIA patients than in controls and so was the prevalence of headache within the last week before TIA and at the time of TIA. A previous headache that worsens and a new type of headache can be a warning of impending TIA.

Abbreviations

CT: Computed tomography; DWI: Diffusion weighted imaging; MRI: Magnetic resonance imaging; TIA: Transient ischemic attack; OR: Odd ratio; CI: Confidence interval; ICHD-3: International Classification of Headache Disorders; TTH: Tension-type headache

Funding

No financial support.
This study was based exclusively on voluntary work.

Authors' contributions

NMG collected the data and made statistical analysis. ERL elaborated design of the study and wrote the manuscript. JO elaborated design of the study and corrected the manuscript. All authors read and approved the manuscript.

Competing interests

The authors declare that they have no competing interest.

Author details

[1]Department of Neurology and Neurosurgery, The Ural State Medical University, Repina 3, Yekaterinburg 620028, Russia. [2]International Headache Center "Europe-Asia", Yekaterinburg, Russia. [3]Medical Union "New Hospital", Yekaterinburg, Russia. [4]Danish Headache Center, Department of Neurology, Rigshospitalet-Glostrup, University of Copenhagen, Copenhagen, Denmark.

References

1. Portenoy RK, Abissi CJ, Lipton RB, Berger AR, Mebler MF, Baglivo J et al (1984) Headache in cerebrovascular disease. Stroke 15:1009–1012
2. Tentschert S, Wimmer R, Greisenegger S, Lang W, Lalouschek W (2005) Headache at stroke onset in 2196 patients with ischemic stroke or transient ischemic attack. Stroke 36:e1–e3
3. Arboix A, Massons J, Oliveres M, Arribas MP, Titus F (1994) Headache in acute cerebrovascular disease: a prospective clinical study in 240 patients. Cephalalgia 14:37–40
4. Koudstaal PJ, van Gijn J, Kappelle LJ (1991) Headache in transient or permanent cerebral ischemia. Dutch TIA study group. Stroke 22:754–759
5. Ferro JM, Costa I, Melo TP, Canhão P, Oliveira V, Salgado AV, Crespo M, Pinto AN (1995) Headache associated with transient ischemic attacks. Headache 35:544–548
6. Carolei A, Sacco S (2010) Headache attributed to stroke, TIA, intracerebral haemorrhage, or vascular malformation. Handb Clin Neurol 97:517–528
7. Gorelick PB, Hier DB, Caplan LR, Langenberg P (1986) Headache in acute cerebrovascular disease. Neurology 36:1445–1450
8. Medina JL, Diamond S, Rubino FA (1975) Headaches in patients with transient ischemic attacks. Headache 15:194–197
9. Edmeads J (1979) The headaches of ischemic cerebrovascular disease. Headache 19:345–349
10. Loeb C, Gandolfo C, Dall'Agata D (1985) Headache in transient ischemic attacks (TIA). Cephalalgia 5(Suppl 2):17–19
11. Classification committee of the international headache society (2018) The international classification of headache disorders. Cephalalgia 38:1–211
12. Easton JD, Saver JL, Albers GW et al (2009) Definition and evaluation of transient ischemic attack. Stroke 40:2276–2293
13. Lebedeva ER, Gurary NM, Gilev DV, Olesen J (2018) Prospective testing of ICHD-3 beta diagnostic criteria for migraine with aura and migraine with typical aura in patients with transient ischemic attacks. Cephalalgia 38:561–567
14. Lebedeva ER, Gurary NM, Gilev DV, Christensen AF, Olesen J (2017) Explicit diagnostic criteria for transient ischemic attacks to differentiate it from migraine with aura. Cephalalgia. https://doi.org/10.1177/0333102417736901
15. Kruit MC, Launer LJ, Ferrari MD, Van Buchem MA (2006) Brain stem and cerebellar hyperintense lesions in migraine. Stroke 37:1109–1112
16. Nozari A, Dilekoz E, Sukhotinsky I, Stein T, Eikermann-Haerter K, Liu C et al (2010) Microemboli may link spreading depression, migraine aura, and patent foramen ovale. Ann Neurol 67:221–229
17. Afridi S, Goadsby PJ (2003) New onset migraine with a brain stem cavernous angioma. J Neurol Neurosurg Psychiatry 74:680–681

18

Exploration of intrinsic brain activity in migraine with and without comorbid depression

Mengmeng Ma[1†], Junran Zhang[2,3†], Ning Chen[1], Jian Guo[1], Yang Zhang[1] and Li He[1*]

Abstract

Background: Major depressive disorder is a common comorbidity in migraineurs. Depression may affect the progression and prognosis of migraine. Few studies have examined the brain function in migraineurs that may cause this comorbidity. Here, we aimed to explore depression-related abnormalities in the intrinsic brain activity of interictal migraineurs with comorbid depression using resting-state functional magnetic resonance imaging.

Results: Significant main effects of migraine and depression provided evidence that migraine and depression jointly affected the left medial prefrontal cortex, which was thought to be the neural basis of self-referential mental activity in previous studies. Abnormalities in this region may contribute to determining the common symptoms of migraine and depression and even result in comorbidity. Additionally, migraineurs with comorbid depression had different developmental trajectories in the right thalamus and fusiform, which were associated with recognizing, transmitting, controlling and remembering pain and emotion.

Conclusions: Based on our findings, the abnormal mPFC which may contribute to determining the common symptoms in migraine and depression and may be a therapeutic target for migraineurs comorbid depression. The different developmental trajectory in thalamus and fusiform indicates that the comorbidity may arise through a specific mechanism rather than simple superposition of migraine and depression.

Keywords: Migraine, Psychiatric comorbidity, Depression, Neuroimaging, Amplitude of low frequency fluctuation patterns

Background

Migraine is often accompanied by emotional dysfunction. The depression comorbidity has high prevalence which is the most common comorbidity in migraineurs. The incidence of depression in migraineurs ranges from 8.6% to 47.9%, according to a meta-analysis of 12 studies [1]. Depression in migraineurs is a significant risk factor for migraine chronification, refractoriness to migraine treatments, overuse of medication, increased migraine-related disability, affective temperament dysregulation and suicidal behaviors which contribute to the psychosocial impairment and altered quality of life [2–6]. However, the depression comorbidity is often overlooked in migraineurs. Therefore, it is imperative to attach importance to this comorbidity to prevent, identify and treat depression in patients with migraine.

The combination of migraine and depression has been associated with smaller brain tissue volume than that in patients with one or neither of these conditions [7]. The brains of migraineurs with comorbid depression differed from patients with migraine only or depression only. Many migraine neuroimaging studies explored alterations of the brain, identified abnormal functions of specific brain regions and speculated that these regions may contribute to determining the depressive symptoms of migraine in migraine without aura [8–11]. However, previous researches have bot clearly determined whether these brain regions differ in migraineurs with depression compared with patients diagnosed with migraine only or depression only. We postulate that migraine and depression exert different effects in brain state, particularly the

* Correspondence: heli2003new@126.com
†Mengmeng Ma and Junran Zhang contributed equally to this work.
[1]Department of Neurology, West China Hospital, Sichuan University, No. 37, Wainan Guoxue Xiang, Chengdu 610041, Sichuan, China
Full list of author information is available at the end of the article

functions of specific brain regions that might be associated with clinical symptom and the shared etiological risk factors of the migraine-depression comorbidity.

The amplitude of low-frequency fluctuation (ALFF) is a way of measuring regional intrinsic brain activity to explore the pathophysiology underlying neurological and psychiatric diseases [12, 13]. We aimed to explore depression-related abnormalities in the intrinsic brain activity of interictal migraineurs with comorbid depression using resting-state functional magnetic resonance imaging (RS-fMRI) and compare the findings among four groups, including migraineurs with depression (dMIG), migraineurs without depression (ndMIG), patients with major depressive disorder (MDD) and healthy controls (HC).

Results

Demographic and neuropsychological characteristics

Subject demographics and clinical characteristics are shown in Table 1. With the exception of the HRSD scores, no significant differences were observed among the four groups ($F = 18.494$, $P < 0.001$). A post hoc test was applied to the mean 24-HRSD scores of the four groups; higher scores were recorded for in the groups of dMIG and MDD than in the groups of ndMIG or HC ($P < 0.001$).

Significant main effects

The two-way ANOVA on ALFF reveled three significant brain regions with a main effect of migraine: the bilateral posterior cingulate cortex/precuneus (PCC/precuneus) ($F = 13.10$; $P < 0.001$) (Fig. 1a), the right gyrus rectus (REC) ($F = 11.83$; $P < 0.001$) and left medial prefrontal cortex (mPFC) ($F = 16.0$; $P < 0.001$) (Fig. 1b). The only region which was observed with a significant main effect of depression was the left mPFC ($F = 71.57$, $P < 0.001$) (Fig. 1c). The details of these brain regions were shown in the Table 2. Post hoc analysis showed significantly decreased ALFF values in the right REC and increased values in the bilateral PCC/precuneus and left mPFC in dMIG and ndMIG compared with the MDD and HC groups, as well assignificantly increased ALFF values in the left mPFC in dMIG and MDD groups compared with those in ndMIG and HC groups. No significant differences were observed in any other comparison.

Interaction effects

Significant interaction effects were observed in the right thalamus ($F = 10.89$; $P < 0.001$) (Fig. 2a) and right fusiform ($F = 16.56$; $P < 0.001$) (Fig. 2b). The details of these brain regions were shown in the Table 2. According to the post hoc analysis, the ALFF values in the right thalamus were decreased in the dMIG group comparing with those in ndMIG group ($P = 0.006$, Bonferroni corrected) and MDD group ($P = 0.01$, Bonferroni corrected). Furthermore, in the fusiform, the dMIG group displayed increased ALFF values compared with those in the ndMIG group ($P = 0.005$, Bonferroni corrected), and the ALFF values of the ndMIG group were decreased compared with those in HC group ($P = 0.004$, Bonferroni

Table 1 Demographic and clinical characteristics of all subjects

	dMIG ($n = 10$)	ndMIG ($n = 22$)	MDD ($n = 13$)	HC ($n = 27$)	P value
Age, y, mean (SD)	27.8 (9.25)	33.59 (8.07)	30.92 (9.1)	29.48 (7,18)	0.206[a]
Male	3 (30%)	5 (22.7%)	3 (23%)	10 (37%)	0.685[b]
Education, y, mean (SD)	13.6 (3.41)	19 (3.28)	13.65 (2.93)	16.11 (3.02)	0.531[a]
Clinical characters of migraine					
With/without aura	0/10	0/22	NA	NA	
Duration of migraine, y, mean (SD)	7.2 (5.55)	9.82 (7.14)	NA	NA	0.314[c]
Attack frequency, per month, mean (SD)	8.52 (7.02)	4.5 (3.50)	NA	NA	0.08[c]
Attack duration, h, mean (SD)	18.65 (14.39)	12.75 (16.79)	NA	NA	0.42[c]
VAS score (0–10), mean (SD)	6.55 (1.17)	5.88 (1.31)	NA	NA	0.174[c]
HIT-6, mean (SD)	65.1 (6.26)	60 (5.77)	NA	NA	0.081[c]
MoCA, mean (SD)	27.5 (2.88)	27.82 (1.5)	27.92 (1.66)	30.59 (1.83)	0.620[a]
24-HRSD, mean (SD)	26.9 (6.67)	3 (2.23)	27.85 (6.49)	2.48 (2.12)	< 0.001[a d]
14-HAMA, mean (SD)	6 (1.826)	3.82 (2.59)	5.23 (2.28)	4.19 (2.69)	0.088[a]

[a]P value for the age, MoCA and neuropsychological scores distribution in the four groups were obtained using a separate one-way ANCOVA tests. Post-hoc tests were then performed using the t-test
[b]P value for the gender distribution and sleep disturbance in the four groups were obtained using a chi-squared test
[c]P value for the clinical characters distribution for dMIG and ndMIG group were obtained using two sample t-test
[d]Post-hoc paired comparisons showed significant differences between dMIG versus ndMIG and HC, depression versus ndMIG and HC, $P < 0.001$
dMIG migraine with depression, *ndMIG* migraine without depression group, *MDD* major depressive disorder, *HC* health control group, *VAS* visual analogue scale, *HIT-6* Headache Impact Test, *MoCA* Montreal Cognitive Assessment, *24-HRSD* 24-Hamilton Rating Scale for Depression, *14-HAMA* Hamilton Anxiety Rating Scale
Values are represented as the mean (standard deviation)

Table 2 Brain regions showing significant main and interaction effects among four groups

	Region	Hemi	Voxel	BA	Peak voxel MNI coordinates			T value
					x	y	z	
Main effect of migraine								
Cluster 1	PCC/Precuneus	L/R	20	23	-3	−36	33	3.62
Cluster 2	REC	R	35	11	6	39	−18	−3.44
Cluster 3	mPFC	L	20	10	−36	45	9	4
Main effect of depression								
Cluster 1	mPFC	L	752	10	−30	51	6	8.46
Interaction effect								
Cluster 1	Thalamus	R	10	NA	12	−12	6	3.30
Cluster 2	fusiform	R	38	37	27	−3	−42	−4.07

Hemi hemisphere, *L* left, *R* right, *BA* Brodmann Area, *MNI* Montreal Neurological Institute, x, y, z, coordinates of primary peak locations in the MNI space, *T value* statistical value of peak voxel showing ALFF differences among the four groups, *PCC* posterior cingulated cortex, *REC* rectus gyrus, *mPFC* medial prefrontal cortex

corrected), but no difference in any other comparison were observed between the groups.

Clinical correlations

As these analyses were exploratory, we used a statistical significance level of $P < 0.01$. Significant correlations were observed between the ALFF values for other ROIs and clinical characteristics.

Discussion

In the current study, we examined the effect of depression on intrinsic brain activity, as reflected by ALFF in migraineurs and HCs among the four groups. Compared with persons without migraine, migraineurs exhibited significantly decreased activity in the right REC and increased intrinsic brain activity in the bilateral PCC/precuneus. Additionally, migraine and depression affected the left mPFC with increasing ALFF simultaneously and exerted different effects in right thalamus and fusiform. Taken together, these findings may yield insights into the comorbidity and provide a basis for developing novel imaging biomarkers for gauging the impact of therapeutics.

Although many studies have shown a clear relationship between migraine and depression, most of them were based on clinical observations, case studies, and genetic epidemiology. Based on these studies, it was speculated that many factors, including serotonergic disorders, hypothalamic-pituitary-adrenal axis hyperactivity, inflammation, and environmental or genetic risk factors for inflammation may converge to result in an altered brain state that could predispose individuals to both migraine and depression [1, 9, 14, 15]. However, the specific changes in brain regions function have not yet been reported in the literature. Therefore, we examined the effect of depression on intrinsic brain activity, reflected by ALFF in migraine and HC among four groups.

Consistent with the findings of previous studies, the current study observed that the depressive patients had increased intrinsic brain activity in the left mPFC. As the anterior node of the default mode network (DMN), the mPFC was highly active at rest but had suppressed activity during cognitive and emotional processing [16, 17]. Converging evidence suggested altered mPFC functional connectivity involved in the development of MDD and the mPFC had long been suspected to be the neural basis of self-referential mental activity [18, 19]. In this study, migraineurs also exhibited increased intrinsic brain activity in the left mPFC. Neuroimaging studies have identified frontal cortical abnormalities in migraineurs [20, 21]. Neuropsychological investigations have highlighted PFC related cognitive impairments in migraineurs, including working memory and executive function deficits [22, 23]. Based on these findings, we speculate that abnormalities in the mPFC region contribute to determining the common symptoms of migraine and depression, even results in the comorbidity and may be a therapeutic target for migraineurs comorbid depression.

In this study, compared with persons without migraine, migraineurs exhibited significantly decreased activity in the right REC and increased intrinsic brain activity in the bilateral PCC/precuneus which has been reported to be dysfunctional in previous studies, particularlythe PCC/precuneus. The REC exhibits a reduced volume in patients with schizophrenia and depression, but relatively fewer studies have reported similar findings in migraine. The REC is part of a circuit that mediates some specific cognitive and emotional functions in humans and plays an important role in the pathogenesis of behavioral addiction combined with substance abuse [24, 25]. Thus, we speculated that the abnormalities in the right REC in migraine may suggest that migraineurs are prone to emotional disorders and drug addiction. The bilateral PCC/ precuneus are the key nodes of

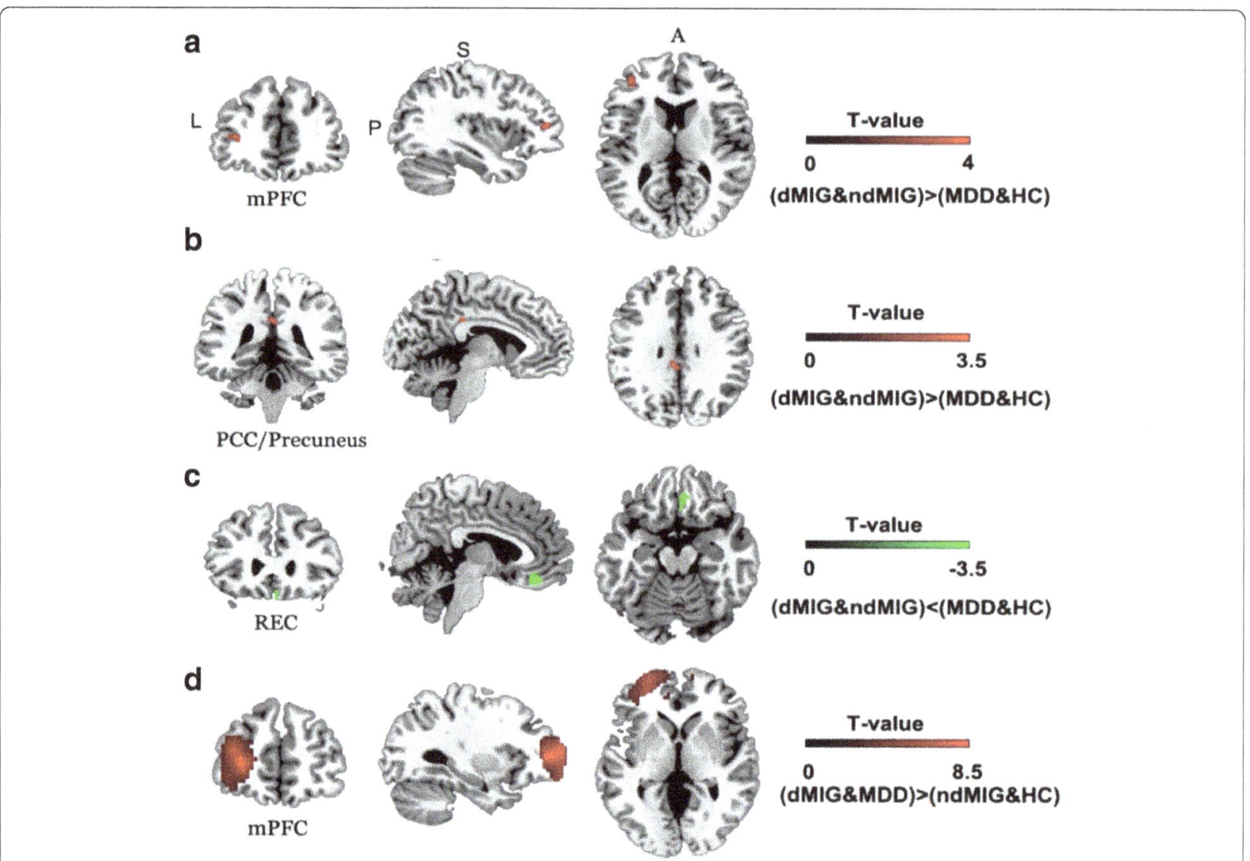

Fig. 1 Significant main effect of migraine. Significant main effect of migraine in left medial prefrontal cortex (**a**), the bilateral posterior cingulate cortex/ precuneus (**b**) and the right rectus gyrus (**c**) and main effect of depression in left medial prefrontal cortex (**d**); mPFC: medial prefrontal cortex; REC: rectus gyrus; PCC: posterior cingulate cortex. dMIG: migraineurs with depression; ndMIG: migraineurs without depression; MDD: patients with major depressive disorderand; HC: healthy controls; mPFC: medial prefrontal cortex; PCC: posterior cingulate cortex; REC: rectus gyrus

DMN and have been observed dysfunction in previous study. There were few reports about activation alteration in migraine. The regions had a high baseline metabolic rate measured by PET. They reduced metabolism and functional connectivity in healthy aging and neurodegenerative diseases like Alzheimier's disease [26, 27]. However, it was reported that the region increased metabolism and altered functional connectivity in MDD [28, 29]. So we speculated that the altered activity of PCC/ precuneus in migraine might be associated with the depressive tendency. It need more neuroimaging study to verify.Migraineurs with comorbid depression showed decreased intrinsic brain activity in the thalamus compared with ndMIG and MDD and increased activity in the fusiform compared with ndMIG. As a critical multifunctional relay center, the thalamus is considered the transmission control center of emotion and is thought to play an important role in the transmission of nociceptive inputs to cortical structures that are speculated to be involved in the migraine-depression comorbidity, as depression may affect the homeostasis of the transmission of headache-related nociceptive signals from the thalamus to the cortex [30, 31]. Thalamic neurons must adjust to constantly changing physiological (sleep, wakefulness, food intake, body temperature, heart rate, and blood pressure), behavioral (addiction and isolation), cognitive (attention, learning, and memory use), and affective (stress, anxiety, depression, and anger) parameters to maintain homeostasis [32]. The current finding of decreased activity in the thalamus may support the hypothesis that the habituation deficit in migraineurs with depression is due to a reduced preactivation level of sensory cortices and not to increased excitability or reduced intracortical inhibition. Moreover, the ALFF of the right fusiform negatively correlated with the mean headache degree of migraine in ndMIG. Vey fewstudies of fusiform activity have been conducted, and they have found divergent results concerning migraine [33, 34]. The divergence in finding from migraine may be due to differences in the course of migraine or a lack of consideration of the emotional effect. The function of the fusiform has been linked to various neural pathways related to recognition, cognitive pain processing and various neurological phenomena such as synesthesia,

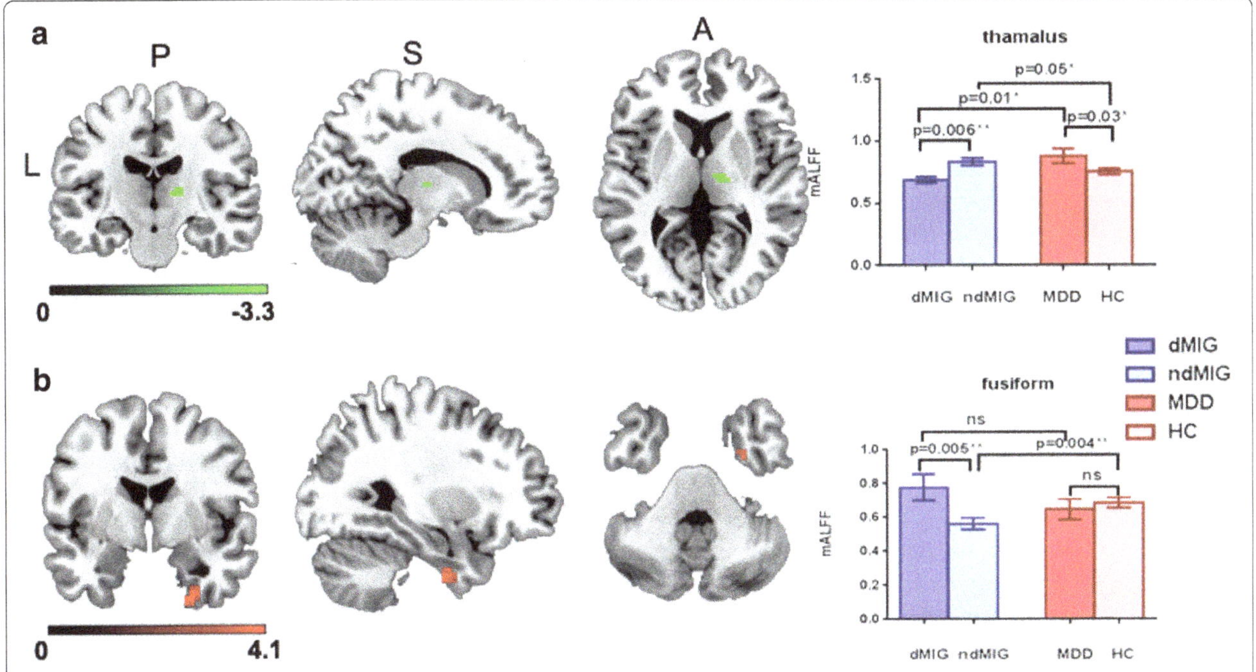

Fig. 2 Significant interaction effects. Significant interaction effects in right thalamus (**a**) and the right fusiform (**b**); * uncorrected, $P < 0.05$. ** indicated Bonfornni corrected. *dMIG* migraineurs with depression, *ndMIG* migraineurs without depression, *MDD* patients with major depressive disorder and, *HC* healthy controls

dyslexia, and prosopagnosia [35]. Atypical functions and structure of the fusiform gyrus have been identified in chronic low back pain, fibromyalgia, and cluster headache patients [35, 36]. Depression combined with migraine may recruit additional neural resources to improve task performance and enhance the mental imagery of pain based on memories of recurrent migraine headaches, raising the possibility of migraine chronification [37].

Migraineurs with comorbid depression showed significantly decreased intrinsic brain activity in the thalamus and increased activity in the fusiform compared with ndMIG. According to genetic studies, migraine may be a symptom or consequence of MDD in at least a subset of migraine patients with depression as the comorbid depression and migraine were genetically most similar to depression patient [38]. Although our results revealed that migraineurs with comorbid depression exhibit significant changes in brain activity in the thalamus and fusiform gyrus (indicated Bonfornni corrected) with those migraineurs and patients with depression. We speculate that these changes determine the different symptoms. This finding highlights the abnormal developmental patterns of intrinsic brain activity in migraine-depression comorbidity as opposed to migraine or depression alone.

Recently, the functional organization of white matter (WM) in resting-state has received greater attention. Several studies demonstrated the existence of functional brain activity in the WM in normal controls and insufficient or ineffective communication associated with WM abnormalities in many brain disorders, including schizophrenia, epilepsy, Alzheimer's and Parkinson's disease [39–43]. In particular, diffusion tensor imaging (DTI) can offer a unique noninvasive insight into the microstructure of WM tracts in the living brain. The DTI studies have revealed abnormal WM integrity in patients with migraine and depression. Solid evidence has been shown that patients with migraine and depression show abnormal diffusion characteristics in several WM tracts such as frontal WM cluster, corpus callosum, optic radiation and internal capsule [44–47]. In current study, it can be found that the partials of the regions of main effect were located in the white matter (WM), especially the with matter in mPFC which has been detected increased radial diffusivity in migraine and depression [45, 48]. Converging the considerable evidence and current results, the mPFC may be the key region of migraineurs cormobid depression.

Based on the results from this study, migraine and depression selectively affect the function of the posterior and anterior nodes of the DMN [49–51]. The DMN is highly related to cognitive processes and influences behavior in response to the environment in a predictive manner [52]. The network reduces its activation during task-related activities or those that require executive function in the healthy human brain. Previous studies have demonstrated that the DMN is dysfunctional in a resting state in various neurological and neuropsychiatric disorders, such as migraine, epilepsy and depression [50, 53, 54]. Studies of functional connectivity and the DMN are necessary to further examine the comorbidity of migraine and depression. Moreover, the relationship between the intrinsic brain activity and cortical thickness has been shown that the spatial distribution of cortical thickness was negatively correlated with surface-based intrinsic brain activity at whole-brain level in epilepsy [55]. This finding contributes to the analysis clinical application of the current results and combine with previous studies of cortical thickness in migraine or depression. But there is no study reporting the cortical thickness in migraine comorbid with depression. Thus, it may be a good direction to research the cortical thickness and elucidate its associate with intrinsic brain activity to aware the brain function of migraineur comorbid with depression.

Similar to most clinical studies, the present study has several limitations. First,, we only included the patients who had never taken any antidepressants or durgs to prevent migraine before the RS-fMRI scan in order to avoid the effects of drugs for migraine and depression on brain activation and the possible withdrawal effect. Therefore, only 10 of 120 migraineurs with depression completed the fMRI scan. The small number of patients could leave our study too underpowered to reveal more subtle findings, such as correlations between clinical features, although our research used rigorous statistical methods with appropriate corrections. Second, as this study employed a cross-sectional design, we were unable to easily estimate whether this abnormal intrinsic brain activity exhibited dynamic changes with follow-up. In the future, it is necessary to conduct prospective longitudinal studies with large sample sizes to assess the associations between migraine with depression and changes in brain activation. An fMRI assessment of changes in functional connectivity might help clarify the association between migraine headache and MDDand elucidate the direction of comorbidity development.

Conclusions

This study explored intrinsic brain activity in migraine with comorbid depression in four groups. As expected, migraine and depression jointly affected left mPFC, which is thought to be the neural basis of self-referential mental activity and has been shown the increased ALFF in depression patients. We speculated the abnormal mPFC may contribute to determining the common symptoms in migraine and depression and may be a therapeutic target for migraineurs comorbid depression. Besides, it was found that migraine and depression had apparently different developmental trajectory in the right thalamus and right fusiform, which are associated with recognizing, transmitting, controlling and remembering pain and emotion. The abnormalities in these regions may be relevant to the special phenotype of the migraine and depression comorbidity, and our results suggest that the comorbidity arises through a specific mechanism rather than a mere superposition of migraine and depression. In the future, migraine studies may need to consider depression when interpreting fMRI data.

Methods

Study population

All the patients were recruited from the Department of Neurology or Psychiatry of West China Hospital between June 2016 and February 2017 and were evaluated by at least two neurologists and two psychiatrists. The diagnosis of migraine without aura was made according to the International Classification of Headache Disorders, 3rd edition (beta version) (ICHD-3 beta). The diagnosis of migraine without aura in ICHD-3 beta is not different from the diagnosis based on ICHD-3 [56]. Depression was diagnosed according to the Diagnostic and Statistical Manual of Mental Disorders, 5th Edition (DSM-5) criteria. The inclusion criteria of all subjects were (1) Han ethnicity (the predominant ethnic group in China), (2) 18–60 years of age, (3) right-handed, and (4) first came to the clinic seeking medical help for migraine and depression. The exclusion criteria were (1) a history of systemic disease, chronic pain disorders and serious neurological disorders; (2) a history of analgesic overuse, as we aimed to avoid recruiting patients with common secondary headache-medication overused headache; (3) the presence of intracranial lesions detected in previous MRI or CT scans; (4) had the contraindications for MRI scanning, including metal implant or psychiatric disorders, such as anxiety (claustrophobia), that prevented patients from completing the MRI scanning; (5) a headache attack during RS-fMRI or within 24 h after scanning.

The dMIG group

The subjects were diagnosed with migraine without aura and comorbid depression according to the criteria of ICHD-3 beta and the DSM-5. They were all initially diagnosed with migraine and depression and had not used any antidepressants or drugs to preventing migraine. All the patients in this group had scores of greater than 24 on 24-item Hamilton Rating Scale for Depression (24-HRSD). The patients had no history of other types of headache, anxiety or other psychiatric disorders.

The ndMIG group

The patients in this group were recruited from the Department of Neurology and diagnosed with migraine without aura and had no history of any psychiatric disorders including MDD or depressive mood. The patients were all initially diagnosed with migraine and had not previously used any drugs to prevent migraine. All the patients in this group had scores of less than 8 on the 24-HRSD.

The MDD group

The patients in the MDD group were diagnosed according to the DSM-5 by at least two psychiatrists. They had no history of migraine, other types of headache, anxiety or other psychiatric disorders. The patients were all first diagnosed with depression and had never used any antidepressant.

The HC group

HC were recruited in June 2016 and February 2017. They were evaluated by two neurologists and two psychiatrists and had no history of migraine, depression, alcohol dependence or of using medications. Besides, they had no family history of migraine and psychiatric disorders.

The subjects in the four groups were matched for sex, mean age, and years of education. After evaluating the potential subjects, we established 4 groups, including 10 dMIG, 22 ndMIG (migraineurs with no depressive mood), 13 MDD and 27 HC. The demographic data of all the subjects and clinical characteristics of migraineurs were obtained, including age, gender, years of education, migraine duration, attack frequency and attack duration of migraine, headache degree, the Headache Impact Test-6 (HIT-6) and scores on the 24-HRSD, 14-Hamilton Anxiety Rating Scale (14-HAMA) and Montreal Cognitive Assessment (MoCA).

MRI data acquisition

All the scans were performed on a 3.0-T MRI scanning system (Siemens Trio Tim, Erlangen, Germany) at the Department of Radiology, West China Hospital of Sichuan University. Earplugs and tight padded clamps were used to minimize noise exposure and head motion. The participants were instructed to remain still, close their eyes, remain awake and let their minds wander. Scanning was terminated if the participant complained of any discomfort. Images of structures were obtained using routine T1 weighted imaging, and the RS-fMRI was conducted using an echo-planar imaging (EPI) sequence (TR 2000 ms, TE 30 ms, voxel size 3.75 × 3.75 × 5 mm3, flip angle 90°, slice thickness 5 mm, matrix 64 × 64, FOV 24 × 24 cm^2). Each resting-state scan lasted for 6 min and 180 volumes were collected. Two experienced neuroradiologists performed all scan and checked the images to exclude brain tissue abnormalities in the four groups.

RS-fMRI image preprocessing

Functional images were preprocessed with the software Data Processing Assistant for Resting-State fMRI, Advanced Edition (DPARSF A, http://rfmri.org/DPARSF) in MATLAB (R2010b). The first 10 volumes were removed for each subject. The remaining images were corrected by slicing time and realigned. No subjects displayed head movement i.e., head motions exceeding 2.0 mm of translation or 2.0 degrees of rotation during the scanning process to disqualify them from the study. The subsequent processing steps included normalizing the scans into the standard stereotactic space using the Montreal Neurological Institute EPI template; smoothing with an 8 × 8 × 8 mm^3 full width at half-maximum kernel; and removing covariates by linear regression, including head motion parameters, averaged signal from the white matter and signal from the cerebrospinal fluid, to further reduce the effects of confounding factors. Finally, the functional images were detrended by bandpass filtering (0.01–0.08 Hz) to reduce low-frequency drift and physiological high-frequency respiratory and cardiac noise.

ALFF analysis

We computed the ALFF value for each voxel using DPARSF software (Advanced Edition, http://rfmri.org/DPARSF) to construct the intrinsic brain activity map of each subject, The power spectrum was obtained after the time series of each voxel was transformed to the frequency domain. The average square root of the power spectrum was regarded as the ALFF. For the purpose of reducing the global effects of variability across subjects, the ALFF value of each voxel was normalized to the global mean ALFF value [49].

Statistical analysis

The values are reported as absolute numbers with percentages for categorical variables and as means with SDs for continuous variables. $\chi 2$ tests, t-tests and analysis of variance (ANOVA) were performedto compare categorical variables between groups, continuous variables between two groups, and continuous variables among four groups, respectively. The level of statistical significance was defined as combined $P < 0.01$.

Two-way ANOVA with migraine and depression as between-subject factors was performed on the individual normalized ALFF maps using statistical parametric mapping (SPM 8, www.fil.ion.ucl.ac.uk/spm). Comparisons of the main effects and interaction effect were corrected using AlphaSim correction. The level of statistical significance was defined as combined $P < 0.05$ (combined height threshold $P < 0.001$ and a minimum cluster size of 10 voxels with AlphaSim correction).The brain regions with significant main effects and interaction effects were designated as regions of interest (ROIs). Post hoc tests were then performed on the ROIs using Bonferroni correction ($P < 0.05/4 = 0.0125$). We computed Pearson correlation coefficients of average ROI ALFF values versus clinical factors of migraine (duration, mean attack frequency, duration of daily attack, mean visual analogue scale score (VAS score) and HIT-6) and neuropsychological variables (MoCA, 14-HRSD and 14-HAMA) separately for dMIG, ndMIG and MDD groups to explore the relationship between intrinsic brain activity and the clinical characteristics.

Abbreviations

14-HAMA: 14-item Hamilton Anxiety Rating Scale; 24-HRSD: 24-item Hamilton Rating Scale for Depression; ALFF: the amplitude of low-frequency fluctuation; ANOVA: Analysis of variance; dMIG: Migraineurs with depression; DMN: Default mode network; DPARSF A: Data Processing Assistant for Resting-State fMRI, Advanced Edition; DSM-5: The Diagnostic and Statistical Manual of Mental Disorders, 5th edition; EPI: Echo-planar imaging; HC: Healthy controls; HIT-6: Headache Impact Test-6; ICHD– 3: The International Classification of Headache Disorders, 3-rd; MDD: Major depressive disorder; mFPC: Medial prefrontal cortex; MoCA: Montreal Cognitive Assessment; ndMIG: Migraineurs without depression; PCC: Posterior cingulate cortex; REC: Right gyrus rectus; ROIs: Regions of interest; RS-fMRI: Resting-state functional magnetic resonance imaging; SPM 8: Statistical parametric mapping 8

Acknowledgments

We would like to thank Wei Wei and Jing Zhang for diagnosiing depression in the enrolling patients and Gui Fu for providing technical assistance during MRI scanning.

Funding

This work was supported by grants from the National Natural Science Foundation of China.
(Grant Nos. 81071140, 81500959, 81000605 and 81110108007).

Authors' contributions

MMM and JRZ were responsible for analyzing the data, revising and drafting the manuscript and they contributed equally to this work. NC, JG and YZ were responsible for data acquisition and interpretation. LH conceived and designed the study. All authors read and approved the final manuscript.

Competing interests

The authors declare that they have no competing interests.

Author details

[1]Department of Neurology, West China Hospital, Sichuan University, No. 37, Wainan Guoxue Xiang, Chengdu 610041, Sichuan, China. [2]Department of Radiology, Huaxi MR Research Center (HMRRC), West China Hospital, Sichuan University, Chengdu, China. [3]Department of Medical Information Engineering, School of Electrical Engineering and Information, Sichuan University, Chengdu, China.

References

1. Antonaci F, Nappi G, Galli F, Manzoni GC, Calabresi P, Costa A (2011) Migraine and psychiatric comorbidity: a review of clinical findings. J Headache Pain 12(7):115–125. https://doi.org/10.1007/s10194-010-0282-4.
2. Ashina S, Serrano D, Lipton RB, Maizels M, Manack AN, Turkel CC, Reed ML, Buse DC (2012) Depression and risk of transformation of episodic to chronic migraine. J Headache Pain 13(8):615–624. https://doi.org/10.1007/s10194-012-0479-9.
3. Lantéri-Minet M, Radat F, Chautard MH, Lucas C (2005) Anxiety and depression associated with migraine: influence on migraine subjects' disability and quality of life, and acute migraine management. Pain 118(3): 319–326. https://doi.org/10.1016/j.pain.2005.09.010.
4. Peck KR, Smitherman TA, Baskin SM (2015) Traditional and alternative treatments for depression: implications for migraine management. Headache 55(2):351–355. https://doi.org/10.1111/head.12521.
5. Radat F, Creac'h C, Swendsen JD, Lafittau M, Irachabal S, Dousset V, Henry P (2005) Psychiatric comorbidity in the evolution from migraine to medication overuse headache. Cephalalgia 25(7):519–522. https://doi.org/10.1111/j.1468-2982.2005.00910.x
6. Serafini G, Pompili M, Innamorati M, Gentile G, Borro M, Lamis DA, Lala N, Negro A, Simmaco M, Girardi P, Martelletti P (2012) Gene variants with suicidal risk in a sample of subjects with chronic migraine and affective temperamental dysregulation. Eur Rev Med Pharmacol Sci 16(10):1389–1398.
7. Gudmundsson LS, Scher AI, Sigurdsson S, Geerlings MI, Vidal JS, Eiriksdottir G, Garcia MI, Harris TB, Kjartansson O, Aspelund T, van Buchem MA, Gudnason V, Launer LJ (2013) Migraine, depression, and brain volume: the AGES-Reykjavik study. Neurology 80(23):2138–2144. https://doi.org/10.1212/WNL.0b013e318295d69e.
8. Li XL, Fang YN, Gao QC, Lin EJ, Hu SH, Ren L, Ding MH, Luo BN (2011) A diffusion tensor magnetic resonance imaging study of corpus callosum from adult patients with migraine complicated with depressive/anxious disorder. Headache 51(2):237–245. https://doi.org/10.1111/j.1526-4610.2010.01774.x.
9. Tietjen GE, Buse DC, Fanning KM, Serrano D, Reed ML, Lipton RB (2015) Recalled maltreatment, migraine, and tension-type headache: results of the AMPP study. Neurology 84(2):132–140. https://doi.org/10.1212/WNL.0000000000001120.
10. Valfrè W, Rainero I, Bergui M, Pinessi L (2008) Voxel-based morphometry reveals gray matter abnormalities in migraine. Headache 48(1):109–117. https://doi.org/10.1111/j.1526-4610.2007.00723.x.
11. Xue T, Yuan K, Zhao L, Yu D, Zhao L, Dong T, Cheng P, von DKM, Qin W, Tian J (2012) Intrinsic brain network abnormalities in migraines without aura revealed in resting-state fMRI. PLoS One 7(12):e52927. https://doi.org/10.1371/journal.pone.0052927.
12. Duff EP, Johnston LA, Xiong J, Fox PT, Mareels I, Egan GF (2008) The power of spectral density analysis for mapping endogenous BOLD signal fluctuations. Hum Brain Mapp 29(7):778–790. https://doi.org/10.1002/hbm.20601.
13. Fox MD, Raichle ME (2007) Spontaneous fluctuations in brain activity observed with functional magnetic resonance imaging. Nat Rev Neurosci 8(9):700–711. https://doi.org/10.1038/nrn2201.
14. Lipton RB, Silberstein SD (1994) Why study the comorbidity of migraine. Neurology 44(10 Suppl 7):S4–S5.
15. Minen MT, De Dhaem OB, Van Diest AK, Powers S, Schwedt TJ, Lipton R, Silbersweig D (2016) Migraine and its psychiatric comorbidities. J Neurol Neurosurg Psychiatry 87(7):741–749. https://doi.org/10.1136/jnnp-2015-312233.
16. Lui S, Wu Q, Qiu L, Yang X, Kuang W, Chan RC, Huang X, Kemp GJ, Mechelli A, Gong Q (2011) Resting-state functional connectivity in treatment-resistant depression. Am J Psychiatry 168(6):642–648. https://doi.org/10.1176/appi.ajp.2010.10101419.
17. Greicius MD, Flores BH, Menon V, Glover GH, Solvason HB, Kenna H, Reiss AL, Schatzberg AF (2007) Resting-state functional connectivity in major depression: abnormally increased contributions from subgenual cingulate cortex and thalamus. Biol Psychiatry 62(5):429–437. https://doi.org/10.1016/j.biopsych.2006.09.020.
18. Ferenczi EA, Zalocusky KA, Liston C, Grosenick L, Warden MR, Amatya D, Katovich K, Mehta H, Patenaude B, Ramakrishnan C, Kalanithi P, Etkin A,

Knutson B, Glover GH, Deisseroth K (2016) Prefrontal cortical regulation of brainwide circuit dynamics and reward-related behavior. Science 351(6268): aac9698. https://doi.org/10.1126/science.aac9698.
19. Liu J, Ren L, Womer FY, Wang J, Fan G, Jiang W, Blumberg HP, Tang Y, Xu K, Wang F (2014) Alterations in amplitude of low frequency fluctuation in treatment-naïve major depressive disorder measured with resting-state fMRI. Hum Brain Mapp 35(10):4979–4988. https://doi.org/10.1002/hbm.22526.
20. Bender S, Oelkers-Ax R, Resch F, Weisbrod M (2006) Frontal lobe involvement in the processing of meaningful auditory stimuli develops during childhood and adolescence. Neuroimage 33(2):759–773. https://doi.org/10.1016/j.neuroimage.2006.07.003.
21. Rocca MA, Ceccarelli A, Falini A, Tortorella P, Colombo B, Pagani E, Comi G, Scotti G, Filippi M (2006) Diffusion tensor magnetic resonance imaging at 3.0 tesla shows subtle cerebral grey matter abnormalities in patients with migraine. J Neurol Neurosurg Psychiatry 77(5):686–689. https://doi.org/10.1136/jnnp.2005.080002.
22. Schmitz N, Arkink EB, Mulder M, Rubia K, Admiraal-Behloul F, Schoonman GG, Kruit MC, Ferrari MD, van Buchem MA (2008) Frontal lobe structure and executive function in migraine patients. Neurosci Lett 440(2):92–96. https://doi.org/10.1016/j.neulet.2008.05.033.
23. Shallice T, Burgess PW (1991) Deficits in strategy application following frontal lobe damage in man. Brain 114(Pt 2):727–741.
24. Andreasen NC, O'Leary DS, Cizadlo T, Arndt S, Rezai K, Watkins GL, Ponto LL, Hichwa RD (1995) Remembering the past: two facets of episodic memory explored with positron emission tomography. Am J Psychiatry 152(11): 1576–1585. https://doi.org/10.1176/ajp.152.11.1576.
25. Chen X, Wang Y, Zhou Y, Sun Y, Ding W, Zhuang Z, Xu J, Du Y (2014) Different resting-state functional connectivity alterations in smokers and nonsmokers with internet gaming addiction. Biomed Res Int 2014:825787. https://doi.org/10.1155/2014/825787.
26. Leech R, Sharp DJ (2014) The role of the posterior cingulate cortex in cognition and disease. Brain 137(Pt 1):12–32. https://doi.org/10.1093/brain/awt162.
27. Irish M, Halena S, Kamminga J, Tu S, Hornberger M, Hodges JR (2015) Scene construction impairments in Alzheimer's disease - a unique role for the posterior cingulate cortex. Cortex 73:10–23. https://doi.org/10.1016/j.cortex.2015.08.004.
28. Serra-Blasco M, de Vita S, Rodríguez MR, de Diego-Adeliño J, Puigdemont D, Martín-Blanco A, Pérez-Egea R, Molet J, Álvarez E, Pérez V, Portella MJ (2015) Cognitive functioning after deep brain stimulation in subcallosal cingulate gyrus for treatment-resistant depression: an exploratory study. Psychiatry Res 225(3):341–346. https://doi.org/10.1016/j.psychres.2014.11.076.
29. Lozano AM, Mayberg HS, Giacobbe P, Hamani C, Craddock RC, Kennedy SH (2008) Subcallosal cingulate gyrus deep brain stimulation for treatment-resistant depression. Biol Psychiatry 64(6):461–467. https://doi.org/10.1016/j.biopsych.2008.05.034.
30. Kupers R, Kehlet H (2006) Brain imaging of clinical pain states: a critical review and strategies for future studies. Lancet Neurol 5(12):1033–1044. https://doi.org/10.1016/S1474-4422(06)70624-X.
31. Noseda R, Kainz V, Borsook D, Burstein R (2014) Neurochemical pathways that converge on thalamic trigeminovascular neurons: potential substrate for modulation of migraine by sleep, food intake, stress and anxiety. PLoS One 9(8):e103929. https://doi.org/10.1371/journal.pone.0103929.
32. Noseda R, Borsook D, Burstein R (2017) Neuropeptides and neurotransmitters that modulate Thalamo-cortical pathways relevant to migraine headache. Headache 57(Suppl 2):97–111. https://doi.org/10.1111/head.13083.
33. Schwedt TJ, Chong CD, Chiang CC, Baxter L, Schlaggar BL, Dodick DW (2014) Enhanced pain-induced activity of pain-processing regions in a case-control study of episodic migraine. Cephalalgia 34(12):947–958. https://doi.org/10.1177/0333102414526069.
34. Wang JJ, Chen X, Sah SK, Zeng C, Li YM, Li N, Liu MQ, Du SL (2016) Amplitude of low-frequency fluctuation (ALFF) and fractional ALFF in migraine patients: a resting-state functional MRI study. Clin Radiol 71(6):558–564. https://doi.org/10.1016/j.crad.2016.03.004.
35. Glass JM, Williams DA, Fernandez-Sanchez ML, Kairys A, Barjola P, Heitzeg MM, Clauw DJ, Schmidt-Wilcke T (2011) Executive function in chronic pain patients and healthy controls: different cortical activation during response inhibition in fibromyalgia. J Pain 12(12):1219–1229. https://doi.org/10.1016/j.jpain.2011.06.007.
36. Yang FC, Chou KH, Fuh JL, Huang CC, Lirng JF, Lin YY, Lin CP, Wang SJ (2013) Altered gray matter volume in the frontal pain modulation network in patients with cluster headache. Pain 154(6):801–807. https://doi.org/10.1016/j.pain.2013.02.005.
37. Yetkin FZ, Rosenberg RN, Weiner MF, Purdy PD, Cullum CM (2006) FMRI of working memory in patients with mild cognitive impairment and probable Alzheimer's disease. Eur Radiol 16(1):193–206. https://doi.org/10.1007/s00330-005-2794-x.
38. Ligthart L, Hottenga JJ, Lewis CM, Farmer AE, Craig IW, Breen G, Willemsen G, Vink JM, Middeldorp CM, Byrne EM, Heath AC, Madden PA, Pergadia ML, Montgomery GW, Martin NG, Penninx BW, McGuffin P, Boomsma DI, Nyholt DR (2014) Genetic risk score analysis indicates migraine with and without comorbid depression are genetically different disorders. Hum Genet 133(2): 173–186. https://doi.org/10.1007/s00439-013-1370-8.
39. Ji GJ, Liao W, Chen FF, Zhang L, Wang K (2017) Low-frequency blood oxygen level-dependent fluctuations in the brain white matter: more than just noise. Sci Bull (Beijing) 62(9):656–657.
40. Bohnen NI, Albin RL (2011) White matter lesions in Parkinson disease. Nat Rev Neurol 7(4):229–236. https://doi.org/10.1038/nrneurol.2011.21.
41. Caso F, Agosta F, Mattavelli D, Migliaccio R, Canu E, Magnani G, Marcone A, Copetti M, Falautano M, Comi G, Falini A, Filippi M (2015) White matter degeneration in atypical Alzheimer disease. Radiology 277(1):162–172. https://doi.org/10.1148/radiol.2015142766.
42. Dong D, Wang Y, Chang X, Jiang Y, Klugah-Brown B, Luo C, Yao D (2017) Shared abnormality of white matter integrity in schizophrenia and bipolar disorder: a comparative voxel-based meta-analysis. Schizophr Res 185:41–50. https://doi.org/10.1016/j.schres.2017.01.005.
43. Xue K, Luo C, Zhang D, Yang T, Li J, Gong D, Chen L, Medina YI, Gotman J, Zhou D, Yao D (2014) Diffusion tensor tractography reveals disrupted structural connectivity in childhood absence epilepsy. Epilepsy Res 108(1): 125–138. https://doi.org/10.1016/j.eplepsyres.2013.10.002.
44. Rocca MA, Colombo B, Pagani E, Falini A, Codella M, Scotti G, Comi G, Filippi M (2003) Evidence for cortical functional changes in patients with migraine and white matter abnormalities on conventional and diffusion tensor magnetic resonance imaging. Stroke 34(3):665–670. https://doi.org/10.1161/01.STR.0000057977.06681.11.
45. Szabó N, Kincses ZT, Párdutz A, Tajti J, Szok D, Tuka B, Király A, Babos M, Vörös E, Bomboi G, Orzi F, Vécsei L (2012) White matter microstructural alterations in migraine: a diffusion-weighted MRI study. Pain 153(3):651–656. https://doi.org/10.1016/j.pain.2011.11.029.
46. Nobuhara K, Okugawa G, Sugimoto T, Minami T, Tamagaki C, Takase K, Saito Y, Sawada S, Kinoshita T (2006) Frontal white matter anisotropy and symptom severity of late-life depression: a magnetic resonance diffusion tensor imaging study. J Neurol Neurosurg Psychiatry 77(1):120–122. https://doi.org/10.1136/jnnp.2004.055129.
47. Mettenburg JM, Benzinger TL, Shimony JS, Snyder AZ, Sheline YI (2012) Diminished performance on neuropsychological testing in late life depression is correlated with microstructural white matter abnormalities. Neuroimage 60(4):2182–2190. https://doi.org/10.1016/j.neuroimage.2012.02.044.
48. Li L, Ma N, Li Z, Tan L, Liu J, Gong G, Shu N, He Z, Jiang T, Xu L (2007) Prefrontal white matter abnormalities in young adult with major depressive disorder: a diffusion tensor imaging study. Brain Res 1168:124–128. https://doi.org/10.1016/j.brainres.2007.06.094.
49. Zang YF, He Y, Zhu CZ, Cao QJ, Sui MQ, Liang M, Tian LX, Jiang TZ, Wang YF (2007) Altered baseline brain activity in children with ADHD revealed by resting-state functional MRI. Brain and Development 29(2):83–91. https://doi.org/10.1016/j.braindev.2006.07.002.
50. Sheline YI, Barch DM, Price JL, Rundle MM, Vaishnavi SN, Snyder AZ, Mintun MA, Wang S, Coalson RS, Raichle ME (2009) The default mode network and self-referential processes in depression. Proc Natl Acad Sci U S A 106(6): 1942–1947. https://doi.org/10.1073/pnas.0812686106.
51. Zhang J, Su J, Wang M, Zhao Y, Yao Q, Zhang Q, Lu H, Zhang H, Wang S, Li GF, Wu YL, Liu FD, Shi YH, Li J, Liu JR, Du X (2016) Increased default mode network connectivity and increased regional homogeneity in migraineurs without aura. J Headache Pain 17(1):98. https://doi.org/10.1186/s10194-016-0692-z.
52. Hamilton JP, Farmer M, Fogelman P, Gotlib IH (2015) Depressive rumination, the default-mode network, and the dark matter of clinical neuroscience. Biol Psychiatry 78(4):224–230. https://doi.org/10.1016/j.biopsych.2015.02.020.
53. Hsiao FJ, Yu HY, Chen WT, Kwan SY, Chen C, Yen DJ, Yiu CH, Shih YH, Lin YY (2015) Increased intrinsic connectivity of the default mode network in temporal lobe epilepsy: evidence from resting-state MEG recordings. PLoS One 10(6):e0128787. https://doi.org/10.1371/journal.pone.0128787.

19

Chronic and intermittent administration of systemic nitroglycerin in the rat induces an increase in the gene expression of CGRP in central areas: potential contribution to pain processing

Rosaria Greco[1*], Chiara Demartini[1], Anna Maria Zanaboni[1,2] and Cristina Tassorelli[1,2]

Abstract

Background: Calcitonin gene related peptide (CGRP) is a key neuropeptide involved in the activation of the trigeminovascular system and it is likely related to migraine chronification. Here, we investigated the role of CGRP in an animal model that mimics the chronic migraine condition via repeated and intermittent nitroglycerin (NTG) administration. We also evaluated the modulatory effect of topiramate on this experimental paradigm. Male Sprague-Dawley rats were injected with NTG (5 mg/kg, i.p.) or vehicle, every 2 days over a 9-day period (5 total injections). A group of animals was injected with topiramate (30 mg/kg, i.p.) or saline every day for 9 days. Twenty-four hours after the last administration of NTG or vehicle, animals underwent tail flick test and orofacial Von Frey test. Rats were subsequently sacrificed to evaluate c-Fos and CGRP gene expression in medulla-pons region, cervical spinal cord and trigeminal ganglia.

Results: NTG administration induced spinal hyperalgesia and orofacial allodynia, together with a significant increase in the expression of CGRP and c-Fos genes in trigeminal ganglia and central areas. Topiramate treatment prevented NTG-induced changes by reversing NTG-induced hyperalgesia and allodynia, and inhibiting CGRP and c-Fos gene expression in all areas evaluated.

Conclusions: These findings point to the role of CGRP in the processes underlying migraine chronification and suggest a possible interaction with gamma-aminobutyrate (GABA) and glutamate transmission to induce/maintain central sensitization and to contribute to the dysregulation of descending pain system involved in chronic migraine.

Keywords: Nitroglycerin, Topiramate, CGRP, Trigeminal nociception

Background

Pain persistence is associated with peripheral and central nervous system reorganization involving neuronal and glial changes [1]. Migraine chronification may result from maladaptive neuroplasticity along the nociceptive pathway [2]. Repeated trigeminal activation at the meningeal neurovascular endings indeed, with the associated neurogenic inflammation, may induce peripheral and central sensitization, which in turn predisposes patients to develop more migraine attacks in a vicious cycle that, in some migraineurs, leads to chronic migraine [3]. The mechanisms involved in migraine chronification are largely elusive; however, a major role seems to be played by the neuropeptide calcitonin gene-related peptide (CGRP), a vasodilatory peptide released by trigeminovascular endings to cause vasodilation, neurogenic inflammation and peripheral sensitization [4]. The role of CGRP in migraine attacks is reinforced by the efficacy of CGRP antagonism in animal models of migraine pain [5–7] and by promising reports on the efficacy of CGRP-related drugs

* Correspondence: rosaria.greco@mondino.it
[1]Laboratory of Neurophysiology of Integrative Autonomic Systems, Headache Science Centre, IRCCS Mondino Foundation, Pavia, Italy
Full list of author information is available at the end of the article

in clinical trials, e.g. telcagepant or LY2951742 [8–10]. Recently, monoclonal antibodies directed against CGRP have proved effective in the preventive treatment of chronic migraine [11]. The precise mechanisms and sites where CGRP may act to favor chronification of migraine are still to be identified. CGRP receptors are largely distributed also in the brain, providing a wide range of possible CGRP targets and sites of interactions with other systems [12]. Topiramate is an antiepileptic drug with established efficacy in chronic migraine prevention [13, 14]. The drug likely acts on the cell excitatory mechanisms via its influence on the receptor/channel protein complexes [15–17].

Nitroglycerin (NTG) is a nitric oxide (NO) donor that has been used for years as a provocative test in migraine for diagnostic and research purposes [18, 19]. In rodents, NTG induces an increased sensitivity to pain stimuli [20–22] and its chronic and intermittent administration causes acute plantar mechanical hyperalgesia with a progressive and sustained hyperalgesia [23, 24]. This behavior nicely reflects the increased sensitivity to painful stimuli in migraineurs [25] and therefore may be relevant for understanding the mechanism underlying migraine. Here, we aimed at gathering more insights into the role and mechanisms of CGRP in migraine chronification by chronic migraine-like rat model that mimics the condition of chronic migraine. In this model we evaluated: a) CGRP and c-Fos gene expression in areas involved in trigeminal nociception; b) the nociceptive threshold at the tail flick; c) orofacial mechanical allodynia; d) the modulatory effect of the migraine preventive drug topiramate.

Methods

Animals

We used adult male Sprague-Dawley rats (weight 200-250 g, Charles River, s.r.l, Calco, Lecco, Italy) at the Centralized Animal Facility of the University of Pavia. The animals were housed under standard laboratory conditions in plastic boxes in groups of 2 with water and food available ad libitum and kept on a 12:12 h light-dark cycle, at room temperature of 19–21 °C with relative humidity of 70–80%. All procedures were conducted in accordance with the European Convention for Care and Use of Laboratory Animals and with the IASP's guidelines for pain research in animals [26]. The experimental protocols were approved by the Italian Ministry of Health (Document number 1239/2015PR).

Drugs

Nitroglycerin (NTG) (Bioindustria L.I.M. Novi Ligure (AL), Italy) was prepared from a stock solution of 5.0 mg/1.5 mL dissolved in 27% alcohol and 73% propylene glycol. For the injections, NTG was further diluted in saline (0.9% NaCl) to reach the final concentration of alcohol 6% and propylene glycol 16%. The diluted NTG is injected intraperitoneally (i.p.) at the dose of 5 mg/Kg [24, 27]. An equivalent volume of saline (0.9% NaCl), alcohol 6% and propylene glycol 16%) was used as vehicle. Topiramate (Topamax, Janssen-Cilag Cologno Monzese (MI), Italy) was dissolved in saline and administered i.p. at the dose of 30 mg/Kg [28]. Before baseline testing, rats were assigned to treatment groups according to a randomization list to ensure blinding to treatments of the researchers who performed the behavioral testing (tail flick test and Von Frey test, see below). Before testing the animals, the blinded examiners were instructed to observe the animal behavior, in order to evaluate the possible impact of topiramate on sedation or locomotor activities.

Experimental design and experimental groups

An a priori power analysis was conducted to determine the minimal sample size needed to obtain a statistical power of 0.80 at an alpha level of 0.05. On the basis of our previous studies in rats evaluating the latency to the tail flick (sec.) before and after NTG, we calculated an effect size of 1.6 for this variable (GPower 3.1.9.2), estimating a sample size of at least 5 rats for experimental group. Rats were injected with NTG or vehicle, every 2 days over a 9-day total period (5 total injections). A group of animals was also injected with topiramate (TOP) or vehicle (saline) every day for 9 days. At baseline (day 0) and 24 h after the last administration of NTG (day 10), the animals belonging to the different experimental groups (see below) underwent the evaluation of the nociceptive threshold by means of the tail flick test and of the orofacial mechanical allodynia by means of the Von Frey test. The schedule of drug treatments is reported in Fig. 1.

Experimental Groups: CT = NTG vehicle + TOP vehicle (N = 10–13 per group); NTG = NTG + TOP vehicle (N = 9–12 per group); TOP = NTG vehicle + Topiramate (N = 5–8 per group); NTG + TOP = NTG + Topiramate (N = 5–8 per group).

Behavioral tests

Rats underwent tail flick test and Von Frey test 30 min apart from each other at baseline and on day 10.

Tail flick test

To determine thermal sensitivity, rats were gently restrained while an infrared light beam with a temperature of 50 °C was focused on the animal's tail. The latency of retraction of the tail from the window of the light beam was automatically captured and measured (in seconds) by means of a sensor (Ugo Basile, model 7360, Varese, Italy) [20, 21]. A cut-off limit of exposure of 20 s was set to avoid tissue damage. The final latency value for each animal was

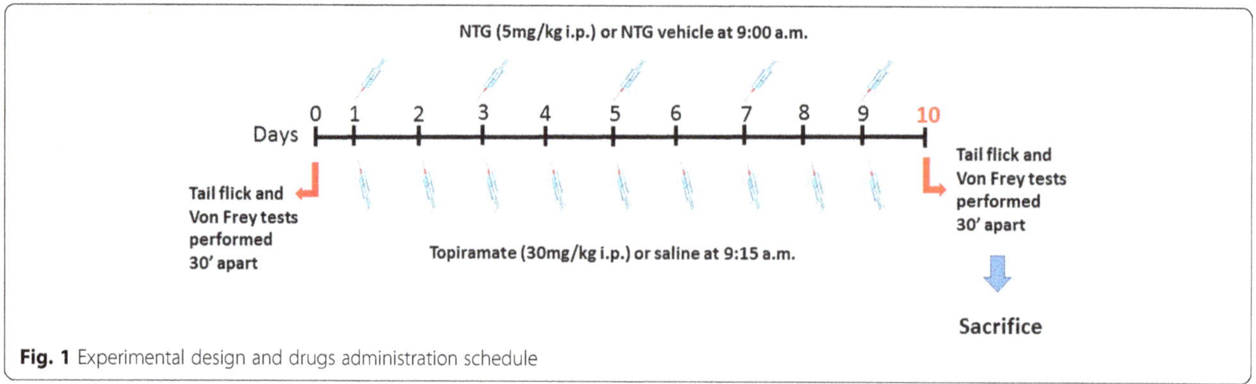

Fig. 1 Experimental design and drugs administration schedule

calculated as the mean of four measurements in 4 different parts of the tail, specifically at 1, 3, 5 and 7 cm from the tip.

Von Frey test

For three consecutive days, prior to baseline testing, the rats were habituated to the behavioral test procedure. Rats were put in clear acrylic cages (30 × 30 × 20 cm) and the orofacial area of the animal was stimulated with a series of Von Frey filaments (bending force ranging from 0.02 to 6 g). Progressively increasing filament forces were applied (each of them 5 times every 30 s) to the cutaneous area on both the left and right sides of the face, over the rostral portion of the eye for periorbital testing and on the skin over the masseter muscle for jaw testing until we obtained a positive response, defined as one of the following: head withdrawal, face wipe, escape/attack. In the absence of a positive response to the starting filament (0.4 g), a heavier filament was applied whereas, with a positive response a lighter filament was tested. The mechanical threshold corresponded to the force of the filament that induced three positive responses [29, 30].

CGRP and c-Fos gene expression

On day 10, immediately after undergoing the Von Frey test, all rats were sacrificed and their medulla-pons region, cervical spinal cord (C1-C2) and trigeminal ganglia were immediately chopped into parts for the evaluation of CGRP and c-Fos gene expression. mRNA levels were analyzed by real-time polymerase chain reaction (RT-PCR) as previously described [22, 31]. Primer sequences of Calca gene, coding for CGRP, (forward primer: CAGT CTCAGCTCCAAGTCATC; reverse primer: TTCC AAGGTTGACCTCAAAG) and c-Fos (forward primer: TACGCTCCAAGCGGAGAC; reverse primer: TTTCCTTCTCTTTCAGTAGATTGG) were obtained from the AutoPrime software (http://www.autoprime.de/AutoPrimeWeb). We used glyceraldehyde 3-phosphate dehydrogenase (GAPDH; forward primer: AACCTGCCA AGTATGATGAC; reverse primer: GGAGTTGCTGTTGA AGTCA) as housekeeping gene. All samples were assayed in triplicate. Gene expression was calculated using the ΔΔCt method.

Data analysis and statistical evaluation

Our data showed a normal distribution when analyzed with the Kolmogorov–Smirnov (KS) normality tests. For the behavioral tests the inter-groups and within groups differences between baseline and post-treatment timings were analyzed using the Two-way ANOVA for repeated measures followed by Bonferroni post hoc test. For gene expression, the differences between groups were analyzed by One-way ANOVA followed by Newman–Keuls multiple comparison test. A p value < 0.05 was considered statistically significant. The results were reported in the figures and all data were expressed as the mean + standard error of the mean. The Statistical analysis was performed using GraphPad Prism 5.02.

Results

Behavioral testing

No distinctive pattern of behavior was identified in the different experimental groups by comparing the reports of the blinded observers after treatment unblinding.

Tail Flick test

No significant difference among CT, NTG and NTG + TOP groups was observed at baseline (Fig. 2a). Chronic NTG administration caused a state of hyperalgesia, which was detected as a reduction in the latency at the tail flick test performed on day 10 as compared with both baseline value and CT group. The chronic administration of topiramate did not influence the tail flick latency, but it prevented NTG-induced hyperalgesic state. Data are reported in Fig. 2a.

Von Frey test

We did not detect any significant difference in baseline mechanical sensitivity among experimental groups (Fig. 2b). Chronic and intermittent NTG administration caused orofacial allodynia with a reduction in the mechanical pain threshold compared to the baseline value and to

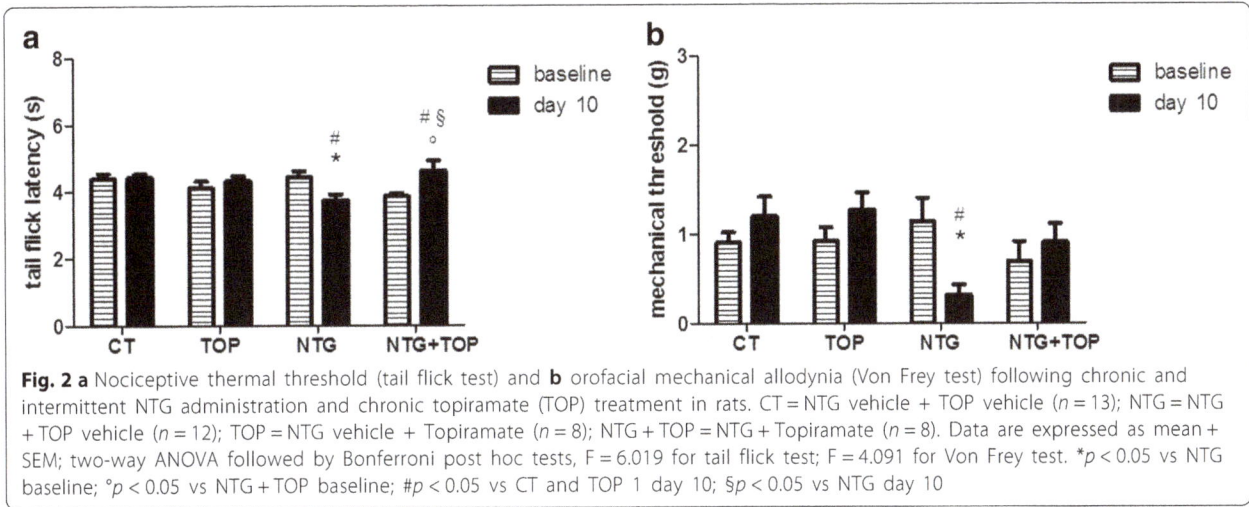

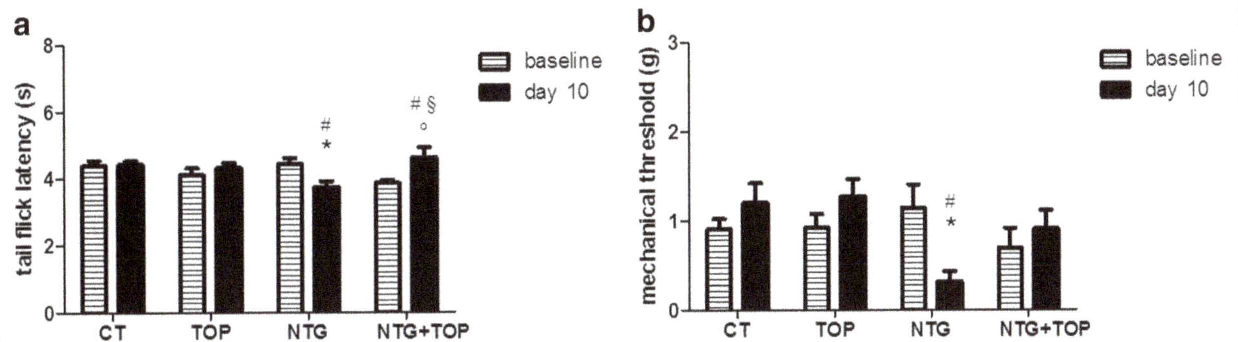

Fig. 2 a Nociceptive thermal threshold (tail flick test) and **b** orofacial mechanical allodynia (Von Frey test) following chronic and intermittent NTG administration and chronic topiramate (TOP) treatment in rats. CT = NTG vehicle + TOP vehicle ($n = 13$); NTG = NTG + TOP vehicle ($n = 12$); TOP = NTG vehicle + Topiramate ($n = 8$); NTG + TOP = NTG + Topiramate ($n = 8$). Data are expressed as mean + SEM; two-way ANOVA followed by Bonferroni post hoc tests, F = 6.019 for tail flick test; F = 4.091 for Von Frey test. *$p < 0.05$ vs NTG baseline; °$p < 0.05$ vs NTG + TOP baseline; #$p < 0.05$ vs CT and TOP 1 day 10; §$p < 0.05$ vs NTG day 10

the CT group. Topiramate did not change the mechanical pain threshold when compared to the baseline value and to the CT group, but it prevented the development of NTG-induced allodynia. The mechanical threshold of NTG + TOP was increased compared to NTG group, although it did not reach a statistical significant level, probably because of the great variability of data. Data are reported in Fig. 2b.

mRNA expression of CGRP and c-Fos genes

NTG administration induced a significant increase in the expression of c-Fos and CGRP mRNA in the medulla-pons region, cervical spinal cord and trigeminal ganglia (Fig. 3). Topiramate did not modify genes expression in these areas when used alone, but it markedly attenuated CGRP and c-Fos gene expression induced by NTG in all the areas under evaluation (Fig. 3).

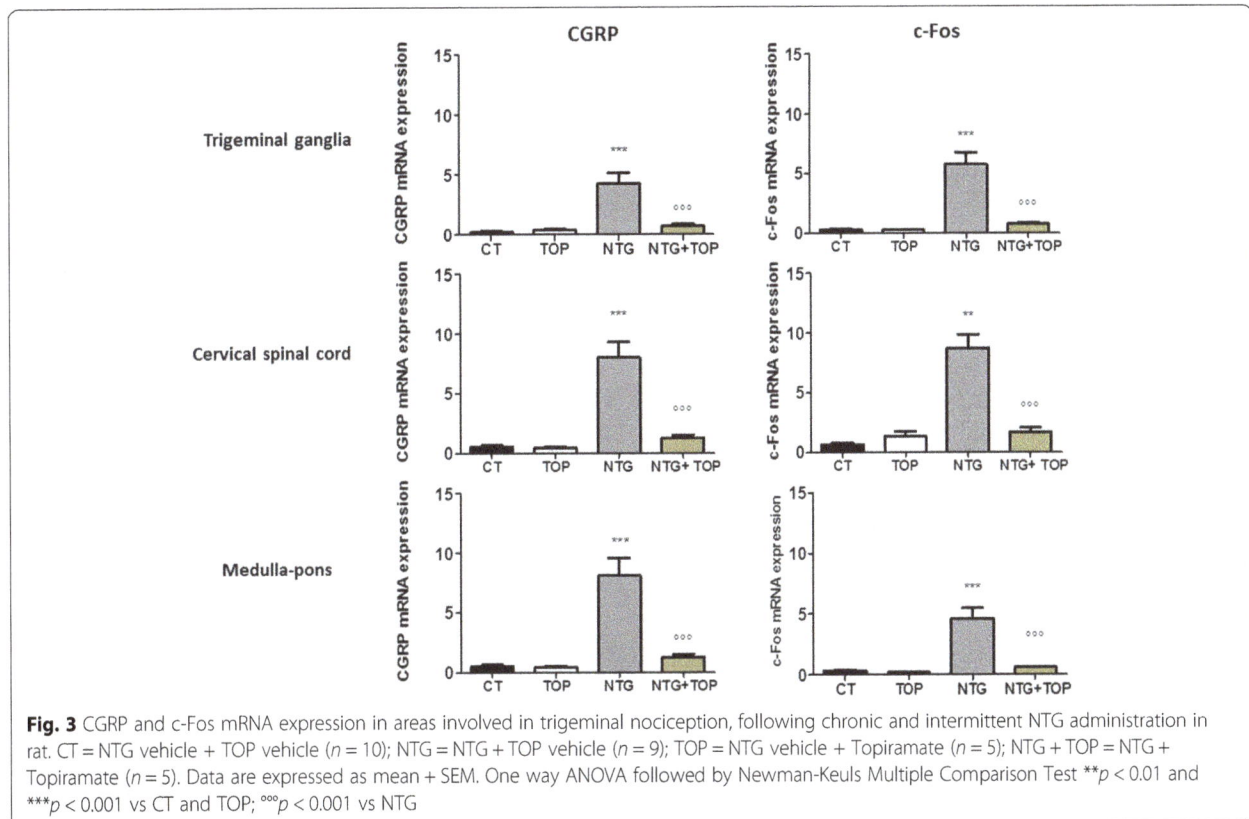

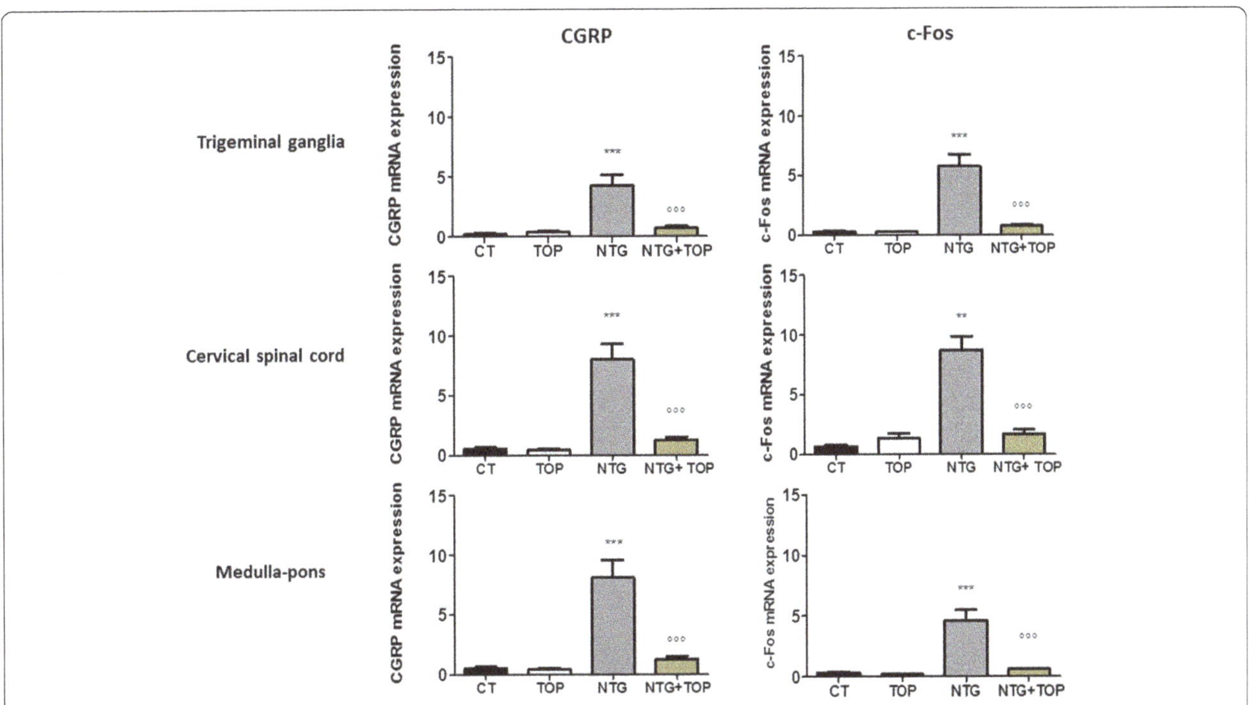

Fig. 3 CGRP and c-Fos mRNA expression in areas involved in trigeminal nociception, following chronic and intermittent NTG administration in rat. CT = NTG vehicle + TOP vehicle ($n = 10$); NTG = NTG + TOP vehicle ($n = 9$); TOP = NTG vehicle + Topiramate ($n = 5$); NTG + TOP = NTG + Topiramate ($n = 5$). Data are expressed as mean + SEM. One way ANOVA followed by Newman-Keuls Multiple Comparison Test **$p < 0.01$ and ***$p < 0.001$ vs CT and TOP; °°°$p < 0.001$ vs NTG

Discussion

Migraine is a highly disabling condition [32] that manifests with recurring attacks. In 2–3% of the general population it becomes chronic (≥ 15 days/months) and therefore even more disabling. Progressive changes in nociceptive thresholds and subsequent central sensitization due to recurrent migraine headaches in vulnerable subjects contribute to the chronic migraine state. Understanding the mechanisms of chronification seems therefore extremely useful. The role of CGRP in the precipitation of migraine attacks is nowadays well accepted [33]. Less known is CGRP role in the processes that lead to migraine chronification.

Several studies indicate that NTG administration in rodents is a predictive model of migraine in humans [24, 34, 35]. In this study we aimed at developing and testing a chronic migraine-like model in rats, based on chronic and intermittent administration of NTG. In this model the animals become hyperalgesic and allodynic, which nicely mimics the clinical picture on one side [25, 36–39], and, on the other, parallels the findings obtained by Pradhan et al. in the animal model of chronic migraine devised in mice [24]. The availability of an animal model of chronic migraine in rats provides a precious opportunity for investigating the pathophysiological mechanisms involved in chronic migraine for a dual reason: 1) rat models have technical and practical advantages [40] and 2) the rat-based migraine model of acute NTG administration is well-established and has already yielded a wealth of data from several groups [41, 42].

Using this chronic migraine-like model we showed that the observed changes in pain perception – namely a reduction in the latency of the tail flick test and orofacial mechanical allodynia - are paralleled by an increased expression in CGRP mRNA in the trigeminal ganglia. CGRP is involved in the maintenance of ongoing sensitization and the increased gene expression observed in our model may be interpreted as a compensatory mechanism for reintegrating CGRP released at the trigeminovascular endings [43–45]. In agreement, Farajdokht et al. [46] demonstrated that the increase in CGRP gene expression in trigeminal ganglia is associated with increased transient receptor potential vanilloid type-1 mRNA levels in the same area 48 h after NTG injection. Previous reports have suggested that NTG induces hyperalgesia via complex mechanisms that involve also sensitization of the trigeminovascular system at the meningeal level [47–49]. Previously, we reported that acute NTG administration did not cause any change in CGRP-immunoreactivity in the lumbar dorsal horns, whereas it increased SP staining intensity in both the cervical and lumbar spinal cord 1 h after NTG administration [43]. Thus, though the effect of NTG administration seems relevant for processes that take place in the cervical spinal cord, we cannot rule out the occurrence of systemic NTG effects on other neuronal subpopulations and other areas of the nervous system. Of note, in a previous study Edelmeyer et al. [50] showed that inflammatory mediators applied to the dura of non-anesthetized rats caused strong and time-related facial and hindpaw allodynia, thus suggesting that the alterations in pain sensitivity associated with primary headache, probably reflect a more generalized condition of central sensitization [50].

In a previous study, we showed that acute NTG administration induces an increase in CGRP gene expression in the trigeminal ganglia, cervical spinal cord and medulla-pons area 5 h after the administration [31, 51]. Here, we show that the levels of CGRP mRNA are elevated in the same areas 24 h after the last dose of NTG administration. These findings are consistent with the synthesis and release of CGRP in these central areas, where the peptide can modulate nociceptive transmission [52]. Indeed, CGRP mRNA signal has been detected in the nucleus trigeminal caudalis (NTC) and other brain structures of naïve rats [53, 54], which include the nucleus tractus solitarius, receiving inhibitory baroreceptor afferents, the ventrolateral medulla, a key structure in the descending pain modulation, and the pontine parabrachial nucleus (PBN) that contributes to nociceptive transmission with its projections to the central nucleus of the amygdala (CeA) [55]. More importantly, CGRP and its receptor antagonists act on neurons in the ventrolateral periaqueductal gray to influence nociceptive transmission in the nucleus tractus caudalis. Functional CGRP receptors are present as well in other regions of the brain that are involved in the modulation of migraine pain [56]. Taken together, these observations support the contribution of CGRP in central sensitization and in the functioning of descending pain pathways, both of which are implicated in chronic migraine [57].

To further test the relevance of our animal model of chronic migraine we evaluated the effect of chronic administration of topiramate, one of the few drugs that have proved effective in the preventive treatment of chronic migraine in randomized controlled trials [58, 59].

Topiramate reduces brain hyperexcitability, a hallmark of migraine [60], via multiple mechanisms: blockade of voltage dependent sodium channels, increased activity of the neurotransmitter gamma-aminobutyrate (GABA) and antagonism of the α-amino-3-hydroxy-5-methyl-4-isoxazolepropionic acid (AMPA)/kainate subtype of the glutamate receptor and inhibition of the carbonic anhydrase enzyme [61, 62]. An in vitro study demonstrated that topiramate is able to attenuate neurogenic dural vasodilation by inhibiting the release of CGRP from prejunctional trigeminal neurons, thus suggesting an interaction with this neuropeptide [15].

Chronic treatment with topiramate in our model reduced trigeminal spinal hyperalgesia and mechanical allodynia, while diminishing CGRP mRNA levels in the areas under investigation. This finding seems in agreement with preclinical studies showing that topiramate has an anti-allodynic effect in neuropathic pain at doses of 20–50 mg/kg [28, 63–65]. Chronic administration of topiramate (50 mg/kg/day, i.p.) to neuropathic rats diminished the mechanical sensitivity and shortened the period of allodynia to 8 days [28].

CGRP can directly activate the nociceptors or facilitate their firing, thus causing peripheral sensitization and hyperalgesia [1]. In this frame, it is possible that the anti-hyperalgesic effect of topiramate observed in the present study is related to the inhibitory activity on the neuronal firing within the trigeminocervical complex and the ventroposteromedial thalamic nucleus, as reported by Andreou and Goadsby [66].

Topiaramate blocks voltage-dependent sodium channel in spinal cord neurons, which prompts a possible mechanism for reducing afferent input to the NTC [67]. Other mechanisms could be involved such as anti-inflammatory and immunomodulatory effects or inhibition of neurotransmitters release [68, 69]. Central sensitization involves an increased sensitivity of second-order neurons to afferent inputs, the augmentation of receptive fields and an increased excitability; furthermore, it involves long-term effects related to transcriptional changes and dysfunctions in the descending pain system [70]. The maintenance of central sensitization may be related to the activation of the glutamate N-methyl-D-aspartate (NMDA), AMPA and metabotropic receptors. Thus, AMPA/kainate receptors inhibition by topiramate treatment could decrease neuronal hyperexcitability within the NTC and brain structures receiving inputs from second order neurons [68]. Glutamate-like immunoreactivity has been indeed detected in tooth pulp neurons that project to the NTC in the rat [71].

It is worth noting that in our experimental paradigm, topiramate treatment significantly reduced CGRP gene expression in cervical spinal cord and medulla-pons. In agreement, topiramate treatment repressed KCl stimulated CGRP release in a time and concentration dependent manner in trigeminal cultures [72]. However, since GABAergic mechanisms have been shown to be implicated in the trigeminocervical complex, it is stimulating to hypothesize that GABA potentiation due to topiramate treatment may interfere with CGRP synthesis in the NTC, as well as in the areas involved in the descending pain system [34, 35, 57, 73]. Synaptic contacts between CGRP-positive terminals and GABAergic neurons were found within the CeA, which may underlie the pain-related neural pathway from PBN to CeA, in chronic pain modulation.

The increased c-Fos mRNA levels found 24 h after NTG treatment, confirms that NTG-induced transcriptional changes are not limited to peripheral areas, but rather affect central structures, directly or indirectly, thus reflecting a widespread, peripheral and central diffusion of sensitization phenomena consistent with the observed alterations in pain responses. While a large body of information has been collected over the years by our group and others on the acute NTG model, the mechanisms responsible for c-Fos gene expression after chronic NTG are almost completely unknown. At this time, we can only speculate that the model proposed in this study actually engages the CNS with persisting functional and morphological changes associated to chronic sensitization.

Limitations of the study

The design of study foresaw the chronic administration of topiramate. Data from the literature suggest that acute administration of topiramate reduces neuronal firing in the trigeminovascular complex [66] therefore the chronic administration used in our design might not have been necessary. In the absence of reliable evidence, we selected the chronic administration for several reasons. First, this treatment schedule reflects more closely the clinical scenario, where topiramate is used daily over months to prevent migraine attacks. Second, data is lacking on the serum/plasma concentration of topiramate in the rat. Human studies show that the plasma half-life of the drug is 20–30 h after a single oral administration [74, 75], while it is shorter in rats [76], thus posing the issue of unstable blood levels of topiramate. This could have been addressed by increasing the dose of the single administration, but also the possibility that the sedative effect of such a higher dose might interfere with the nocifensive behavior of the rat [77]. The lack of precise pharmacokinetics studies on repeated dosing in the laboratory animal ultimately suggested the selection of dose regimens based on a best-guess modality, guided by careful evaluation of available evidence.

Future studies are needed to address topiramate serum/plasma concentrations in our model, together with the evaluation of the potential impact of topiramate-induced locomotor activity in the nocifensive behavior of chronically NTG-treated rats using specific behavioral testing.

Conclusions

The present findings, obtained in a novel chronic migraine-like model in the rat, suggest that CGRP pathway activation is involved in the facilitation of nociceptive transmission and is likely to contribute to central sensitization and dysfunction in descending pain control, via modulatory effects that encompass the modulation of voltage dependent sodium channels, GABA activity and the glutamate pathway. A fuller understanding of CGRP effects and CGRP network in brain regions will provide powerful insights for understanding the complex circuitry of migraine and for the improvement of migraine therapies.

Abbreviations

AMPA: α-amino-3-hydroxy-5-methyl-4-isoxazolepropionic acid; CeA: Central nucleus of the amygdala; CGRP: Calcitonin gene-related peptide;

GABA: Gamma-aminobutyrate; GAPDH: Glyceraldehyde 3-phosphate dehydrogenase; NMDA: N-methyl-D-aspartate; NO: Nitric oxide; NTC: trigeminal nucleus caudalis; NTG: Nitroglycerin; PBN: Pontine parabrachial nucleus; RT-PCR: Real-time polymerase chain reaction; TOP: Topiramate

Funding

This work was supported by a grant of the Italian Ministry of Health (Ricerca Corrente 2016) to the IRCCS Mondino Foundation.

Authors' contributions

RG designed the experiments and drafted the manuscript. CD and AZ performed the experiments. RG analyzed and interpreted the data. CT revised the manuscript. All authors read and approved the final manuscript.

Competing interests

The authors declare that they have no competing interests.

Author details

[1]Laboratory of Neurophysiology of Integrative Autonomic Systems, Headache Science Centre, IRCCS Mondino Foundation, Pavia, Italy. [2]Department of Brain and Behavioral Sciences, University of Pavia, Pavia, Italy.

References

1. Basbaum AI, Bautista DM, Scherrer G, Julius D (2009) Cellular and molecular mechanisms of pain. Cell 139(2):267–284
2. Latremoliere A, Woolf CJ (2009) Central sensitization: a generator of pain hypersensitivity by central neural plasticity. J Pain 10(9):895–926
3. Bernstein C, Burstein R (2012) Sensitization of the trigeminovascular pathway: perspective and implications to migraine pathophysiology. J Clin Neurol 8(2):89–99
4. Iyengar S, Ossipov MH, Johnson KW (2017) The role of calcitonin gene-related peptide in peripheral and central pain mechanisms including migraine. Pain 158(4):543–559
5. Greco R, Mangione AS, Siani F, Blandini F, Vairetti M, Nappi G, Sandrini G, Buzzi MG, Tassorelli C (2014) Effects of CGRP receptor antagonism in nitroglycerin-induced hyperalgesia. Cephalalgia 34(8):594–604
6. Cornelison LE, Hawkins JL, Durham PL (2016) Elevated levels of calcitonin gene-related peptide in upper spinal cord promotes sensitization of primary trigeminal nociceptive neurons. Neuroscience 339:491–501
7. Filiz A, Tepe N, Eftekhari S, Boran HE, Dilekoz E, Edvinsson L, Bolay H (2017) CGRP receptor antagonist MK-8825 attenuates cortical spreading depression induced pain behavior. Cephalalgia. https://doi.org/10.1177/0333102417735845
8. Ho TW, Connor KM, Zhang Y, Pearlman E, Koppenhaver J, Fan X, Lines C, Edvinsson L, Goadsby PJ, Michelson D (2014) Randomized controlled trial of the CGRP receptor antagonist telcagepant for migraine prevention. Neurology 83(11):958–966
9. Ho TW, Ho AP, Ge YJ, Assaid C, Gottwald R, MacGregor EA, Mannix LK, van Oosterhout WP, Koppenhaver J, Lines C, Ferrari MD, Michelson D (2016) Randomized controlled trial of the CGRP receptor antagonist telcagepant for prevention of headache in women with perimenstrual migraine. Cephalalgia 36(2):148–161
10. Dodick DW, Goadsby PJ, Spierings EL, Scherer JC, Sweeney SP, Grayzel DS (2014) Safety and efficacy of LY2951742, a monoclonal antibody to calcitonin gene-related peptide, for the prevention of migraine: a phase 2, randomised, double-blind, placebo-controlled study. Lancet Neurol 13(9):885–892
11. Silberstein SD, Dodick DW, Bigal ME, Yeung PP, Goadsby PJ, Blankenbiller T, Grozinski-Wolff M, Yang R, Ma Y, Aycardi E (2017) Fremanezumab for the preventive treatment of chronic migraine. N Engl J Med 377(22): 2113–2122
12. Russo AF (2015) Calcitonin gene-related peptide (CGRP): a new target for migraine. Annu Rev Pharmacol Toxicol 55:533–552
13. Brandes JL, Saper JR, Diamond M, Couch JR, Lewis DW, Schmitt J, Neto W, Schwabe S, Jacobs D, MIGR-002 Study Group (2004) Topiramate for migraine prevention: a randomized controlled trial. JAMA 291(8):965–973
14. Silberstein SD (2017) Topiramate in migraine prevention: a 2016 perspective. Headache 57(1):165–178
15. Akerman S, Goadsby PJ (2005) Topiramate inhibits trigeminovascular activation: an intravital microscopy study. Br J Pharmacol 146(1):7–14
16. Motaghinejad M, Motevalian M (2016) Involvement of AMPA/kainate and GABAA receptors in topiramate neuroprotective effects against methylphenidate abuse sequels involving oxidative stress and inflammation in rat isolated hippocampus. Eur J Pharmacol 784:181–191
17. Curia G, Aracri P, Colombo E, Scalmani P, Mantegazza M, Avanzini G, Franceschetti S (2007) Phosphorylation of sodium channels mediated by protein kinase-C modulates inhibition by topiramate of tetrodotoxin-sensitive transient sodium current. Br J Pharmacol 150(6):792–797
18. Sances G, Tassorelli C, Pucci E, Ghiotto N, Sandrini G, Nappi G (2004) Reliability of the nitroglycerin provocative test in the diagnosis of neurovascular headaches. Cephalalgia 24(2):110–119
19. Ashina M, Hansen JM, Olesen J (2013) Pearls and pitfalls in human pharmacological models of migraine: 30 years' experience. Cephalalgia 33(8):540–553
20. Greco R, Tassorelli C, Armentero MT, Sandrini G, Nappi G, Blandini F (2008) Role of central dopaminergic circuitry in pain processing and nitroglycerin-induced hyperalgesia. Brain Res 1238:215–223
21. Greco R, Bandiera T, Mangione AS, Demartini C, Siani F, Nappi G, Sandrini G, Guijarro A, Armirotti A, Piomelli D, Tassorelli C (2015) Effects of peripheral FAAH blockade on NTG-induced hyperalgesia–evaluation of URB937 in an animal model of migraine. Cephalalgia 35(12):1065–1076
22. Greco R, Siani F, Demartini C, Zanaboni A, Nappi G, Davinelli S, Scapagnini G, Tassorelli C (2016) Andrographis Paniculata shows anti-nociceptive effects in an animal model of sensory hypersensitivity associated with migraine. Funct Neurol 31(1):53–60
23. Farajdokht F, Babri S, Karimi P, Alipour MR, Bughchechi R, Mohaddes G (2017) Chronic ghrelin treatment reduced photophobia and anxiety-like behaviors in nitroglycerin- induced migraine: role of pituitary adenylate cyclase-activating polypeptide. Eur J Neurosci 45(6):763–772
24. Pradhan AA, Smith ML, McGuire B, Tarash I, Evans CJ, Charles A (2014) Characterization of a novel model of chronic migraine. Pain 155(2):269–274
25. Perrotta A, Serrao M, Tassorelli C, Arce-Leal N, Guaschino E, Sances G, Rossi P, Bartolo M, Pierelli F, Sandrini G, Nappi G (2011) Oral nitric-oxide donor glyceryl-trinitrate induces sensitization in spinal cord pain processing in migraineurs: a double-blind, placebo-controlled, cross-over study. Eur J Pain 15(5):482–490
26. Zimmerman M (1983) Ethical guidelines for investigations of experimental pain in conscious animals. Pain 16:109–110
27. Tassorelli C, Greco R, Cappelletti D, Sandrini G, Nappi G (2005) Comparative analysis of the neuronal activation and cardiovascular effects of nitroglycerin, sodium nitroprusside and L-arginine. Brain Res 1051(1–2):17–24
28. Wieczorkiewicz-Płaza A, Płaza P, Maciejewski R, Czuczwar M, Przesmycki K (2004) Effect of topiramate on mechanical allodynia in neuropathic pain model in rats. Pol J Pharmacol 56(2):275–278
29. Martin YB, Avendaño C (2009) Effects of removal of dietary polyunsaturated fatty acids on plasma extravasation and mechanical allodynia in a trigeminal neuropathic pain model. Mol Pain 5:8
30. Oshinsky ML, Sanghvi MM, Maxwell CR, Gonzalez D, Spangenberg RJ, Cooper M, Silberstein SD (2012) Spontaneous trigeminal allodynia in rats: a model of primary headache. Headache 52(9):1336–1349
31. Demartini C, Tassorelli C, Zanaboni AM, Tonsi G, Francesconi O, Nativi C, Greco R (2017) The role of the transient receptor potential ankyrin type-1 (TRPA1) channel in migraine pain: evaluation in an animal model. J Headache Pain 18(1):94
32. GBD 2015 Neurological Disorders Collaborator Group (2017) Global, regional, and national burden of neurological disorders during 1990–2015: a

systematic analysis for the Global Burden of Disease Study 2015. Lancet Neurol 16(11):877–897
33. Bigal ME, Walter S, Rapoport AM (2013) Calcitonin gene-related peptide (CGRP) and migraine current understanding and state of development. Headache 53(8):1230–1244
34. Moye LS, Pradhan AAA (2017) Animal model of chronic migraine-associated pain. Curr Protoc Neurosci 80:9.60.1–9.60.9
35. Farkas S, Bölcskei K, Markovics A, Varga A, Kis-Varga Á, Kormos V, Gaszner B, Horváth C, Tuka B, Tajti J, Helyes Z (2016) Utility of different outcome measures for the nitroglycerin model of migraine in mice. J Pharmacol Toxicol Methods 77:33–44
36. de Tommaso M, Ambrosini A, Brighina F, Coppola G, Perrotta A, Pierelli F, Sandrini G, Valeriani M, Marinazzo D, Stramaglia S, Schoenen J (2014) Altered processing of sensory stimuli in patients with migraine. Nat Rev Neurol 10(3):144–155
37. Sandrini G, Tassorelli C, Cecchini AP, Alfonsi E, Nappi G (2002) Effects of nimesulide on nitric oxide-induced hyperalgesia in humans–a neurophysiological study. Eur J Pharmacol 450(3):259–262
38. Burstein R, Jakubowski M, Rauch SD (2011) The science of migraine. J Vestib Res 21(6):305–314
39. Louter MA, Bosker JE, van Oosterhout WP, van Zwet EW, Zitman FG, Ferrari MD, Terwindt GM (2013) Cutaneous allodynia as a predictor of migraine chronification. Brain 136(Pt 11):3489–3496
40. Ellenbroek B, Youn J (2016) Rodent models in neuroscience research: is it a rat race? Dis Model Mech 9(10):1079–1087
41. Valença MM (2017) Commentary: the effect of systemic nitroglycerin administration on the kynurenine pathway in the rat. Front Neurol 8:518
42. Ramachandran R, Pedersen SH, Amrutkar DV, Petersen S, Jacobsen JM, Hay-Schmidt A, Olesen J, Jansen-Olesen I (2017) Selective cephalic upregulation of p-ERK, CamKII and p-CREB in response to glyceryl trinitrate infusion. Cephalalgia Jan 1:333102417722511
43. Greco R, Tassorelli C, Sandrini G, Di Bella P, Buscone S, Nappi G (2008) Role of calcitonin gene-related peptide and substance P in different models of pain. Cephalalgia 28(2):114–126
44. Pardutz A, Multon S, Malgrange B, Parducz A, Vecsei L, Schoenen J (2002) Effect of systemic nitroglycerin on CGRP and 5-HT afferents to rat caudal spinal trigeminal nucleus and its modulation by estrogen. Eur J Neurosci 15(11):1803–1809
45. Capuano A, Greco MC, Navarra P, Tringali G (2014) Correlation between algogenic effects of calcitonin-gene-related peptide (CGRP) and activation of trigeminal vascular system, in an in vivo experimental model of nitroglycerin-induced sensitization. Eur J Pharmacol 740:97–102
46. Farajdokht F, Mohaddes G, Shanehbandi D, Karimi P, Babri S (2017) Ghrelin attenuated hyperalgesia induced by chronic nitroglycerin: CGRP and TRPV1 as targets for migraine management. Cephalalgia. Jan 1:333102417748563. https://doi.org/10.1177/0333102417748563
47. Tassorelli C, Joseph SA, Buzzi MG, Nappi G (1999) The effects on the central nervous system of nitroglycerin–putative mechanisms and mediators. Prog Neurobiol 57(6):607–624
48. Buzzi MG, Tassorelli C (2010) Experimental models of migraine. Handb Clin Neurol 97:109–123
49. Reuter U, Bolay H, Jansen-Olesen I, Chiarugi A, Sanchez del Rio M, Letourneau R, Theoharides TC, Waeber C, Moskowitz MA (2001) Delayed inflammation in rat meninges: implications for migraine pathophysiology. Brain 124(Pt 12):2490–2502
50. Edelmayer RM, Ossipov MH, Porreca F (2012) An experimental model of headache-related pain. Methods Mol Biol 851:109–120
51. Greco R, Demartini C, Zanaboni AM, Redavide E, Pampalone S, Toldi J, Fülöp F, Blandini F, Nappi G, Sandrini G, Vécsei L, Tassorelli C (2017) Effects of kynurenic acid analogue 1 (KYNA-A1) in nitroglycerin-induced hyperalgesia: targets and anti-migraine mechanisms. Cephalalgia 37(13):1272–1284
52. Raddant AC, Russo AF (2011) Calcitonin gene-related peptide in migraine: intersection of peripheral inflammation and central modulation. Expert Rev Mol Med 13:e36
53. Bhatt DK, Gupta S, Ploug KB, Jansen-Olesen I, Olesen J (2014) mRNA distribution of CGRP and its receptor components in the trigeminovascular system and other pain related structures in rat brain, and effect of intracerebroventricular administration of CGRP on Fos expression in the TNC. Neurosci Lett 559:99–104
54. Kresse A, Jacobowitz DM, Skofitsch G (1995) Detailed mapping of CGRP mRNA expression in the rat central nervous system: comparison with previous immunocytochemical findings. Brain Res Bull 36(3):261–274
55. Bernard JF, Alden M, Besson JM (1993) The organization of the efferent projections from the pontine parabrachial area to the amygdaloid complex: a Phaseolus vulgaris leucoagglutinin (PHA-L) study in the rat. J Comp Neurol 329(2):201–229
56. Eftekhari S, Edvinsson L (2011) Calcitonin gene-related peptide (CGRP) and its receptor components in human and rat spinal trigeminal nucleus and spinal cord at C1-level. BMC Neurosci 12:112
57. Eftekhari S, Gaspar RC, Roberts R, Chen TB, Zeng Z, Villarreal S, Edvinsson L, Salvatore CA (2016) Localization of CGRP receptor components and receptor binding sites in rhesus monkey brainstem: a detailed study using in situ hybridization, immunofluorescence, and autoradiography. J Comp Neurol 524:90–118
58. Silberstein S, Lipton R, Dodick D, Freitag F, Mathew N, Brandes J, Bigal M, Ascher S, Morein J, Wright P, Greenberg S, Hulihan J (2009) Topiramate treatment of chronic migraine: a randomized, placebo-controlled trial of quality of life and other efficacy measures. Headache 49:1153–1162
59. Diener HC, Bussone G, Van Oene JC, Lahaye M, Schwalen S, Goadsby PJ, TOPMAT-MIG-201(TOP-CHROME) Study Group (2007) Topiramate reduces headache days in chronic migraine: a randomized, double-blind, placebo-controlled study. Cephalalgia 27:814–823
60. Ambrosini A, Schoenen J (2006) Electrophysiological response patterns of primary sensory cortices in migraine. J Headache Pain 7:377–388
61. Shank RP, Gardocki JF, Streeter AJ, Maryanoff BE (2000) An overview of the preclinical aspects of topiramate: pharmacology, pharmacokinetics and mechanism of action. Epilepsia 41(Suppl 1):S3–S9
62. Angehagen M, Ben-Menachem E, Rönnbäck L, Hansson E (2003) Novel mechanisms of action of three antiepileptic drugs, vigabatrin, tiagabine, and topiramate. Neurochem Res 28(2):333–340
63. Benoliel R, Tal M, Eliav E (2006) Effects of topiramate on the chronicconstriction injury model in the rat. J Pain 7:878–883
64. Rus NN, Boçşan C, Vesa ŞC, Coadă CA, Buzoianu AD (2013) Topiramate in nociceptive pain - experimental analgesia study. Human & Vet Med Int J Bioflux Soc:70–76
65. Wild KD, Yagel SK, Shank RP (1997) The novel anticonvul-sant topiramate is anti-allodynic in a rat model of neu-ropathic pain. Soc Neurosci Abstr 23:2358 abstr 918.10
66. Andreou AP, Goadsby PJ (2011) Topiramate in the treatment of migraine: a kainate (glutamate) receptor antagonist within the trigeminothalamic pathway. Cephalalgia 31(13):1343–1358
67. McLean MJ, Bukhari AA, Wamil AW (2000) Effects of topiramate on sodium-dependent action-potential firing by mouse spinal cord neurons in cell culture. Epilepsia 41(Suppl 1):S21–SS4
68. Schiffer WK, Gerasimov MR, Marsteller DA, Geiger J, Barnett C, Alexoff DL, Dewey SL (2001) Topiramate selectively attenuates nicotine-induced increases in monoamine release. Synapse 42:196–198
69. Shank RP, Maryanoff BE (2008) Molecular pharmacodynamics, clinical therapeutics, and pharmacokinetics of topiramate. CNS Neurosci Ther Summer 14(2):120–142
70. Benarroch EE (2011) CGRP: sensory neuropeptide with multiple neurologic implications. Neurology 77(3):281–287
71. Bouhassira D, Le Bars D, Villanueva L (1987) Heterotopic activation of ad and C fibres triggers inhibition of trigeminal and spinal convergent neurons in the rat. J Physiol 389:301–317
72. Durham PL, Niemann C, Cady R (2006) Repression of stimulated calcitonin gene-related peptide secretion by topiramate. Headache 46(8):1291–1295
73. Lau BK, Vaughan CW (2014) Descending modulation of pain: the GABA disinhibition hypothesis of analgesia. Curr Opin Neurobiol 29:159–164
74. Johannessen SI (1997) Pharmacokinetics and interaction profile of topiramate: review and comparison with other newer antiepileptic drugs. Epilepsia 38(Suppl 1):S18–S23
75. Matar KM, Tayem YI (2014) Effect of experimentally induced hepatic and renal failure on the pharmacokinetics of topiramate in rats. Biomed Res Int 2014:570910
76. Löscher W (2007) The pharmacokinetics of antiepileptic drugs in rats: consequences for maintaining effective drug levels during prolonged drug administration in rat models of epilepsy. Epilepsia 48(7):1245–1258
77. Motaghinejad M, Motevalian M, Shabab B (2016) Neuroprotective effects of various doses of topiramate against methylphenidate induced oxidative stress and inflammation in rat isolated hippocampus. Clin Exp Pharmacol Physiol 43(3):360–371

Abnormal brain white matter in patients with right trigeminal neuralgia: a diffusion tensor imaging study

Junpeng Liu[1], Jiajia Zhu[2], Fei Yuan[3], Xuejun Zhang[1*] and Quan Zhang[3*]

Abstract

Background: Idiopathic or classical trigeminal neuralgia (TN) is a chronic painful condition characterized by intermittent pain attacks. Enough evidence demonstrates classical TN is related to neurovascular compression (NVC) at the trigeminal root entry zone (REZ), but white matter change secondary to TN are not totally known.

Methods: Visual Analogue Scale (VAS) and diffusion tensor imaging were performed on 29 patients with right TN and 35 healthy individuals. Voxel-wise analyses were performed with TBSS using multiple diffusion metrics, including fractional anisotropy (FA), mean diffusivity (MD), axial diffusivity (AD) and radial diffusivity (RD). Group differences in these parameters were compared between right TN patients and controls using TBSS and correlations between the white matter change and disease duration and VAS in right TN patients were assessed. Multiple comparison correction were applied to test significant correlations.

Results: The right TN patients showed significantly lower FA and higher RD in most left white matter ($P < 0.05$, FWE corrected). Moreover, negative correlations were observed between disease duration and the FA values of left corona radiata, genu of corpus callosum, left external capsule and left cerebral peduncle, and between VAS and the FA values of left corona radiata, left external capsule and left cerebral peduncle ($P < 0.05$). Positive correlations were observed for disease duration and the RD values of left corona radiata, right external capsule, left fornix cerebri and left cerebral peduncle, and for VAS and the RD values of left corona radiata and left external capsule ($P < 0.05$). However, once Bonferroni corrections were applied, these correlations were not statistically significant.

Conclusion: These findings suggest that TN selectively impairs widespread white matter, especially contralateral hemisphere, which may be the hallmark of disease severity in TN patients.

Keywords: Trigeminal neuralgia, Neurovascular compression, Magnetic resonance imaging, Tract-based spatial statistics, White matter

Background

Trigeminal neuralgia (TN) is the most common form of facial neuropathic pain with an annual incidence of 4 to 5 new patients per 100,000 [1]. It is characterized by recurrent episodes of unilateral brief electric shock-like pains localized to the sensory supply areas of trigeminal nerve and has been considered as one of the most serious pains that can experience [2–4]. Idiopathic or classical TN is mainly caused by neurovascular compression of trigeminal nerve at its root entry zone (REZ) and microvascular decompression (MVD) surgery is most effective method for relieving neuralgic pain [3–7]. However, peripheral nerve injury caused by neurovascular compression does not fully explain the persistence of long-term recurrent pain in TN patients [8–11].

Neurovascular compression may result in focal demyelination of the trigeminal nerve at the REZ, which consequently generates ectopic discharges and pathological

* Correspondence: zhangxj@tmu.edu.cn; tj_zhangquan1981@163.com
[1]School of Medical Imaging, Tianjin Medical University, No. 1, Guangdong Road, Hexi District, Tianjin 300203, China
[3]Department of Radiology, Pingjin Hospital, Logistics University of Chinese People's Armed Police Forces, No. 220, Chenglin Road, Hedong District, Tianjin 300162, China
Full list of author information is available at the end of the article

cross-activation between afferent nerve fibers [12]. And pain ensues. What's more, this process may lead to central white matter changes and/or higher brain structures and sensitization of neurons [13–15]. Previous studies have mostly concentrated on abnormalities of trigeminal nerve [16], but the nature of assumed nerve abnormalities is not known. Diffusion tensor imaging (DTI) based on magnetic resonance imaging (MRI) has been considered as a useful and effective examination of the trigeminal nerve system in great detail [8, 12, 17].

Previous studies have demonstrated white matter abnormalities due to chronic pain and peripheral nerve damage in the TN patients [8, 16, 18]. The results of these studies are similar. These studies demonstrate significantly decreased FA and increased AD, RD and MD. However, the mechanism of TN affecting brain white matter remains unclear.

In order to further understand the relationship between TN and brain white matter plasticity, we examined white matter microstructural change and correlation of between white matter abnormality and disease duration and pain intensity in patients with classical TN.

Methods

Participants

Twenty-nine patients (age range 35–77 years; 20 females and 9 males) with right-sided TN and 35 healthy control subjects (age range 41–74 years; 27 females and 8 males) were selected for this study. Patients were enrolled from Department of Functional Neurosurgery of Pingjin Hospital of Logistics University of Chinese People's Armed Police Forces (Additional file 1: Table S1) and control subjects by newspaper advertisement. The patients belonged to a consecutive series of patients who had undergone evaluation for MVD surgery between 2014 and 2016. All these patients had a long duration (more than 1 year) complaint of classical TN according to the International Classification of Headache Disorders criteria (third edition) [19] and had high-resolution imaging to exclude secondary causes of TN. Visual analogue scale (VAS) [20] was used to assess pain intensity in the TN patients. All patients were measured during a painful attack and on medications. Exclusion criteria [18] for both the patients and controls were as follows: (1) other headache disorders; (2) chronic pain elsewhere; (3) previous TN operations; (4) untreated hypertension or diabetes mellitus; (5) left-handed; (6) alcohol or illicit drug abuse, or current intake of psychoactive medications; and (7) MRI contraindications, such as claustrophobia and metallic implants or devices in the body. This study was approved by our institutional review board, and written informed consent was obtained from all patients and control subjects.

MRI data acquisition

DTI data were obtained using a 3.0-T MR scanner (Verio system; Siemens, Erlangen, Germany) with a 12-channel head coil. Comfortable and tight foam padding was used to limit head movement. Diffusion weighted images were obtained using a single-shot echo planar imaging (EPI) sequence. The scanning location was in alignment with the anterior-posterior commissural plane. The integral parallel acquisition technique (iPAT) was used and the acceleration factor was 2, which can decrease image distortion from susceptibility artifacts. Diffusion sensitizing gradients were applied along 64 non-collinear directions ($b = 1000$ s/mm^2) together with an acquisition without diffusion weighting ($b = 0$ s/mm^2). The imaging parameters were applied as follows: 48 continuous axial slices, slice thickness of 3 mm and no gap, field of view (FOV) = 256 mm × 256 mm, repetition time/echo time (TR/TE) = 8000/95 ms, and matrix size = 128 × 128. The reconstruction matrix was 256 × 256 with a voxel dimension of 1 mm × 1 mm × 3 mm.

Data preprocessing

All diffusion weighted images were carefully checked by three radiologists to exclude apparent artifacts resulted from instrument malfunction and subject motion. DTI data was preprocessed using FMRIB's diffusion toolbox (FDT, http://www.fmrib.ox.ac.uk/fsl, FSL 4.0) [21]. First, the eddy current distortions and motion artifacts were corrected by using the affine alignment of each diffusion-weighted image to the image of $b = 0$ s/mm^2 in the DTI dataset. Then, non-brain tissue from the average b0 image was removed using the FMRIB's Brain Extraction Toolbox, BET. The brain mask was applied to the rest of the diffusion-weighted images. Finally, the diffusion tensor was estimated for each voxel using the DTIFIT function via linear regression to derive FA, MD, AD and RD maps.

Tract-based spatial statistics (TBSS)

The following steps were adopted to perform voxel-wise analysis of whole brain white matter measures using the TBSS package (http://www.fmrib.ox.ac.uk/fsl/tbss/index.html) [22]. All subjects' FA images were aligned to a template of the averaged FA images (FMRIB-58) in Montreal Neurological Institute (MNI) space using a nonlinear registration algorithm implemented in FNIRT (FMRIB's nonlinear registration Tool) [23]. After transformation into the MNI space, a mean FA image was generated and thinned to create a mean FA skeleton of white matter tracts. Each subject's aligned FA images were then projected onto the mean FA skeleton according to filling the mean FA skeleton by FA values, resulting in an alignment-invariant representation of the central trajectory of white matter pathways for all subjects. These FA values were obtained by searching perpendicular to the local skeleton structure for maximum value, which was from the nearest relevant tract center. During the former registration step, this second local coregistration step can alleviate the malalignment of diffusion-weighted images. Next, this process was repeated for each subject's MD, AD and RD map using the individual registration and projection vectors obtained in the FA nonlinear registration and skeletonization.

Statistical analyses

Voxel-wise differences in FA, MD, AD and RD values of white matter between TN patients and healthy controls were tested using a permutation-based inference tool by nonparametric statistic ("randomize", part of FSL) and two-sample t-tests. The mean FA skeleton was applied as a mask (thresholded at a mean FA value of 0.2 to include only major fiber bundles and exclude peripheral tracts with significant intersubject variability), and the number of permutations was set to 5000 to allow robust statistical inference. Age and gender were entered into the analysis as confound regressors. The significance threshold for intergroup differences was $P < 0.05$ after correcting for family wise error (FWE) applying the threshold-free cluster enhancement (TFCE) option by permutation-testing tool in FSL. The white matter tracts were identified using the Johns Hopkins University ICBM-DTI-81 White-Matter Labels provided in the FSL toolbox. In addition, significant white matter clusters were described by their coordinates in MNI convention and by their cluster size.

To study the relationship between clinical variables (disease duration and VAS) and each of the DTI measures, region-of-interest- (ROI-) based correlation analyses was performed by using a partial correlation ($P < 0.05$). Regional ROI masks were created for brain sites using clusters determined by voxel-by-voxel intergroup analysis procedures mentioned above. After the extraction of each ROI, the mean FA, MD, AD or RD value of the ROI were calculated. Finally, the correlations were calculated between the DTI measures of each ROI and disease duration and VAS with age and gender as covariates of no interest. Because so many correlations were run, the Bonferroni correction was applied to correct for multiple correlation comparisons.

The demographic and clinical data were compared between the two groups using independent-sample *t*-test for age and Chi-square test for sex distribution, which was conducted with Statistical Package for the Social Sciences version 22.0 (SPSS, Chicago, Ill, USA). Differences were considered significant when P was less than 0.05.

Results

Demographic and clinical data

In our study, 35 patients with right-sided TN were enrolled. Due to the abnormal data quality and no surgery, 6 patients were excluded in this study. Therefore, 29 patients (age range 35–77 years; 20 females and 9 males) and 35 healthy control subjects (age range 41–74 years; 27 females and 8 males) were selected for this study. Demographic and clinical characteristics of each group are summarized in Additional file 1: Table S2. The self-reported duration in TN patients was 10.2 ± 9.6 years (range: 1–30 years) and the VAS was 5.9 ± 3.1 (range: 2–10). There were no significant differences ($P > 0.05$) between TN patients and healthy controls in age and gender.

Comparison of DTI metrics between TN and controls

Compared with the control group, the TN group showed significantly lower FA in the bilateral superior corona radiata, bilateral anterior corona radiata, body of corpus callosum, splenium of corpus callosum, genu of corpus callosum, left cingulum, left superior fronto-occipital fasciculus, bilateral anterior limb of internal capsule, left posterior limb of internal capsule, left external capsule, left fornix cerebri, internal sagittal stratum and left cerebral peduncle ($P < 0.05$, FWE corrected) (Fig. 1; Additional file 1: Table S3). Moreover, the TN group demonstrated higher RD in the bilateral superior corona radiata, bilateral anterior corona radiata, body of corpus callosum, splenium of corpus callosum, left cingulum, left superior fronto-occipital fasciculus, bilateral anterior limb of internal capsule, bilateral posterior limb of internal capsule, bilateral external capsule, left retrolenticular portion, left fornix cerebri, pontine crossing tract, corticospinal tract and left cerebral peduncle ($P < 0.05$, FWE corrected) (Additional file 1: Figure S1, Table S3). However, no significant difference was found in MD and AD between the TN group and control group.

Correlations between clinical variables and altered DTI metrics

In the TN patients, negative correlations were observed between disease duration and the FA values of left anterior corona radiata ($r = 0.211$, $P = 0.012$), genu of corpus callosum ($r = 0.166$, $P = 0.028$), left external capsule ($r = 0.190$, $P = 0.018$), left cerebral peduncle ($r = 0.192$, $P = 0.017$), and between VAS and the FA values of left anterior corona radiata ($r = 0.221$, $P = 0.010$), left external capsule ($r = 0.218$, $P = 0.011$), left cerebral peduncle ($r = 0.168$, $P = 0.027$) (Fig. 2). Positive correlations were observed for disease duration and the RD values of left anterior corona radiata ($r = 0.190$, $P = 0.018$), right external capsule ($r = 0.170$, $P = 0.026$), left fornix cerebri ($r = 0.168$, $P = 0.027$), left cerebral peduncle ($r = 0.156$, $P =$

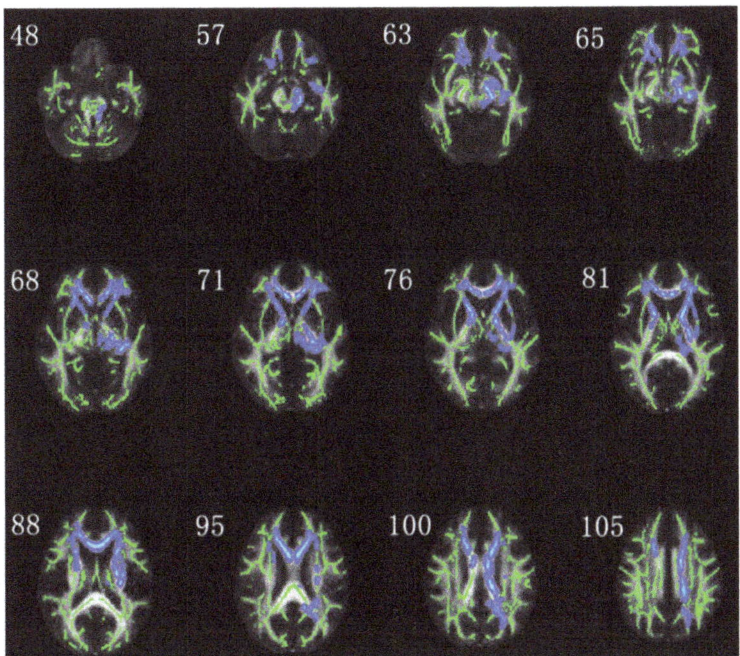

Fig. 1 TBSS shows white matter regions with significant differences in FA between TN patients and healthy subjects ($P < 0.05$, FWE corrected). Green represents mean FA skeleton of all participants; blue represents reduction in right TN patients. Coordinates are in millimeters along z axe

0.034), and for VAS and the RD values of left anterior corona radiata ($r = 0.174$, $P = 0.025$), left external capsule ($r = 0.191$, $P = 0.018$) (Additional file 1: Figure S2). However, once Bonferroni corrections were applied, these correlations were not statistically significant.

Discussion

Methological consideration

Compared with voxel-based analysis (VBA), the TBSS method is applied more and more popularly to reveal microstructural alterations of white matter fibers between groups [24–27]. VBA has two severe limitations about different subjects' alignment of FA images and the self-willed choice of smoothing kernels without any principle or standard [28]. TBSS solve these issues using carefully tuned non-linear registration, and then projecting onto the "mean FA skeleton"(an alignment-invariant tract representation). Moreover, TBSS doesn't need a smoothing process [22]. Therefore, TBSS can avoid the two limitations and provides us with more diffusion metrics [29]. In many disease studies, TBSS has a wide application to research microstructural white matter alterations, such as adiposity, parkinsonism, Alzheimer's disease (AD), genetic disease, type2 diabetes mellitus and so on [30–35]. In this study, we have been showed well results of the diffusion metrics (FA, MD, AD and RD) in TBSS methods between groups.

White matter impairment in TN patients

The primary diffusion metrics (FA and MD) reflect overall white matter health, organization and maturation [36]. In addition, AD reflects axon integrity and RD reflects myelin sheath integrity [31]. Both AD and RD are of great significance in understanding the underlying physiological mechanism [26]. Decreased FA values maybe based on predominantly increase of RD or both RD and AD [30]. The study of DeSouza et al. showed the right-sided TN patients had significantly decreased FA and increased RD, MD, and AD in the brain white matter including the corpus callosum, posterior corona radiata, cingulum, and superior longitudinal fasciculus. Moreover, MD and RD changes of brain white matter in TN patients maybe have relation to central nervous system plasticity, neuroinflammation and edema [18]. In our study, we found the similar results that reduced FA and elevated RD in the corona radiata (mainly concentrating on bilateral superior corona radiate and anterior corona radiata), corpus callosum and left cingulum. Additionally, we found reduced FA and elevated RD in the fronto-occipital fasciculus, internal capsule, external capsule, fornix cerebri and cerebral peduncle in the TN patients. Moreover, altered FA and RD was mainly located in white matter of left hemisphere. However, the differences of MD and AD were not statistically significant. As we all know, TN is involved in trigeminal nerve functional disorders, but other theories of central nervous system pathology is not clear [18, 37]. Due to

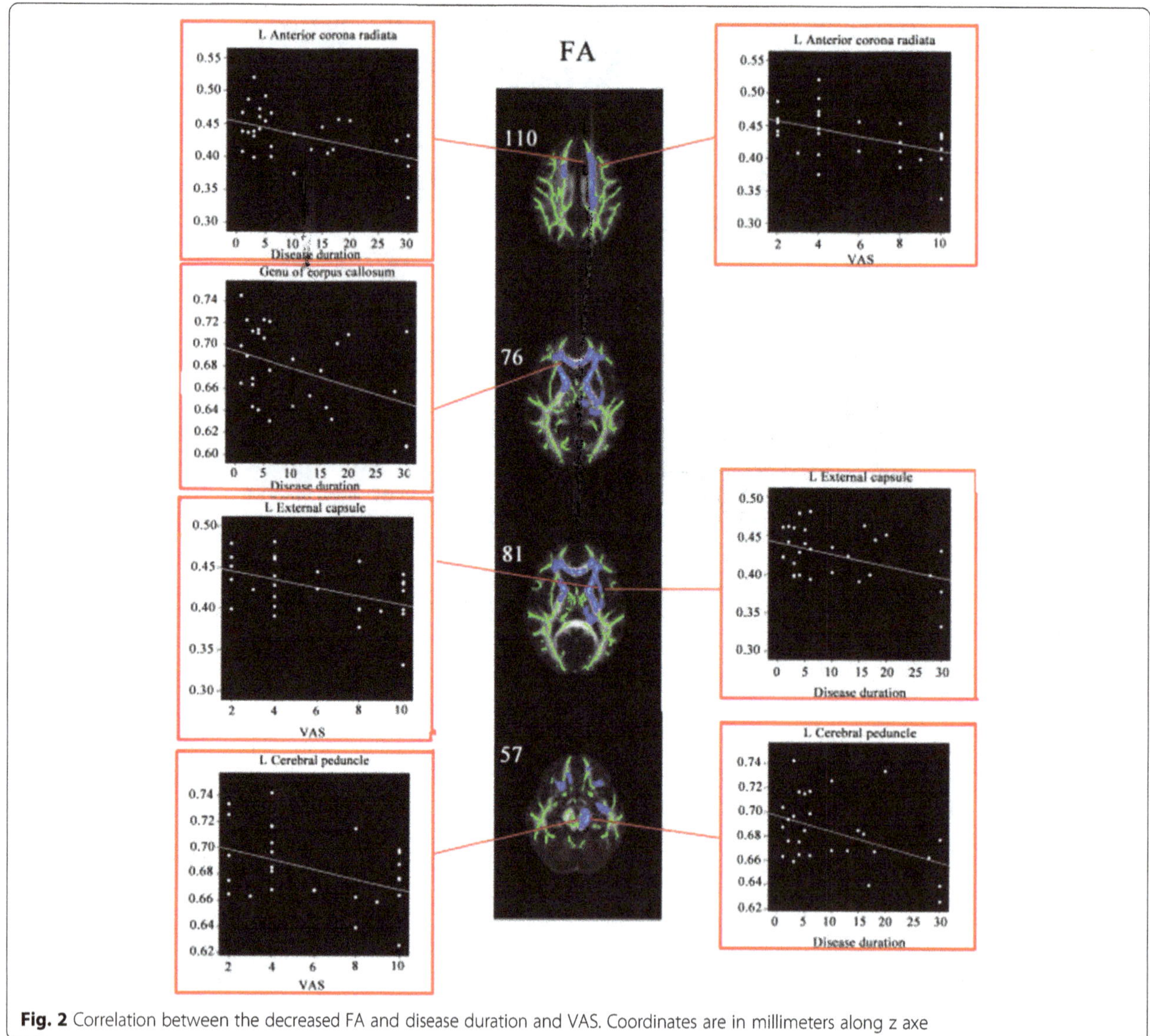

Fig. 2 Correlation between the decreased FA and disease duration and VAS. Coordinates are in millimeters along z axe

peripheral trigeminal nerve injury, central nervous system plasticity will most probably occur [18, 38, 39], including fiber organization changes, astrocyte morphology and angiogenesis [18, 40–42]. In our study, compared with healthy controls, TN patients showed decreased FA. The decreased FA may correspond to less fiber organization, such as more axonal sprouting/branching, larger axons, or more crossing fibers [18, 42]. Besides, neuropathic pain is usually related to chronic painful influence on central nervous system. This leads to central sensitization, a process involving demyelination and neuroinflammation processes [18]. The decreased FA is presumably caused by a significant increase of RD, inferring that demyelination and neuroinflammation processes may lead to the impairment of white matter integrity in the TN patients. The RD abnormalities maybe result from these mechanisms in the white matter of TN patients [8].

Many studies have reported cortical and subcortical gray matter impairment in the cognitive-affective, sensory, modulation of pain, attention and motor regions of TN patients [43–45]. In anatomy and/or function respect, these brain areas are connected [13, 46–48]. In our study, we reported decreased FA and increased RD in the corona radiata, corpus callosum, cingulum, fronto-occipital fasciculus, internal capsule, external capsule, fornix cerebri and cerebral peduncle in the TN patients. These fiber connection of brain regions is related to rapid transmission of pain, attention and motor function [49], and maybe lead to the unique sensory symptoms of TN. Our finding also revealed that altered FA and RD was mainly located in white matter of left hemisphere, suggesting contralateral white matter lesions of TN patients.

Correlation analyses found negative correlations between the disease duration and the FA values of left anterior corona radiata, genu of corpus callosum, left external capsule, left cerebral peduncle, indicating the white matter impairment is more and more severe as the disease progressed. With impairing progression of left anterior corona radiata, left external capsule and left cerebral peduncle, painful sensation is more serious. What is more, we infer these regions are probably related to transmission of pain [50]. The RD and the disease duration also reveal positive correlations in the regions of left anterior corona radiata, right external capsule, left fornix cerebri, left cerebral peduncle, demonstrating the white matter demyelination and neuroinflammation of these regions is aggravated in the disease progression. And as demyelination and neuroinflammation of left anterior corona radiate and left external capsule progresses, painful sensation is also more serious. Regrettably, the results of these correlation analyses had not been able to withstand multiple comparison correction.

Conclusion

In our study, we revealed directly differences between the healthy control and right TN to demonstrate how brain white matter is changed using TBSS methods, suggesting that white matter impairment is the significant hallmark in the right TN. Moreover, the correlation analyses between FA/RD and the disease duration and VAS indicate white matter impairment is more and more severe in the disease progression. And the pain is also more serious with some regions of white matter impairment. The white matter impairment is mostly based on fiber organization, demyelination and neuroinflammation. So we can deeply understand the mechanism of white matter change of TN patients.

Limitations

Several limitations should be considered when interpreting our results. First, the sample size of the present study was not much, which might cause correlation analyses to fail to withstand multiple comparison correction. Second, non-isotropic voxels were used for DTI data acquisition in this study. In terms of the tensor evaluation, isotropic voxels are more accurate than non-isotropic voxels. Finally, all patients in our study were on medications for TN pain and the anticonvulsant carbamazepine is the most common. The influences of antiepileptics on brain structure are not clear. Future studies are needed to collect more sample sizes, adopt more optimized DTI parameters and avoid the effects of drugs.

Additional file

Additional file 1: Table S1. Characteristics and findings in 29 right TN patients who underwent MVD. **Table S2.** Demographic and clinical data for TN patients and healthy controls. **Table S3.** Comparison of DTI metrics between TN and controls. **Figure S1.** TBSS shows white matter regions with significant differences in RD between TN patients and healthy subjects ($P < 0.05$, FWE corrected). Green represents mean FA skeleton of all participants; red denotes increase in right TN patients. Coordinates are in millimeters along z axe. **Figure S2.** Correlation between the increased RD and disease duration and VAS. Coordinates are in millimeters along z axe. (DOC 1102 kb)

Abbreviations

AD: Axial diffusivity; DTI: Diffusion tensor imaging; EPI: Echo planar imaging; FA: Fractional anisotropy; FDT: FMRIB's diffusion toolbox; FOV: Field of view; iPAT: Integral parallel acquisition technique; MD: Mean diffusivity; MNI: Montreal Neurological Institute; MRI: Magnetic resonance imaging; MVD: Microvascular decompression; NVC: Neurovascular compression; RD: Radial diffusivity; REZ: Root entry zone; ROI: Region-of-interest; SPSS: Statistical package for the social sciences; TFCE: Threshold-free cluster enhancement; TN: Trigeminal neuralgia; VAS: Visual analogue scale/score; VBA: Voxel-based analysis

Acknowledgments

We thank Dr. Hongtao Sun (Department of Functional Neurosurgery of Pingjin Hospital, Logistics University of Chinese People's Armed Police Forces, Tianjin, China) for his help in the recruitment of patients; and Dr. Kewen AI (Department of Radiology of Pingjin Hospital, Logistics University of Chinese People's Armed Police Forces, Tianjin, China) for his help in the recruitment of healthy volunteers.

Funding

This study was supported by the Natural Science Foundation of China (No. 81401401), the Natural Science Foundation of Tianjin (Nos. 16JCQNJC10900 and 16JCZDJC36000) and the Science Fund of Tianjin Medical University (No. 2014KYQ11).

Declarations

No financial support has been directly or indirectly received for the ideation, preparation and in writing this paper.

Authors' contributions

QZ was the project leader and contributed to project design and development of the methodology. FY enrolled and evaluated the patients. JL and JZ collected and analyzed the imaging data. JL drafted the manuscript. QZ and XZ revised the manuscript critically. All authors read and approved the final manuscript.

Competing interests

The authors declare that they have no competing interests.

Author details

[1]School of Medical Imaging, Tianjin Medical University, No. 1, Guangdong Road, Hexi District, Tianjin 300203, China. [2]Department of Radiology, The First Affiliated Hospital of Anhui Medical University, Hefei, China. [3]Department of Radiology, Pingjin Hospital, Logistics University of Chinese People's Armed Police Forces, No. 220, Chenglin Road, Hedong District, Tianjin 300162, China.

References

1. Bescos A, Pascual V, Escosa-Bage MMalaga X (2015) Treatment of trigeminal neuralgia: an update and future prospects of percutaneous techniques. Rev Neurol 61:114–124.
2. Zakrzewska JM (2002) Diagnosis and differential diagnosis of trigeminal neuralgia. Clin J Pain 18:14–21.
3. Wankel I, Dietrich U, Oppel FPuchner MJA (2005) Endovascular treatment of trigeminal neuralgia caused by arteriovenous malformation: is surgery really necessary? Zbl Neurochir 66:213–216.
4. Hayashi M (2009) Trigeminal neuralgia. Prog Neurol Surg 22:182–190.
5. Yoshino N, Akimoto H, Yamada I, Nagaoka T, Tetsumura A, Kurabayashi T et al (2003) Trigeminal neuralgia: evaluation of neuralgic manifestation and site of neurovascular compression with 3D CISS MR imaging and MR angiography. Radiology 228:539–545.
6. Tien RD, Wilkins RH (1993) MRA delineation of the vertebral-basilar system in patients with hemifacial spasm and trigeminal neuralgia. AJNR. Am J Neuroradiol 14:34–36.
7. Sens MA, Higer HP (1991) MRI of trigeminal neuralgia: initial clinical results in patients with vascular compression of the trigeminal nerve. Neurosurg Rev 14:69–73.
8. Liu Y, Li J, Butzkueven H, Duan Y, Zhang M, Shu N et al (2013) Microstructural abnormalities in the trigeminal nerves of patients with trigeminal neuralgia revealed by multiple diffusion metrics. Eur J Radiol 82: 783–786.
9. Leclercq D, Thiebaut JB, Heran F (2013) Trigeminal neuralgia. Diagn Interv Imaging 94:993–1001.
10. Fahlstrom A, Laurell K, Ericson H (2014) Trigeminal neuralgia. Lakartidningen 111:2295–2298.
11. Cruccu G (2017) Trigeminal Neuralgia. Continuum (Minneapolis, Minn) 23: 396–420.
12. Neetu S, Sunil K, Ashish A, Jayantee K, Usha Kant M (2016) Microstructural abnormalities of the trigeminal nerve by diffusion-tensor imaging in trigeminal neuralgia without neurovascular compression. Neuroradiol J 29: 13–18.
13. Scrivani S, Moulton E, Pendse G, Morris S, Aiello-Larnmens M, Beccera L et al (2008) Functional magnetic resonance imaging (fMRI) of evoked and spontaneous painful tics in trigeminal neuralgia (tic doloureux). Headache 48:S11–S11.
14. Naegel S, Holle D, Gaul C, Gizewski ER, Diener HC, Katsarava Z et al (2009) Event-related fMRI activation in spontaneous trigeminal neuralgia attacks. Cephalalgia 29:115–116.
15. Blatow M, Nennig E, Sarpaczki E, Reinhardt J, Schlieter M, Herweh C et al (2009) Altered somatosensory processing in trigeminal neuralgia. Hum Brain Mapp 30:3495–3508.
16. Wang Y, Li D, Bao F, Guo C, Ma S, Zhang M (2016) Microstructural abnormalities of the trigeminal nerve correlate with pain severity and concomitant emotional dysfunctions in idiopathic trigeminal neuralgia: a randomized, prospective, double-blind study. Magn Reson Imaging 34:609–616.
17. Lacerda Leal PR, Roch JA, Hermier M, Nobre Souza MA, Cristino-Filho G, Sindou M (2011) Structural abnormalities of the trigeminal root revealed by diffusion tensor imaging in patients with trigeminal neuralgia caused by neurovascular compression: a prospective, double-blind, controlled study. Pain 152:2357–2364.
18. DeSouza DD, Hodaie M, Davis KD (2014) Abnormal trigeminal nerve microstructure and brain white matter in idiopathic trigeminal neuralgia. Pain 155:37–44.
19. Cho SJ, Kim BK, Kim BS, Kim JM, Kim SK, Moon HS et al (2016) Vestibular migraine in multicenter neurology clinics according to the appendix criteria in the third beta edition of the international classification of headache disorders. Cephalalgia 36:454–462.
20. Li X, Lin CN, Liu CC, Ke SJ, Wan Q, Luo HJ et al (2017) Comparison of the effectiveness of resistance training in women with chronic computer-related neck pain: a randomized controlled study. Int Arch Occ Env Hea 90: 673–683.
21. Smith SM, Jenkinson M, Woolrich MW, Beckmann CF, Behrens TEJ, Johansen-Berg H et al (2004) Advances in functional and structural MR image analysis and implementation as FSL. Neuroimage 23:S208–SS19.
22. Smith SM, Jenkinson M, Johansen-Berg H, Rueckert D, Nichols TE, Mackay CE et al (2006) Tract-based spatial statistics: Voxelwise analysis of multi-subject diffusion data. Neuroimage 31:1487–1505.
23. Rueckert D, Sonoda LI, Hayes C, Hill DLG, Leach MO, Hawkes DJ (1999) Nonrigid registration using free-form deformations: application to breast MR images. Ieee T Med Imaging 18:712–721.
24. Sage CA, Van Hecke W, Peeters R, Sijbers J, Robberecht W, Parizel P et al (2009) Quantitative diffusion tensor imaging in amyotrophic lateral sclerosis: revisited. Hum Brain Mapp 30:3657–3675.
25. Huang R, Lu M, Song Z, Wang J (2015) Long-term intensive training induced brain structural changes in world class gymnasts. Brain Struct Funct 220:625–644.
26. Hasan KM, Walimuni IS, Abid H, Hahn KR (2011) A review of diffusion tensor magnetic resonance imaging computational methods and software tools. Comput Biol Med 41:1062–1072.
27. Duan F, Zhao T, He Y, Shu N (2015) Test-retest reliability of diffusion measures in cerebral white matter: a multiband diffusion MRI study. J Magn Reson Imaging 42:1106–1116.
28. Wang D, Qin W, Liu Y, Zhang Y, Jiang T, Yu C (2013) Altered white matter integrity in the congenital and late blind people. Neural Plasticity 2013: 128236.
29. Bach M, Laun FB, Leemans A, Tax CMW, Biessels GJ, Stieltjes B et al (2014) Methodological considerations on tract-based spatial statistics (TBSS). Neuroimage 100:358–369.
30. Squarcina L, Houenou J, Altamura AC, Soares J, Brambilla P (2017) Association of increased genotypes risk for bipolar disorder with brain white matter integrity investigated with tract-based spatial statistics. J Affect Disorders 221:312–317.
31. Rizk MM, Rubin-Falcone H, Keilp J, Miller JM, Sublette ME, Burke A et al (2017) White matter correlates of impaired attention control in major depressive disorder and healthy volunteers. J Affect Disorders 222:103–111.
32. Michielse S, Gronenschild E, Domen P, van Os J, Marcelis M, Genetic Risk Outcome P (2017) The details of structural disconnectivity in psychotic disorder: a family-based study of non-FA diffusion weighted imaging measures. Brain Res 1671:121–130.
33. Lukoshe A, van den Bosch GE, van der Lugt A, Kushner SA, Hokken-Koelega ACWhite T (2017) Aberrant white matter microstructure in children and adolescents with the subtype of Prader-Willi syndrome at high risk for psychosis. Schizophrenia Bull 43:1090–1099.
34. Drew DA, Koo B-B, Bhadelia R, Weiner DE, Duncan S, Mendoza-De la Garza M et al (2017) White matter damage in maintenance hemodialysis patients: a diffusion tensor imaging study. BMC Nephrol 18(1):213.
35. Chen F, Chen F, Shang Z, Shui Y, Wu G, Liu C et al (2017) White matter microstructure degenerates in patients with postherpetic neuralgia. Neurosci Lett 656:152–157.
36. Xie Y, Zhang Y, Qin W, Lu S, Ni CZhang Q (2017) White matter microstructural abnormalities in type 2 diabetes mellitus: a diffusional kurtosis imaging analysis. AJNR Am J Neuroradiol 38:617–625.
37. Siddiqui MN, Siddiqui S, Ranasinghe JS, Furgang FA (2002) Pain Management: Trigeminal Neuralgia. Physician 39:64–70.
38. Taylor KS, Anastakis DJ, Davis KD (2009) Cutting your nerve changes your brain. Brain J. Neurol 132:3122–3133.
39. Davis KD, Taylor KS, Anastakis DJ (2011) Nerve injury triggers changes in the brain. Neuroscientist 17:407–422 A Review Journal Bringing Neurobiology Neurology & Psychiatry.
40. Boretius S, Escher A, Dallenga T, Wrzos C, Tammer R, Brück W et al (2012) Assessment of lesion pathology in a new animal model of MS by multiparametric MRI and DTI. Neuroimage 59:2678–2688.
41. Beaulieu C (2002) The basis of anisotropic water diffusion in the nervous system – a technical review. NMR Biomed 15:435–455.
42. Zatorre RJ, Fields RD, Johansenberg H (2012) Plasticity in gray and white: neuroimaging changes in brain structure during learning. Nat Neurosci 15: 528–536.
43. Parise M, Almodovar Kubo TT, Doring TM, Tukamoto G, Vincent MGasparetto EL (2014) Cuneus and fusiform cortices thickness is reduced in trigeminal neuralgia. J Headache Pain 15:17.
44. Abarca-Olivas J, Feliu-Rey E, Sempere AP, Sanchez-Paya J, Bano-Ruiz E, Angel Caminero-Canas M et al (2010) Volumetric measurement of the posterior fossa and its components using magnetic resonance imaging in idiopathic trigeminal neuralgia. Rev Neurol 51:520–524.

45. DeSouza DD, Moayedi M, Chen DQ, Davis KD, Hodaie M (2013) Sensorimotor and pain modulation brain abnormalities in trigeminal neuralgia: a paroxysmal, sensory-triggered neuropathic pain. PLoS One 8(6): e66340.
46. Obermann M, Rodriguez-Raecke R, Naegel S, Holle D, Mueller D, Yoon M-S et al (2013) Gray matter volume reduction reflects chronic pain in trigeminal neuralgia. Neuroimage 74:352–358.
47. Obermann M, Midler D, Zwarg T, Gizewski ER, Rodriguez-Racke R, Diener H-C et al (2009) Gray matter decrease in patients with trigeminal neuralgia. Neurology 72:A251–AA51.
48. Moisset X, Villain N, Ducreux D, Serrie A, Cunin G, Valade D et al (2011) Functional brain imaging of trigeminal neuralgia. Eur J Pain 15:124–131.
49. Malfliet A, Coppieters I, Van Wilgen P, Kregel J, De Pauw R, Dolphens M et al (2017) Brain changes associated with cognitive and emotional factors in chronic pain: a systematic review. Eur J Pain 21:769–786.
50. Hayes DJ, Chen DQ, Zhong JD, Lin A, Behan B, Walker M et al (2017) Affective circuitry alterations in patients with trigeminal neuralgia. Front Neuroanat 11:73.

21

Upper cervical two-point discrimination thresholds in migraine patients and headache-free controls

Kerstin Luedtke[1,2,3,6*], Waclaw Adamczyk[3,2,5], Katrin Mehrtens[4], Inken Moeller[1], Louisa Rosenbaum[1], Axel Schaefer[4], Janine Schroeder[1], Tibor Szikszay[2], Christian Zimmer[1] and Bettina Wollesen[1]

Abstract

Background: Chronic pain including migraine is associated with structural and functional changes in the somatosensory cortex. Previous reports proposed two-point discrimination (TPD) as a measurement for cortical alterations. Limited evidence exists for tactile acuity in the neck and no data is available for migraine.

Methods: To introduce a standardized protocol for the measurement of TPD in the upper cervical spine, 51 healthy participants were investigated with a newly developed paradigm which was evaluated for intra-rater reliability. The same protocol was applied by two further examiners to 28 migraine patients and 21 age-, and gender-matched healthy controls to investigate inter-rater reliability and between group differences.

Results: Results indicated excellent intra-rater (right $ICC_{(2,4)} = 0.82$, left $ICC_{(2,4)} = 0.83$) and good inter-rater reliability (right $ICC_{(2,4)} = 0.70$, left $ICC_{(2,4)} = 0.75$). Migraine patients had larger TPD thresholds (26.86 ± 7.21) than healthy controls (23.30 ± 6.17) but these became only statistically significant for the right side of the neck ($p = 0.02$). There was a significant, moderate association with age for the right side ($r = 0.42$ $p = 0.002$, $n = 51$), and less strong association for the left side ($r = 0.34$, $p = 0.14$) in healthy individuals. TPD did not correlate with headache days per month or the dominant headache side in migraine patients.

Conclusions: Surprisingly, migraine patients showed increased TPD thresholds in the upper cervical spine interictally. Although a body of evidence supports that hypersensitivity is part of the migraine attack, the current report indicates that interictally, migraine patients showed worse tactile acuity similar to other chronic pain populations. This has been hypothesized to indicate structural and functional re-organisation of the somatosensory cortex.

Keywords: Tactile acuity, Hypersensitivity, Migraine, Headache, Two-point discrimination

Background

Current knowledge on functional and structural cortical alterations following longstanding pain, is mainly based on chronic low back pain populations [1–6] with very limited data for the upper spinal region [7]. However, it has been suggested, that at least structural brain changes are similar for any chronic pain condition including headaches [8] and that the somatosensory cortex is one of the structures typically affected [5, 9, 10].

Two-point discrimination threshold (TPD) assessment is a routine procedure during the neurological examination that has been shown to be associated with such structural brain changes [9, 10]. TPD thresholds indicate the smallest distance between two points of sliding mechanical callipers, that can still be perceived as two distinct points. This paradigm has been used in research to investigate tactile acuity in chronic pain patients and a recent systematic review reported a general tendency to increased TPD thresholds in patients with longstanding pain compared to pain-free controls [11, 12].

* Correspondence: kerstin.luedtke@uni-luebeck.de
[1]Department of Human Movement Science, University of Hamburg, Hamburg, Germany
[2]Academic Physiotherapy, Medical Section, Department of Orthopaedics and Trauma Surgery, University of Luebeck, Luebeck, Germany
Full list of author information is available at the end of the article

Six studies have previously investigated TPD in the neck: Song et al. investigated patients with spinal cord injuries and found multiple sites of reduced sensory discrimination compared to healthy controls that were reported to be particularly distinct in the neck area [13]. Moreira et al. found increased TPD thresholds in patients with idiopathic neck pain but although there was a mean difference between groups of almost 5 mm, values failed to reach statistical significance [14]. Nolan et al. investigated TPD only in healthy participants; the mean TPD at the level of C7 was 55.4 mm [15]. All three studies applied their measurements to the lower cervical area. The only study that included a measurement in the upper cervical spine in patients with mild recurrent neck pain, while observing slightly larger TPD values in the patient group, failed to show any statistically significant difference between patients and controls at C2 and at C7 [16]. The mean two-point discrimination threshold of the included 30 neck pain patients was 29.75 mm at C2 and 32.5 mm at C7. Catley et al. and Harvie et al. conducted reliability studies in healthy participants. The authors examined TPD threshold only at the C7 spinal level and reported a mean of 45.9 mm and of 35 mm, respectively [17, 18].

All six studies showed that tactile acuity can feasibly be measured in the cervical area, two studies confirmed the intra-rater and inter-rater reliability (ICC > 0.75) of the measurement [17, 18]. All studies evaluating patients showed that the patient population had larger TPD values compared to the control group. No study has previously applied TPD to a headache population. However, the test procedures used in the six studies were heterogeneous and reported a wide range of mean threshold in a variety of populations. Only one study investigated the upper cervical region and no data were available for migraine patients.

The aim of the current project was therefore to investigate TPD thresholds in the upper cervical spine in patients with migraine in comparison to healthy controls. Since only one study has investigated this region previously, this current project includes the development and both, intra- and inter-reliability testing of the procedure.

Methods

Study overview

The study was designed in two stages: the initial stage was the development of the test protocol and determination of intra-rater reliability using a test-retest design. The second stage for the inter-rater reliability and the difference between migraine patients and controls was a repeated-measures case-control design with blinded examiners (Fig. 1).

The study was approved by the local ethics committee of the University of Hamburg (AZ 2017_86). It was registered a priori in the German clinical trials register (DRKS00011795). The data collection for the intra-rater stage was conducted between November and December 2016 and for the inter-rater and case control stage between May and June 2017.

Participants

Healthy control participants for the intra-rater reliability phase as well as those serving as controls for the case-control study had to be adults (18+ years old), age and gender matched to the patient group (only for the case-control phase), and right-handed. Patients for the case-control phase were: adults, diagnosed with migraine according to IHS 3 criteria [19], had a minimum of 4 migraine days on average per month, took pain medication on < 10 days per month to exclude medication overuse headache, had no other relevant headache diagnosis (episodic tension-type headache was accepted), had to be headache-free 48 h prior to the assessment. Patients and controls were excluded when they were older than 65 years; to reduce bias and to differentiate between the influence of headache and any other pain condition, they were also excluded when they had acute pain including toothache on the day of testing, had any chronic pain condition, had neck pain in the past 3 months, had a history of cervical pathology or trauma including whiplash associated disorder, disc disease or others requiring medical intervention, suffered from any psychological, neurological or other disease potentially influencing the sensory system, or a skin condition in the area over the upper cervical spine.

Patients were recruited from the University Headache Clinic at the University Medical Center Hamburg-Eppendorf and from local neurology clinics. Control participants were selected from social media and digital network postings and personal contacts.

Measurement procedure

An initial test protocol was developed and piloted in a small convenience sample of healthy participants before it was subsequently applied to the study population. It was based on the most widely used procedure for the lumbar spine of Moberg [20] who introduced a protocol with increasing and decreasing distances between two tips of a mechanical sliding calliper [20] similar to the *method of limits* used in the quantitative sensory testing protocol [21]. Previous publications suggested that the discrimination threshold in the neck will be between 10 and 45 mm [11, 15, 18] and it was reported as 29.75 mm at C2 in patients with neck pain [16]. Therefore, the TPD test started at a distance of 50 mm, a distance that was perceived by all participants as two distinct points. The distance was subsequently decreased by 5 mm until only 1 point was perceived and increased in steps of

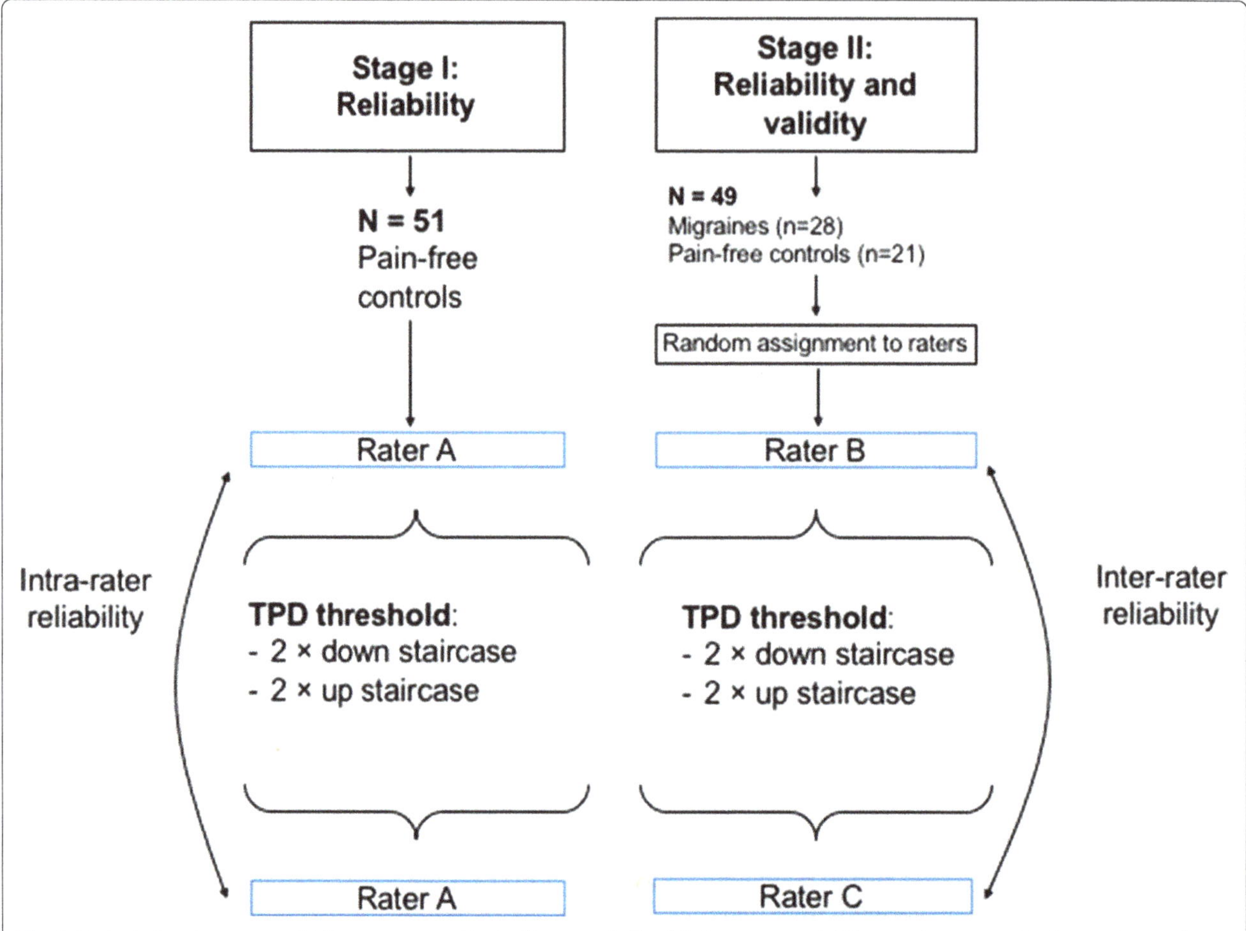

Fig. 1 Study design. Intra-rater reliability was assessed in the first stage (left) while inter-rater and differences between migraines and controls in the second stage of the study. TPD - Two-point discrimination threshold

1 mm until two points were felt. This was followed by decreasing the distance in 1 mm steps until only one point was perceived. This was repeated until 4 values were documented, two from increasing and two from decreasing the distance. The mean of these 4 data points was the TPD threshold for one measurement. For the intra-rater evaluation, the procedure was repeated by the same examiner after a five-minute break. All participants were tested on both sides of the neck in a randomized order.

Participants were positioned on a stool in front of a table with the forehead resting on a folded towel. The third vertebra was located manually and marked with a felt tip pen. The medial tip of the callipers was always within a radius of 2 cm from the midpoint of the 3rd vertebrae. The TPD was always measured horizontally at the level of C3. To standardize the pressure, calliper tips were placed on the test location until the first blanching of the skin. This standardization has been widely applied in previous studies assessing tactile acuity [17, 22].

For the inter-rater reliability and case-control stage, patients and controls were randomly allocated to a first blinded examiner who performed the TPD testing as described above (two measurements on each side of the neck, 1 measurement at the hand). After a resting period of 10 min they changed to the second blinded examiner. During this stage of the study, the lateral border of the dorsal hand was additionally tested as a control region in both groups, healthy controls and migraines. This allowed an indication whether tactile acuity changes are limited to the painful region or can also be identified in remote regions, thereby potentially indicating central sensitization.

Blinding of the examiners was ensured by a third researcher, who contacted potential participants, performed the randomization to the first blinded examiner, distributed the questionnaires and instructed participants to not reveal their status as a patient or a control person during the test procedure. Both examiners were experienced in the physical examination of patients and trained during repeated sessions to perform the test in a standardized manner. In addition to the TPD thresholds, the following parameters were recorded during the test days by a piloted questionnaire: gender, age, number of headache days per month, years since diagnosis and dominant headache side.

Proposed sample size and statistical analysis

The required sample size for the case-control phase was based on data for patients with chronic low back pain [13, 22] pain using 80% power and an alpha value of 0.05. The minimal required sample size per group was minimum of 19, the calculation was conducted in G*Power [23].

Reliability was calculated using the two-way random average measures intraclass-correlation coefficient for absolute agreement ($ICC_{2,4}$). Reliability was interpreted as excellent if the ICC was > 0.75 [24] and good if the ICC was between 0.74–0.50. The variance components (σ^2 patient, σ^2 observer and σ^2 residual) were calculated with VARCOMP-Analysis (Method: ANOVA Type III Sum of Squares) to determine Standard Error of Measurement (SEM) and the smallest detectable difference (SDD) [25]. Differences across groups were calculated using two-sided t-tests for independent samples for each side of the neck and for the reference area (hand) individually. For these calculations, the mean ratings across the two examiners were used.

Since previous research has indicated that age and gender may play a role in the TPD measurement [26, 27], secondary analyses evaluated whether TPD thresholds were significantly different between male and female patients and in younger and older patients. For the analysis of age, a median split was used and significance was tested using t-tests at an alpha level of 0.05. Additionally, Pearson's correlation coefficient was calculated to assess association between age and TPD threshold. Because TPD in the neck region has recently been shown to be associated with the severity of a disease [28], TPD thresholds were correlated in the headache group with headache days per months and with the dominant headache side using Pearson's correlation. All analyses were calculated using the software packages SPSS 23 (IBM, Illinois, USA) and Stata 15 (StataCorp LLC, College Station, Texas, USA).

Results

Intra-rater reliability

Fifty-one healthy participants (26 female) aged between 20 and 65 years (mean 37.8 ± 13 years) were recruited. TPD thresholds ranged between 7.5 and 41 mm (mean 26.7 ± 7.1 mm). Values for male and female as well as older and younger participants are presented in Table 1. The intra-rater reliability was excellent with an $ICC_{(2,4)}$ of 0.83 (95% CI, 0.72–0.90) for the left side of the neck and an $ICC_{(2,4)}$ of 0.82 (95% CI, 0.70–0.89) for the right side of the neck. The SEM was 3.1 mm for both sides with corresponding SDDs of 8.5 (left side) and 8.6 (right side). There was a significant, moderate correlation between age and TPD (left side $r = 0.342$; right side $r = 0.421$).

Inter-rater reliability and case-control

For the inter-rater and case-control phase of the study, 49 participants (28 migraine patients) were recruited. Characteristics for patients and control participants are reported in Table 2. The inter-rater reliability for all measurements on the left ($ICC_{(2,4)}$ 0.75; 95% CI 0.55–0.86; SDD 12.02; SEM 4.34) and the right side ($ICC_{(2,4)}$ 0.70; 95% CI 0.46–0.83; SDD 12.36; SEM 4.46) of the neck and for the measurements on the hand ($ICC_{(2,4)}$ 0.70; 95% CI 0.48–0.83; SDD 6.01; SEM 2.1) was good. Migraine patients had larger TPD thresholds at all test locations including the hand. Statistical significance was only reached for the right side of the neck ($p = 0.02$) (Table 3). There was no correlation with headache days per month for left ($r = -0.09$), or right side ($r = -0.11$) of the neck, and the hand ($r = -0.15$). Neither was a correlation with the dominant headache side revealed for the left (r = – 0,19) or the right side (r = – 0,20) of the neck.

Discussion

This paper aimed to investigate tactile acuity in migraine patients compared to headache-free controls and to develop a standardised test protocol with sufficient intra- and inter-rater reliability. The mean TPD thresholds in healthy participants in this study are in line with those in the only other study on the upper cervical spine [16]. Intra- and inter-rater reliability coefficients were similarly high as those reported by Harvie et al. [28] and Catley et al. [17] for the lower part of the neck, thereby supporting TPD testing as a clinically reliable tool. Also similar to the results reported by Harvie et al. [28], who

Table 1 TPD thresholds for male and female as well as younger and older participants (intra-rater reliability sample)

Between group differences	Male ($n = 25$)	Female ($n = 26$)	*t* - test
Left neck (mean ± SD)	2.75 (0.71) cm	2.6 (0.72) cm	$p = 0.458$
Right neck (mean ± SD)	2.9 (0.73) cm	2.5 (0.53) cm	$p = 0.031$
Between group differences	Age 36 ≥ (n = 26)	Age > 35 (n = 25)	*t* - test
Left neck (mean ± SD)	2.42 (0.64) cm	2.93 (0.7) cm	$p = 0.008$
Right neck (mean ± SD)	2.40 (0.54) cm	3.0 (0.65) cm	$p = 0.001$

SD Standard deviations

Table 2 Characteristics of groups

Variable	Migraine $n = 28$	Control participants $n = 21$
Female: number (%)	27 (93.1%)	17 (85%)
Male: number (%)	2 (6.89%)	3 (15%)
Age (years)	34.4 (11.9)	39.8 (13.6)
Years since diagnosis	19.7 (14.1)	-
Headache days per month	9.4 (9.1)	-
Dominant headache side		
- Left number (%)	7 (24.1)	-
- Right number (%)	7 (24.1)	-
- Bilateral number (%)	15 (51.7)	-

assessed patients with chronic neck pain, migraine patients scored worse, i.e. had larger TPD thresholds than control participants, although the results in this current study were only statistically significant for the right side of the neck. TPD thresholds for the left side of the neck were also larger than in healthy controls but not statistically significant. Furthermore, results did not overcome the SDD and were very close to the SEM and might therefore be in line with Elsig et al. who found no difference between patients with recurrent neck pain and healthy controls [16]. The consistency of the direction of change for all tested body regions and the overwhelming majority of publications in this field showing larger TPD thresholds in pain patients compared to healthy populations, increase the confidence in the current results. Interestingly, although not statistically significant was, that TPD thresholds were also increased when measured outside the area of clinical pain at the right hand, pointing towards central rather than peripheral or region-specific changes. This result is also similar to that reported by Harvie et al. [28]. Older and younger healthy participants (median split at 35 years) showed a statistically significant difference and younger females showed the highest tactile acuity, i.e. smallest TPD thresholds.

Although significance was only reached for the right side of the neck, the generally increased TPD thresholds in migraine patients compared to controls might support the frequently stated hypothesis and that repeated migraine attacks result in similar cortical changes as observed in patients with chronic pain conditions [11]. While not surprising in the context of chronic pain research, the results of the current study are somewhat puzzling considering the prevalence of hypersensitivity and/or allodynia in patients with migraine. Altered sensitivity to external stimuli such as light, noise, smell or touch is one of the trait symptoms and diagnostic criteria for migraine [19]. Numerous studies focused on this phenomenon and reported hypersensitivity and/or allodynia in patients with migraine [29–37]. Smaller TPD thresholds would have been the more intuitive result representing an increased tactile sense and thereby a phenomenon which could be interpreted as hypersensitivity. One explanation for this controversy could be that hypersensitivity and/or allodynia are indeed only present during the pre-ictal and ictal phase of migraine [33], while reports on interictal hypersensitivity are conflicting [38]. A further explanation could be that allodynia and/or hypersensitivity is restricted to the reference area of the trigeminal nerve. Very few studies, additionally to the typically measured supraorbital region, measured hypersensitivity in the neck [34, 39, 40]. This limited evidence is surprising, since neck pain is more common in migraine patients than other typically associated symptoms - such as nausea - and occurs in more than 70% of migraine patients [41]. The 12-item Allodynia Checklist contains items such as "wearing a neckless" which was found to be the second most discriminative item between migraine patients with and without cutaneous allodynia [36]. Based on the trigeminocervical convergence theory, stating that afferent fibres from the trigeminal and the cervical systems connect to the same nuclei in the brainstem, there is a strong anatomical and physiological explanation for a reciprocal influence of the trigeminal system on cervical reference areas and vice versa [42–44]. Furthermore, a study using a neural staining technique in rodents reported a connection between the dura mater and peripheral muscles through the cranial fissures and thereby another possible pathway explaining neck pain or/and sensitivity when the dura mater is sensitized [45].

A final explanation is that tactile acuity and hypersensitivity/allodynia, while fulfilling the same biological role of an increased awareness to potentially damaging stimuli to a diseased or painful body region, are unrelated entities. The most common paradigm to quantify hypersensitivity and/or allodynia is the quantitative sensory testing (QST) protocol where different noxious and non-noxious modalities are applied to the affected body part and perception thresholds, pain thresholds and pain responses are recorded [21]. However, QST requires

Table 3 Mean and standard deviations of two-point discrimination thresholds

Side / location of testing	Migraine patients ($n = 28$)	Healthy control ($n = 21$)	t - test
Left	27.4 (8.2) mm	24.9 (7.1) mm	$p = 0.27$
Right	26.3 (7.3) mm	21.7 (6.2) mm	$p = 0.02$
Hand	8.3 (4.0) mm	6.4 (2.2) mm	$p = 0.05$

equipment not always available to clinicians and the full protocol is extremely time consuming. Whether TPD thresholds can be used as an alternative test paradigm feasible for the use in the daily clinical practice remains to be evaluated in future studies.

A limitation of this study is, that only the neck and the hand but not the reference area of the trigeminal nerve was assessed. Although this was the aim of this project, retrospectively, an additional assessment of the supraorbital area on the side most affected by migraine would have been helpful to at least partially disentangle whether the test location influences results. Furthermore, a second modality, such as thermal thresholds or von Frey hairs would have been interesting to compare the current results with previous publications and to investigate whether TPD thresholds are related to hypersensitivity and/or allodynia. To disentangle responses to tactile stimuli and thereby better understand what the test modalities actually measure would be valuable future projects.

Conclusion

Despite the limited available space in the upper cervical region, TPD thresholds can be measured reliably in healthy participants and in patients with migraine. Younger and female patients have smaller TPD thresholds than older and male patients, future research should take this into account. Patients with migraine show larger TPD thresholds in the upper cervical region, but significance was only reached for the right side of the neck. Remote body parts also showed increased values (but did not reach statistical significance), potentially pointing towards cortical changes similar to those reported for chronic pain conditions.

Abbreviations

ICC: Intraclass correlation coefficient; QTS: Quantitative sensory testing; SD: Standard deviation; SEM: Standard error of measurement; TPD: Two-point discrimination threshold

Funding

WMA is supported by the scholarship awarded within grant #2014/14/E/HS6/00415 funded by the National Science Centre in Poland.

KL received financial support from the Maitland Research Foundation.

Authors' contributions

KL planned and designed the study, supported the analysis and wrote the final manuscript, WA designed the two-point discrimination paradigm, supported the data analysis and corrected the final manuscript. KM, IM, LR, JS and CZ recruited participants, collected the data, analysed the data and prepared a first draft of the manuscript. AS supervised the intra-rater stage and analysed intra-rater data. TS supported the data analysis and helped prepare the final draft of the manuscript, BW supervised the inter-rater stage of the study and helped prepare the final manuscript. All authors read and approved the final manuscript.

Competing interests

The authors declare that they have no competing interests.

Author details

[1]Department of Human Movement Science, University of Hamburg, Hamburg, Germany. [2]Academic Physiotherapy, Medical Section, Department of Orthopaedics and Trauma Surgery, University of Luebeck, Luebeck, Germany. [3]The Jerzy Kukuczka Academy of Physical Education, Department of Physiotherapy, Katowice, Poland. [4]Faculty of Social Science, Degree Course Speech and Language Therapy and Physiotherapy, University of Applied Sciences Bremen, Bremen, Germany. [5]Pain Research Group, Institute of Psychology, Jagiellonian University, Krakow, Poland. [6]Department of Systems Neuroscience, University Medical Center Hamburg-Eppendorf, Hamburg, Germany.

References

1. Apkarian AV, Sosa Y, Sonty S et al (2004) Chronic back pain is associated with decreased prefrontal and thalamic gray matter density. J Neurosci 24: 10410–10415. https://doi.org/10.1523/JNEUROSCI.2541-04.2004
2. Apkarian AV, Hashmi JA, Baliki MN (2010) Pain and the brain: specificity and plasticity of the brain in clinical chronic pain. Pain 152:S49–S64. https://doi.org/10.1016/j.pain.2010.11.010
3. Buckalew N, Haut MW, Morrow L, Weiner D (2008) Chronic pain is associated with brain volume loss in older adults: preliminary evidence. Pain Med Malden Mass 9:240–248. https://doi.org/10.1111/j.1526-4637.2008.00412.x
4. Schmidt-Wilcke T, Leinisch E, Gänßbauer S et al (2006) Affective components and intensity of pain correlate with structural differences in gray matter in chronic back pain patients. Pain 125:89–97. https://doi.org/10.1016/j.pain.2006.05.004
5. Flor H, Braun C, Elbert T, Birbaumer N (1997) Extensive reorganization of primary somatosensory cortex in chronic back pain patients. Neurosci Lett 224:5–8
6. Giesecke T, Gracely RH, Grant MAB et al (2004) Evidence of augmented central pain processing in idiopathic chronic low back pain. Arthritis Rheum 50:613–623. https://doi.org/10.1002/art.20063
7. Mao C, Wei L, Zhang Q et al (2013) Differences in brain structure in patients with distinct sites of chronic pain: a voxel-based morphometric analysis. Neural Regen Res 8:2981–2990. https://doi.org/10.3969/j.issn.1673-5374.2013.32.001
8. May A (2011) Structural brain imaging: a window into chronic pain. Neurosci Rev J Bringing Neurobiol Neurol Psychiatry 17:209–220. https://doi.org/10.1177/1073858410396220
9. Pleger B, Ragert P, Schwenkreis P et al (2006) Patterns of cortical reorganization parallel impaired tactile discrimination and pain intensity in complex regional pain syndrome. Neuroimage 32:503–510. https://doi.org/10.1016/j.neuroimage.2006.03.045
10. Schmidt-Wilcke T, Wulms N, Heba S et al (2018) Structural changes in brain morphology induced by brief periods of repetitive sensory stimulation. Neuroimage 165:148–157. https://doi.org/10.1016/j.neuroimage.2017.10.016
11. Catley MJ, O'Connell NE, Berryman C et al (2014) Is tactile acuity altered in people with chronic pain? A systematic review and meta-analysis. J Pain Off J Am Pain Soc 15:985–1000. https://doi.org/10.1016/j.jpain.2014.06.009
12. Adamczyk W, Luedtke K, Saulicz E (2017) Lumbar tactile acuity in patients with low back pain and healthy controls: systematic review and meta-analysis. Clin J Pain. https://doi.org/10.1097/AJP.0000000000000499
13. Song ZK, Cohen MJ, Ament PA et al (1993) Two-point discrimination thresholds in spinal cord injured patients with dysesthetic pain. Paraplegia 31:425–493. https://doi.org/10.1038/sc.1993.79
14. Moreira C, Bassi AR, Brandão MP, Silva AG (2017) Do patients with chronic neck pain have distorted body image and tactile dysfunction? Eur J Phys 19: 215–221. https://doi.org/10.1080/21679169.2017.1334818
15. Nolan MF (1985) Quantitative measure of cutaneous sensation. Two-point discrimination values for the face and trunk. Phys Ther 65:181–185
16. Elsig S, Luomajoki H, Sattelmayer M et al (2014) Sensorimotor tests, such as movement control and laterality judgment accuracy, in persons with recurrent neck pain and controls. A case-control study. Man Ther 19:555–561. https://doi.org/10.1016/j.math.2014.05.014

17. Catley MJ, Tabor A, Wand BM, Moseley GL (2013) Assessing tactile acuity in rheumatology and musculoskeletal medicine–how reliable are two-point discrimination tests at the neck, hand, back and foot? Rheumatol Oxf Engl 52:1454–1461. https://doi.org/10.1093/rheumatology/ket140
18. Harvie DS, Kelly J, Buckman H et al (2017) Tactile acuity testing at the neck: a comparison of methods. Musculoskelet Sci Pract 32:23–30. https://doi.org/10.1016/j.msksp.2017.07.007
19. International Headache Society (2018) Headache classification Committee of the International Headache Society (IHS) the international classification of headache disorders, 3rd edition. Cephalalgia Int J Headache 38:1–211. https://doi.org/10.1177/0333102417738202
20. Moberg E (1990) Two-point discrimination test. A valuable part of hand surgical rehabilitation, e.g. in tetraplegia. Scand J Rehabil Med 22:127–134
21. Rolke R, Baron R, Maier C et al (2006) Quantitative sensory testing in the German research network on neuropathic pain (DFNS): standardized protocol and reference values. Pain 123:231–243. https://doi.org/10.1016/j.pain.2006.01.041
22. Adamczyk W, Sługocka A, Saulicz O, Saulicz E (2016) The point-to-point test: a new diagnostic tool for measuring lumbar tactile acuity? Inter and intra-examiner reliability study of pain-free subjects. Man Ther 22:220–226. https://doi.org/10.1016/j.math.2015.12.012
23. Faul F, Erdfelder E, Lang A-G, Buchner A (2007) G*power 3: a flexible statistical power analysis program for the social, behavioral, and biomedical sciences. Behav Res Methods:175–191
24. Fleiss JL (2011) Design and analysis of clinical experiments. New Jersey: Wiley. https://doi.org/10.1002/9781118032923
25. Rousson V (2013) Measurement in medicine, by H. C. W. de Vet, C. B. Terwee, L. B. Mokkink, and D. L. Knol. J Biopharm Stat 23:277–279. https://doi.org/10.1080/10543406.2013.737220
26. Kaneko A, Asai N, Kanda T (2005) The influence of age on pressure perception of static and moving two-point discrimination in normal subjects. J Hand Ther Off J Am Soc Hand Ther 18:421–424, quiz 425. https://doi.org/10.1197/j.jht.2005.09.010
27. Won S-Y, Kim H-K, Kim M-E, Kim K-S (2017) Two-point discrimination values vary depending on test site, sex and test modality in the orofacial region: a preliminary study. J Appl Oral Sci Rev FOB 25:427–435. https://doi.org/10.1590/1678-7757-2016-0462
28. Harvie DS, Edmond-Hank G, Smith AD (2018) Tactile acuity is reduced in people with chronic neck pain. Musculoskelet Sci Pract 33:61–66. https://doi.org/10.1016/j.msksp.2017.11.009
29. Schwedt TJ, Krauss MJ, Frey K, Gereau RW (2011) Episodic and chronic migraineurs are hypersensitive to thermal stimuli between migraine attacks. Cephalalgia Int J Headache 31:6–12. https://doi.org/10.1177/0333102410365108
30. Aguggia M (2012) Allodynia and migraine. Neurol Sci Off J Ital Neurol Soc Ital Soc Clin Neurophysiol 33(Suppl 1):S9–S11. https://doi.org/10.1007/s10072-012-1034-9
31. Ashkenazi A, Silberstein S, Jakubowski M, Burstein R (2007) Improved identification of allodynic migraine patients using a questionnaire. Cephalalgia Int J Headache 27:325–329. https://doi.org/10.1111/j.1468-2982.2007.01291.x
32. Ashkenazi A, Young WB (2005) The effects of greater occipital nerve block and trigger point injection on brush allodynia and pain in migraine. Headache 45:350–354. https://doi.org/10.1111/j.1526-4610.2005.05073.x
33. Burstein R, Cutrer MF, Yarnitsky D (2000) The development of cutaneous allodynia during a migraine attack clinical evidence for the sequential recruitment of spinal and supraspinal nociceptive neurons in migraine. Brain J Neurol 123(Pt 8):1703–1709
34. Cooke L, Eliasziw M, Becker WJ (2007) Cutaneous allodynia in transformed migraine patients. Headache 47:531–539. https://doi.org/10.1111/j.1526-4610.2006.00717.x
35. Landy S, Rice K, Lobo B (2004) Central sensitisation and cutaneous Allodynia in migraine. CNS Drugs 18:337–342. https://doi.org/10.2165/00023210-200418060-00001
36. Lipton RB, Bigal ME, Ashina S et al (2008) Cutaneous allodynia in the migraine population. Ann Neurol 63:148–158. https://doi.org/10.1002/ana.21211
37. Lovati C, D'Amico D, Rosa S et al (2007) Allodynia in different forms of migraine. Neurol Sci Off J Ital Neurol Soc Ital Soc Clin Neurophysiol 28(Suppl 2):S220–S221. https://doi.org/10.1007/s10072-007-0781-5
38. Nahman-Averbuch H, Shefi T, Schneider VJ et al (2018) Quantitative sensory testing in patients with migraine: a systemic review and meta-analysis. Pain. https://doi.org/10.1097/j.pain.0000000000001231
39. Gonçalves MC, Chaves TC, Florencio LL et al (2015) Is pressure pain sensitivity over the cervical musculature associated with neck disability in individuals with migraine? J Bodyw Mov Ther 19:67–71. https://doi.org/10.1016/j.jbmt.2014.02.007
40. Florencio LL, Giantomassi MCM, Carvalho GF et al (2015) Generalized pressure pain hypersensitivity in the cervical muscles in women with migraine. Pain Med Malden Mass 16:1629–1634. https://doi.org/10.1111/pme.12767
41. Ashina S, Bendtsen L, Lyngberg AC et al (2015) Prevalence of neck pain in migraine and tension-type headache: a population study. Cephalalgia Int J Headache 35:211–219. https://doi.org/10.1177/0333102414535110
42. Bogduk N (1992) The anatomical basis for cervicogenic headache. J Manip Physiol Ther 15:67–70
43. Bogduk N, Govind J (2009) Cervicogenic headache: an assessment of the evidence on clinical diagnosis, invasive tests, and treatment. Lancet Neurol 8:959–968. https://doi.org/10.1016/S1474-4422(09)70209-1
44. Bartsch T, Goadsby PJ (2003) The trigeminocervical complex and migraine: current concepts and synthesis. Curr Pain Headache Rep 7:371–376
45. Schueler M, Neuhuber WL, De Col R, Messlinger K (2014) Innervation of rat and human dura mater and pericranial tissues in the parieto-temporal region by meningeal afferents. Headache 54:996–1009. https://doi.org/10.1111/head.12371

Effects of sildenafil and calcitonin gene-related peptide on brainstem glutamate levels: a pharmacological proton magnetic resonance spectroscopy study at 3.0 T

Samaira Younis[1], Anders Hougaard[1], Casper Emil Christensen[1], Mark Bitsch Vestergaard[2], Esben Thade Petersen[3], Olaf Bjarne Paulson[4], Henrik Bo Wiberg Larsson[2] and Messoud Ashina[1*]

Abstract

Background: Studies involving human pharmacological migraine models have predominantly focused on the vasoactive effects of headache-inducing drugs, including sildenafil and calcitonin gene-related peptide (CGRP). However, the role of possible glutamate level changes in the brainstem and thalamus is of emerging interest in the field of migraine research bringing forth the need for a novel, validated method to study the biochemical effects in these areas.

Methods: We applied an optimized in vivo human pharmacological proton (^{1}H) magnetic resonance spectroscopy (MRS) protocol (PRESS, repetition time 3000 ms, echo time 37.6–38.3 ms) at 3.0 T in combination with sildenafil and CGRP in a double-blind, placebo-controlled, randomized, double-dummy, three-way cross-over design. Seventeen healthy participants were scanned with the ^{1}H-MRS protocol at baseline and twice (at 40 min and 140 min) after drug administration to investigate the sildenafil- and CGRP-induced glutamate changes in both brainstem and thalamus.

Results: The glutamate levels increased transiently in the brainstem at 40–70 min after sildenafil administration compared to placebo (5.6%, $P = 0.039$). We found no sildenafil-induced glutamate changes in the thalamus, and no CGRP-induced glutamate changes in the brainstem or thalamus compared to placebo. Both sildenafil and CGRP induced headache in 53%–62% of participants. We found no interaction in the glutamate levels in the brainstem or thalamus between participants who developed sildenafil and/or CGRP-induced headache as compared to participants who did not.

Conclusions: The transient sildenafil-induced glutamate change in the brainstem possibly reflects increased excitability of the brainstem neurons. CGRP did not induce brainstem or thalamic glutamate changes, suggesting that it rather exerts its headache-inducing effects on the peripheral trigeminal pain pathways.

Keywords: MRS, Glutamate, Glx, Lactate, Migraine, Brainstem, Thalamus, CGRP, Sildenafil

Background

Human pharmacological migraine models have been used for the past two decades with great success to study migraine attack mechanisms using vasoactive drugs such as calcitonin gene-related peptide (CGRP) and sildenafil [1–7]. The models have been pivotal in the development of new anti-migraine therapy [8]. Human pathophysiological studies applying these models have predominantly focused on the cerebrovascular effects of the headache-inducing substances. However, emerging evidence suggests that metabolic changes, especially of brain glutamate levels [9, 10], in the brainstem [11–15] and thalamus [15] are key processes for the initiation of migraine headache attacks and thereby potentially important effects of the headache-inducing drugs. At present, methods for the study of pharmacologically induced biochemical effects on the brainstem glutamate levels have not been validated.

* Correspondence: ashina@dadlnet.dk
[1]Danish Headache Center, Department of Neurology, Rigshospitalet Glostrup, University of Copenhagen, Copenhagen, Denmark
Full list of author information is available at the end of the article

Pharmacological proton (^{1}H) magnetic resonance spectroscopy (MRS) provides the ability to non-invasively study drug-induced biochemical changes in the brain. Imaging of the deep brain structures, especially the brainstem by magnetic resonance imaging (MRI), is challenging due to the small size of the region of interest, location in areas of relatively high magnetic field inhomogeneity and potential physiological artifacts. Thus, it is essential to systematically investigate the quality and reproducibility of ^{1}H-MRS measurements in these areas before application of the method in patients. Only a few ^{1}H-MRS studies of the brainstem have previously been conducted. One such study, of patients with amyotrophic lateral sclerosis, did not report data on the reproducibility or variability of the glutamate measurements [16], while other ^{1}H-MRS brainstem studies did not measure the glutamate concentrations at all [17–20] .

The headache-inducing drugs, CGRP and sildenafil, were selected for the study based on their different modes of action. CGRP is generally considered to exert its primary effect outside of the central nervous system (CNS), in the meningeal vasculature and the first order trigeminal neurons [21, 22], while sildenafil, as a lipophilic molecule, readily crosses the blood-brain barrier [23].

Here, we conducted a double-blind, placebo-controlled, randomized, double-dummy, three-way cross-over pharmacological ^{1}H-MRS study to investigate the sildenafil- and CGRP-induced glutamate concentration changes in healthy participants. Our null-hypothesis was that the glutamate levels are not altered in the brainstem of healthy participants after administration of sildenafil and CGRP when compared to placebo. Additionally, we assessed the spectral quality and variability of the glutamate measurements over time in the brainstem based on our ^{1}H-MRS protocol.

Methods

Participants

Healthy volunteers were recruited through announcement on a Danish website for recruitment of participants to health research (www.forsoegsperson.dk). Inclusion criteria were: age 18–50 years and weight 50–100 kg. Exclusion criteria were: history of any primary headache disorders (except episodic tension-type headache for < 2 day per month during the last year) according to the diagnostic criteria of the beta version of the third International Classification of Headache Disorders (ICHD-3 beta) [24], first-degree family members with migraine or other primary headache disorders according to ICHD-3 beta (except episodic tension-type headache for < 6 days per month), daily intake of medication (except oral contraceptives), no usage of safe contraception, cardiovascular, cerebrovascular, or psychiatric disease, and drug abuse. Participants were excluded if there were any contraindications to MRI such as metal implants, pacemaker, insulin pump, claustrophobia and/or surgical procedure during the last 6 weeks before inclusion. We also excluded participants with braces and teeth implants of metal, which are normally regarded MRI compatible, to avoid potential MR scan artifacts in the deep brain structures of interest.

Experimental design

All participants were randomly allocated to receive sildenafil, CGRP and placebo on three separate study days. On each study day, participants underwent an MRI scan protocol consisting of three scan sessions: a baseline MRI scan, followed by two additional post drug administration MRI scan sessions. The first post drug scan was initiated at 40 min (scan 1), and the second scan was initiated at 140 min (scan 2) after administration of sildenafil, CGRP or placebo (Fig. 1). MR spectra were obtained from brainstem and thalamus during each scan.

On the sildenafil day, the participants received sildenafil as two 50 mg tablets (STADA, Bad Vilbel, Germany) in two non-transparent capsules, combined with placebo isotonic saline infusion into the cubital vein for 20 min (Pressure tubes, Argon Medical Devices, The Hague, the Netherlands), at the time of infusion start. On the CGRP day, the participants received 1.5 µg/min human-alfa-CGRP (PolyPeptide, Strasbourg, France) via infusion for 20 min combined with placebo calcium in two non-transparent capsules. On the placebo day, the participants received placebo isotonic saline infusion for 20 min combined with placebo calcium in two non-transparent capsules. The sildenafil and CGRP dosages for the study were

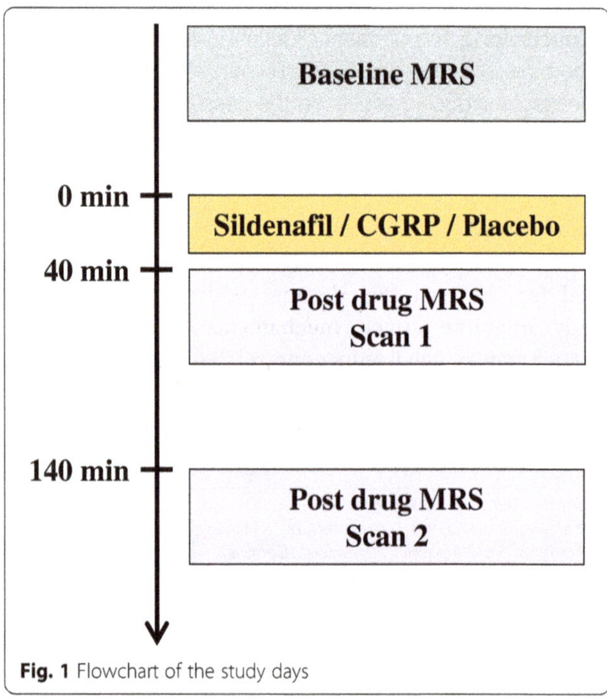

Fig. 1 Flowchart of the study days

determined based on findings of previous studies, which reported sildenafil- and CGRP-induced headache in healthy volunteers, and migraine-like attack in migraine patients [1–7]. The randomization was administrated by the Hospital Pharmacy of the Capital Region of Denmark.

All participants were headache-free for at least 72 h before each study day. The participants were not allowed coffee, tea, cocoa, soft drinks, alcohol or tobacco for 12 h before study start on each study day, and fasted for all food and beverages (except for water), for 4 h before study start. Between scan 1 and scan 2, all participants were offered a standardized small meal consisting of soft bread with cheese, banana, and water. Other criteria for the study days were no intake of any medication four half-lives before the start of the study day, except for oral contraception. After insertion of a peripheral venous catheter (18G Vasofix® Safety, B.Braun, Melsungen, Germany) into a cubital vein, the participants were instructed to rest in a hospital bed for approximately 30 min before the baseline scans.

We aimed to initiate the scan sessions at the same time of the day on all three study days for each participant, allowing for a maximum time deviation of 1 h, to account for metabolite concentration variations due to the circadian rhythm [25, 26]. In addition, the timing of scan 1 and scan 2 was fixed according to the baseline scan. The ^{1}H-MRS sequences were part of a larger study (results of these will be presented elsewhere). Before and after each scan sequence it was ensured that participants remained awake, and data were excluded in case they fell asleep during the scans as this could affect the measurements [27]. Participants were instructed to remain still and avoid any head motion during the scan sessions to ensure stable measurements from the regions of interest.

Headache characteristics

Data on headache characteristics were acquired on each study day, i.e. intensity, quality, aggravation by physical activity, location and associated symptoms (nausea, photophobia, and phonophobia). The headache intensity was rated on a numeric rating scale ranging from 0 to 10, where '0' translated to no headache and '10' to the worst imaginable headache. The headache data were obtained between all scans. All participants were asked to register headache hourly in a standardized questionnaire after the last scan session until 24 h, starting from the time of study drug administration.

Vital signs

The vital variables were registered and monitored at baseline, and during the scan sessions after study drug administration. Systolic and diastolic blood pressure were measured with an interval of 10 min, and heart rate, blood oxygen saturation and nostril end-tidal CO_2 tension (water trap and gas sample line, Medrad, Warrendale, PA) (Veris Monitor, Medrad, Warrendale, PA) were monitored continuously.

Data acquisition and imaging protocol

All MRI scans were performed on a 3.0 T Philips Achieva MRI scanner (Philips Medical Systems, Best, The Netherlands) using a 32-channel phase array head coil.

Anatomical scan

High-resolution anatomical scans were obtained with a 3D T1-weighted turbo field echo sequence (field of view $240 \times 240 \times 170$ mm^3; voxel size $1.00 \times 1.08 \times 1.10$ mm^3; echo time 3.7 ms; repetition time 8.0 ms; flip angle 8°). The reconstruction software on the scanner was used to additionally obtain the axial and coronal anatomical views of the scan to ensure correct placement of the volumes-of-interest (VOIs) for brainstem and thalamus.

Magnetic resonance spectroscopy

We used proton (^{1}H) magnetic resonance spectroscopy (MRS) to measure the combined concentration of glutamate and glutamine (reported as 'glutamate'), lactate, *N*-Acetylaspartate (NAA) and the total concentration of creatine i.e. phosphocreatine and creatine. The water-suppressed point-resolved spectroscopy (PRESS) pulse sequence was used in brainstem (repetition time 3000 ms; echo time 38.3 ms, voxel size $10.5 \times 12.5 \times 22$ mm^3; 480 acquisitions; total duration 24 min) and thalamus (repetition time 3000 ms; echo time 37.6 ms; voxel size 16 mm × 12 mm × 12 mm; 192 acquisitions; total duration 9 min 36 s). High number of acquisitions was used to ensure sufficient signal-noise-ratio. Voxel size based shimming was performed using first-order pencil beam to reduce the inhomogeneity in the chosen VOIs. The protocol was thus optimized to precisely target small VOIs in deep brain structures and to avoid cerebrospinal fluid contributions and partial volume artifacts. The repetition time was 3000 ms to ensure sufficient relaxation. The unsuppressed water signal was measured from the VOIs and used as internal reference for quantification [28]. The first VOI was placed unilaterally in the right side of the brainstem, and the second VOI was placed in the left, contralateral thalamus, following the anatomical and functional trigeminal pain pathways.

Metabolite quantification and analysis

Post-processing and quantification of the spectral data were performed by LCModel (Version 6.3-1F, Toronto, Canada). Representative ^{1}H-MRS spectra obtained from brainstem and thalamus are illustrated in Fig. 2. Spectra were evaluated in a blinded manner and abnormal

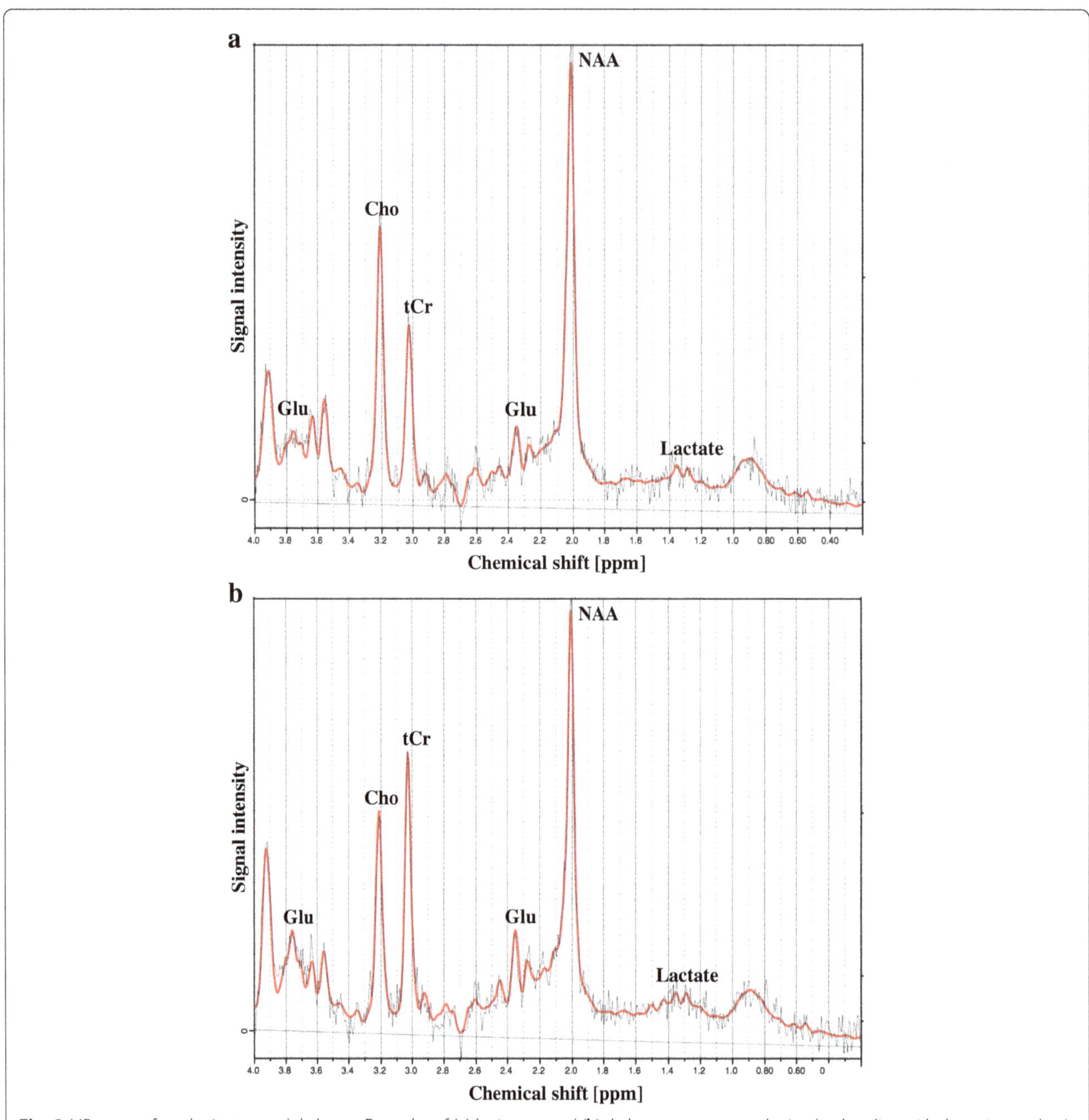

Fig. 2 MR spectra from brainstem and thalamus. Examples of (**a**) brainstem and (**b**) thalamus spectra are obtained at baseline with the point-resolved spectroscopy (PRESS) pulse sequence at 3.0 T. The spectra are acquired from LCModel. The red line represents the fit, and the horizontal linear line represents the baseline as estimated by LCModel. Cho: Choline, Glu: Glutamate, tCr: Total creatine, NAA: *N*-Acetylaspartate

spectra were excluded. The quality of the included spectra was estimated based on the signal-noise-ratio (SNR) and full-width of half-maximum (FWHM) of the spectra peaks as provided by LCModel. The means and standard deviations of the SNR and FWHM for the brainstem and thalamus spectra were calculated.

Statistical analysis

The primary endpoint was glutamate, lactate, NAA and total creatine concentration changes in brainstem and thalamus from baseline to after sildenafil and CGRP administration, compared to the corresponding placebo changes. A linear mixed model was used for each metabolite with interaction between scans (baseline, scan 1 and scan 2) and drug days (sildenafil, CGRP and placebo) and with subjects and study day (5 levels) nested within subjects as random effects. The placebo day baseline scan was set as the reference parameter in the model.

The secondary endpoint was changes in the metabolite concentrations in participants who developed pharmacologically induced headache during the scan sessions after sildenafil and CGRP, compared to participants who did not. A linear mixed model was used for each metabolite on the sildenafil and CGRP day with interaction between scans and headache and the random effects: subjects and study day nested within subjects. The data did not allow for correlation analyses between metabolite concentration and headache characteristics. The headache frequencies after sildenafil and CGRP were compared to placebo using McNemar's test.

For explorative vital parameter analyses, we included data from the following time points: 0, 20, 70, 120, and 170 min after infusion. Changes from baseline after sildenafil and CGRP were compared to placebo using a linear mixed model with interaction between drug days and the selected time points with subjects as random effects.

The variability structure of the glutamate measurements in the brainstem and thalamus was estimated in an explorative analysis based on baseline, scan 1, and scan 2 data acquired on the placebo day, and baseline data acquired on the sildenafil and CGRP day, using a linear mixed model with no fixed effects, and the random effects: subjects and study day (5 levels) nested within subjects.

All statistical analyses were performed using R (Version 3.4.2). P values were reported as two-tailed with a level of significance of 5%.

Results

Participants

Seventeen healthy volunteers participated in the study (10 women and 7 men) with mean age 22.9 (SD ± 3.4 and range 18–30 years) (Fig. 3). Vitals signs are presented in Fig. 4.

Alterations in metabolite concentration

Brainstem

The glutamate concentration significantly increased from baseline to scan 1 after sildenafil compared to the corresponding change after placebo ($P = 0.039$) (Table 1, Fig. 5). The lactate concentration decreased from baseline to scan 1 ($P = 0.017$), but not to scan 2 ($P = 0.156$) after sildenafil, compared to corresponding changes after placebo. In the brainstem, we did not detect changes in the metabolite concentrations from baseline to scan 1 or scan 2 after CGRP, compared to placebo.

Thalamus

We did not detect changes in the glutamate, lactate or NAA concentrations in the thalamus from baseline to scan 1 or scan 2 after sildenafil or CGRP, compared to placebo. The increase in the total creatine concentration from baseline to scan 2 after CGRP (3.3%, $P = 0.028$) was significant in comparison to placebo ($P = 0.004$).

Headache vs. no headache

The proportion of participants who developed headache during scan 1 and scan 2, and after the scan sessions and until 24 h from drug administration, is reported in Fig. 6. We found no interaction in the glutamate, lactate, NAA or total creatine concentrations in the brainstem or thalamus between participants who developed sildenafil- and/or CGRP-induced headaches as compared to participants who did not.

Quality of spectra

The brainstem spectra had mean SNR of 17.56 (± 2.33), and mean FWHM of 0.05 ppm (± 0.01) / 6.39 Hz (± 1.28). In thalamus, the mean SNR was 15.30 (± 1.86) and the mean FWHM was 0.04 ppm (± 0.01) / 5.11 Hz (± 1.28). In addition, the Cramér–Rao lower bound was < 12% for glutamate measurements in the brainstem and thalamus, except for 12–13% in four brainstem spectra and one thalamus spectrum in different subjects.

Glutamate variability in brainstem and thalamus

From the linear mixed model, we obtained separate brainstem glutamate concentration variations, where 6.9% was due to residual measurement error with additional 2.1% due to inter-subject variation, and 6.0% due to between day variations. The thalamic glutamate concentration variations were 6.8% due to residual measurement error with 2.7% inter-subject and 0% between day variations.

The mean time difference from day 1 to day 2 of the study days was 12.5 days (± 9.2) and 10.7 days (± 6.0) between day 2 and day 3. Participants were mainly scanned from afternoon time on all three scan days. The scans were initiated in the morning for three subjects, whereof one subject completed all three study days.

Discussion

The major outcome of the present study was an increase in the glutamate concentration in the brainstem after administration of sildenafil when compared to placebo. We did not detect any changes in the glutamate concentration in the brainstem after CGRP infusion.

Sildenafil-induced biochemical changes

Glutamate, as the major excitatory neurotransmitter in the brain, promotes neuronal depolarization [29]. Extracellular glutamate levels are directly correlated to levels of neuronal hyperexcitability and seizure intensity in animal models of epilepsy [30, 31]. Here, we evaluated the combined concentration of the glutamate and glutamine as these metabolites are not differentiable at 3.0 T ^{1}H-MRS. In healthy volunteers, the majority of the combined concentration consists of glutamate (~ 80%) [32] and 13%–22% of the glutamate concentration in the healthy brain is present in the

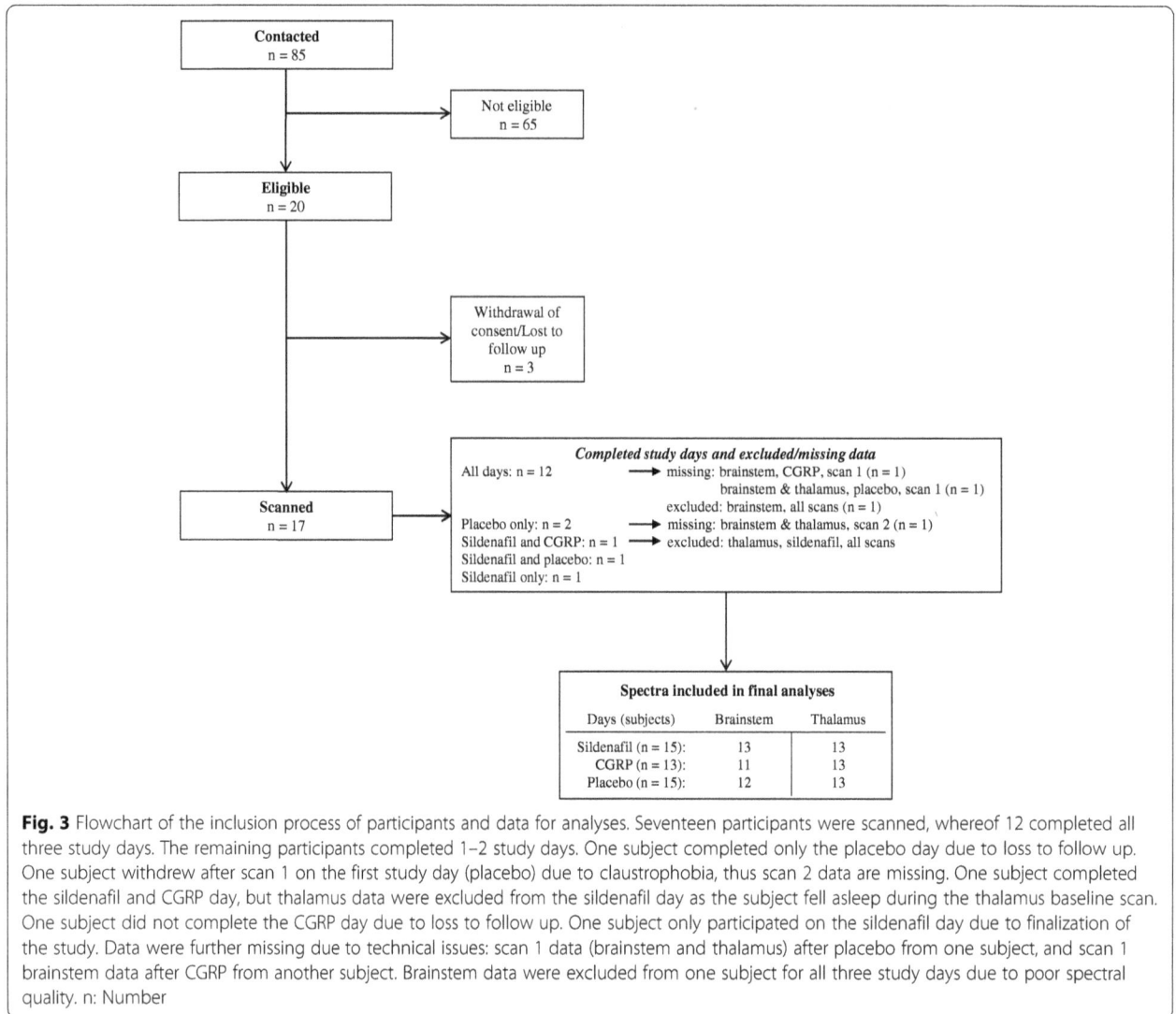

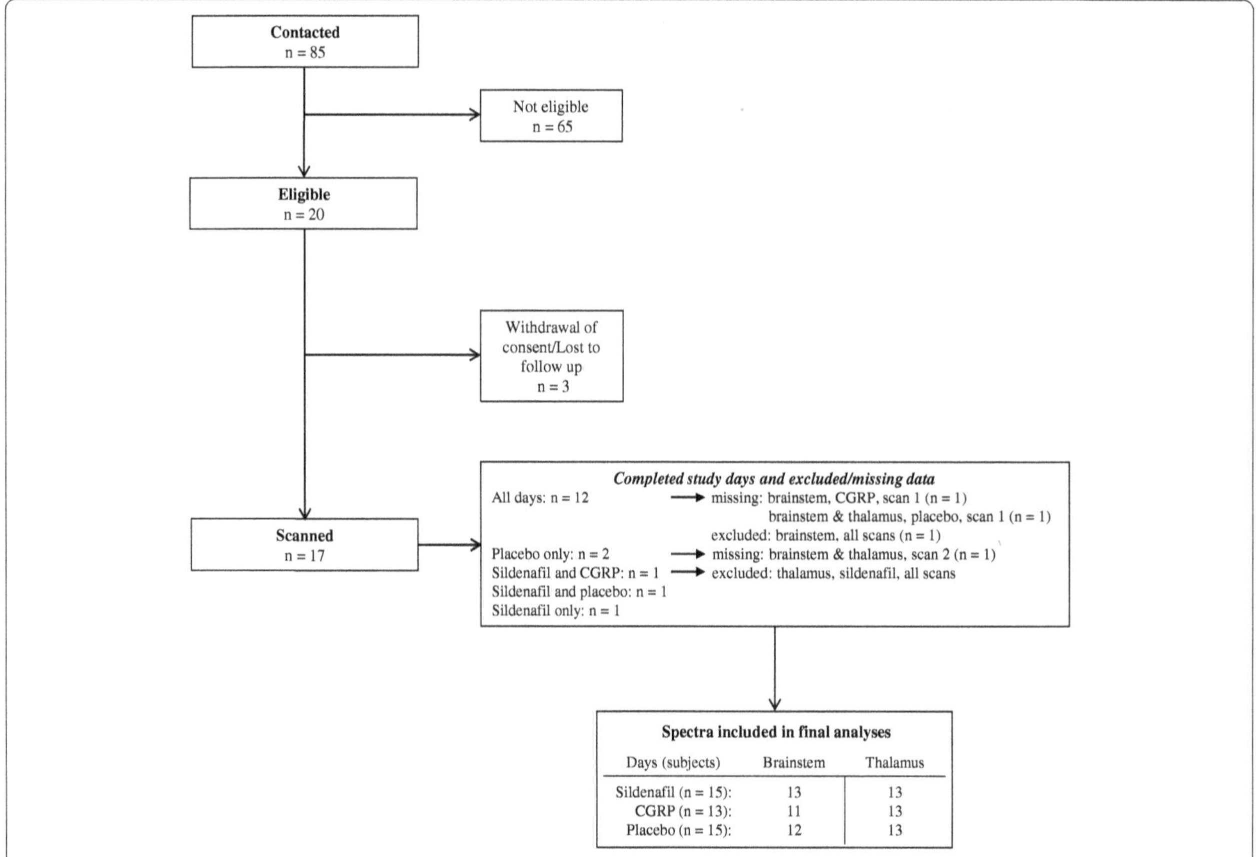

Fig. 3 Flowchart of the inclusion process of participants and data for analyses. Seventeen participants were scanned, whereof 12 completed all three study days. The remaining participants completed 1–2 study days. One subject completed only the placebo day due to loss to follow up. One subject withdrew after scan 1 on the first study day (placebo) due to claustrophobia, thus scan 2 data are missing. One subject completed the sildenafil and CGRP day, but thalamus data were excluded from the sildenafil day as the subject fell asleep during the thalamus baseline scan. One subject did not complete the CGRP day due to loss to follow up. One subject only participated on the sildenafil day due to finalization of the study. Data were further missing due to technical issues: scan 1 data (brainstem and thalamus) after placebo from one subject, and scan 1 brainstem data after CGRP from another subject. Brainstem data were excluded from one subject for all three study days due to poor spectral quality. n: Number

extracellular space [29]. Most likely, the glutamate concentrations measured by ^{1}H-MRS largely reflect the extracellular glutamate levels. In support of this, a ^{1}H-MRS study reported lower glutamate levels in amyotrophic lateral sclerosis patients treated with riluzole, a drug that increases glutamate uptake in central nervous system (CNS) neurons, compared to riluzole-naive amyotrophic lateral sclerosis patients and healthy controls [16]. The transient sildenafil-induced increase of glutamate in the brainstem in the present study thus likely reflects increased extracellular glutamate levels and possibly increased neuronal excitability. In support, sildenafil is able to cross the blood-brain barrier [23, 33] and some individuals report CNS side effects, such as dizziness and confusion [33–36]. Thus, sildenafil may be able to directly affect the neurons in deep brain structures such as the brainstem. In contrast, a functional MRI (fMRI) study of the visual cortex suggested that oral sildenafil intake did not change the neuronal activation threshold either at 1 or 2 h after administration [2]. The plasma t_{max} of oral 100 mg sildenafil is about 1 h with a close to 4 h half-life in the fasting state [36]. Here, we detected an increased glutamate level at scan 1 (40–70 min after sildenafil), around the time of t_{max}, but not at scan 2 (140–170 min after sildenafil). Possibly, plasma concentrations of sildenafil above a certain level are needed to alter the glutamate levels. Another possibility is that the transient changes may be attributed to adaptation of sildenafil's effect at scan 2.

We detected no difference in the glutamate levels between groups of participants developing headache vs. no headache. It should be noted that the participants were healthy with no family history of migraine developing merely a mild to moderate non-migraine headache after the drug administration. Therefore, we speculate that a "healthy" trigeminonociceptive system would not be sufficiently activated to produce detectable changes in the glutamate level. This may also explain the lack of changes in the glutamate levels after CGRP as well as in the thalamus.

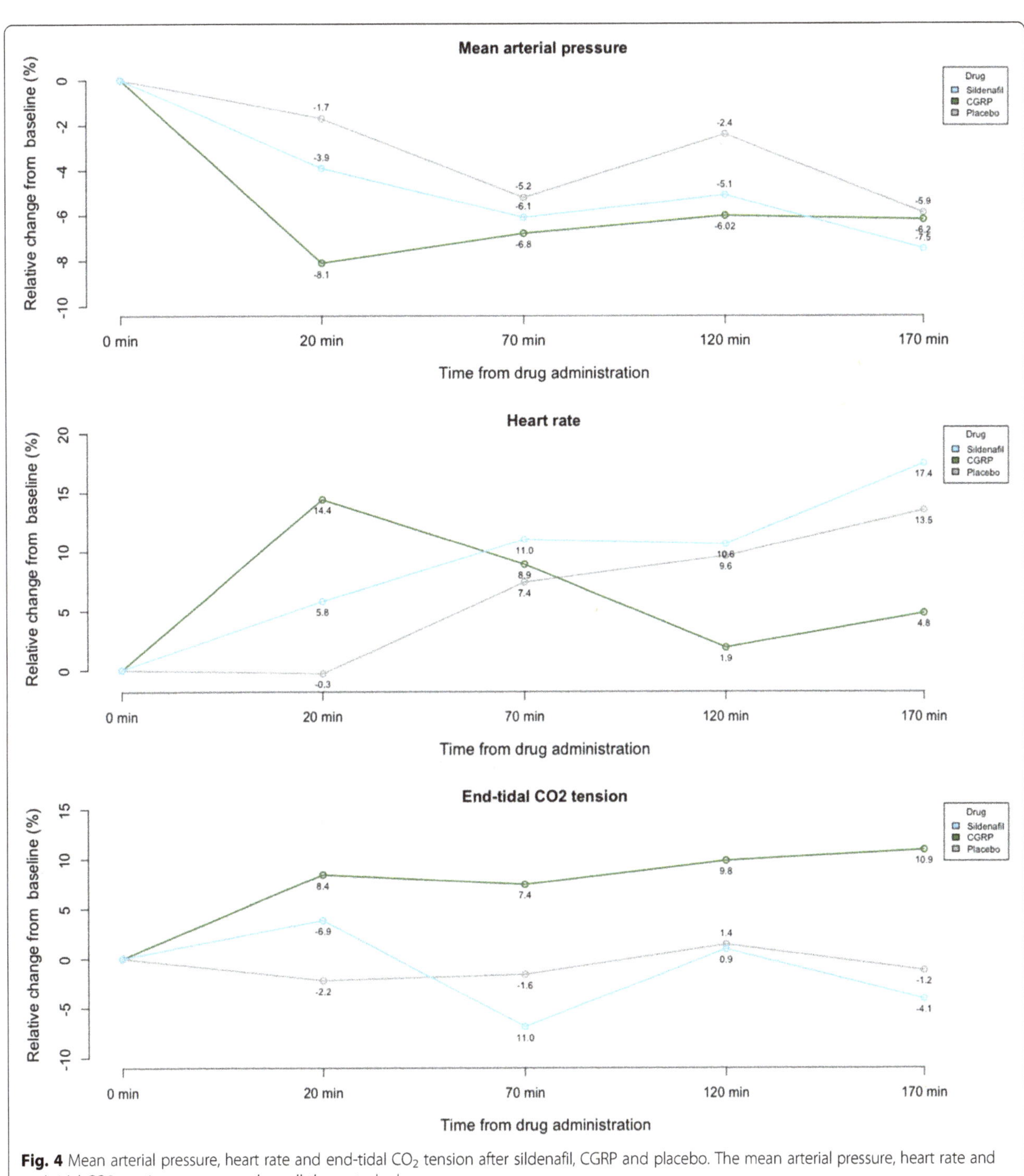

Fig. 4 Mean arterial pressure, heart rate and end-tidal CO_2 tension after sildenafil, CGRP and placebo. The mean arterial pressure, heart rate and end-tidal CO2 tension were normal on all three study days

Given the transient glutamate changes and lack of correlation to headache status, it is likely that the observed changes are related to the pharmacological effects of the drug rather than the headache per se.

The lactate concentration was decreased in the brainstem at scan 1 after sildenafil compared to the corresponding placebo change. This observation is very interesting since brain lactate levels under normal conditions increase during neuronal activation [37]. Therefore, we would expect the brainstem lactate levels to increase following sildenafil administration, along with the observed increase in glutamate. A possible explanation could be that the lactate decrease reflects a neuronal energy consumption via conversion to pyruvate [38]. The lactate concentration finding in the present study should be interpreted with caution due to the relatively large standard deviations. Also of note, the

Table 1 Summary of metabolite concentrations in brainstem after sildenafil, CGRP and placebo

	Baseline		Scan 1				Scan 2			
	Mean mmol/L	SD	Mean mmol/L	SD	% change from baseline	*P*	Mean mmol/L	SD	% change from baseline	*P*
Glutamate										
Sildenafil	7.77	0.65	8.21	0.53	5.6	0.039*	8.06	0.77	3.7	0.101
CGRP	7.92	1.11	7.49	0.88	−5.4	0.639	8.08	0.73	−2.0	0.228
Placebo	7.96	0.50	7.72	0.61	−3.0	–	7.70	0.65	−3.3	–
Lactate										
Sildenafil	0.90	0.21	0.45	0.41	−50.0	0.017*	0.43	0.33	− 51.9	0.156
CGRP	0.71	0.51	0.49	0.44	−30.9	0.151	0.42	0.41	−40.6	0.494
Placebo	0.75	0.65	0.89	0.68	21.6	–	0.62	0.42	−15.6	–
NAA										
Sildenafil	7.73	0.79	7.93	0.79	2.8	0.236	7.95	0.69	3.0	0.370
CGRP	7.58	0.72	7.56	0.68	−0.2	0.821	8.06	0.82	6.3	0.127
Placebo	7.61	0.63	7.64	0.58	0.4	–	7.73	0.72	1.6	–
Total creatine										
Sildenafil	4.25	0.35	4.33	0.32	1.0	0.978	4.23	0.28	−0.3	0.735
CGRP	4.38	0.38	4.39	0.53	0.03	0.562	4.50	0.33	2.7	0.170
Placebo	4.24	0.33	4.33	0.47	2.0	–	4.21	0.32	−0.7	–

$^*P<0.05$. *P* values reported for delta change from baseline to scan 1 and 2 after sildenafil and CGRP, compared to the corresponding change from baseline after placebo
NAA N-Acetylaspartate, *SD* standard deviation

lactate concentration is very low in the healthy brain (below 1.0 mmol/L) [39]. This contributes to the risk of lactate signal loss in the spectrum due to chemical shift displacement or J-modulations deviations during the MRS measurements, which are known issues [39].

CGRP-induced biochemical changes

We detected no alterations in the glutamate levels after CGRP infusion in either brainstem or thalamus in healthy participants. This suggests that CGRP does *not* modify the neuronal excitability in these key CNS structures involved in pain processing in healthy subjects. The blood-brain barrier is believed to have no permeability to CGRP [4, 40], and thus little or no direct effects on central brain regions, which our findings support.

In line with previous reports [3, 4], we found that participants developed more headache after CGRP, compared to placebo, demonstrating that CGRP is able to activate the trigeminal pain pathway. Given that systemic CGRP is unlikely to cross the blood-brain barrier, the present findings support the notion that CGRP acts on perivascular afferents [22] or the trigeminal ganglion [21, 41]. Interestingly, an fMRI study reported no change in the neuronal activation of the visual cortex of healthy volunteers after CGRP infusion [42]. Increased neuronal response to visual stimulation has previously been

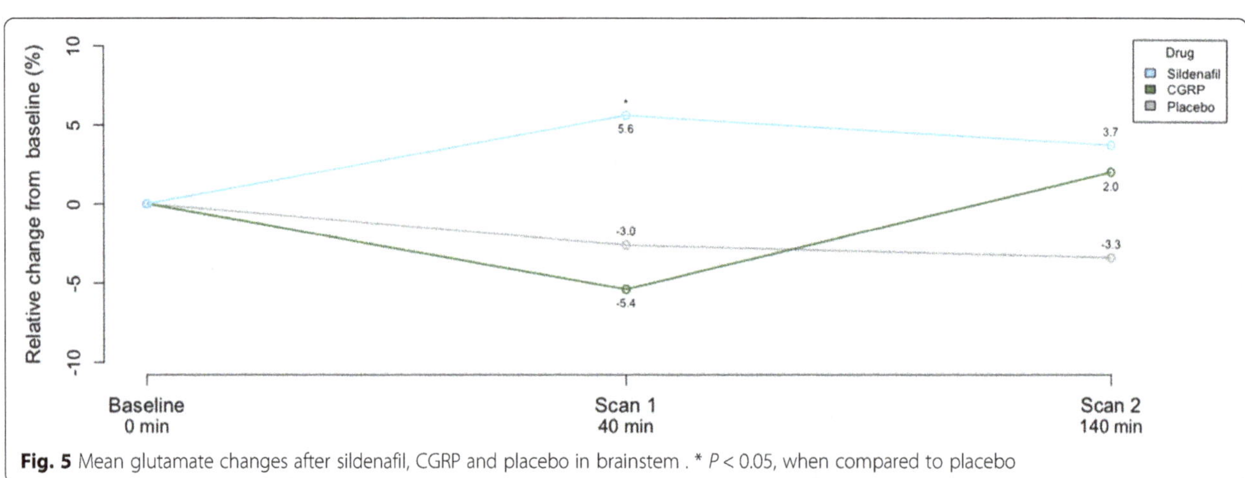

Fig. 5 Mean glutamate changes after sildenafil, CGRP and placebo in brainstem . * $P < 0.05$, when compared to placebo

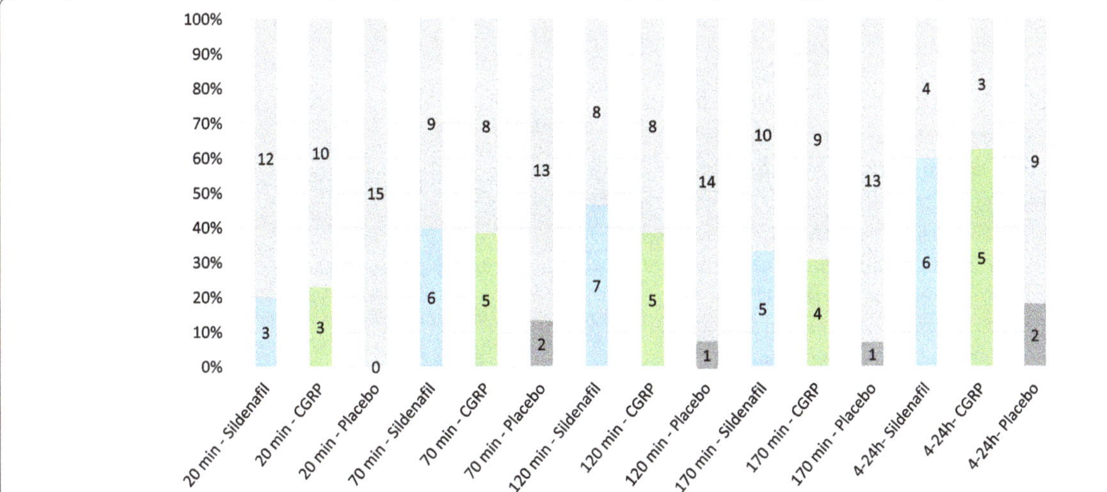

Fig. 6 Proportion of healthy participants who developed headache after sildenafil, CGRP and placebo. Blue, green and dark grey bars indicate headache. Light grey bars indicate no headache. During the scan sessions (0–4 h), 8 of 13 participants (62%) developed headache after CGRP ($P = 0.041$, compared to placebo), 8 of 15 (53%) developed headache after sildenafil ($P = 0.131$, compared to placebo), and 2 of 13 (13%) developed headache after placebo.

shown to be correlated with an increase in the glutamate levels [43, 44]. Another fMRI study involving application of heat pain to the forehead of healthy volunteers reported altered blood-oxygenation-level-dependent signal 40 min after administration of CGRP in pain associated brain regions, including the brainstem and thalamus, with no changes during placebo [45]. This observation suggests that CGRP may be capable of modulating the neuronal response indirectly (i.e. outside the CNS) given that the pain pathway is already activated [45].

Reliability of glutamate measurements

With our ^{1}H-MRS protocol, we obtained high quality spectra from the brainstem and thalamus with narrow line widths and relatively high SNR allowing for reliable quantification. A previous 3.0 T ^{1}H-MRS study measured glutamate changes in the brainstem without reporting the SNR or spectral line widths, but visual inspection of the brainstem spectrum reveals more noise compared to the brainstem spectra obtained in the present study [16]. Other ^{1}H-MRS brainstem studies reported relatively wider mean line widths of 8.1 Hz (± 0.9) [18], and 10.04 Hz (± 4.64) [17] at 3.0 T, and 7 Hz at 4.0 T [19] indicating spectra of lower quality. One of the studies reported the SNR as well, which was relatively high, 21(± 3), most likely due to the larger VOI used in the study [18]. None of the studies reported glutamate findings and the VOIs were larger than in the present study [17–19]. While large VOIs can improve the spectral quality, it also restricts the possibility of targeting a brain area with precision.

A previous 3.0 T ^{1}H-MRS study of thalamus used a larger VOI with fewer acquisitions, and reported a mean line width similar to the present study findings, but did not report the SNR value for comparison [17]. One 1.5 T ^{1}H-MRS thalamus study reported reduced mean line width of 3.2 Hz (± 0.5), however, the SNR of 3.9 (± 1.2) was much lower [46].

The brainstem ^{1}H-MRS spectra reveal a different metabolite composition compared to the conventional spectra obtained from e.g. the thalamus and occipital lope, as the choline peak is higher than the total creatine peak (Fig. 2), which is commonly reported [16, 17, 19].

To our knowledge, our study is the first ^{1}H-MRS study to provide information on the variability of glutamate levels in both brainstem and thalamus, based on repeated measurements, on the same day and on three separate days. In the present study, the overall variability of the glutamate measurements was low. For comparison, a previous 3.0 T ^{1}H-MRS study reported a higher inter-subject glutamate variability of 15.4%–16.3% in the deep brain area of the amygdala, based on two scans obtained 1 week apart [47]. Another 3.0 T ^{1}H-MRS study of repeated measurements on three consecutive days reported residual measurement error as the main contributor to the glutamate variability in a small hippocampus VOI [48]. Finally, one previous 7.0 T ^{1}H-MRS study reported higher glutamate variability of 11.48% (± 8.87) within day (based on two scans), and 6.56% (± 4.69) between day, measured in the visual cortical area of healthy subjects [49]. However, the study did not report a separate inter-subject and residual measurement error variability [49].

The present study has several major strengths to account for the measurement error variation, as all participants were scanned at fixed time points on each scan day, accounting for possible changes due to the metabolic circadian rhythm [25, 26]. In addition, we maintained identical and stable study conditions for all participants on all three study days, including detailed dietary restrictions before and during the scan sessions. All participants were carefully instructed to avoid any head motion during the scans. However, we cannot exclude the possibility of motion affecting our findings during the scan sessions. We estimated that the high acquisition number for the ^{1}H-MRS sequences was appropriate and feasible to obtain a sufficient signal noise ratio from the spectral VOIs. Additionally, as our primary aim was to investigate and compare relative changes from baseline within subjects, these issues were unlikely to affect our results.

Conclusion

Here we present a protocol for pharmacological ^{1}H-MRS at 3.0 T in the brainstem and thalamus, with good spectral quality, and overall low measurement variability. We demonstrated that sildenafil induces transiently increased glutamate levels in the brainstem, which suggest transiently increased excitability of the brainstem neurons. CGRP does not induce glutamate changes in the brainstem or thalamic neurons, suggesting that its headache-inducing effects are not mediated by biochemical changes in deep brain structures, but rather its effects on the peripheral trigeminal pain pathways.

Abbreviations

^{1}H: proton; CGRP: calcitonin gene-related peptide; CNS: central nervous system; fMRI: functional magnetic resonance imaging; FWHM: full-width of half-maximum; ICHD-3 beta: The diagnostic criteria of the beta version of the third International Classification of Headache Disorders; MRI: magnetic resonance imaging; MRS: magnetic resonance spectroscopy; NAA: *N*-Acetylaspartate; PRESS: point-resolved spectroscopy pulse sequence; SNR: signal-noise-ratio; VOI: volume-of-interest

Funding

We thank the Lundbeck Foundation [grant number R155–2014-171] and the Research Foundation of Rigshospitalet [grant number E-23327-02]. Funding sources played no role in study design, data collection, analysis, interpretation, manuscript preparation, or submission.

Authors' contributions

SY drafted and revised the paper and contributed to study design, protocol development, participant enrolment, acquisition and processing of data, statistical analysis and interpretation of data. AH contributed to study design, protocol development, interpretation of data and revising manuscript for content. CEC contributed to protocol development, participant enrolment, acquisition of data, and revising manuscript for content. MBV contributed to study design, processing of data, statistical analysis, and revising manuscript for content. ETP and OBP contributed to study design and revising manuscript for content. HBWL contributed to study design, protocol development, statistical analysis, and revising manuscript for content. MA initiated the study and contributed to study design, protocol development, data interpretation, and revision of the manuscript. All authors read and approved the final manuscript.

Competing interests

MA reports personal fees from Alder BioPharmaceuticals, Allergan, Amgen, Alder, Eli Lilly, Novartis and Teva. MA participated in clinical trials as the principal investigator for Alder ALD403-CLIN-011 (Phase 3b), Amgen 20,120,178 (Phase 2), 20,120,295 (Phase 2), 20,130,255 (OLE), 20,120,297 (Phase 3), GM-11 gamma-Core-R trials, Novartis CAMG334a2301 (Phase 3b), Amgen PAC1 20,150,308 (Phase 2a), Teva TV48125-CNS-30068 (Phase 3). MA has no ownership interest and does not own stocks of any pharmaceutical company. MA serves as associated editor of Cephalalgia, co-editor of the Journal of Headache and Pain. MA is President-elect of the International Headache Society and General Secretary of the European Headache Federation. The remaining authors report no conflicts of interest.

Author details

[1]Danish Headache Center, Department of Neurology, Rigshospitalet Glostrup, University of Copenhagen, Copenhagen, Denmark. [2]Functional Imaging Unit, Department of Clinical Physiology, Nuclear Medicine and PET, Rigshospitalet Glostrup, University of Copenhagen, Copenhagen, Denmark. [3]Danish Research Centre for Magnetic Resonance, Centre for Functional and Diagnostic Imaging and research, Copenhagen University Hospital Hvidovre, Copenhagen, Denmark. [4]Neurobiology Research Unit, Department of Neurology, Rigshospitalet, University of Copenhagen, Copenhagen, Denmark.

References

1. Kruuse C, Thomsen LL, Jacobsen TB, Olesen J (2002) The phosphodiesterase 5 inhibitor sildenafil has no effect on cerebral blood flow or blood velocity, but nevertheless induces headache in healthy subjects. J Cereb Blood Flow Metab 22:1124–1131
2. Kruuse C, Hansen AE, Larsson HBW, Lauritzen M, Rostrup E (2009) Cerebral haemodynamic response or excitability is not affected by sildenafil. J Cereb Blood Flow Metab 29:830–839
3. Asghar MS, Hansen AE, Kapijimpanga T, van der Geest RJ, van der Koning P, Larsson HBW et al (2010) Dilation by CGRP of middle meningeal artery and reversal by sumatriptan in normal volunteers. Neurology 75:1520–1526
4. Petersen KA, Lassen LH, Birk S, Lesko L, Olesen J (2005) BIBN4096BS antagonizes human alpha-calcitonin gene related peptide-induced headache and extracerebral artery dilatation. Clin Pharmacol Ther 77:202–213
5. Kruuse C, Thomsen LL, Birk S, Olesen J (2003) Migraine can be induced by sildenafil without changes in middle cerebral artery diameter. Brain 126:241–247
6. Lassen LH, Haderslev PA, Jacobsen VB, Iversen HK, Sperling B, Olesen J (2002) CGRP may play a causative role in migraine. Cephalalgia 22:54–61
7. Asghar MS, Hansen AE, Amin FM, van der Geest RJ, Van Der KP, Larsson HBW et al (2011) Evidence for a vascular factor in migraine. Ann Neurol 69:635–645
8. Ashina M, Hansen JM, á Dunga BO, Olesen J (2017) Human models of migraine — short-term pain for long-term gain. Nat Rev Neurol 13:713–724
9. Hoffmann J, Charles A (2018) Glutamate and its receptors as therapeutic targets for migraine. Neurotherapeutics 15:361-370
10. Younis S, Hougaard A, Vestergaard MB, Larsson HBW, Ashina M (2017) Migraine and magnetic resonance spectroscopy : a systematic review. Curr Opin Neurol 30:246–262
11. Weiller C, May A, Limmroth V, Jüptner M, Kaube H, Schayck RV et al (1995) Brain stem activation in spontaneous human migraine attacks. Nat Med 1: 658–660
12. Afridi SK, Matharu MS, Lee L, Kaube H, Friston KJ, Frackowiak RSJ et al (2005) A PET study exploring the laterality of brainstem activation in migraine using glyceryl trinitrate. Brain 128:932–939
13. Stankewitz A, May A (2011) Increased limbic and brainstem activity during migraine attacks following olfactory stimulation. Neurology 77:476–482
14. Hougaard A, Amin FM, Christensen CE, Younis S, Wolfram F, Cramer SP et al (2017) Increased brainstem perfusion, but no blood- brain barrier disruption, during attacks of migraine with aura. Brain 140:1633–1642
15. Afridi SK, Giffin NJ, Kaube H, Friston KJ, Ward NS, Frackowiak RSJ et al (2005) A positron emission tomographic study in spontaneous migraine. Arch Neurol 62:1270–1275

16. Foerster BR, Pomper MG, Callaghan BC, Petrou M, Edden RAE, Mohamed MA et al (2013) An imbalance between excitatory and inhibitory neurotransmitters in amyotrophic lateral sclerosis revealed by use of 3-T proton magnetic resonance spectroscopy. JAMA Neurol 70:1009–1016
17. Baker EH, Basso G, Barker PB, Smith MA, Bonekamp D, Horská A (2010) Regional apparent metabolite concentrations in young adult brain measured by 1H MR spectroscopy at 3 tesla. J Magn Reson Imaging 27: 489–499
18. Adanyeguh IM, Henry P-G, Nguyen TM, Rinaldi D, Jauffret C, Valabregue R et al (2015) In vivo neurometabolic profiling in patients with spinocerebellar ataxia types 1, 2, 3, and 7. Mov Disord 30:662–670
19. Öz G, Tkáč I (2011) Short-echo, single-shot, full-intensity proton magnetic resonance spectroscopy for neurochemical profiling at 4 T: validation in the cerebellum and brainstem. Magn Reson Med 65:901–910
20. Zielman R, Teeuwisse WM, Bakels F, Van der Grond J, Webb A, van Buchem MA et al (2014) Biochemical changes in the brain of hemiplegic migraine patients measured with 7 tesla 1H-MRS. Cephalalgia 34:959–967
21. Eftekhari S, Salvatore CA, Calamari A, Kane SA, Tajti J, Edvinsson L (2010) Differential distribution of calcitonin gene-related peptide and its receptor components in the human trigeminal ganglion. Neuroscience 169:683–696
22. Miller S, Liu H, Warfvinge K, Shi L, Dovlatyan M, Xu C et al (2016) Immunohistochemical localization of the calcitonin gene-related peptide binding site in the primate trigeminovascular system using functional antagonist antibodies. Neuroscience 328:165–183
23. Gómez-Vallejo V, Ugarte A, García-Barroso C, Cuadrado-Tejedor M, Szczupak B, Dopeso-Reyes IG et al (2016) Pharmacokinetic investigation of sildenafil using positron emission tomography and determination of its effect on cerebrospinal fluid cGMP levels. J Neurochem 136:403–415
24. Headache Classification Committee of the International Headache Society (IHS) (2013) The international classification of headache disorders, 3rd edition (beta version). Cephalalgia 33:629–808
25. Peng S-L, Dumas JA, Park DC, Liu P, Filbey FM, McAdams CJ et al (2014) Age-related increase of resting metabolic rate in the human brain. Neuroimage 98:176–183
26. Soreni N, Noseworthy MD, Cormier T, Oakden WK, Bells S, Schachar R (2006) Intraindividual variability of striatal 1H-MRS brain metabolite measurements at 3 T. Magn Reson Imaging 24:187–194
27. Lopez-Rodriguez F, Medina-Ceja L, Wilson CL, Jhung D, Morales-Villagran A (2007) Changes in extracellular glutamate levels in rat orbitofrontal cortex during sleep and wakefulness. Arch Med Res 38:52–55
28. Christiansen P, Henriksen O, Stubgaard M, Gideon P, Larsson HBW (1993) In vivo quantification of brain metabolites by 1H-MRS using water as an internal standard. Magn Reson Imaging 11:107–118
29. Danbolt NC (2001) Glutamate uptake. Prog Neurobiol 65:1–105
30. Hunsberger HC, Konat GW, Reed MN (2017) Peripheral viral challenge elevates extracellular glutamate in the hippocampus leading to seizure hypersusceptibility. J Neurochem 141:341–346
31. Hunsberger HC, Wang D, Petrisko TJ, Alhowail A, Setti SE, Suppiramaniam V et al (2016) Peripherally restricted viral challenge elevates extracellular glutamates and enhances synaptic transmission in the hippocampus. J Neurochem 138:307–316
32. Tkáč I, Öz G, Adriany G, Uğurbil K, Gruetter R (2009) In vivo 1H NMR spectroscopy of the human brain at high magnetic fields: metabolite quantification at 4T vs. 7T. Magn Reson Med 62:868–879
33. Milman HA, Arnold SB (2002) Neurologic, psychological, and aggressive disturbances with sildenafil. Ann Pharmacother 36:1129–1134
34. Moreira SG, Brannigan RE, Spitz A, Orejuela FJ, Lipshultz LI, Kim ED (2000) Side-effect profile of sildenafil citrate (Viagra) in clinical practice. Urology 4295:474–476
35. Schultheiss D, Müller SV, Nager W, Stief CG, Schlote N, Jonas U et al (2001) Central effects of sildenafil (Viagra) on auditory selective attention and verbal recognition memory in humans: a study with event-related brain potentials. World J Urol 19:46–50
36. Nichols DJ, Muirhead GJ, Harness JA (2002) Pharmacokinetics of sildenafil after single oral doses in healthy male subjects: absolute bioavailability, food effects and dose proportionality. Br J Clin Pharmacol 53:5S–12S
37. Mangia S, Giove F, Tkáč I, Logothetis NK, Henry P-G, Olman CA et al (2009) Metabolic and hemodynamic events after changes in neuronal activity: current hypotheses, theoretical predictions and in vivo NMR experimental findings. J Cereb Blood Flow Metab 29:441–463
38. Lemire J, Mailloux RJ, Appanna VD (2008) Mitochondrial lactate dehydrogenase is involved in oxidative-energy metabolism in human astrocytoma cells (CCF-STTG1). PLoS One 3:1–10
39. Lange T, Dydak U, Roberts TPL, Rowley HA, Bjeljac M, Boesiger P (2006) Pitfalls in lactate measurements at 3T. Am J Neuroradiol 27:895–901
40. Petersen KA, Birk S, Lassen LH, Kruuse C, Jonassen O, Lesko L et al (2005) The CGRP-antagonist, BIBN4096BS does not affect cerebral or systemic haemodynamics in healthy volunteers. Cephalalgia 25:139–147
41. Eftekhari S, Salvatore CA, Johansson S, Chen T, Zeng Z, Edvinsson L (2015) Localization of CGRP, CGRP receptor, PACAP and glutamate in trigeminal ganglion. Relation to the blood–brain barrier. Brain Res 1600:93–109
42. Asghar MS, Hansen AE, Larsson HBW, Olesen J, Ashina M (2012) Effect of CGRP and sumatriptan on the BOLD response in visual cortex. J Headache Pain 13:159–166
43. Bednařík P, Tkáč I, Giove F, DiNuzzo M, Deelchand DK, Emir UE et al (2015) Neurochemical and BOLD responses during neuronal activation measured in the human visual cortex at 7 tesla. J Cereb Blood Flow Metab 35:601–610
44. Schaller B, Xin L, O'Brien K, Magill AW, Gruetter R (2014) Are glutamate and lactate increases ubiquitous to physiological activation? A 1H functional MR spectroscopy study during motor activation in human brain at 7 tesla. Neuroimage 93:138–145
45. Asghar MS, Becerra L, Larsson HBW, Borsook D, Ashina M (2016) Calcitonin gene-related peptide modulates heat nociception in the human brain - an fMRI study in healthy volunteers. PLoS One 11:1–20
46. Helms G, Piringer A (2001) Restoration of motion-related signal loss and line-shape deterioration of proton MR spectra using the residual water as intrinsic reference. Magn Reson Med 46:395–400
47. Nacewicz BM, Angelos L, Dalton KM, Fischer R, Anderle MJ, Alexander AL et al (2012) Reliable non-invasive measurement of human neurochemistry using proton spectroscopy with an anatomically defined amygdala-specific voxel. Neuroimage 59:2548–2559
48. Allaïli N, Valabrègue R, Auerbach EJ, Guillemot V, Yahia-Cherif L, Bardinet E et al (2015) Single-voxel 1H spectroscopy in the human hippocampus at 3 T using the LASER sequence: characterization of neurochemical profile and reproducibility. NMR Biomed 28:1209–1217
49. Cai K, Nanga RPR, Lamprou L, Schinstine C, Elliott M, Hariharan H et al (2012) The impact of gabapentin administration on brain GABA and glutamate concentrations: a 7T 1H-MRS study. Neuropsychopharmacology 37:2764–2771

23

Evaluation of gray matter perfusion in episodic migraine using voxel-wise comparison of 3D pseudo-continuous arterial spin labeling

Zhiye Chen[1,2,3†], Xiaoyan Chen[3†], Mengyu Liu[1†], Mengqi Liu[1,2], Lin Ma[1*] and Shengyuan Yu[3*]

Abstract

Background: Although previous studies have demonstrated that structural and functional abnormalities in episodic migraine (EM), less is known about altered brain perfusion in the EM. The aim of this study is to investigate altered gray matter perfusion in EM using a 3D volumetric perfusion imaging.

Methods: Fifteen EM patients and 15 normal controls (NC) underwent structural and 3D pseudo-continuous arterial spin labeling (3D pc-ASL). The structural images were segmented using DARTEL methods and the generated normalized T1 tissue probability maps were used to coregister the cerebral blood flow (CBF) images, which would further be performed with standardization using Fisher Z Transformation. Voxel-wise analysis was applied to CBF map with Z standardization, and the Z value of the abnormal brain region was extracted and performed with correlation with the clinical variables.

Results: The increased CBF value located in the left Brodmann 38 (BA38) and no significantly decreased CBF value were detected in EM. HAMD scores presented significantly positive correlation with the CBF value of the left BA38.

Conclusion: The current study indicated that the pattern of cerebral hyperperfusion may elucidate the neurogenic mechanism in the EM genesis, and 3D pc-ASL technique would non-invasively provide valuable cerebral perfusion information for the further pathophysiological and neuropsychological study in EM.

Keywords: Brain, Episodic migraine, Gray matter, Magnetic resonance imaging, 3D pseudo-continuous arterial spin labeling

Background

Migraine is a common primary headache disorder, which was the second largest contributors of disability-adjusted life-years in the Global Burden of Disease Study [1]. Migraine episodes are characterized classically by unilateral, throbbing headache, frequently associated with nausea, vomiting, photophobia, phonophobia, or allodynia [2]. The pathogenesis of migraine is not completely understood. Cortical spreading depression (CSD) has been considered to account for migraine aura and to be a migraine trigger via trigeminal sensory afferents activation [3]. Cerebral or meningeal vasodilation and potential perivascular release of vasoactive substances may lead to headache generation in migraine [4]. Advanced imaging studies have provided more insights into migraine pathophysiology and migraine-related dysfunctions. The brainstem has been considered to play a pivotal role in the first phase of a migraine attack. Limbic pathways and cognitive processing network have participated in migraine processing. Hyperexcitability of visual cortex and thalamus in migraine may be associated with photophobia and allodynia respectively. Interictal abnormalities such as altered grey volume, white matter lesions, altered

* Correspondence: cjr.malin@vip.163.com; yusy1963@126.com
†Zhiye Chen, Xiaoyan Chen and Mengyu Liu contributed equally to this work.
[1]Department of Radiology, Chinese PLA General Hospital, 28 Fuxing Road, Beijing 100853, China
[3]Department of Neurology, Chinese PLA General Hospital, 28 Fuxing Road, Beijing 100853, China
Full list of author information is available at the end of the article

neural activity and functional connectivity in migraine and their correlation with migraine duration/frequency suggested migraine may be a progressive brain disorder [5, 6]. However, whether the altered structure and function is the cause or the result of migraine attack is still a debate.

Previous perfusion imaging studies using xenon 133 intra-arterial injection method, single photon emission computed tomography (SPECT), CT perfusion, and perfusion-weighted MR imaging (PWI) have been conducted for migraine research. The hypoperfusion during aura in hemisphere contralateral to neural deficit did not fulfill vascular distribution, supporting a neurogenic rather than vascular explanation for migraine aura [7–10]. However, The perfusion status of interictal migraine were inconsistent [11–13]. The previous perfusion studies were generally case reports or small sample-sized, perhaps limited by the radioactivity or contrast of the scanning.

3D pseudo-continuous ASL (3D pc-ASL) was a novel non-enhancement perfusion sequence on MR750 3.0 T(GE Healthcare, Milwaukee, WI, USA). Advantage of this technique included 3D acquisition, spiral k-space filling, FSE pulse sequence and non-invasive labelling technique without MRI contrast injection, which would further expand the clinical application range of ASL. ASL has been adopted for migraine aura and hypoperfusion was detected, consistent with former perfusion studies [14, 15]. However, so far, very few studies used ASL for interictal migraine research and the results differed [16–18].

The aim of this study is detect the pattern of altered cerebral perfusion at interictal stage of episodic migraine (EM) without aura. We prospectively obtained high resolution structural images and 3D pc-ASL images from 15 EM patients and 15 normal controls(NC). Voxel-wise comparison of CBF maps were performed between EM and NC, and the correlation analysis were applied between the CBF values of the abnormal brain regions and the clinical variables.

Methods

Subjects

Fifteen EM patients and 15 normal controls (NC) were recruited from the International Headache Center, Department of Neurology, Chinese PLA General Hospital. The inclusion criteria should be fulfilled as follows: 1) EM is defined as migraine attack days being less than 15 days per month. The definition of migraine refers to 1.1 Migraine without aura in ICHD 3beta [2]; 2) no migraine preventive medication used in the past 3 months; 3) absence of other subtypes of headache, chronic pain other than headache, severe anxiety or depression preceding the onset of headache, psychiatric diseases, etc.; 4) absence of alcohol, nicotine, or other substance abuse; and 5) patient's willingness to engage in the study. NCs were recruited from the hospital's staff and their relatives. Inclusion criteria were similar to those of patients, except for the first items. NCs should never have had any primary headache disorders or other types of headache in the past year. The exclusion criteria were the following: cranium trauma, illness interfering with central nervous system function, psychotic disorder, and regular use of a psychoactive or hormone medication. General demographic and headache information were entered in our headache database. All the patients were given with the Visual Analogue Scale (VAS) and the migraine disability assessment scale (MIDAS), and all the subjects received anxiety and depression evaluation by using the Hamilton Anxiety Scale (HAMA) [19], the Hamilton Depression Scale (HAMD) [20], respectively.

The study protocols were approved by the Ethical Committee of Chinese PLA General Hospital and complied with the Declaration of Helsinki. Written informed consent was obtained from all participants according to the approval of the ethics committee of the local institutional review board. MRI scans were taken in the interictal stage at least three days after a migraine attack for EM patients. All the subjects were right-handed and underwent conventional MRI examination to exclude the subjects with cerebral infarction, malacia, or occupying lesions. Alcohol, nicotine, caffeine, and other substances were avoided for at least 12 h before MRI examination.

MRI acquisition

Images were acquired on a GE 3.0 T MR system (DISCOVERY MR750, GE Healthcare, Milwaukee, WI, USA) and a conventional eight-channel quadrature head coil was used. All subjects were instructed to lie in a supine position, and formed padding was used to limit head movement. The structural images were acquired by a three-dimensional T1-weighted fast spoiled gradient recalled echo (3D T1-FSPGR) sequence generating 360 contiguous axial slices [TR (repetition time) = 7.0 ms, TE (echo time) = 3.0 ms, flip angle = 15°, FOV (field of view) = 25.6 cm × 25.6 cm, Matrix = 256 × 256, NEX (number of acquisition) = 1]. Volumetric perfusion imaging was obtained using a pseudo-continuous ASL tagging scheme with a 3D interleaved spiral FSE readout (3D spiral FSE ASL) with parameters as: TR/TE = 5128/15.9 ms, flip angle = 111°, FOV = 20 cm × 20 cm, x, y matrix = 1024 × 8 (spiral acquisition), slice thickness = 3.0 mm. The labeling duration was 1.5 s, and post-labeling delay time (PLD) was 1.5 s.Oblique axial T2-weighted imaging (T2WI), T1 fluid-attenuated inversion recovery (T1-FLAIR) and diffusion weighted imaging (DWI) were also acquired. All imaging protocols were identical for all subjects. No obvious structural damage and T2-visible lesion were observed on the conventional MR images.

MR image processing

Generating CBF maps

3D pc-ASL data, including perfusion weighted images and proton density-weighted images, was processed using Functional tools (version:9.4.05) on GE Advanced Workstation 4.5. Fifty axial CBF images were acquired based on the following equation according to the reported lieratures [21–26]:

$$f = \frac{\lambda}{2\alpha T_{1b}(1-e^{\frac{\tau}{T_{1b}}})} \frac{(s_{con} \; - \; S_{lbe})(1-e^{\frac{t_{sat}}{T_{1g}}})}{S_{ref}} e^{\frac{w}{T_{1b}}}$$

f, flow; $\lambda = 0.9$ (brain–blood partition coefficient); $\alpha = 0.85$ (labeling efficiency); $T_{1b} = 1.6$ s (the T1 value ofblood); $T_{1g} = 1.2$ s (the T1 value of gray matter); $\tau = 1.5$ s (labeling duration); S_{con}, S_{lbe} and S_{ref}, the singnal of control, label and reference images, respectively; $t_{sat} = 2$ s (the saturation time for proton density images); w, post-labeling delay.

3D structural segmentation and CBF maps normalization

All MR image data were processed using Statistical Parametric Mapping 12 (SPM 12) (http://www.fil.ion.ucl.ac.uk/spm/) running under MATLAB 7.6 (The Mathworks, Natick, MA, USA) to perform structural segment [27] and CBF maps normalization [28, 29]. The image processing included following steps: (1) The structural images were segmented into grayand white matter tissue probability maps (GM-TPM and WM-TPM) using DARTEL methods, which simultaneously generated the normalized T1 tissue probabilitymaps (T1-TPM); (2) All the T1-TPM wereused to generate average T1-TPM and further generate brain mask; (3) The individual CBF maps were spatially normalize into standard Montreal Neurologic Institute (MNI) stereotaxic space by coregistering with the individual T1-TPM and resampled into $1.5 \times 1.5 \times 1.5$ mm^3 isotropic size, which would generated individual normalized CBF maps (nCBF); (4) The individual nCBF maps were warped by the brain mask to extract brain tissue; (5) The individual normalized CBF maps with brain extraction (bet_nCBF)were performed Z transformation to avoid individual hemodynamic variation, and spatially smoothed with a 6-mm isotropic Gaussian kernel (Fig. 1).

All the individual GM-TPM (including EM and NC) were used to generate customized GM template using DARTEL tool software package. The customized GM template was transformed as GM mask (Fig. 2), which

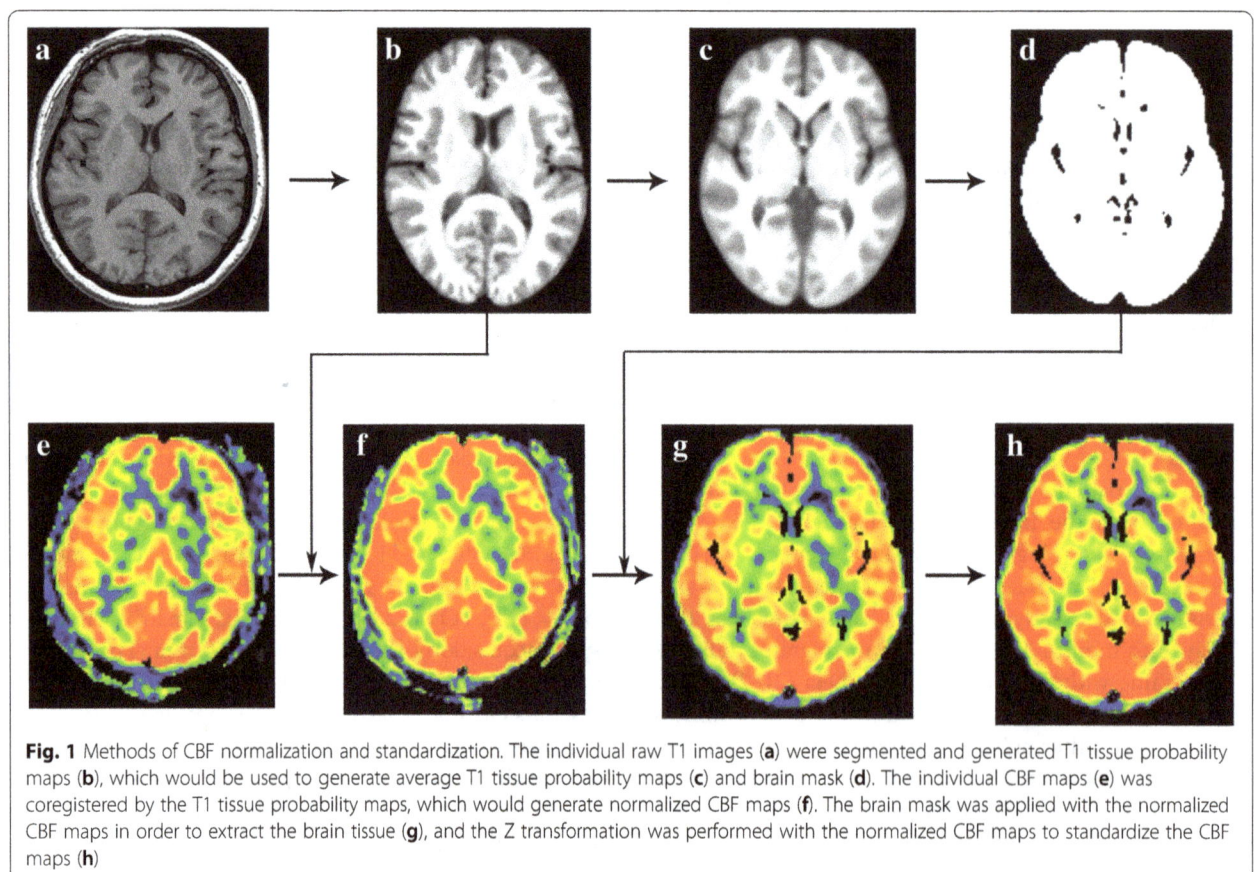

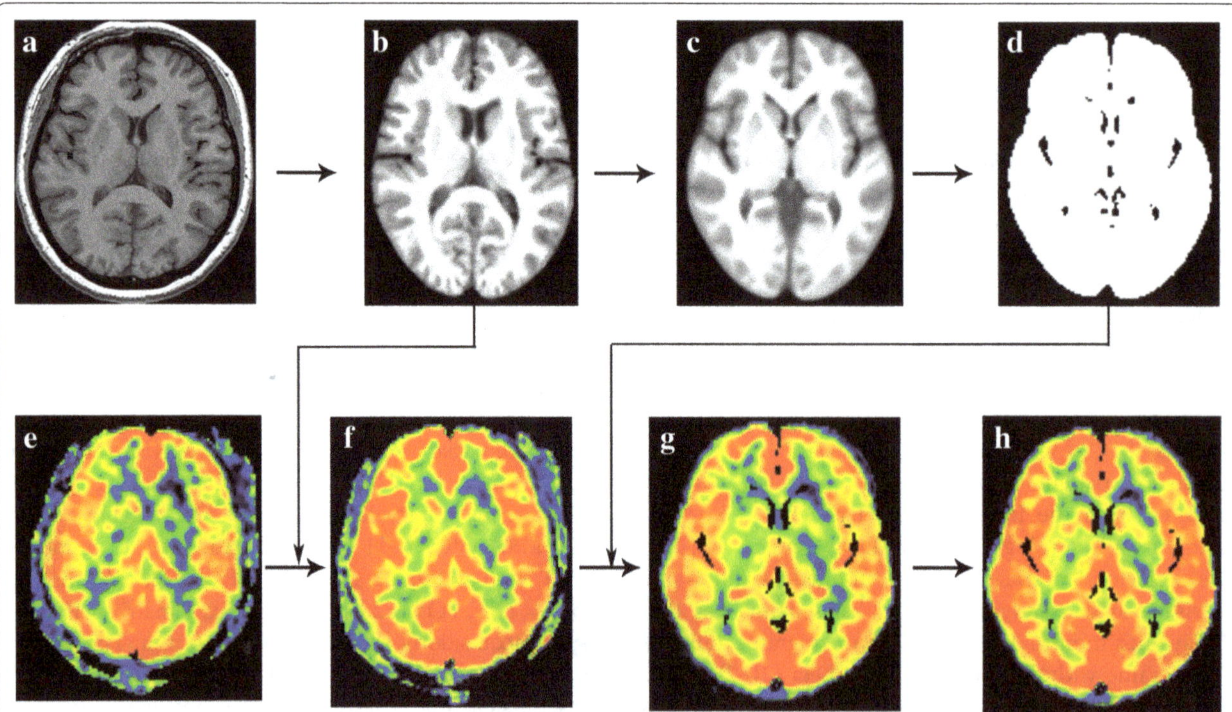

Fig. 1 Methods of CBF normalization and standardization. The individual raw T1 images (**a**) were segmented and generated T1 tissue probability maps (**b**), which would be used to generate average T1 tissue probability maps (**c**) and brain mask (**d**). The individual CBF maps (**e**) was coregistered by the T1 tissue probability maps, which would generate normalized CBF maps (**f**). The brain mask was applied with the normalized CBF maps in order to extract the brain tissue (**g**), and the Z transformation was performed with the normalized CBF maps to standardize the CBF maps (**h**)

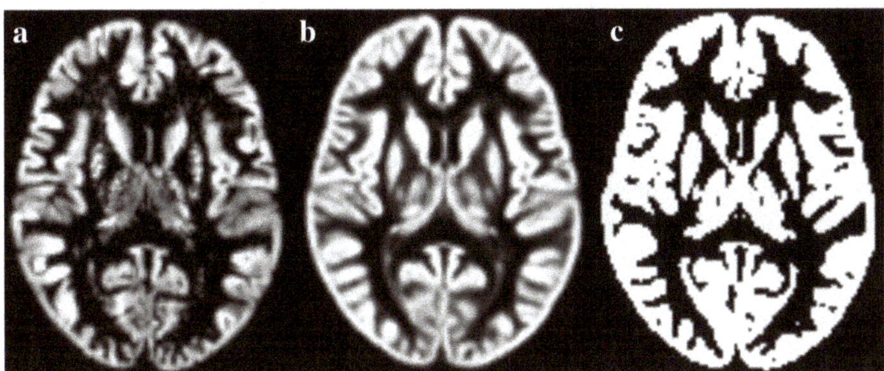

Fig. 2 The generation of customized gray matter mask. **a**, individual gray matter tissue probability maps; **b**, customized gray matter template; **c**, customized gray matter mask

was used as an explicit mask in the voxel-based analysis for 3D pc-ASL data.

Statistical analysis

The statistical analysis was performed by using PASW Statistics 18.0. The data with non-normal distribution presented by median (minimum, maximum) and the data with normal distribution presented as mean ± standard deviation. The quantitative data (including age, HAMA, HAMD) was performed with independent samples T test, and the qualitative data (including sex) was applied with Chi-Square test. The Pearson correlation was performed with the data with normal distribution, and the Spearman correlation was performed with the data with non-normal distribution. Significant difference was set at a P value of < 0.05.

Voxel-wise comparison of volumetric perfusion was performed by the SPM 12 software. The factorial design was set as Two-sample t-test with age and sex as covariates. The customized gray matter mask was selected as the explicit mask, and all the voxels in the customized gray matter mask were performed with voxel-wise comparison. The minimal number of contiguous voxels was based on the expected cluster size.

Results

Demography and neuropsychological test

The current study included 15 EM patients (F/M = 11/4) and 15 NC (F/M = 11/4). The age (EM, 32 ± 10.62 years old; NC, 38 ± 9.56 years old) and sex presented no significant difference between EM and NC. The headache variables of EM were listed as follows: the disease duration 10(0.5,21) years, headache frequence 3(1,10) per month, the mean interictal time 10.27 ± 4.73 days after last migraine attack at scanning, VAS 8(6,10), sleep quality 1(0,3) and MIDAS 11.53 ± 12.44. The HAMA and HAMD score significantly increased in EM patients (16.13 ± 10.51 and 15.73 ± 2.91, respectively) compared with that in NC (9.73 ± 3.39 and 11.4 ± 7.52, respectively) (P = 0.001 and 0.000, respectively).

Comparison of gray matter perfusion between EM and NC

The brain region with increased perfusion located in the left Brodmann 38 (BA38) (the left superior temporal) (MNI coordinate, 57 5–2; P_{uncorr} value, 0.000; cluster size, 143) (Fig. 3). There was no significant decreased perfusion in EM compared with NC.

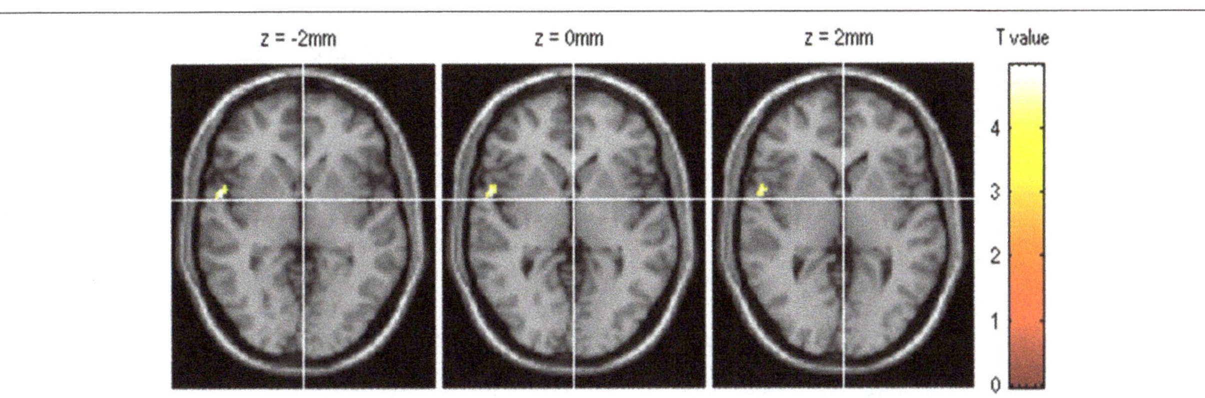

Fig. 3 The brain region with hyperperfusion located in the left superior temporal (BA 38)in EM patients compared with NC

Correlation analysis between CBF value of positive brain regions and clinical variables

HAMD scores were positively related with the CBF value of the left BA38 ($r = 0.529$, P value = 0.043). The other clinical variables, including VAS scores, disease duration, MIDAS score, headache frequency, sleep quality and HAMA scores, showed no significant correlation with the CBF value of the left BA38 (Table 1).

Discussion

This study adopted 3D pc-ASL, a novel non-enhancement perfusion sequence to detect the pattern of altered cerebral perfusion in interictal phase of EM in a China headache center. By this method, we found increased perfusion in the left BA38 (the left superior temporal) in EM compared with NC and a positive correlation of HAMD scores with the CBF value of the left BA38.

Perfusion imaging studies have been conducted for migraine research for decades. For migraine with aura (MA), hypoperfusion during aura in hemisphere with posterior predominance contralateral to neural deficit was usually detected by using xenon 133 intra-arterial injection method [10],single photon emission computed tomography (SPECT) [7], CT perfusion [9], perfusion-weighted MR imaging (PWI) [8], and ASL [8, 14, 15] followed by hyperperfusion at headache phase [7, 10, 14]. For prolonged hemiplegic migraine, hemispheric hyperperfusion [30] and normal perfusion [31] have also been observed using PWI method. The perfusion status during headache attack of migraine without aura (MO) varied more [32, 33], which may largely depend on when the imaging is done and the course of the migraine attack.

The interictal perfusion studies varied too. One study using 133Xe inhalation method showed that a derangement of the cerebral perfusion was present in both MA and MO, suggesting they were due to the same disease process [12] while another study only found abnormal mean hemispheric blood flows or disturbed intra-hemispheric rCBF patterns in MA rather than MO [13].Later studies using SPECT found decreased CBF in patients at interictal phase of MA, which often corresponded to the site of headache and the topography of transient neurological symptoms [34, 35]. In a recent study using PWI, interictal hyperperfusion was observed in the inferior and middle temporal gyrus in MO patients, hypoperfusion was seen in the postcentral gyrus and in the inferior temporal gyrus in MA patients and in the inferior frontal gyrus in MO patients [11].A research group using pc-ASL found increased rCBF within the primary somatosensory cortex (S1) in adult migraineurs as well as in pediatric and young adult migraineurs [17]. However, other two ASL studies did not find differences in resting CBF between MA, MO and NC [16, 18].

Table 1 Correlation analysis between the CBF value of the brain region with hyperperfusion and the clinical variables

	Left BA38	
	r value	*P* value
VAS[a]	− 0.479	0.071
DD[a]	−0.333	0.225
MIDAS[b]	−0.082	0.772
HF[a]	0.093	0.742
SQ[a]	0.462	0.083
HAMA[b]	−0.286	0.302
HAMD[b]	0.529	0.043
MoCA[a]	0.422	0.117

VAS visual analogue scale, *DD* disease duration (years), *MIDAS* migraine disability assessment scale, *HF* headache frequency (per month), *SQ* sleep quality, *HAMA* Hamilton Anxiety Scale, *HAMD*, Hamilton Depression Scale, *MoCA* Montreal Cognitive Assessment.[a], Spearman correlation analysis, [b], Pearson correlation analysis

Most of previous perfusion studies were case reports and few were small cohorts. The diversity of disease severity and accompanied disorders, the scanning methods and timing of examination may lead to the inconsistency of perfusion studies at headache and interictal phase. Compared to the earlier perfusion techniques for migraine research using xenon 133 intra-arterial injection, SPECT, CT perfusion, PET, newer techniques using PWI and ASL have advantages in superior spatial resolution, increased sensitivity, and being nonradioactive. ASL has advantages over PWI in that no contrast is needed [36, 37] and has high spatial resolution. Therefore, ASL may be an ideal technique for migraine research since repeated ASL can be acquired during each phase of migraine attack without harm to patients.

Areas with altered interictal perfusion may reflect local interictal differences in neuronal metabolism or activity, or the presence of some degree of interictal cerebrovascular dysregulation in migraineurs [11].Like some previous perfusion studies, this study observed regional CBF alteration in interictal phase of MO which did not fulfill vascular distribution, supporting that migraine was a primary neurogenic disorder. In this study, we found only one brain region with hyperperfusion: left BA38(the left superior temporal gyrus) in EM patients.

The left BA38 is located in temporal pole(TP), which is supposed to be a convergence zone integrating information from auditory, somato-sensorimotor, visual, olfactory, language, paralimbic structures and default-semantic network, suggesting its participation in autonomic regulation, multisensory, memory, and emotional processing [38]. Neuroimaging studies have provided much evidence supporting an important role of TP in migraine pathophysiology. Gray matter density within left TP significantly decreased interictally and increased ictally for MO compared with NC [39], implicating a key role in cyclical recurrence of migraine attacks. The TP was hyperexcitable with painful heat stimulation and showed increased resting-state connectivity with hypothalamic in interictal migraine patients, indicating that TP may be involved in the interictal hypersensitivity to pain, smell and light [40, 41].In another fMRI study, increased average regional homogeneity values in TP showed significantly positive correlations with disease duration of MO [42]. During odour stimulation in a H(2)(15)O-PET study, migraineurs showed significantly higher activation than controls in the left TP, suggesting a role in olfactory hypersensitivity of migraine [43].A recent study found that enhancing excitability of the TP with non-invasive anodal transcranial direct current stimulation normalized abnormal interictal visual information processing in migraineurs [44], supporting TP as a possible therapeutic target to relieve hypersensitivity of migraine. Our study further provides evidence of TP perfusion abnormality in interictal migraine and this structure needs deeper investigation. TP and superior temporal gyrus have been shown to be involved in major depressive disorders [45, 46]. In our study, the hyperperfusion of left BA38 and its positive correlation with HAMD may be associated with the genesis of multisensory hypersensitivity and mood disorder of migraine.

The interictal perfusion alteration in this study supported migraine as a central nervous dysfunction and may provide biomarkers for migraine diagnosis and treatment. The mechanism of how the perfusion in this region changed is still unknown and needs to be further investigated. In addition to the alteration of the left BA38 as reported by this study, previous interictal studies usually found volume and functional alteration in brain stem, thalamus, anterior cingulate cortex, insula, prefrontal cortex, etc., indicating the involvement of multiple brain regions in migraine processing network [5, 6]. However, we did not find perfusion changes in those regions. Aa a matter of fact, the perfusion may not necessarily change in consistent with grey volume or neural function [47].

This study has some limitations. Firstly, we only included MO patients in interictal phase, thus we could not speculate whether there's difference of the interictal brain between MO and MA patients. Secondly, we only scanned once for a patient and the dynamic perfusion changes during different phase of a migraine attack and post-attack were not presented. In the future, we may repeatedly scan migraine patients at more timing points. Thirdly, the sample size was not large enough, thus we did not analyze the influence to positive brain areas by some clinical parameters such as headache laterality and headache-free time. Lastly, masking of the CBF maps with the segmented T1 image did not sufficiently address the issue of partial volume correction (PVC) in ASL data because of the sensitive to noise and errors in the partial volume estimates, and the further advanced PVC methods should be performed to balance the spatial and smooth effect in the PV estimates [48].

Conclusion

In conclusion, this study revealed that the interictal hyperperfusion in left temporal pole and vlPFC may reflect the neural metabolism abnormality regarding multi-dimensional pain processing in migraine. The pattern of cerebral hyperperfusion at interictal migraine may elucidate the neurogenic mechanism in the EM genesis. 3D pc-ASL technique would non-invasively provide valuable cerebral perfusion information for the further pathophysiological and neuropsychological study in EM.

Abbreviations

3D pc-ASL: 3D pseudo-continuous arterial spin labeling; BA38: Brodmann 38; bet_nCBF: normalized CBF maps with brain extraction; CBF: cerebral blood flow; EM: episodic migraine; GM-TPM: gray matter tissue probability map; HAMA: Hamilton Anxiety Scale; HAMD: Hamilton Depression Scale; MA: migraine with aura; MIDAS: migraine disability assessment scale; MO: migraine without aura; NC: normal controls; nCBF: normalized CBF maps; PWI: perfusion-weighted imaging; SPECT: single photon emission computed tomography; T1-TPM: T1 tissue probability maps; TP: temporal pole; VAS: visual analogue scale; WM-TPM: white matter tissue probability map

Funding

This work was supported by supported by Hainan Provincial Natural Science Foundation of China (818MS153), the Special Financial Grant from the China Postdoctoral Science Foundation (2014 T70960), the Foundation for Medical and health Sci & Tech innovation Project of Sanya (2016YW37),and the Nursery Fund of Chinese PLA General Hospital(12KMM39).

Authors' contributions

Category 1: (a) Conception and Design: LM; SYY. (b) Acquisition of Data: ZYC; MQL; MYL; XYC. (c) Analysis and Interpretation of Data: ZYC, MQL. MYL; Category 2: (a) Drafting the Article: ZYC, XYC. (b) Revising It for Intellectual Content: LM; SYY. All authors read and approved the final manuscript.

Competing interests

The authors declare that they have no competing interests.

Author details

[1]Department of Radiology, Chinese PLA General Hospital, 28 Fuxing Road, Beijing 100853, China. [2]Department of Radiology, Hainan Branch of Chinese PLA General Hospital, Beijing 100853, China. [3]Department of Neurology, Chinese PLA General Hospital, 28 Fuxing Road, Beijing 100853, China.

References

1. Group GBDNDC (2017) Global, regional, and national burden of neurological disorders during 1990-2015: a systematic analysis for the global burden of disease study 2015. Lancet Neurol 16:877–897
2. Headache Classification Committee of the International Headache S (2013) The international classification of headache disorders, 3rd edition (beta version). Cephalalgia 33:629–808
3. Eikermann-Haerter K, Ayata C (2010) Cortical spreading depression and migraine. Curr Neurol Neurosci Rep 10:167–173
4. Asghar MS, Hansen AE, Amin FM, van der Geest RJ, Koning P, Larsson HB et al (2011) Evidence for a vascular factor in migraine. Ann Neurol 69:635–645
5. Lakhan SE, Avramut M, Tepper SJ (2013) Structural and functional neuroimaging in migraine: insights from 3 decades of research. Headache 53:46–66
6. Russo A, Silvestro M, Tedeschi G, Tessitore A (2017) Physiopathology of migraine: what have we learned from functional imaging? Curr Neurol Neurosci Rep. 17:95
7. Cheng MF, Wu YW, Tang SC (2010) Cerebral perfusion changes in hemiplegic migraine: illustrated by Tc-99m ECD brain perfusion scan. Clin Nucl Med 35:456–458
8. Kim S, Kang M, Choi S (2016) A case report of sporadic hemiplegic migraine associated cerebral hypoperfusion: comparison of arterial spin labeling and dynamic susceptibility contrast perfusion MR imaging. Eur J Pediatr 175:295–298
9. Martinez E, Moreno R, Lopez-Mesonero L, Vidriales I, Ruiz M, Guerrero AL, Telleria JJ (2016) Familial hemiplegic migraine with severe attacks: a new report with ATP1A2 mutation. Case Rep Neurol Med 2016:3464285
10. Norris JW, Hachinski VC, Cooper PW (1975) Changes in cerebral blood flow during a migraine attack. Br Med J 3:676–677
11. Arkink EB, Bleeker EJ, Schmitz N, Schoonman GG, Wu O, Ferrari MD et al (2012) Cerebral perfusion changes in migraineurs: a voxelwise comparison of interictal dynamic susceptibility contrast MRI measurements. Cephalalgia 32:279–288
12. Cavestri R, Arreghini M, Longhini M, Ferrarini F, Gori D, Ubbiali A et al (1995) Interictal abnormalities of regional cerebral blood flow in migraine with and without aura. Minerva Med 86:257–264
13. Lagreze HL, Dettmers C, Hartmann A (1988) Abnormalities of interictal cerebral perfusion in classic but not common migraine. Stroke 19:1108–1111
14. Burns R, De Malherbe M, Chadenat ML, Pico F, Buch D (2017) Arterial spin-labeled MR imaging detecting biphasic neurovascular changes in migraine with persistent Aura. Headache 57:1627–1628
15. Cadiot D, Longuet R, Bruneau B, Treguier C, Carsin-Vu A, Corouge I, et al. (2017) Magnetic resonance imaging in children presenting migraine with aura: association of hypoperfusion detected by arterial spin labelling and vasospasm on MR angiography findings. Cephalalgia. https://doi.org/10.1177/0333102417723570
16. Datta R, Aguirre GK, Hu S, Detre JA, Cucchiara B (2013) Interictal cortical hyperresponsiveness in migraine is directly related to the presence of aura. Cephalalgia 33:365–374
17. Youssef AM, Ludwick A, Wilcox SL, Lebel A, Peng K, Colon E et al (2017) In child and adult migraineurs the somatosensory cortex stands out ... Again: an arterial spin labeling investigation. Hum Brain Mapp 38:4078–4087
18. Zhang Q, Datta R, Detre JA, Cucchiara B (2017) White matter lesion burden in migraine with aura may be associated with reduced cerebral blood flow. Cephalalgia 37:517–524
19. Maier W, Buller R, Philipp M, Heuser I (1988) The Hamilton anxiety scale: reliability, validity and sensitivity to change in anxiety and depressive disorders. J Affect Disord 14:61–68
20. Hamilton M (1967) Development of a rating scale for primary depressive illness. Br J Soc Clin Psychol 6:278–296
21. Jarnum H, Steffensen EG, Knutsson L, Frund ET, Simonsen CW, Lundbye-Christensen S et al (2010) Perfusion MRI of brain tumours: a comparative study of pseudo-continuous arterial spin labelling and dynamic susceptibility contrast imaging. Neuroradiology 52:307–317
22. Alsop DC, Detre JA (1996) Reduced transit-time sensitivity in noninvasive magnetic resonance imaging of human cerebral blood flow. J Cereb Blood Flow Metab 16:1236–1249
23. Wang J, Zhang Y, Wolf RL, Roc AC, Alsop DC, Detre JA (2005) Amplitude-modulated continuous arterial spin-labeling 3.0-T perfusion MR imaging with a single coil: feasibility study. Radiology 235:218–228
24. Garcia DM, Duhamel G, Alsop DC (2005) Efficiency of inversion pulses for background suppressed arterial spin labeling. Magn Reson Med 54:366–372
25. Dai W, Garcia D, de Bazelaire C, Alsop DC (2008) Continuous flow-driven inversion for arterial spin labeling using pulsed radio frequency and gradient fields. Magn Reson Med 60:1488–1497
26. Herscovitch P, Raichle ME (1985) What is the correct value for the brain–blood partition coefficient for water? J Cereb Blood Flow Metab 5:65–69
27. Ashburner J, Friston KJ (2000) Voxel-based morphometry–the methods. NeuroImage 11:805–821
28. Hu F, Li T, Wang Z, Zhang S, Wang X, Zhou H et al (2017) Use of 3D-ASL and VBM to analyze abnormal changes in brain perfusion and gray areas in nasopharyngeal carcinoma patients undergoing radiotherapy. Biomed Res 28:7879–7885
29. Kaneta T, Katsuse O, Hirano T, Ogawa M, Shihikura-Hino A, Yoshida K et al (2017) Voxel-wise correlations between cognition and cerebral blood flow using arterial spin-labeled perfusion MRI in patients with Alzheimer's disease: a cross-sectional study. BMC Neurol 17:91
30. Mourand I, Menjot de Champfleur N, Carra-Dalliere C, Le Bars E, Roubertie A, Bonafe A, Thouvenot E (2012) Perfusion-weighted MR imaging in persistent hemiplegic migraine. Neuroradiology 54:255–260
31. Gutschalk A, Kollmar R, Mohr A, Henze M, Ille N, Schwaninger M et al (2002) Multimodal functional imaging of prolonged neurological deficits in a patient suffering from familial hemiplegic migraine. Neurosci Lett 332:115–118
32. Gil-Gouveia R, Pinto J, Figueiredo P, Vilela PF, Martins IP (2017) An arterial spin labeling MRI perfusion study of migraine without Aura attacks. Front Neurol 8:280
33. Kato Y, Araki N, Matsuda H, Ito Y, Suzuki C (2010) Arterial spin-labeled MRI study of migraine attacks treated with rizatriptan. J Headache Pain 11:255–258
34. Calandre EP, Bembibre J, Arnedo ML, Becerra D (2002) Cognitive disturbances and regional cerebral blood flow abnormalities in migraine patients: their relationship with the clinical manifestations of the illness. Cephalalgia 22:291–302
35. Schlake HP, Bottger IG, Grotemeyer KH, Husstedt IW, Vollet B, Schober O, Brune GG (1990) Single photon emission computed tomography with technetium-99m hexamethyl propylenamino oxime in the pain-free interval of migraine and cluster headache. Eur Neurol 30:153–156
36. Aksoy FG, Lev MH (2000) Dynamic contrast-enhanced brain perfusion imaging: technique and clinical applications. Semin Ultrasound CT MR 21:462–477
37. Alsop DC, Detre JA, Golay X, Gunther M, Hendrikse J, Hernandez-Garcia L et al (2015) Recommended implementation of arterial spin-labeled perfusion MRI for clinical applications: a consensus of the ISMRM perfusion study group and the European consortium for ASL in dementia. Magn Reson Med 73:102–116
38. Pascual B, Masdeu JC, Hollenbeck M, Makris N, Insausti R, Ding SL, Dickerson BC (2015) Large-scale brain networks of the human left temporal pole: a functional connectivity MRI study. Cereb Cortex 25:680–702
39. Coppola G, Di Renzo A, Tinelli E, Iacovelli E, Lepre C, Di Lorenzo C et al (2015) Evidence for brain morphometric changes during the migraine cycle: a magnetic resonance-based morphometry study. Cephalalgia 35:783–791
40. Moulton EA, Becerra L, Johnson A, Burstein R, Borsook D (2014) Altered hypothalamic functional connectivity with autonomic circuits and the locus coeruleus in migraine. PLoS One 9:e95508
41. Moulton EA, Becerra L, Maleki N, Pendse G, Tully S, Hargreaves R et al (2011) Painful heat reveals hyperexcitability of the temporal pole in interictal and ictal migraine states. Cerebral cortex (New York NY : 1991) (21):435–448
42. Zhao L, Liu J, Dong X, Peng Y, Yuan K, Wu F et al (2013) Alterations in regional homogeneity assessed by fMRI in patients with migraine without aura stratified by disease duration. J Headache Pain. 14:85
43. Demarquay G, Royet JP, Mick G, Ryvlin P (2008) Olfactory hypersensitivity in migraineurs: a H(2)(15)O-PET study. Cephalalgia 28:1069–1080
44. Cortese F, Pierelli F, Bove I, Di Lorenzo C, Evangelista M, Perrotta A et al (2017) Anodal transcranial direct current stimulation over the left temporal pole restores normal visual evoked potential habituation in interictal migraineurs. J Headache Pain. 18:70
45. Peng J, Liu J, Nie B, Li Y, Shan B, Wang G, Li K (2011) Cerebral and cerebellar gray matter reduction in first-episode patients with major depressive disorder: a voxel-based morphometry study. Eur J Radiol 80:395–399
46. Takahashi T, Yucel M, Lorenzetti V, Walterfang M, Kawasaki Y, Whittle S et al (2010) An MRI study of the superior temporal subregions in patients with current and past major depression. Prog Neuro-Psychopharmacol Biol Psychiatry 34:98–103

Use and overuse of triptans in Austria – a survey based on nationwide healthcare claims data

Karin Zebenholzer[1*], Walter Gall[2] and Christian Wöber[1]

Abstract

Background: To evaluate triptan use and overuse as well as prescription patterns in Austria based on a nationwide healthcare database because data on triptan use and overuse in Austria is missing.

Methods: We included all persons insured with one of 19 Austrian social security institutions in 2007. Inclusion criteria comprised an age of 18–99 years, known sex, and receipt of insurance benefits. We defined triptan use as ≥1 package of a triptan dispensed in 2007 and triptan overuse as ≥30 defined daily doses dispensed in at least one quarter.

Results: Out of 8.295 million inhabitants in Austria, 7,426,412 persons (89.5%) were insured with a social insurance carrier and 5,918,487 persons of those insured (79.7%) fulfilled the inclusion criteria. Among the latter 33,062 persons (0,56%) were triptan users and 1970 (0.033%) were triptan overusers. The estimated proportion of persons with migraine using a triptan was less than 6%. Among users 5.9% were overusers of whom 55% overused triptans in ≥2 quarters of 2007. The median number of days of sick-leave was higher in triptan users than in non-users: due to any reason of sick-leave 12 vs. 10, $p < 0.001$, due to migraine 3 vs. 2, $p < 0.001$. The proportion of hospital admissions did not differ between triptan users and non-users.

Conclusion: The rate of triptan use is low in Austria but triptan users are at risk for triptan overuse. In triptan users more days of sick-leave and the same proportion of hospital admissions as in the older non-users suggest poorer health.

Keywords: Triptan, Migraine, Medication overuse headache, Triptan overuse

Background

Migraine shows one-year prevalence rates of 10–18% and is associated with a substantial burden [1]. In the Global Burden of Disease Study, migraine was the second most common disorder after tension-type headache and the second largest contributor to disability-adjusted life years (DALYs) after stroke [2]. Annual direct and indirect costs per person caused by migraine were estimated at 1222 Euros rising to 3700 Euros in chronic migraine in 2008 and 2009 [3, 4]. These costs are largely due to sick leave and presenteeism [3].

The management of migraine comprises treatment of acute attacks and prophylaxis. Acute migraine attacks are treated with analgesics, nonsteroidal anti-inflammatory drugs (NSAIDS), or triptans [5]. Triptans are selective serotonin agonists acting at 5-HT1B/1D receptors. Non-pharmacological and pharmacological prophylaxis is required in patients with three or more migraine attacks per month [5]. It is particularly important in patients with frequent use of acute migraine medication to prevent medication overuse headache which affects approximately 1% of the general population [6]. In specialized headache centres in Austria more than 40% of the patients with chronic headache had (probable) medication overuse headache [7].

Furthermore, the management of migraine requires considering comorbidities such as depression and anxiety disorders [8]. Their prevalence in patients with migraine was estimated two to 10 times that of the general population with higher rates in chronic migraine [8]. Depression and anxiety have a negative impact on

* Correspondence: karin.zebenholzer@meduniwien.ac.at
[1]Department of Neurology, Medical University of Vienna, Waehringer Guertel 18-20, 1090 Vienna, Austria
Full list of author information is available at the end of the article

migraine [8, 9], and the use of antidepressants was reported in 4–49% of the patients with migraine [10–12]. Persons using triptans together with serotonergic antidepressants or other serotonergic drugs may be at risk of a serotonin syndrome [13].

In previous pharmacoepidemiological studies, the proportion of triptan users was low whereas triptan overuse was not uncommon: In recent studies from the Netherlands, Italy, and France the proportion of triptan users ranged from 0.7–2.3% of the examined populations of whom 3.3–10% were overusers [10, 14, 15]. Older studies reported triptan use in 0.55–1.4% of the populations and overuse in 0.9–14.3% of the users [16–20]. However, these older studies were restricted to certain regions or certain insurance requirements or were based on pharmacies' datasets.

In Austria, data on the use and overuse of triptans is missing. A nationwide research database allowed to overcome this lack of information. The General Approach for Patient-oriented outpatient-based Diagnosis Related Groups (GAP-DRG) database of the Main Association of Austrian Social Security Institutions (Hauptverband der Österreichischen Sozialversicherungsträger) provides anonymous data on dispensed drugs, sex, age, and other details for particular years. The database covers the vast majority of Austria's population as each inhabitant, with minor exceptions, has to be insured with a social security institution. The responsible carrier is set by law and cannot be chosen freely. We used the GAP-DRG database to assess the use and overuse of triptans and to explore differences between the nine provinces as well as between urban and rural regions. In addition, we analysed the prescription of migraine prophylactics, antidepressants, and serotonergic drugs, as well as sick leave and hospital admissions in non-users of triptans and users with and without triptan overuse.

Methods

The study was approved by the ethics committee of the Medical University of Vienna. In order to analyse triptans and co-medications dispensed in 2007, we used the GAP-DRG database which includes data from 19 social security institutions in Austria. The analysis was based on prescriptions billed by pharmacies to the social security institutions. The GAP-DRG database includes all prescriptions covered by the insurances. For each package dispensed in 2007, the patients had to pay a prescription charge which was 4.70 Euros. The database does not include over-the-counter medication and prescription medication paid by the patients from their own pocket or dispensed free of charge to patients with severe chronic diseases or low income.

Characteristics of subjects

For each insured person the following descriptors were available: anonymized unique identifiers of the patient receiving the drug and of the prescribing physician, the patients' date of birth and sex, the postal code of her/his physical address, the Anatomical Therapeutic Chemical code (ATC) and the pharmacy article identifier of the dispensed drug (Pharmazentralnummer), the number of packages, details of sick leave (date and diagnosis) as well as the number of hospital admissions.

Triptan use and overuse

We identified triptans and other medications by the ATC code and package size (units per package), dose per unit, and route of administration by the pharmacy article identifier. The first prescription of a triptan must be made by a neurologist; further prescriptions can be done by general practitioners and other physicians. In 2007, sumatriptan tablets, zolmitriptan tablets, melting tablets as well as nasal spray, eletriptan, and frovatriptan were available and reimbursed. Rizatriptan, naratriptan, sumatriptan injections, and sumatriptan suppositories were available but reimbursed in exceptional cases only. Sumatriptan nasal spray and almotriptan were not available.

We defined triptan use as ≥1 package of a triptan dispensed in 2007 and triptan overuse as ≥30 defined daily doses (DDD) dispensed in at least one quarter. According to the World Health Organisation (WHO) the DDD is defined as "the assumed average maintenance dose per day for a drug used for its main indication in adults" [21]. For acute medications the DDD is the average initial adult dose recommended [21]. Table 1 shows the specific DDD for each triptan according to these guidelines. The cut-off dose of 30 DDD was chosen in line with the International Classification of Headache Disorders (ICHD-3 beta) that requires the use of a triptan on 10 or more days per month over a period of three months for diagnosing triptan overuse headache [22]. As triptan use in the individual patient may be fluctuating over time, we assessed triptan overuse in one, two, three, and four quarters of 2007.

We compared the number of triptan users and overusers between the nine provinces of Austria as well as between predominantly urban, predominantly rural, and intermediate regions. These regions are categorised by the Statistik Austria based on the NUTS3 criteria (Nomenclature des unités territoriales statististiques) developed by the European Commission [23]. Furthermore, we assessed whether the prescribing physician was a general practitioner, neurologist, or other specialist.

Use of other medications

We analysed the prescription of drugs used for migraine prophylaxis, antidepressants, and other serotonergic drugs in users and non-users of triptans. Migraine

Table 1 Defined daily doses for each triptan available in Austria according to WHO guidelines [21]

	Formulation	Defined daily dose
Sumatriptan	50 mg tablet	1 tablet
	100 mg tablet	1 tablet
	10 mg nasal spray	not available
	20 mg nasal spray	not available
	25 mg suppository	1 suppository
	6 mg subcutaneous injection	1 injection
Zolmitriptan	2.5 mg tablet	1 tablet
	2.5 mg melting tablet	1 melting tablet
	5 mg nasal spray	1 spray
Eletriptan	20 mg tablet	2 tablets
	40 mg tablet	1 tablet
Frovatriptan	2.5 mg tablet	1 tablet
Rizatriptan	5 mg tablet	2 tablets[a]
	5 mg lyotablet	2 tablets[a]
	10 mg tablet	1 tablet
	10 mg lyotablet	1 tablet
Naratriptan	2.5 mg tablet	1 tablet

[a] 1 tablet for patients taking propranolol therapy and for patients with mild to moderately decreased kidney or liver function

prophylactics comprised betablockers (propranolol, metoprolol, bisoprolol, atenolol), flunarizine, and antiepileptic drugs (topiramate, valproate). The inclusion of antidepressants had three reasons. First, some of them (e. g. amitriptyline and venlafaxine) are used as second-line migraine prophylactics. Second, comorbidity of migraine and depressive or anxiety disorders is common [2, 7, 9]. Third, the use of triptans together with serotonergic antidepressants may be associated with a serotonin syndrome [13]. For this reason, we included also other serotonergic drugs, namely fluanxol, ziprasidon, saquonavir, and lithium.

General health status

To assess the general health status we compared the number of days of sick-leave and the number of hospital admissions in users and non-users of triptans comparing triptan overusers and non-overusers in the former group. The sick-leave diagnoses were made by general practitioners.

Statistical analysis

Data was extracted from the GAP-DRG database and transferred into SPSS 24.0 (IBM SPSS Statistics, IBM Group 2016). We analysed data for all persons as well as for non-users and users of triptans separately, with the differentiation of triptan users into non-overusers and overusers. None of the continuous variables was normally distributed, therefore we used medians and quartiles (Q1, Q3) for descriptive analyses and Mann-Whitney-U tests for comparisons of different study groups. We calculated Chi^2-tests for categorical variables and odds ratios (OR) for comparing the prescription of co-medication and hospital admissions in non-users of triptans and users without overuse (using non-users as reference) as well as in users without and with overuse (using users without overuse as reference).

Results

Triptan use and overuse

The database provided data of 7,426,412 million insured persons, covering 89.5% of all 8,295,189 inhabitants in Austria in 2007 [24]. The research population of persons aged 18–99 years with known sex and with insurance benefits in 2007 comprised 5,918,487 persons (90% of the inhabitants aged 18–99 years). Triptans were used by 33,062 persons (0.56% of the research population and 0.45% of all insured persons in the database) and overused by 1970 persons (i.e. 5.96% of all triptan users and 0.033% of the research population). Triptan users were significantly younger than non-users (median 44 vs. 47 years; $p < 0.001$) and they were more often female (82% vs. 54%; p < 0.001). Further details are given in Table 2. Comparisons between triptan users without and with overuse are given in Table 3. Triptan users without overuse refilled a median of 12 DDD per year, whereas triptan overusers refilled a median of 102 DDD per year ($p < 0.001$). Triptan overusers were significantly older than users without overuse (median 47 vs. 44 years; p < 0.001). Although triptans are not licensed for the use in persons older than 65 years we identified 1779

Table 2 Demographic data of triptan non-users and triptan users

	Triptan non-users n = 5,885,425		Triptan users n = 33,062		Statistics p-value
Age (years)					
Median	47		44		< 0.001[#]
Lower quartile	34		35		
Upper quartile	63		52		
Age group (years)	n	%	n	%	
18–35	1,619,098	27.5	8343	25.2	< 0.001[§]
36–50	1,698,601	28.9	15,134	45.8	
51–65	1,284,461	21.8	7806	23.6	
66–99	1,283,265	21.8	1779	5.4	
Sex					< 0.001[§]
Female	3,160,117	53.7	27,254	82.4	
Male	2,725,308	46.3	5808	17.6	

[#]Mann-Whitney-U-Test, [§]Chi-Square Test

Table 3 Comparison of triptan users without and with overuse

	Triptan users without overuse $n = 31{,}092$		Triptan overusers $n = 1970$		Statistics *p*-value
Triptans DDD/year					
Median	12		102		< 0.001[#]
Lower quartile	6		84		
Upper quartile	32		132		
Range	1–106		30–762		
Age (years)					
Median	44		47		< 0.001[#]
Lower quartile	35		40		
Upper quartile	52		55		
Age group (years)	n	%	n	%	
18–35	8051	25.9	292	14.8	< 0.001[§]
36–50	14,216	45.7	918	46.6	
51–65	7210	23.2	396	30.3	
66–99	1615	5.2	164	8.3	
Sex					
Female	25,623	82.4	1631	82.8	0.666
Male	5469	17.6	339	17.2	

[#]Mann-Whitney-U-Test, [§]Chi-Square Test, DDD/year defined daily doses per year

Table 4 Comparison of triptan overuse in one quarter and in two or more quarters of 2007

	Overuse in 1 quarter $n = 886$		Overuse in ≥2quarters $n = 1084$		Statistics p-value
Triptan DDD/year					
Median	80		132		< 0.001[#]
Lower quartile	64		110.3		
Upper quartile	90		162		
Range	30–132		60–762		
Age (years)					
Median	47		48		< 0.001[#]
Lower quartile	39		41		
Upper quartile	54		56		
Range	18–87		19–95		
Age group (years)	n	%	n	%	
18–35	153	17.3	139	12.8	0.002[§]
36–50	427	48.2	491	45.3	
51–65	245	27.7	351	32.4	
66–99	61	6.9	103	9.5	
Sex					0.761
Female	731	82.5	900	83	
Male	155	17.5	184	17	

[#]Mann-Whitney-U-Test, [§]Chi-Square Test. *ns* not significant

triptan users (5.4% of all users) and 164 overusers (8.3% of all overusers) in this age group. Triptan overuse in one, two, three or four quarters was found in 886 (45%), 409 (20.8%), 313 (15.9%), and 362 (18.4%) persons, whereas the corresponding median DDD (Q1; Q3) per year were 80 (64; 90), 108 (96; 117.5), 132 (120; 148.5), 174 (150; 220). The comparison of an overuse in one quarter to an overuse in two or more quarters showed an older age and – expectedly – a larger number of DDD in the latter (Table 4).

Regional differences

On the whole, the number of triptan users per 100,000 persons was 559 in Austria. In the nine provinces it ranged from 474 in Upper Austria to 640 in Vienna. The difference between the nine provinces was statistically significant (Chi^2-test, $p < 0.001$). The proportion of triptan overusers was highest in Salzburg (10.7%) and lowest in Styria (3.0%). Triptan use was more common in urban than in rural and intermediate regions (Chi^2-test, $p < 0.001$), whereas overuse did not differ between these regions (Chi^2-test, $p = 0.31$); (Table 5).

Prescription patterns

Out of a total of 904,063 DDD of triptans dispensed in 2007, 95.7% were tablets, 1.3% were sumatriptan injections, 2.5% zolmitriptan nasal spray, and 0.4% sumatriptan suppositories; 675,146 DDDs (74.7%) were dispensed to non-overusers and 228,917 (25.3%) to overusers. Of 155,403 billed prescriptions, 91.4% were made for packages with six single doses, 41.2% for zolmitriptan, 32.5% for eletriptan, 14.8% for sumatriptan, 10% for frovatriptan, 1.2% for rizatriptan, and 0.4% for naratriptan.

In accordance with prescription rules, the majority of triptans was prescribed by general practitioners (113,649 prescriptions; 73.1%), followed by neurologists (23,139 prescriptions; 14.9%), and other specialists or hospital physicians (16,578 prescriptions; 10.7%). The prescriber could not be identified in 2037 (1.3%) of the prescriptions. In triptan overusers, 28,018 of 36,912 prescriptions (76.1%) were made by general practitioners, 5045 (13.7%) by neurologists and 3323 (9%) by other specialists.

Co-medication

The drugs dispensed most often and second most often were betablockers and SSRI in non-users of triptans as well as SSRI and betablockers both in users without and with triptan overuse (Table 6). Any of the migraine prophylactics, antidepressants, and other serotonergic drugs specified in Table 6 were dispensed to 37% of the triptan users without overuse and to 54% of the overusers. All single drugs (Table 6) showed the same prescription pattern: Triptan users had a higher risk of being dispensed any of these co-medications than non-users, and triptan

Table 5 Research population and triptan use and overuse in the nine provinces and in rural, urban and intermediate regions

	Research population $n = 5,918,487$		Triptan users $n = 33,062$		Triptan overusers $n = 1970$		Users / 100,000 persons	Overusers among users
Province	n	%	n	%	n	%		%
Vienna	1,242,072	21.0	7956	24.1	348	17.7	640.5	4.4
Lower Austria	1,111,474	18.8	5722	17.3	560	28.4	514.8	9.8
Styria	874,749	14.8	4729	14.3	141	7.2	540.6	3.0
Upper Austria	922,842	15.6	4374	13.2	180	9.1	474.0	4.1
Tyrol	510,347	8.6	2989	9.0	140	7.1	585.7	4.7
Carinthia	406,493	6.9	2498	7.6	235	11.9	614.5	9.4
Salzburg	407,978	6.9	2363	7.1	253	12.8	579.2	10.7
Burgenland	194,083	3.3	1196	3.6	43	2.2	616.2	3.6
Vorarlberg	237,738	4.0	1201	3.6	68	3.5	505.2	5.7
Unknown	10,711	0.1	34	0.1	2	0.1	na	na
Region								
Rural	2,517,891	42.5	12,961	39.2	804	40.8	514.8	6.2
Urban	2,334,651	39.4	14,615	44.2	851	43.2	626.0	5.8
Intermediate	1,055,234	17.8	5452	16.5	313	15.9	516.7	5.7
Unknown	10,711	0.2	34	0.1	2	0.1	na	na

na not applicable

overusers had a higher risk than non-overusers. Looking at overusers more closely, 448 (50.6%) of those with an overuse in one quarter of 2007 and 611 (56.3%) of those with an overuse in ≥ two quarters had any of these co-medications (Chi^2-test, $p = 0.008$).

Sick leave

The number of days with sick leave due to any diagnosis as well as due to migraine (Table 7) was significantly greater in triptan users than in non-users (Mann-Whitney-U test, $p < 0.001$ for both). In contrast, days with sick leave in general and due to migraine did not differ between triptan users without overuse and triptan overusers. Similarly, the number of hospital admissions did not differ in the three subgroups (Table 7).

Discussion

This is the first study that examined the prevalence of triptan use and overuse in the Austrian general population based on a nationwide healthcare database. Among people older than 18 years 0.56% were triptan users of whom nearly 6% were triptan overusers (0.033% of the general Austrian population). Triptan users were younger than non-users and they were more often female. Triptan overusers were older than non-overusers,

Table 6 Co-medications dispensed to triptan non-users and to users without and with overuse

	Triptan non-users $n = 5,885,425$		Triptan users without overuse $n = 31,092$				Triptan users with overuse $n = 1970$			
	n	%	n	%	OR#	95% CI	n	%	OR#	95% CI
Betablockers	493,457	8.4	3455	11.1	1.4	1.3–1.4	376	19.1	1.9	1.7–2.1
Flunarizine	10,617	0.2	1425	4.6	26.6	25.1–28.6	162	8.2	1.9	1.6–2.2
Topiramate or valproate	26,605	0.4	1381	4.4	10.2	9.7–10.8	240	12.2	3.0	2.6–3.5
Tricyclic antidepressants	49,935	0.9	1319	4.2	5.2	4.9–5.5	166	8.4	2.1	1.8–2.5
SSRI	459,917	7.8	5596	18.0	2.6	2.5–2.7	444	22.5	1.3	1.2–1.5
SNRI	63,009	1.1	1412	4.5	4.4	4.2–4.6	116	5.9	1.3	1.1–1.6
NaSSA	85,402	1.5	1019	3.3	2.3	2.2–2.5	84	4.3	1.3	1.0–1.6
Other antidepressants or serotonergic drugs	168,020	2.9	2360	7.6	2.8	2.7–2.9	189	9.6	1.3	1.1–1.5

OR, odds ratio. *CI*, confidence interval. #Odds ratios for triptan users without overuse refer to non-users (OR = 1) and odds ratios for triptan users with overuse refer to users without overuse (OR = 1) *SSRI*, selective serotonin re-uptake inhibitors, *SNRI*, serotonin-noradrenalin re-uptake inhibitors, *NaSSA*, noradrenergic and specific serotonergic antidepressants

Table 7 Sick-leave and hospital admissions in triptan non-users and in users without and with overuse

	Triptan non-users n = 5,885,425			Triptan users without overuse n = 31,092			Triptan users with overuse n = 1970		
	Median	Q1	Q3	Median	Q1	Q3	Median	Q1	Q3
Sick-leave for									
any reason (days)	10	4	23	12	5	29	12	5	27.3
migraine (days)	2	1	4	3	1	7	4	1	9
	n	%		n	%	OR (CI)[a]	n	%	OR (CI)[#]
Hospital admissions	1,124,587	19.1		6082	19.6	1.0 (1.0–1.1)	386	19.6	1.0 (0.9–1.1)

Q1: 25% Quartile, Q3: 75% Quartile. *OR*, odds ratio. *CI*, confidence interval. [a]Odds ratios for triptan users without overuse refer to non-users (OR = 1) and odds ratios for triptan users with overuse refer to users without overuse (OR = 1)

whereas the female to male ratio was similar in the two groups. The prescription rates for triptans differed in the nine provinces of Austria and between urban, rural, and intermediate regions. The prescription of co-medications was lowest in triptan non-users, higher in users without overuse, and highest in triptan overusers. General health was poorer in triptan users and overusers than in non-users in terms of days of sick leave but not in terms of hospital admission rates.

Triptan use

The rate of triptan use in Austria was lower than in other studies based on insurance claims. The rate of triptan overuse was comparable with other countries. A Dutch study found 1.3% triptan users and 0.1% overusers in the general population. The rate of triptan overusers among users was 10% according to IHS criteria and 3.3% according to more restrictive criteria requiring 18 DDD per month over a period of 3 months [14]. An Italian study found 0.7–1% triptan users of whom 10% – using at least 10 DDD per month – were classified as overusers [15]. Braunstein et al. [10] reported a rate of 2.3% triptan users in France; the proportion of overusers was 2.3% among all users and 5.4% among regular users. Differences between countries may be explained by methodological issues as well as by divergent insurance systems and prescription habits. In accordance with previous findings, the majority of triptan users was in the younger and middle age groups whilst triptan overusers were significantly older than non-overusers [10, 14, 15, 25]. Although triptans are not licensed in persons older than 65 years, 5.4% of the triptan users in our study were beyond this age. This finding is comparable with previous studies reporting triptan use in three to 10 % of people older than 65 years [10, 14, 15, 26]. In clinical practice, the use of triptans in this age group is not limited to otherwise healthy persons. Biagi et al. [27] found a substantial number of triptan users above 65 years with concomitant vascular risk factors. Even though the vascular risk of triptans is still under debate, triptans are contraindicated in vascular disorders [28, 29]. In addition, triptan overuse is not uncommon in persons older than 65 years. This age group accounted for 8.3% of all overusers in our study and for 12% of the overusers in the study from France [10].

The definition of triptan overuse varies in pharmacoepidemiological studies from ≥10, ≥ 15, ≥ 18, or ≥ 20 DDD per month to ≥30 DDD per quarter, or a conversion into ≥216 or ≥ 120 DDD per year, respectively [14–16]. We used quarterly DDD as a compromise between monthly DDD which may overestimate triptan overuse and annual DDD which may underestimate overuse if it is not present continuously [14, 15]. The fluctuation of triptan overuse is mirrored in our findings as well as in a previous study [15]. We found triptan overuse in one quarter of 2007 in 45% of the overusers and in two or more quarters in 55%. In the Dutch study, 63% to 65% of those who overused triptans in the first quarter of the year showed an overuse in at least one more quarter [14]. Defining triptan overuse by 30 or more DDD per quarter may still overestimate triptan overuse because patients may use more than one single dose per day. Therefore, the cut-off of 10 days of triptan use per month [22] may not be reached in each month. In our study. The lower quartile of DDD per quarter was 64 and the 5th percentile was 36. That suggests a low risk of overestimating triptan overuse in Austria.

The relation of 0.56% triptan users in our study to a migraine prevalence of 10% reported for Austria many years ago [30] suggests that less than 6% of the patients with migraine are using triptans in our country. This may reflect a low awareness of the options for treating acute migraine attacks among physicians and patients, and it may point out that some patients with migraine (but probably not 94%) respond well to analgesics and NSAIDS. A median of 12 DDD per year, i.e. one DDD per month, suggests a low to moderate use of triptans. A probable underuse of triptans in Austria is even more pronounced in men. The male to female ratio in the one-year-prevalence of migraine of 1:2.5 in Austria [30] contrasts with a ratio of 1:4.5 in the use of triptans in our analysis. This supports previous studies which showed that migraine is underdiagnosed and undertreated in men [31].

The low rate of triptan use contrasts with a considerable number of persons who overuse triptans. Triptan overusers accounted for 5.9% of all triptan users and for 25% of all dispensed triptans. This highlights the need of improving education about medication overuse headache for both patients and physicians.

Regional differences

Our data cannot explain the differences in triptan use and overuse between the provinces as well as between urban and rural regions. In Burgenland and Carinthia, high rates of triptan users contrast with few available neurologists whereas in urban regions the higher rates of triptan users seem to be in line with a better availability of neurologists. For the treatment of migraine, patients may travel to another province or from rural to urban regions. In addition, socioeconomic differences not assessed in this study may play a role. Similar to our findings, DaCas et al. [15] showed a wide range of triptan use in different Italian regions without giving a specific explanation for the differences.

Prescription patterns

The triptans prescribed most often in the present study were zolmitriptan and eletriptan. The same two were reported in France, whereas sumatriptan and rizatriptan ranked on top in the Netherlands as well as almotriptan and rizatriptan in Italy [10, 14, 15]. These prescription patterns may reflect differences in availability and reimbursement and suggest a common trend towards triptans with a faster onset of action [10, 14, 15]. In accordance with prescription rules and due to easier access, general practitioners prescribed the vast majority of triptans followed by neurologists. Compared to other countries, triptans were more often prescribed by neurologists [10, 14]. This may reflect an easier access to neurologists in Austria and may contribute to the lower rate of triptan overuse but also suggests that, compared to other countries, neurologists in Austria are more reluctant to prescribe triptans.

Co-medication

Any of the migraine prophylactics, antidepressants, or other serotonergic drugs specified in Table 6 was dispensed to 37% of the triptan users without overuse and to 54% of the overusers. Hereby, physicians try to get in control of high- frequent headaches. However, patients with medication overuse headache have a higher prevalence of psychiatric comorbidity [6, 8, 25, 32]. Selective serotonin re-uptake inhibitors were most often dispensed presumably for depression or anxiety disorders. Among possible prophylactic drugs, betablockers were most often dispensed followed by flunarizine and tricyclic antidepressants. In triptan overusers, antiepileptic drugs came second. This supports findings of previous studies with prescriptions of antidepressants, prophylactics, and benzodiazepines in about one third of triptan users and even more often in triptan overusers [10, 14]. Although psychopharmacologic drugs may lead to a serotonin syndrome in combination with triptans [13], in everyday routine a substantial number of patients got triptans in combination with serotonergic drugs.

Sick leave and hospital admissions

The number of days with sick leave for any reason as well as for migraine was higher in triptan users than in non-users. This supports the necessity of treating migraine and comorbid diseases adequately. The days with sick leave due to migraine should be interpreted with caution. Experience in daily practice suggests that patients may pretend other complaints due to the fear of losing their job if they miss work too often because of migraine. General practitioners are not allowed to share medical diagnoses with the employers but pressure amongst colleagues to tell about reasons for sick leave is high. Comparable to findings of Braunstein et al. [10], the days with sick leave did not differ between triptan users without and with overuse. The proportion of hospital admissions did not differ between triptan users and non-users although triptan users were significantly younger than non-users. This may indirectly point to a poorer health status in triptan users.

Limitations of the study

Our study is limited by inhabitants not included in the research population, delays in billing dispensed drugs, the uncertainty if dispensed drugs were actually taken, and the fact that the database does not include diagnoses for outpatient treatments.

The findings in this study may have been biased because four small social security institutions are not included in the GAP-DRG database. These institutions, however, account for only 3% of all insured persons in Austria. The basis for our analysis comprised 89.5% of the general population in 2007. The study may have been biased by the fact that persons who were waived from prescription charges in 2007 could not be included. Usually, these are persons with lower socioeconomic status which was found to be associated with high frequency migraine, medication overuse headache, and psychiatric comorbidity [2, 26, 33].

Dispensed drugs were billed to the insurance by the pharmacies by the end of each quarter of the year. This may have led to missing data in one quarter and to carry-over effects in the next quarter. These deferrals are evened out over 12 months, but it may have influenced the DDD count for triptan overuse. Furthermore, we did not know, if the dispensed triptans were actually taken by the patients. Nevertheless, the finding that most patients refilled their prescription suggests that the dispensed triptans were taken.

Since the database does not include diagnoses for outpatient treatments or indications for medications, our inferences on migraine diagnoses were indirect. We may have misclassified cluster headache for migraine. Patients with cluster headache use triptans very frequently without being an overuser [34, 35]. The low prevalence of cluster headache and the finding that the triptans of choice for treating cluster headache, i.e. subcutaneous sumatriptan and zolmitriptan nasal spray, accounted for less than 4 % of the DDD suggest a low (if any) impact on our findings. In addition, we could not determine if persons fulfilling our definition of triptan overuse had medication overuse headache.

We analysed data from 2007 because at the time of the analysis this was the most recent complete data available. This data still reflects the current situation: In Austria no new formulations of triptans, other triptans, or other new groups of acute medications relevant for migraine have been marketed since 2007. In addition, a study by Fischer et al. found that in a tertiary care outpatient headache clinic in Innsbruck 73% of the migraineurs were triptan naive at their first consultation at the clinic in the years 2009 to 2012 [36].

Strengths of the study

This is the first study in Austria and one of few nationwide studies in the literature looking at triptan use and overuse. In contrast to previous studies, the study covers the vast majority of the general population and is representative of the population structure as it includes nearly 90% of the inhabitants in the predefined age range of 18 to 99 years [10, 14–20]. In addition to the examination of triptan use and overuse, we were able to assess regional differences, prescription patterns of triptans, prescriptions of co-medications as well as data on sick leave and hospital admissions, and to compare these findings in non-users, users, and overusers of triptans.

Conclusion

Overall triptan use and consequently overall triptan overuse was low in Austria but triptan users were at risk of overuse. Citing Leonard Cohen's "Bird on the Wire", some migraineurs may need the advice "Why not ask for more?" whereas others "You must not ask for so much".

Abbreviations

ATC code: Anatomical therapeutic chemical code; DALYs: Disability adjusted life years; DDD: Defined daily dose; GAP-DRG: General approach patient-oriented outpatient-based diagnosis related groups; ICHD-3: International Classification of Headache Disorders, 3rd version; NSAIDS: Non-steroidal antiiflammatory drugs; NUTS3: Nomenclature des unites territoriales statistiques; WHO: World Health Organisation

Acknowledgements

We thank Dr. Gottfried Endel from the Hauptverband der Österreichischen Sozialversicherungsträger for allowing us to analyse data of the GAP-DRG database. We thank Mag. Matthias Deckert for his corrections of grammar and punctuation.

Authors' contributions

K. Zebenholzer conceived the study, contributed to data acquisition, the statistical analysis, and drafted the manuscript. W. Gall conceived the study, contributed to data acquisition and statistical analysis. C. Wöber conceived the study and contributed to the drafting of the manuscript. All authors revised the manuscript and approved the final manuscript.

Competing interests

All authors declare no conflict of interest.

Author details

[1]Department of Neurology, Medical University of Vienna, Waehringer Guertel 18-20, 1090 Vienna, Austria. [2]Center for Medical Statistics, Informatics and Intelligent Systems, Institute of Medical Information Management, Medical University of Vienna, Waehringer Guertel 18-20, 1090 Vienna, Austria.

References

1. Stovner LJ, Andree C (2010) Prevalence of headache in Europe: a review for the Eurolight project. J Headache Pain 11:289–299
2. GBD (2015) Neurological disorders collaborator group (2017) global, regional, and national burden of neurological disorders during 1990-2015: a systematic analysis for the global burden of disease study 2015. Lancet Neurol 16(11):877–897
3. Linde M, Gustavsson A, Stovner LJ, Steiner TJ, Barré J (2012) The cost of headache disorders in Europe: the Eurolight project. Eur J Neurol 19(5):703–711
4. Bloudek LM, Stokes M, Buse DC, Scher A, Stewart WF, Lipton RB (2012) Cost of healthcare for patients with migraine in five European countries: results from the international burden of migraine study (IBMS). J Headache Pain 13(5):361–378
5. DGN https://www.dgn.org/images/red_leitlinien/LL_2012/pdf/030-057l_S1_Migraene_Therapie_2012_verlaengert.pdf . Accessed 19 December 2017
6. Diener HC, Holle D, Solbach K, Gaul C (2016) Medication-overuse headache: risk factors, pathophysiology and management. Nat Rev Neurol 22:375–583
7. Zebenholzer K, Andree C, Lechner A, Broesner G, Lampl C, Luthringshause G et al (2015) Prevalence, management and burden of episodic and chronic headaches – a cross-sectional multicentre study in eight Austrian headache centres. J Headache Pain 16:531
8. Buse DC, Silberstein SD, Manack AN, Papapetropoulos S, Lipton RB (2013) Psychiatric comorbidities of episodic and chronic migraine. J Neurol 260 88: 1960–1969
9. Zebenholzer K, Lechner A, Broessner G, Lampl C, Luthringshause G, Wuschitz A (2016) Impact of depression and anxiety on burden and management of episodic and chronic headaches – a cross-sectional multicentre study in eight Austrian headache centres. J Headache Pain 17:15
10. Braunstein D, Donnet A, Pradel V (2015) Triptans use and overuse: a pharmacoepidemiology study from the French health insurance system database covering 4.1 million people. Cephalalgia 35(13):1172–1180
11. Oedegaard KJ, Riise T, Dilsaver SC, Lund A, Akuskal HS, Fasmer OB, Hundal O (2001) A pharmaco-epidemiological study of migraine and antidepressant medications: complete one year data from the Norwegian population. J Affect Disord 129(1–3):198–2014

12. Lafata JE, Tunceli O, Cerghet M, Sharma KP, Lipton RB (2010) The use of migraine preventive medications among patients with and without migraine headaches. Cephalalgia 30(1):97–104
13. Tepper SJ, Shapiro RE, Sun-Edelstein C (2012) Triptans and serotonin syndrome – a response. Headache 52(7):1185–1188
14. Dekker F, Wiendels NJ, de Valk V, van der Vliet C, Knuistingh Neven A, Assendelft WJ, Ferrari MD (2011) Triptan overuse in the Dutch general population: a nationwide pharmaco-epidemiology database analysis in 6.7 million people. Cephalalgia 31(8):937–946
15. Da Cas R, Nigro A, Terrazzino S, Sances G, Viana M, Tassorelli C et al (2014) Triptan use in Italy: insights from administrative databases. Cephalalgia 35(7):619–626
16. Gaist D, Andersen M, Aarup AL, Hallas J, Gram LF (1997) Use of sumatriptan in Denmark in 1994-5: an epidemiological analysis of nationwide prescription data. Br J Clin Pharmacol 43:429–433
17. Søndergaard J, Foged A, Kragstrup J, Gaist D, Gram LF, Sindrup SH et al (2006) Intensive community pharmacy intervention had little impact on triptan consumption: a randomized controlled trial. Scand J Prim Health Care 24:16–21
18. Lohman JJ, van der Kuy-de Ree MM, Group of Co-operating Pharmcists Sittard-Geleen and its environs (2005) Patterns of specific antimigraine drug use – a study based on the records of 18 community pharmacies. Cephalalgia 25:214–218
19. Lugardon S, Roussel H, Sciortino V, Montastruc JL, Lapeyre-Mestre M (2007) Triptan use and risk of cardiovascular events: a nested-case-control study from the French health system database. Eur J Clin Pharmacol 63:801–807
20. Pavone E, Banfi R, Vaiani M, Panconcesi A (2007) Patterns of triptan use: a study based on the records of a community pharmaceutical department. Cephalalgia 27:1000–1004
21. World Health Organization. WHO Collaborating Centre for Drug Statistics Methodology, Guidelines for ATC classification and DDD assignment 2013, http://www.whocc.no. Accessed 17 April 2017
22. Headache Classification Subcommittee of the International Headache Society (2013) The international classification of headache disorders, 3rd edition (beta version). Cephalalgia 33(9):629–808
23. Eurostat Statistics explained. Urban rural typology. http://www.ec.europe.eu. Accessed 17 April 2017
24. Statistik Austria. http://statistik.at. Accessed 26 July 2017
25. Katsarava Z, Obermann M (2013) Medication-overuse headache. Curr Opin Neurol 26:276–281
26. Bigal ME, Serrano D, Buse D, Scher A, Stewart WF, Lipton RB (2008) Acute migraine medications and evolution from episodic to chronic migraine: a longitudinal population-based study. Headache 48:1157–1168
27. Biagi C, Poluzzi E, Roberto G, Puccini A, Vaccheri A, D'Alessandro R et al (2011) Pattern of triptan use and cardiovascular coprescription: a pharmacoepidemiological study in Italy. Eur J Clin Pharmacol 67:1283–1289
28. Roberto G, Piccinni C, D'Alessandro R, Poluzzi E (2014) Triptans and serious adverse vascular events: data mining of the FDA adverse event reporting system database. Cephalalgia 34:5–13
29. Dodick D, Lipton RB, Martin V, Papademetriou V, Rosamond W, Maassen VanDenBrink A at al. (2004) Consensus statement: cardiovascular safety profile of triptans (5-HT agonists) in the acute treatment of migraine. Headache 44:414–425
30. Lampl C, Buzath A, Baumhackl U, Klingler D (2002) One-year prevalence of migraine in Austria: a nation-wide survey. Cephalalgia 23(4):280–286
31. Buse DC, Loder EW, Gorman JA, Stewart WF, MI R, Fanning KM et al (2013) Sex differences in the prevalence, symptoms, and associated features of migraine, probable migraine and other severe headache: results of the American migraine prevalence and prevention (AMPP) study. Headache 53(8):1278–1289
32. Minen MT, Begasse De Dhaem O, Kroon Van Diest A, Powers S, Schwedt TJ et al (2016) Migraine and its psychiatric comorbidities. J Neurol Neurosurg Psychiatry 87(7):741–749
33. Ng-Mak DS, Chen YT, Ho TW, Stanford B, Roset M (2012) Results of a 2-year retrospective cohort study of newly prescribed triptans users in European nationwide databases. Cephalalgia 32:875–887
34. Ekbom K, Waldenlind E, Cole J, Pilgrim A, Kirkham A (1992) Sumatriptan in chronic cluster headache: results of continuous treatment for eleven months. Cephalalgia 12:254–256
35. Dahlof C, Ekbom K, Persson L (1994) Clinical experiences from Sweden on the use of subcutaneously administered sumatriptan in migraine and cluster headache. Arch Neurol 51:1256–1261
36. Fischer M, Frank F, Wille G, Klien S, Lackner P, Broessner G (2016) Triptans for acute migraine headache: current experience with triptan use and prescription habits in a tertiary care headache outpatient clinic: an observational study. Headache 56(6):952–960

25

Effectiveness of transcutaneous electrical nerve stimulation for the treatment of migraine

Huimin Tao, Teng Wang, Xin Dong, Qi Guo, Huan Xu and Qi Wan*

Abstract

Background: Migraine is now ranked as the second most disabling disorder worldwide reported by the Global Burden of Disease Study 2016. As a noninvasive neurostimulation technique, transcutaneous electrical nerve stimulation(TENS) has been applied as an abortive and prophylactic treatment for migraine recently. We conduct this meta-analysis to analyze the effectiveness and safety of TENS on migraineurs.

Methods: We searched Medline (via PubMed), Embase, the Cochrane Library and the Cochrane Central Register of Controlled Trials to identify randomized controlled trials, which compared the effect of TENS with sham TENS on migraineurs. Data were extracted and methodological quality assessed independently by two reviewers. Change in the number of monthly headache days, responder rate, painkiller intake, adverse events and satisfaction were extracted as outcome.

Results: Four studies were included in the quantitative analysis with 161 migraine patients in real TENS group and 115 in sham TENS group. We found significant reduction of monthly headache days (SMD: -0.48; 95% CI: -0.73 to −0.23; $P < 0.001$) and painkiller intake (SMD: -0.78; 95% CI: -1.14 to − 0.42; $P < 0.001$). Responder rate (RR: 4.05; 95% CI: 2.06 to 7.97; $P < 0.001$) and satisfaction (RR: 1.85; 95% CI: 1.31 to 2,61; $P < 0.001$) were significantly increased compared with sham TENS.

Conclusion: This meta-analysis suggests that TENS may serve as an effective and well-tolerated alternative for migraineurs. However, low quality of evidence prevents us from reaching definitive conclusions. Future well-designed RCTs are necessary to confirm and update the findings of this analysis.

Systematic review registration: Our PROSPERO protocol registration number: CRD42018085984. Registered 30 January 2018.

Keywords: Migraine, Transcutaneous electrical nerve stimulation, TENS, Meta-analysis

Background

Migraine is now ranked as the second most disabling disorder worldwide reported by the Global Burden of Disease Study 2016 [1], which is characterized by recurrent moderate to severe unilateral throbbing head pain accompanied by photophobia, phonophobia, nausea and vomiting [2]. Therapeutic strategies are mainly based on both preventive and abortive drug therapy. However, conventional pharmacological therapies are partially effective and have unpleasant adverse effects inevitably. Overuse of symptomatic medication for headaches may lead to drug resistance and even transformation into refractory medication overuse headache [3]. Therefore, nonpharmacological therapeutic strategies with better efficacy and tolerance are pressingly needed.

Transcutaneous electrical nerve stimulation (TENS) is the delivery of pulsed low voltage electrical currents across the intact surface of the skin to stimulate peripheral nerves principally for pain relief [4]. As a

* Correspondence: chinaqiwan@126.com
Department of Neurology, The First Affiliated Hospital of Nanjing Medical University, 300 Guangzhou Road, Nanjing 210029, Jiangsu Province, China

noninvasive neurostimulation technique, TENS has gradually been the subject of extensive research in the treatment of headache disorders. Cefaly® is the first medical device approved by the FDA as a prophylactic treatment for episodic migraine, which stimulates the supratrochlear and supraorbital nerves [5]. Another novel non-invasive transcutaneous vagal nerve stimulation device, nVNS gammaCore, has been developed and is CE marked for acute and prophylactic treatment of primary headache disorders including cluster headache and migraine [6–8].

Although several clinical trials applying TENS as an abortive or prophylactic treatment for migraine have been carried out, there is no rigorous systematic review, to the best of our knowledge, investigating the effectiveness and safety of TENS in migraineurs. Therefore, the aim of this meta-analysis was to assess the evidence from randomized controlled clinical trials that used TENS for pain relief in migraine patients.

Methods

This meta-analysis was conducted according to the guidance of the Preferred Reporting Items for Systematic Reviews and Meta-analysis statement [9]. The review protocol was registered in the International Prospective Register of Systematic Reviews and the registration number was CRD42018085984.

Eligibility criteria

Studies were identified based on the following criteria: (1) participants over 18 years old diagnosed with migraine according to the International Classification of Headache Disorders (ICHD-II or ICHD-III beta version); (2) comparing real TENS with sham TENS; (3) reporting migraine days, headache days, migraine attacks, pain intensity, painkiller intakes, adverse events or satisfaction as outcomes; (4) randomized controlled trials.

The exclusion criteria were as follows: (1) comparison with other therapies such as drugs or psychotherapy; (2) applying invasive electrical nerve stimulation; (3) other types of trials such as cross-over designs, self-contrast trials and healthy controlled trials.

Literature search and study selection

Two reviewers (Tao and Wang) independently searched the following electronic databases up to December 2017: MEDLINE (via PubMed), Embase, the Cochrane Library and the Cochrane Central Register of Controlled Trials without language restrictions. The search strategies used can be found in Additional file 1. To avoid omitting relevant trials, conference abstracts and reference lists of all identified related publications were also searched. The computer search was supplemented with manual searches of the reference to expand potentially relevant articles. When multiple reports describing the same population were published, the most complete report was included.

Data extraction and outcome measures

Data extraction was performed independently by two authors. The following information was extracted from the included RCTs: first author; publication year; country; study design; sample size; study population (age range, gender split, baseline characteristics); intervention (stimulation site, parameters and duration of stimulation); adverse events and outcomes. We contacted to the corresponding authors when the related data were incomplete. Those who did not reply to our data request were excluded from the meta-analysis.

The primary outcomes included changes in monthly headache days between real and sham TENS, evaluated by headache diaries. Percentage of 'responders', i.e., of subjects having at least 50% reduction of monthly migraine days between the run-in period and the end of treatment was also investigated as primary outcome measures. Secondary outcomes were painkiller intake, satisfaction and adverse events during or after stimulation.

Assessment of risk of bias

Risk of bias assessment was performed independently by two authors (Tao and Wang) and adjudicated by a third investigator (Dong) in the event of disagreement, according to Cochrane Collaboration's tool for assessing bias in randomized trials [10]. The domains assessed were sequence generation (selection bias), allocation sequence concealment (selection bias), blinding of participants and personnel (performance bias), blinding of outcome assessment (detection bias), incomplete outcome data (attrition bias), selective outcome reporting (reporting bias) and other potential sources of bias.

Data analysis

The data synthesis was performed by Review Manager 5.3 (Cochrane Collaboration, Oxford, UK). The standardized mean difference (SMD) and relative risk (RR) were used to compare continuous and dichotomous variables, respectively. All results were reported with 95% confidence intervals (CIs). For studies that presented continuous data as means and range values, the standard deviations were calculated based on the principles of the Cochrane Handbook for Systematic Reviews of Interventions [11].

Heterogeneity was tested using the chi-square test ($P < 0.1$) and quantified with the I^2 statistic, which described the variation of effect size that was attributable to heterogeneity across studies [12]. I^2 values smaller than 50% indicate no significant heterogeneity and are acceptable. The fixed-effect model of analysis is the appropriate. Otherwise, the random-effect model is considered.

Prespecified subgroup analysis was performed according to migraine attack frequency (episodic or chronic). Sensitivity analysis was also performed to determine effect size when low-quality studies were excluded. Owing to the limited number ($n < 10$) of included studies, publication bias was not assessed.

Finally, we assessed the quality of evidence by GRADE profiler, considering risk of bias, inconsistency, indirectness, imprecision, and publication bias [13].

Results

Study selection and inclusion

The flow chart for the selection process and detailed identification was presented in Fig. 1. Search strategies identified 368 potentially relevant publications. After the removal of duplicates, 294 articles were spotted, but only 22 remained after screening titles and abstracts. In the eligible articles, one trial enrolled both tension-type headache patients and migraineurs [14], and we were unable to extract data of migraineurs separately. We failed to contact the authors for the detail data until the end of this review. Ultimately, four RCTs, enrolling a total of 276 patients were included in the meta-analysis [15–18].

Study characteristics

The characteristics of the studies included are summarized in Table 1. The four studies were published between 2013 and 2017 in English. Two of them were multicenter trials in Belgium [15] and the USA [16], the others were monocenter trials in China [17, 18]. Patients with at least 2 migraine attacks each month or chronic migraine were recruited in the trials. The four included studies ranged in size from 59 to 88 subjects and from 1 to 8 months in duration. Different TENS manufacturers applied pulsed electrical stimulation to supraorbital nerves (the branch of the trigeminal nerve), vagus nerves, occipital nerves and Taiyang (EX-HN 5)

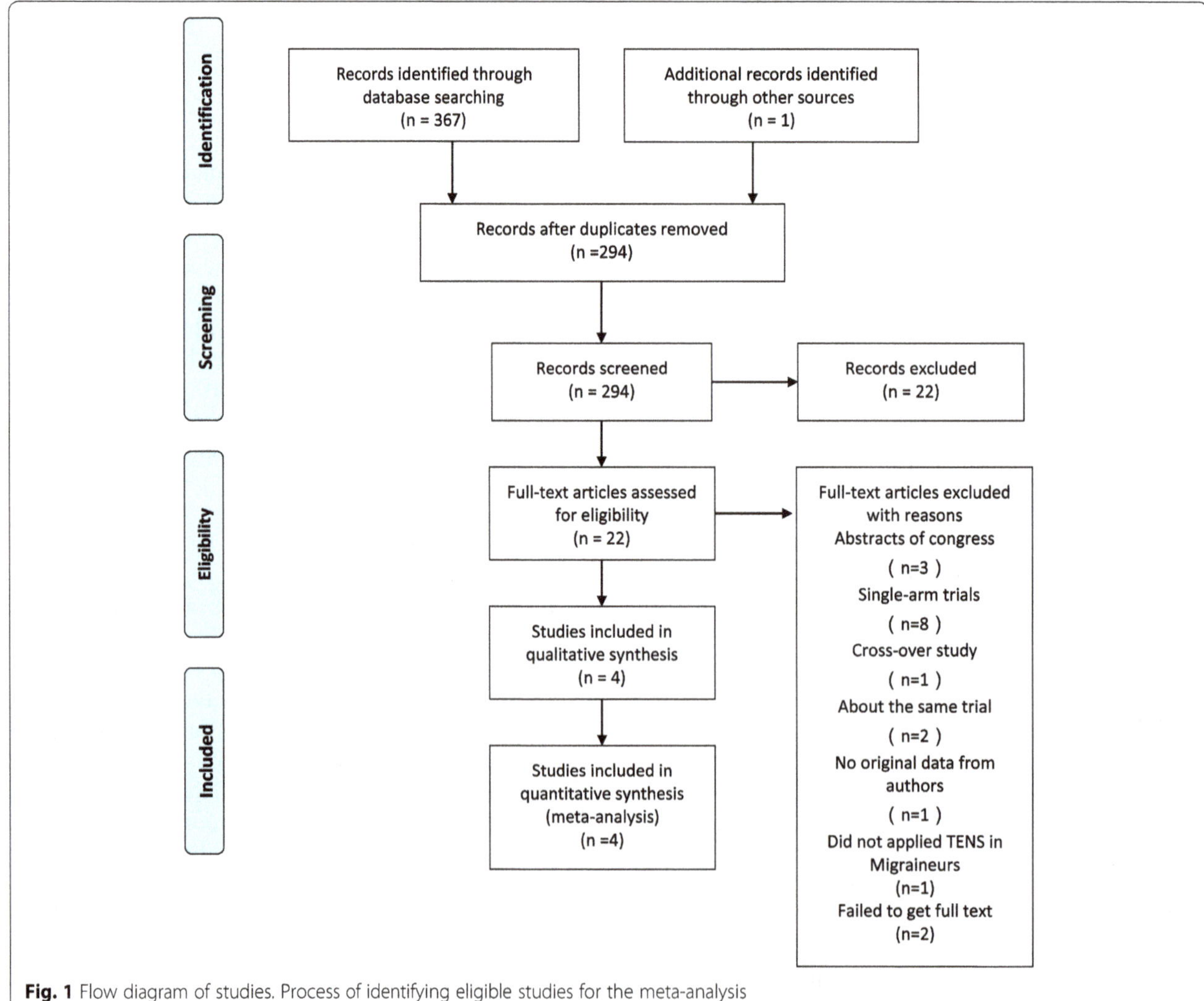

Fig. 1 Flow diagram of studies. Process of identifying eligible studies for the meta-analysis

Table 1 Characteristics of included studies

Included studies	Country	Groups (n)	Gender female/ male	Age	Headache days during baseline	Stimulation location	Parameters	Device/manufacturer	Duration and frequency	Adverse events	ITT	Outcomes (Assessment Tool)
Li et al. 2017	China	EG = 31 CG = 31	EG 28/3 CG 2/29	EG = 35.9 ± 10.6 CG = 37.1 ± 11.4	EG = 7.6 ± 3.7 CG = 7.2 ± 3.3	Bilateral Taiyang acupoints. (trigeminal nerve indirectly)	EG: frequency 2/ 100 Hz; CG: deliver no electrical stimulation	LH202H Han Electrostimulator, Jinghua Wei Industry Development Company, Beijing, China	5 times weekly for 12 weeks	No	Yes	Change in monthly migraine days, migraine attacks, headache days and acute antimigraine drug intake between run-in and third month of treatment
Schoenen et al. 2013	Belgium	EG = 34 CG = 33	EG 31/3 CG 30/3	EG = 34.6 ± 11.0 CG = 39.1 ± 9.9	EG = 7.8 ± 4.0 CG = 6.7 ± 2.6	Bilateral supratrochlear and supraorbital nerves	EG: biphasic rectangular impulses, pulse width 250 µs, frequency 60 Hz, intensity 16 mA; CG: pulse width 30 µs, frequency 1 Hz, intensity 1 mA	Cefaly, STX-Med., Herstal, Belgium	20 min daily for 3 months	No	Yes	Change in monthly migraine days, 50%response rate, change in monthly migraine attacks, headache days, mean headache severity per migraine day, acute antimigraine drug use between run-in and third month of treatment; satisfaction
Silberstein et al. 2016	USA	EG = 30 CG = 29	EG 26/4 CG 27/2	EG = 40.5 ± 14.2 CG = 38.8 ± 11.1	EG = 20.8 ± 5.0 CG = 22.3 ± 4.9	Vagus nerve	EG: voltage peak 24 V, maximum current of 60 mA; CG: deliver no electrical stimulation	GammaCore®, electroCore, LLC, Basking Ridge, NJ	Two 2-min 3 times a day for 8 months	EG: 12 AEs CG: 8 AEs	Yes	Safety and tolerability, Change of headache days per 28 days, 75% response rate, 50%response rate, acute medication use
Liu et al. 2017	China	EG = 66 CG = 22	EG 52/14 CG 18/4	EG = 37.6 ± 10.4 CG = 44.3 ± 8.3	EG = 11.5 ± 7.2 CG = 9.9 ± 3.9	Bilateral occipital nerves	EG: intensity 10 mA Group A 2 Hz, Group B 100 Hz, Group C 2/ 100 Hz CG: deliver no electrical stimulation	HANS-200A machine, JiSheng Medical Technology Limited Company, China	30 min daily for 1 month	EG: Group A 1 AE	Yes	50% responder rate, changes in headache days monthly, headache intensity (measured using the VAS), headache duration, scores on SDS、SAS、HIT-6, percentage of satisfaction

EG experimental group, *CG* control group, *ITT* intension-to-treat, *AE* adverse event

acupoints (trigeminal nerve indirectly) respectively. Parameters including frequency and amplitude were different among the trials in real TENS groups. In three studies [16–18], the sham group had the same device applied but received no electrical stimulation. In the one study [15], the intensity of sham simulation was far less than the real group. The outcome measurement methods were common across all studies, using headache diaries. One study had a high dropout rate [16] and all studies had an intention-to-treat analysis.

Risk of bias

Figure 2 summarized the risk of bias of four selected studies considering main outcomes. For the criteria sequence generation, we judged one trial as having an uncertain risk of bias [15], because it didn't provide sufficient information about randomization. All studies reported allocation concealment, therefore, we judged these studies as having low bias. It was noteworthy that, although all the studies claimed to be double-blind trials, it is difficult for patients to achieve a true blindness. For the sham protocol, three studies delivered no stimulation to devices [16–18], thus establishing blinding of participants is difficult. Only in one study both stimulators buzzed identically during treatment [15], and thus it was not possible to distinguish a sham from a real stimulator without testing both devices in parallel. Therefore, we deemed it at low risk of bias and the other three studies at a high risk of bias with respect to blinding of participants. All four studies used the headache diary to evaluate pain control, hence, evaluators could not influence this outcome measure. Therefore, we consider the studies as low risk of with regard to detection bias. One study had high dropout rate and we judge it as having a high risk of bias in terms of incomplete outcome data [16]. All studies utilized intention-to-treat analyses. Reporting bias and other potential sources of bias were judged as low in all included studies.

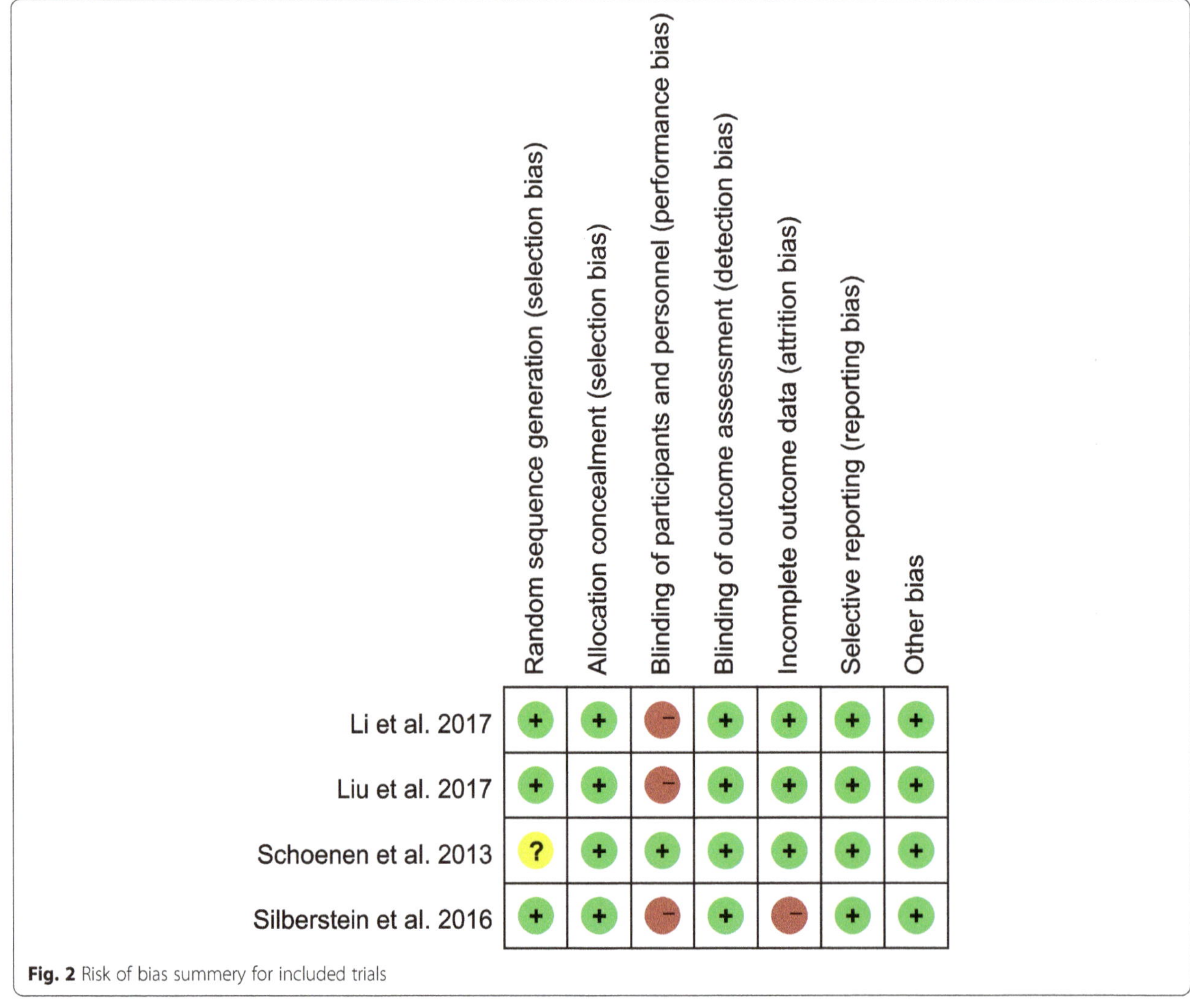

Fig. 2 Risk of bias summery for included trials

Primary outcomes

Change in the number of monthly headache days

The outcome data was analyzed with a fixed-effect model, and the pooled estimate of the four included RCTs suggested that compared with placebo group in migraine patients, real TENS was found to significantly reduce the number of monthly headache days (SMD: -0.48; 95% CI: -0.73 to – 0.23; $P < 0.001$), with moderate heterogeneity among the studies ($I^2 = 40\%$) (Fig. 3). Sensitivity analysis showed that heterogeneity was most likely because of the study by Li et al. [18], without which the heterogeneity reduced to zero with little change to the summary estimate (Fig. 4). The heterogeneity might be caused by the intervention. In the trial by Li et al. [18], percutaneous electrical nerve stimulation therapy utilized acupuncture-like needle probes insertion into the soft tissues to stimulate trigeminal nerves instead of electrodes.

Responder rate

All four studies with a total of 276 patients reported the number of responders. Responder rate was significantly higher in real TENS group than in sham TENS group (32.9% and 7.8%; RR: 4.05; 95% CI: 2.06–7.97; $P < 0.001$) (Fig. 5). Furthermore, the meta-analysis result of the included trials found a low level of heterogeneity ($I^2 = 0$). Thus, we did not perform sensitivity analysis.

Secondary outcomes

Painkiller intake

Only two studies included reported painkiller intake as an outcome [15, 18]. The pooled estimate of two included RCTs suggested that compared with sham TENS in migraine patients, real TENS yielded significantly decreased monthly painkiller intake (SMD: -0.78; 95% CI: -1.14 to – 0.42; P < 0.001), presented in Fig. 6.

Adverse events

All studies included mentioned adverse events or side effects related to TENS or sham TENS therapy during the trials. Only one study aimed to assess the feasibility, safety, and tolerability of TENS and reported adverse events in detail [16]. The tolerability profile of noninvasive vagus nerve stimulation (nVNS) was satisfactory and generally similar to that of sham treatment. Most adverse events were mild or moderate and transient. The most commonly reported adverse events were upper respiratory tract infections, facial pain and gastrointestinal symptoms. Two studies explicitly reported no adverse events associated with TENS treatment [15, 18]. In the other study [17], only one patient reported one adverse event in the 2 Hz group. It was a form of pinch pain and the uncomfortable feeling subsided when the intensity of the stimulation was reduced.

Satisfaction

Three studies reported the number of people satisfied with the TENS treatment [15–17]. Compared with sham TENS in migraine patients, real TENS yielded significant satisfaction rate. The pooled data of the 104 patients in these three studies showed significantly higher satisfaction rate in the real TENS group than the sham group (RR:1.85; 95% CI: 1.31 to 2.61; $P < 0.001$), with no heterogenicity ($I^2 = 0\%$) across the studies (Fig. 7).

GRADE analysis

The quality of evidence for outcomes evaluated in this review was assessed according to GRADE guidelines (Fig. 8) For the outcome of change in monthly headache days, the evidence quality was rated as low. We rated down one level for risk of bias. As samples size was smaller than optimal information size, the quality of evidence was downgraded once again for imprecision. The prevalence of small studies increases the risk of publication bias. There is a propensity for small negative studies not to reach full publication, and this might lead to an exaggerated estimate of effect [19]. We found that some of the trials were registered on clinicaltrials.gov, but the results were not updated in time. However, we did not downgrade for the publication bias as we had no direct evidence of this. For the outcome of responder rate, the evidence quality was rated as 'low' similar to change in monthly headache days.

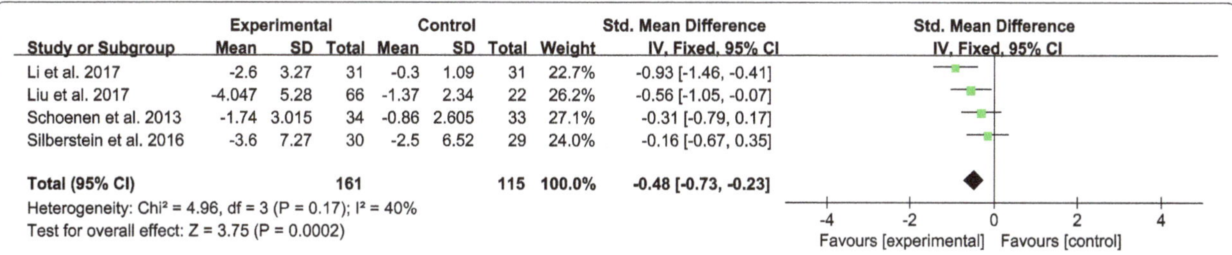

Experimental
Control
Std. Mean Difference
Std. Mean Difference
Study or Subgroup Mean SD Total Mean SD Total Weight IV, Fixed, 95% CI
IV, Fixed, 95% CI
Li et al. 2017 -2.6 3.27 31 -0.3 1.09 31 22.7% -0.93 [-1.46, -0.41]
Liu et al. 2017 -4.047 5.28 66 -1.37 2.34 22 26.2% -0.56 [-1.05, -0.07]
Schoenen et al. 2013 -1.74 3.015 34 -0.86 2.605 33 27.1% -0.31 [-0.79, 0.17]
Silberstein et al. 2016 -3.6 7.27 30 -2.5 6.52 29 24.0% -0.16 [-0.67, 0.35]
Total (95% CI) 161 115 100.0% -0.48 [-0.73, -0.23]
Heterogeneity: Chi² = 4.96, df = 3 (P = 0.17); I² = 40%
Test for overall effect: Z = 3.75 (P = 0.0002)
-4 -2 0 2 4
Favours [experimental] Favours [control]

Fig. 3 Change in the number of monthly headache days. Forest plot of the meta-analysis showed a significant decrease in the number of monthly headache days after therapy with TENS compared with sham TENS

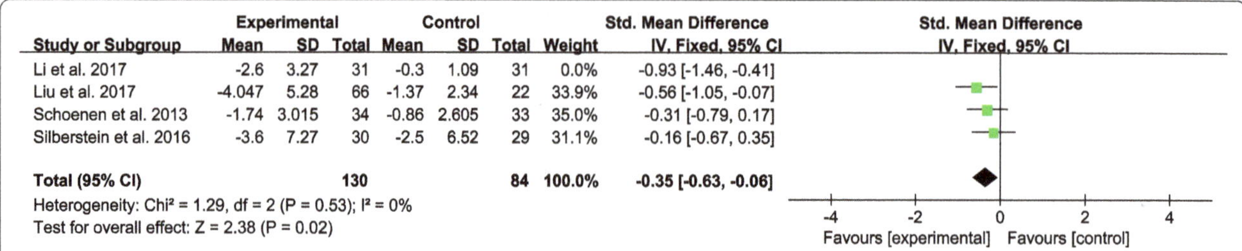

Fig. 4 Change in the number of monthly headache days (sensitivity analysis). Sensitivity analysis showed that heterogeneity was most likely because of the study by Li et al., without which the heterogeneity reduced to zero with little change to the summary estimate

Discussion

This meta-analysis of 4 RCTs including 276 patients provides evidence that TENS could be an effective and well-tolerated technique in increasing responder rate, reducing headache days and painkiller intake when compared with sham treatment. All the enrolled patients in the included studies didn't use prophylaxis drugs during the treatment and for 1 month prior to the treatment, which reduced the interference of prophylaxis drugs to a certain degree. However, the quality of the evidence was judged as 'low' GRADE due to the methodological limitations of the included studies, and overall small study sizes. Further research is very likely to have an important impact on our confidence in the estimate of effect and is likely to change the estimate.

This is the first meta-analysis, to the best of our knowledge, to investigate the effectiveness and safety of TENS for the treatment of migraine. This result is similar to a 2017 Cochrane review by Gibson et al. [20] and a 2015 Cochrane review by Johnson et al. [4], which were unable to makes definitive conclusions of TENS for acute and neuropathic pain largely because of inadequate sample sizes and unsuccessful blinding of treatment interventions in the included studies.

TENS induced analgesia is thought to be multifactorial and the 'gate control theory' is in fact the most conceivable view [21]. Neurostimulation may work by activating large fiber sensory afferents, which may secondarily inhibit nociceptive inputs from small fibers and elevate pain thresholds. Moreover, central descending pain inhibitory systems may be engaged as demonstrated by both animal studies and functional imaging studies [22]. GammaCore may reduce pain through restoration of brainstem monoaminergic neurotransmission [23], suppression of glutamate levels and cortical spreading depression [24, 25]. Cefaly may exert beneficial effects via normalization of orbitofrontal and rostral anterior cingulate cortices hypometabolism [26]. Occipital neurostimulation may active Aβ fibers of trigeminocervical complex in the neck in order to inhibit the pain transmission [17] and restore central descending pain modulatory tone at the same time [22]. Electrical stimulation to Taiyang acupoints, which indirectly stimulates the branch of the trigeminal nerve, improves the endogenous morphine like substance and serotonin in the central nervous system to relieve pain [27, 28]. Despite their unique mechanisms, all stimulated are peripheral nerves, and they have a common basic theory– 'gate control theory'. In the future, with the increase in the number of studies, subgroup analysis can be performed according to the type of stimulated nerves to reduce heterogeneity to some extent.

Maintaining blinding is a major methodological challenge in studying TENS. Various types of sham TENS have been proposed including units that are identical in appearance but just deliver an initial brief period of stimulation at the start and then faded out [29]. In some studies, sham stimulation parameters are set below levels

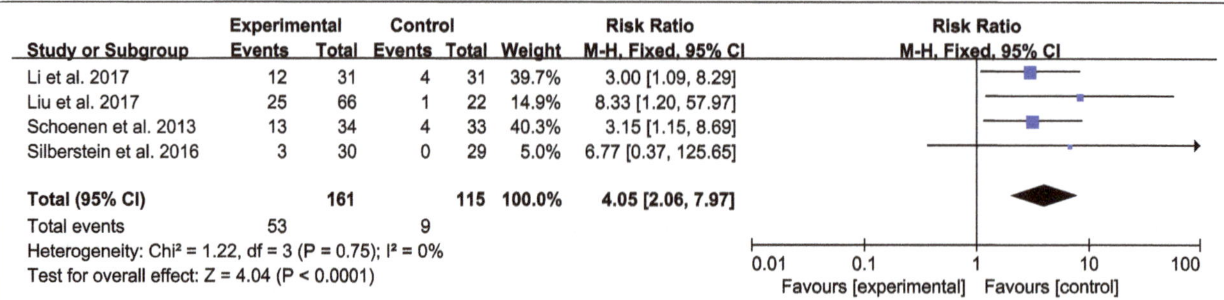

Experimental
Control
Risk Ratio
Risk Ratio
Study or Subgroup Events Total Events Total Weight M-H, Fixed, 95% CI
M-H, Fixed, 95% CI
Li et al. 2017 12 31 4 31 39.7% 3.00 [1.09, 8.29]
Liu et al. 2017 25 66 1 22 14.9% 8.33 [1.20, 57.97]
Schoenen et al. 2013 13 34 4 33 40.3% 3.15 [1.15, 8.69]
Silberstein et al. 2016 3 30 0 29 5.0% 6.77 [0.37, 125.65]
Total (95% CI) 161 115 100.0% 4.05 [2.06, 7.97]
Total events 53 9
Heterogeneity: Chi² = 1.22, df = 3 (P = 0.75); I² = 0%
Test for overall effect: Z = 4.04 (P < 0.0001)
0.01 0.1 1 10 100
Favours [experimental] Favours [control]

Fig. 5 Responder rate. Forest plot of the meta-analysis showed significant increase in 50% responder rate after therapy with TENS compared with sham TENS

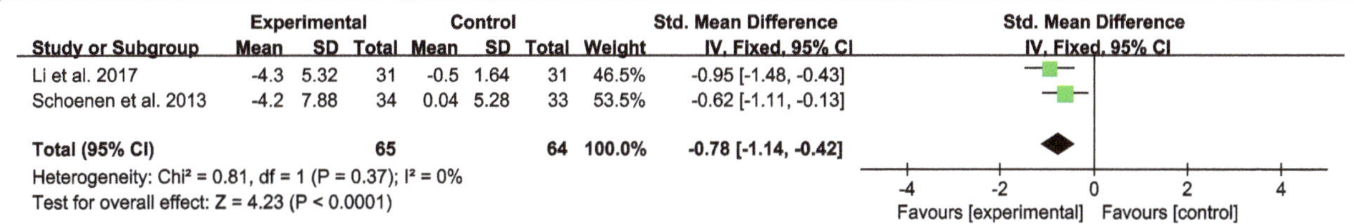

Study or Subgroup	Experimental Mean	SD	Total	Control Mean	SD	Total	Weight	Std. Mean Difference IV, Fixed, 95% CI
Li et al. 2017	-4.3	5.32	31	-0.5	1.64	31	46.5%	-0.95 [-1.48, -0.43]
Schoenen et al. 2013	-4.2	7.88	34	0.04	5.28	33	53.5%	-0.62 [-1.11, -0.13]
Total (95% CI)			**65**			**64**	**100.0%**	**-0.78 [-1.14, -0.42]**

Heterogeneity: Chi² = 0.81, df = 1 (P = 0.37); I² = 0%
Test for overall effect: Z = 4.23 (P < 0.0001)

Fig. 6 Painkiller intake. Forest plot of the meta-analysis showed a significant decrease in the number of painkiller intake after therapy with TENS compared with sham TENS

needed for therapeutic or even no current is delivered in control group [16–18]. However, active stimulation elicits strong sensations and a true sham treatment that establishes robust blinding of participants is challenge [30].

TENS technique has been applied for both acute treatment of migraine [31, 32] and migraine prevention [15, 17]. Even though some single-arm trials demonstrate the effectiveness of TENS for migraine [8, 31–35], the reliability is downgraded considering the placebo effect. Given that sham TENS methodologies may be inherently flawed, further studies can focus on assessing TENS versus preventive anti-migraine drugs, botulinum neurotoxin, or other nonpharmacologic treatments like neurofeedback and transcranial magnetic stimulation. Assessing conventional therapy versus conventional therapy plus active TENS can also be taken into consideration.

Limitations

Several limitations should be taken into account. Firstly, our analysis was based on only four RCTs and all of them had a relatively small sample size ($n < 100$). One trial enrolled both tension-type headache patients and migraineurs, and we failed to contact the authors for the detail data until the review was completed. The included studies varied in the number of sessions, stimulation parameters and stimulated nerve types particularly, which increased the potential biases in the studies. Secondly, no subgroup analysis was performed based on the stimulated nerve types owing to the small number of studies included. Thirdly, since only two trials reported headache intensity as outcomes and they differed in measuring method, classified as mild, moderate, severe pain and visual analogue (VAS) scale respectively, thus we didn't perform a pooled analysis. Finally, the follow-up period was generally short, so long-term outcomes of TENS remain to be proved.

Conclusions

This meta-analysis indicates that TENS may be effective in increasing responder rate, reducing headache days and painkiller intake, serving as a well-tolerated alternative for migraineurs. Nevertheless, despite our rigorous methodology, the inherent limitations of included studies make it impossible for us to draw definitive conclusions. Blinding of participants should be emphasized in future TENS trials to explore the efficacy of TENS as a sole or adjuvant therapy in patients with migraine, especially suffering from refractory migraine. TENS could be of help also in patients with (or at risk for) medication overuse and in fragile migraine populations, namely children, adolescents, pregnants and elderly. Future large-scale, well-designed RCTs with extensive follow-up are necessary to provide evidence-based efficacy data, optimize our knowledge concerning patient selection, stimulation parameters and update the findings of this analysis.

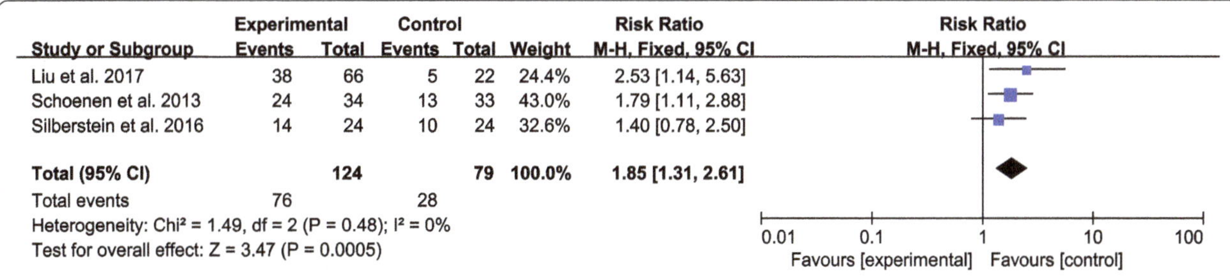

Study or Subgroup	Experimental Events	Total	Control Events	Total	Weight	Risk Ratio M-H, Fixed, 95% CI
Liu et al. 2017	38	66	5	22	24.4%	2.53 [1.14, 5.63]
Schoenen et al. 2013	24	34	13	33	43.0%	1.79 [1.11, 2.88]
Silberstein et al. 2016	14	24	10	24	32.6%	1.40 [0.78, 2.50]
Total (95% CI)		**124**		**79**	**100.0%**	**1.85 [1.31, 2.61]**
Total events	76		28			

Heterogeneity: Chi² = 1.49, df = 2 (P = 0.48); I² = 0%
Test for overall effect: Z = 3.47 (P = 0.0005)

Fig. 7 Satisfaction. Forest plot of the meta-analysis showed a significant increase in satisfaction after therapy with TENS compared with sham TENS

TENS compared to sham TENS for Migraine

Patient or population: patients with Migraine
Settings:
Intervention: TENS
Comparison: sham TENS

Outcomes	Illustrative comparative risks* (95% CI)		Relative effect (95% CI)	No of Participants (studies)	Quality of the evidence (GRADE)	Comments
	Assumed risk	Corresponding risk				
	Sham TENS	TENS				
Change in the number of monthly headache days Headache diary		The mean change in the number of monthly headache days in the intervention groups was **0.48 standard deviations lower** (0.73 to 0.23 lower)		276 (4 studies)	⊕⊕⊖⊖ **low**[1,2]	SMD -0.48 (-0.73 to -0.23)
Responder rate Headache diary	**Study population**		**RR 4.05** (2.06 to 7.97)	276 (4 studies)	⊕⊕⊖⊖ **low**[3,4]	
	78 per 1000	**317 per 1000** (161 to 624)				
	Moderate					
	83 per 1000	**336 per 1000** (171 to 662)				

*The basis for the **assumed risk** (e.g. the median control group risk across studies) is provided in footnotes. The **corresponding risk** (and its 95% confidence interval) is based on the assumed risk in the comparison group and the **relative effect** of the intervention (and its 95% CI).

CI: Confidence interval; **RR:** Risk ratio;

GRADE Working Group grades of evidence
High quality: Further research is very unlikely to change our confidence in the estimate of effect.
Moderate quality: Further research is likely to have an important impact on our confidence in the estimate of effect and may change the estimate.
Low quality: Further research is very likely to have an important impact on our confidence in the estimate of effect and is likely to change the estimate.
Very low quality: We are very uncertain about the estimate.

[1] One study had incomplete outcome data and the blinding to participants in three studies was easy to broken. Final decision: we rated down one level for risk of bias.
[2] Despite short confidence interval, total studies samples were smaller than OIS(optimal information size). Final decision: we rated down one level for imprecision.
[3] One study had incomplete outcome data and the blinding to participants in three studies was easy to broken. Final decision: we rated down one level for risk of bias.
[4] Despite short confidence interval, total studies samples were smaller than OIS(optimal information size). Final decision: we rated down one level for imprecision.

Fig. 8 Quality of evidence assessment. Quality of evidence assessment for pain control outcomes performed by GRADE profiler

Clinical implications

This is the first meta-analysis investigating the effectiveness and safety of TENS for the treatment of migraine.

There is low quality evidence suggesting that TENS may be effective in increasing responder rate, reducing headache days and painkiller intake, serving as a well-tolerated alternative for migraineurs.

Future well-designed RCTs with extensive follow-up are necessary to provide evidence-based efficacy data, optimize our knowledge concerning patient selection and stimulation parameters.

Abbreviations

AE: Adverse event; CG: Control group; CI: Confidence interval; EG: Experimental group; ICHD: the International classification of headache disorders; ITT: Intension-to-treat; M-H: Mantel-Haenszel; TENS: Transcutaneous electrical nerve stimulation

Acknowledgements

The authors thank Dr. Shu Min Tao (Department of Medical Imaging, Affiliated Hospital of Nantong University, Nantong, Jiangsu 226001, China) for reviewing the manuscript.

Authors' contributions

Study concept and design: QW, HT. Acquisition of data: HT, TW. Analysis and interpretation of data: HT, TW, XD, QG. Drafting of the manuscript: HT, HX. Critical revision of the manuscript for important intellectual content: QW, XD. All authors read and approved the final manuscript.

Competing interests

The authors declare that they have no competing interests.

References

1. GBD (2016) Disease, injury incidence, prevalence collaborators (2017) global, regional, and national incidence, prevalence, and years lived with disability for 328 diseases and injuries for 195 countries, 1990-2016: a systematic analysis for the global burden of disease study 2016. Lancet 390(10100): 1211–1259
2. Akerman S, Romero-Reyes M, Holland PR (2017) Current and novel insights into the neurophysiology of migraine and its implications for therapeutics. Pharmacol Ther 172:151–170
3. Kristoffersen ES, Lundqvist C (2014) Medication-overuse headache: epidemiology, diagnosis and treatment. Ther Adv Drug Saf 5(2):87–99
4. Johnson MI, Paley CA, Howe TE, Sluka KA (2015) Transcutaneous electrical nerve stimulation for acute pain. Cochrane Database Syst Rev 6:CD006142. https://doi.org/10.1002/14651858.CD006142.pub3

5. Peroutka SJ (2015) Clinical trials update 2014: year in review. Headache 55(1):149–157
6. Gaul C, Diener HC, Silver N, Magis D, Reuter U, Andersson A, Liebler EJ, Straube A, Group PS (2016) Non-invasive vagus nerve stimulation for PREVention and acute treatment of chronic cluster headache (PREVA): a randomised controlled study. Cephalalgia 36(6):534–546
7. Kinfe TM, Pintea B, Muhammad S, Zaremba S, Roeske S, Simon BJ, Vatter H (2015) Cervical non-invasive vagus nerve stimulation (nVNS) for preventive and acute treatment of episodic and chronic migraine and migraine-associated sleep disturbance: a prospective observational cohort study. J Headache Pain 16:101
8. Barbanti P, Grazzi L, Egeo G, Padovan AM, Liebler E, Bussone G (2015) Non-invasive vagus nerve stimulation for acute treatment of high-frequency and chronic migraine: an open-label study. J Headache Pain 16:61
9. Moher D, Liberati A, Tetzlaff J, Altman DG, Group P (2009) Preferred reporting items for systematic reviews and meta-analyses: the PRISMA statement. BMJ 339:b2535
10. Higgins JP, Altman DG, Gotzsche PC, Juni P, Moher D, Oxman AD, Savovic J, Schulz KF, Weeks L, Sterne JA, Cochrane Bias Methods G, Cochrane Statistical Methods G (2011) The Cochrane Collaboration's tool for assessing risk of bias in randomised trials. BMJ 343:d5928
11. Higgins J, Green S (2011) Cochrane Handbook for Systematic Reviews of Interventions Version 5.1.0 Wiley-Blackwell,2011:102–8
12. Higgins JP, Thompson SG, Deeks JJ, Altman DG (2003) Measuring inconsistency in meta-analyses. BMJ 327(7414):557–560
13. Guyatt GH, Oxman AD, Vist GE, Kunz R, Falck-Ytter Y, Alonso-Coello P, Schunemann HJ, Group GW (2008) GRADE: an emerging consensus on rating quality of evidence and strength of recommendations. BMJ 336(7650):924–926
14. Bono F, Salvino D, Mazza MR, Curcio M, Trimboli M, Vescio B, Quattrone A (2015) The influence of ictal cutaneous allodynia on the response to occipital transcutaneous electrical stimulation in chronic migraine and chronic tension-type headache: a randomized, sham-controlled study. Cephalalgia 35(5):389–398
15. Schoenen J, Vandersmissen B, Jeangette S, Herroelen L, Vandenheede M, Gerard P, Magis D (2013) Migraine prevention with a supraorbital transcutaneous stimulator: a randomized controlled trial. Neurology 80(8): 697–704
16. Silberstein SD, Calhoun AH, Lipton RB, Grosberg BM, Cady RK, Dorlas S, Simmons KA, Mullin C, Liebler EJ, Goadsby PJ, Saper JR, Group ES (2016) Chronic migraine headache prevention with noninvasive vagus nerve stimulation: the EVENT study. Neurology 87(5):529–538
17. Liu Y, Dong Z, Wang R, Ao R, Han X, Tang W, Yu S (2017) Migraine prevention using different frequencies of transcutaneous occipital nerve stimulation: a randomized controlled trial. J Pain 18(8):1006–1015
18. Li H, Xu QR (2017) Effect of percutaneous electrical nerve stimulation for the treatment of migraine. Medicine (Baltimore) 96(39):e8108
19. Dechartres A, Trinquart L, Boutron I, Ravaud P (2013) Influence of trial sample size on treatment effect estimates: meta-epidemiological study. BMJ 346:f2304
20. Gibson W, Wand BM, O'Connell NE (2017) Transcutaneous electrical nerve stimulation (TENS) for neuropathic pain in adults. Cochrane Database Syst Rev 9:CD011976. https://doi.org/10.1002/14651858.CD011976.pub2
21. Treede RD (2016) Gain control mechanisms in the nociceptive system. Pain 157(6):1199–1204
22. Robbins MS, Lipton RB (2017) Transcutaneous and percutaneous Neurostimulation for headache disorders. Headache 57 Suppl 1:4–13
23. Yuan H, Silberstein SD (2016) Vagus nerve and Vagus nerve stimulation, a comprehensive review: part III. Headache 56(3):479–490
24. Oshinsky ML, Murphy AL, Hekierski H Jr, Cooper M, Simon BJ (2014) Noninvasive vagus nerve stimulation as treatment for trigeminal allodynia. Pain 155(5):1037–1042
25. Chen SP, Ay I, de Morais AL, Qin T, Zheng Y, Sadeghian H, Oka F, Simon B, Eikermann-Haerter K, Ayata C (2016) Vagus nerve stimulation inhibits cortical spreading depression. Pain 157(4):797–805
26. Magis D, D'Ostilio K, Thibaut A, De Pasqua V, Gerard P, Hustinx R, Laureys S, Schoenen J (2017) Cerebral metabolism before and after external trigeminal nerve stimulation in episodic migraine. Cephalalgia 37(9):881–891
27. Ahmed HE, White PF, Craig WF, Hamza MA, Ghoname ES, Gajraj NM (2000) Use of percutaneous electrical nerve stimulation (PENS) in the short-term management of headache. Headache 40(4):311–315
28. Heidland A, Fazeli G, Klassen A, Sebekova K, Hennemann H, Bahner U, Di Iorio B (2013) Neuromuscular electrostimulation techniques: historical aspects and current possibilities in treatment of pain and muscle waisting. Clin Nephrol 79(Suppl 1):S12–S23
29. Rakel B, Cooper N, Adams HJ, Messer BR, Law LAF, Dannen DR, Miller CA, Polehna AC, Ruggle RC, Vance CGT (2010) A new transient sham TENS device allows for investigator blinding while delivering a true placebo treatment. J Pain Official J Am Pain Soc 11(3):230
30. Sluka KA, Bjordal JM, Marchand S, Rakel BA (2013) What makes transcutaneous electrical nerve stimulation work? Making sense of the mixed results in the clinical literature. Phys Ther 93(10):1397–1402
31. Chou DE, Gross GJ, Casadei CH, Yugrakh MS (2017) External trigeminal nerve stimulation for the acute treatment of migraine: open-label trial on safety and efficacy. Neuromodulation 20(7):678–683
32. Grazzi L, Egeo G, Liebler E, Padovan AM, Barbanti P (2017) Non-invasive vagus nerve stimulation (nVNS) as symptomatic treatment of migraine in young patients: a preliminary safety study. Neurol Sci 38(1):197–199
33. Russo A, Tessitore A, Conte F, Marcuccio L, Giordano A, Tedeschi G (2015) Transcutaneous supraorbital neurostimulation in "de novo" patients with migraine without aura: the first Italian experience. J Headache Pain 16:69
34. Straube A, Ellrich J, Eren O, Blum B, Ruscheweyh R (2015) Treatment of chronic migraine with transcutaneous stimulation of the auricular branch of the vagal nerve (auricular t-VNS): a randomized, monocentric clinical trial. J Headache Pain 16:543
35. Vikelis M, Dermitzakis EV, Spingos KC, Vasiliadis GG, Vlachos GS, Kararizou E (2017) Clinical experience with transcutaneous supraorbital nerve stimulation in patients with refractory migraine or with migraine and intolerance to topiramate: a prospective exploratory clinical study. BMC Neurol 17(1):97

Novel capsaicin-induced parameters of microcirculation in migraine patients revealed by imaging photoplethysmography

Alexei A. Kamshilin[1*], Maxim A. Volynsky[1], Olga Khayrutdinova[2], Dilyara Nurkhametova[3,4], Laura Babayan[5], Alexander V. Amelin[5], Oleg V. Mamontov[1,6] and Rashid Giniatullin[1,3,4]

Abstract

Background: The non-invasive biomarkers of migraine can help to develop the personalized medication of this disorder. In testing of the antimigraine drugs the capsaicin-induced skin redness with activated TRPV1 receptors in sensory neurons associated with the release of the migraine mediator CGRP has already been widely used.

Methods: Fourteen migraine patients (mean age 34.6 ± 10.2 years) and 14 healthy volunteers (mean age 29.9 ± 9.7 years) participated in the experiment. A new arrangement of imaging photoplethysmography recently developed by us was used here to discover novel sensitive parameters of dermal blood flow during capsaicin applications in migraine patients.

Results: Blood pulsation amplitude (BPA) observed as optical-intensity waveform varying synchronously with heartbeat was used for detailed exploration of microcirculatory perfusion induced by capsicum patch application. The BPA signals, once having appeared after certain latent period, were progressively rising until being saturated. Capsaicin-induced high BPA areas were distributed unevenly under the patch, forming "hot spots." Interestingly the hot spots were much more variable in migraine patients than in the control group. In contrast to BPA, a slow component of waveforms related to the skin redness changed significantly less than BPA highlighting the latter parameter as the potential sensitive biomarker of capsaicin-induced activation of the blood flow. Thus, in migraine patients, there is a non-uniform (both in space and in time) reaction to capsaicin, resulting in highly variable openings of skin capillaries.

Conclusion: BPA dynamics measured by imaging photoplethysmography could serve as a novel sensitive non-invasive biomarker of migraine-associated changes in microcirculation.

Keywords: Migraine, Capsaicin, Microcirculation, CGRP, TRPV1, Dermal blood flow, Imaging photoplethysmography

Background

One of the main trends in migraine studies is to find out the most sensitive and preferably non-invasive biomarkers serving for the diagnostic and personalized treatments of this often-intractable disorder. Application of capsaicin to the skin is widely used to monitor the reactiveness of local blood flow following activation of capsaicin-sensitive TRPV1 receptors [1, 2]. The underlying mechanism of redness (flare) is mainly associated with the release of the neuropeptide CGRP from nociceptive C-fibers expressing TRPV1 receptors in membrane [3]. Several recent studies in animals and humans suggested the role of TRPV1 receptors in migraine [4, 5]. Accumulated evidence also suggested that CGRP is the main neuropeptide implicated in migraine pathology [6–8]. Many modern approaches for migraine treatment are based on inhibition of CGRP driven pro-nociceptive activity [7, 9]. This requires simple tests to evaluate the release of CGRP in humans. Thus, capsaicin-induced increase in dermal blood flow (DBF) is widely used to test the activity of potential anti-migraine medicines [2]. Apart from general

* Correspondence: alexei.kamshilin@yandex.ru
[1]Department of Computer Photonics and Videomatics, ITMO University, St. Petersburg, Russia
Full list of author information is available at the end of the article

pharmaceutical significance, this DBF method could be attractive to develop personalized approaches for migraine treatments, for instance, to test the sensitivity of the particular individual to capsaicin as a prognostic of CGRP mediated component in his/her vascular reactions. In this regard, it is worth noting that people with TRPV1 rs8065080 polymorphism are differentially sensitive to capsaicin [1] providing a genetic background for the distinct reactivity.

A recent study has shown that migraine patients reported higher level of capsaicin-induced feeling of pain and larger areas of flare [10]. In most studies simple measurement of the flare size is commonly used as the index of activation of capsaicin receptors [4, 10] although it is clear that this general reaction is determined by many non-specific factors such as the thickness of skin, its native color and, importantly, the level of CGRP released from the skin nerves [2].

Laser Doppler imaging systems are commonly used for assessment of the cutaneous microcirculation [11, 12]. However, these systems provide sequential scanning of the area under study, which increases the time needed to collect information from the area under study when its size is big and high spatial resolution is required. In contrast, imaging photoplethysmography (IPPG) systems acquire information from multiple points in parallel and simultaneously thus providing high spatial and temporal resolution [13]. It was shown recently that these systems are capable to visualize capillary blood flow [14, 15] making IPPG method more preferable for detailed study of spatial-temporal variations of microcirculation. Previously we suggested the non-invasive IPPG technique to evaluate the vascular reactions in migraine [16, 17]. Recently we advanced this technique by linking peripheral changes in pulsatile blood flow with heart rate, which largely increased the sensitivity of this combined approach [18]. In the current study, we used IPPG to monitor parameters of local blood circulation in the skin during capsaicin applications in patients with migraine and compared those with microcirculation in control group. With this technique we find out highly heterogeneous (both in time and space) reaction of migraine patients to stimulation of TRPV1 receptors that control local microcirculation. We also show that BPA does not always coincide with redness (or skin flare) and can serve as potential biomarker of blood flow changes associated with migraine and probably with other cardiovascular diseases.

Methods

General description of participants

The study was conducted in St. Petersburg and Kazan in accordance with ethical standards presented in the 2013 Declaration of Helsinki. The Ethics Committees of the Pavlov First Saint-Petersburg State Medical University and Kazan Federal University prior the research approved the protocol of this study. The study involved 14 patients with migraine and 14 healthy volunteers. Both groups were comparable in age, main constitutional, and hemodynamic parameters (see Table 1). An informed consent was obtained from all participants prior to enrollment.

Patients' selection

The diagnosis of migraine was established according to the International classification of headache disorder (third edition, beta version, ICHD-III3-beta) [19]. Patients meeting the following criteria were included in the study: previously diagnosed migraine with/without aura (as defined in ICHD-3-beta), age from 18 to 55. Exclusion criteria included chronic diseases in stage of decompensation, oncology, pregnancy, breast feeding, intolerance or allergic reaction to lidocaine or capsaicin, treatment by CGRP neutralizing antibodies or antibodies blocking the function of CGRP receptors in the history. In total 48 patients were evaluated for inclusion and exclusion criteria. Twelve patients were excluded due to oncological diseases, pregnancy or breast feeding. Thirty-six patients met the inclusion criteria. Twenty-two people declined to participate in the study. Fourteen patients and 14 healthy volunteers provided informed consent to take part in the study and had undergone the intervention. Most patients with migraine had experienced an episodic form of disease (Table 2). An aura during an attack occurred in a third of patients. None of the patients used CGRP neutralizing antibodies or antibodies blocking the function of CGRP receptors. The frequency of attacks was varying from one to fifteen per month (4.6 ± 4.1) and disease duration from 6 to 30 years (14.7 ± 9.2). The duration of the attack varied from 24 to 72 h. Six patients used triptans, 10 used NSAIDs, while three patients used both types of medications to reverse symptoms. In all patients, the examinations were conducted during the interictal period, at least one day after the last episode of headaches. A

Table 1 Healthy subjects and migraine patients

Parameter	Control group	Migraine patients	Significance of differences
Population	14	14	$p > 0.05$
Female/male	6/6	10/4	$p > 0.05$
Age, years	33.7 ± 9.8	34.6 ± 10.2	$p > 0.05$
Body mass index, kg/m^2	23.1 ± 2.8	22.5 ± 2.6	$p > 0.05$
Systolic blood pressure, mmHg	122 ± 11	121 ± 12	$p > 0.05$
Diastolic blood pressure, mmHg	77 ± 7	79 ± 7	$p > 0.05$
Heart rate	78 ± 13	74 ± 14	$p > 0.05$

Table 2 Clinical characteristics of patients with migraine

Index	Value
Form of migraine, rare / frequent / chronic	11 / 2 / 1
Aura, n (%)	4 (28.6%)
Cupping migraine attack by triptans, n (%)	6 (42.9%)
Frequency of attacks, per month	4.6 ± 4.1
Duration of the disease, years, age	14.7 ± 9.2

period of ten days minimum had passed since the last use of triptan medication.

Experimental technique

Parameters of the cutaneous blood flow were measured at the upper arm of each subject by using imaging photoplethysmography (IPPG) method [18]. Figure 1 shows the schematic presentation of the experimental setup. During the experiment, the subject was laid in horizontal position. His upper arm was illuminated by the green light (at the wavelength of 530 ± 25 nm) generated by eight light-emitted diodes (LEDs) as shown in Fig. 1b. The imaging lens of a digital black-and-white CMOS camera (8-bit model GigE uEye UI-5220SE of the Imaging Development Systems GmbH) was situated in the central part of the LEDs ring. Cross polarizing films were attached ahead of the lens and LEDs to eliminate superficial reflection from the skin [20]. All images were recorded at the frame rate of 39 frames per second with the resolution of 752 × 480 pixels, and transferred frame-by-frame in the PNG format into a personal computer for subsequent off-line analysis. An electrocardiogram (ECG) was recorded simultaneously and synchronously with video frames to improve the quality of data processing [18]. All video recordings were carried out in a dark laboratory room at the temperature of 23 ± 1 °C whereas subject's eyes were protected by special glasses that do not transmit the green light.

Protocol of the study

The experimental protocol included the following steps.

1. Before measurements, each subject was asked to relax in the laboratory during 15 min. After relaxation, his/her blood pressure was measured. Thereafter, subject took the recumbent position for video recording of an area of the upper arm during 20 s by means of the IPPG system (Fig. 1). This recording was used to estimate the baseline of blood circulation parameters.
2. In the next step, local anesthesia with 10% lidocaine was applied in an area on the upper arm for 1 h by using gauze patch. During this period, the subject was free in movements. After removal of the lidocaine patch, the subject was asked to take recumbent position again for the recording of 20-s video using IPPG system.
3. Then the patch (5 × 5 cm^2) containing 8% capsaicin (officinal Quatenza patch) was applied to the upper-arm area recorded by the IPPG system in the previous steps. Application of the Quatenza patch lasted from 15 to 25 min during which the subject was asked to keep the recumbent position and refrain from movements. Video images of the area with Quatenza patch were recorded during 20 s repeating the recording about every minute. Since the Quatenza patch is transparent for the green light, we were able to estimate parameters of blood circulation and their evolution under the patch.
4. In the last step, the Quatenza patch was removed, and the study area was cleaned by a special gel.

By this way, we obtained a series of video frames for each subject before and after topical application of the capsaicin to the upper arm. Processing of simultaneously

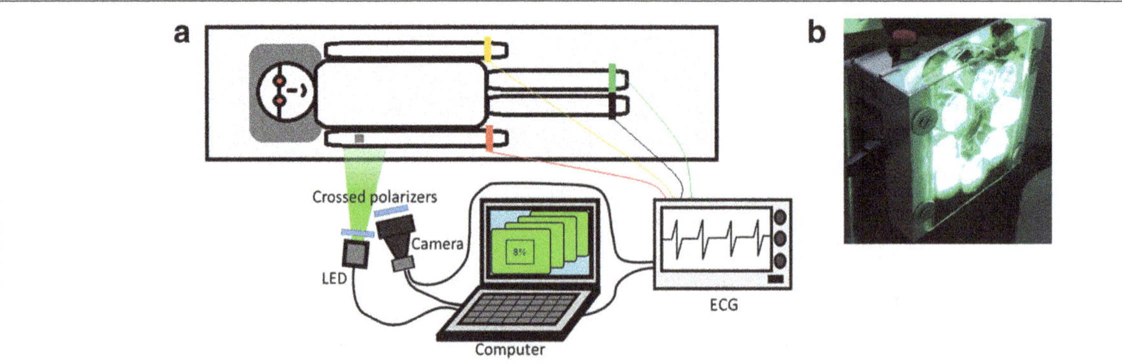

Fig. 1 Experimental technique. **a** Layout of the setup for photoplethysmographic image acquisition simultaneously with ECG and **b** photograph of the unit containing digital camera and illuminator with eight green LEDs

recorded video and ECG data allowed us to reveal the parameters of microcirculation in each point of the area under study and their evolution during the experiment.

Data processing

Each series of recorded video frames was processed off-line by using custom-made software implemented in the MATLAB platform. First, we calculated the spatial distribution of the blood pulsations amplitude (BPA) by using the algorithm described in details in our previous paper [18]. Briefly, the technique includes the following steps. (i) in the recorded image of subject's upper arm, we manually selected an area slightly larger than the Quatenza patch. It was automatically covered by small non-overlapping regions of interest (ROI) sizing 5 × 5 pixels (1.5 × 1.5 mm^2 in the arm). (ii) in every ROI we calculated frame-by-frame evolution of average pixel values to evaluate a PPG waveform. Typical waveform consisted of alternative component (AC) modulated at the heartbeat frequency, which was superimposed with the slowly varying component (DC). After calculation of AC-to-DC ratio, deducing the unity, and inverting the sign, we obtained a PPG waveform. Examples of the waveforms are shown in Fig. 2a, c. (iii) we defined the beginning of each cardiac cycle by the position of every R-peak in ECG, summarized all PPG pieces recorded during 20 s to evaluate the mean PPG shape of one cycle (shown in Fig. 2b, d), and calculated blood pulsation amplitude (BPA) as difference between maximal and minimal values of the mean PPG waveform.

The typical PPG waveform before Quatenza patch application is shown in Fig. 2a. One can see that the signal modulation is of a noise-like type. In addition, the heartbeat related modulation is hidden in the waveform shown in Fig. 2a. It can be revealed after averaging the PPG signal over 20 or more cardiac cycles if the beginning of each cardiac cycle is known (that is achieved by synchronous recording of PPG and EGC). Thick red curve in Fig. 2b shows the mean shape of one cardiac cycle whereas thin colored curves show the signals during every cycle presented in phase with R-peaks of ECG. Mean PPG waveform contains heartbeat related modulation affected by physiological noise [18]. The algorithm of BPA estimation allowed us to calculate the spatial distribution of BPA over subject's arm. Typical examples of BPA maps are shown in Fig. 3.

Statistical analysis

Statistical analysis was performed using the STATISTICA 10 software. All continuous variables were expressed as the mean ± standard deviation of the mean

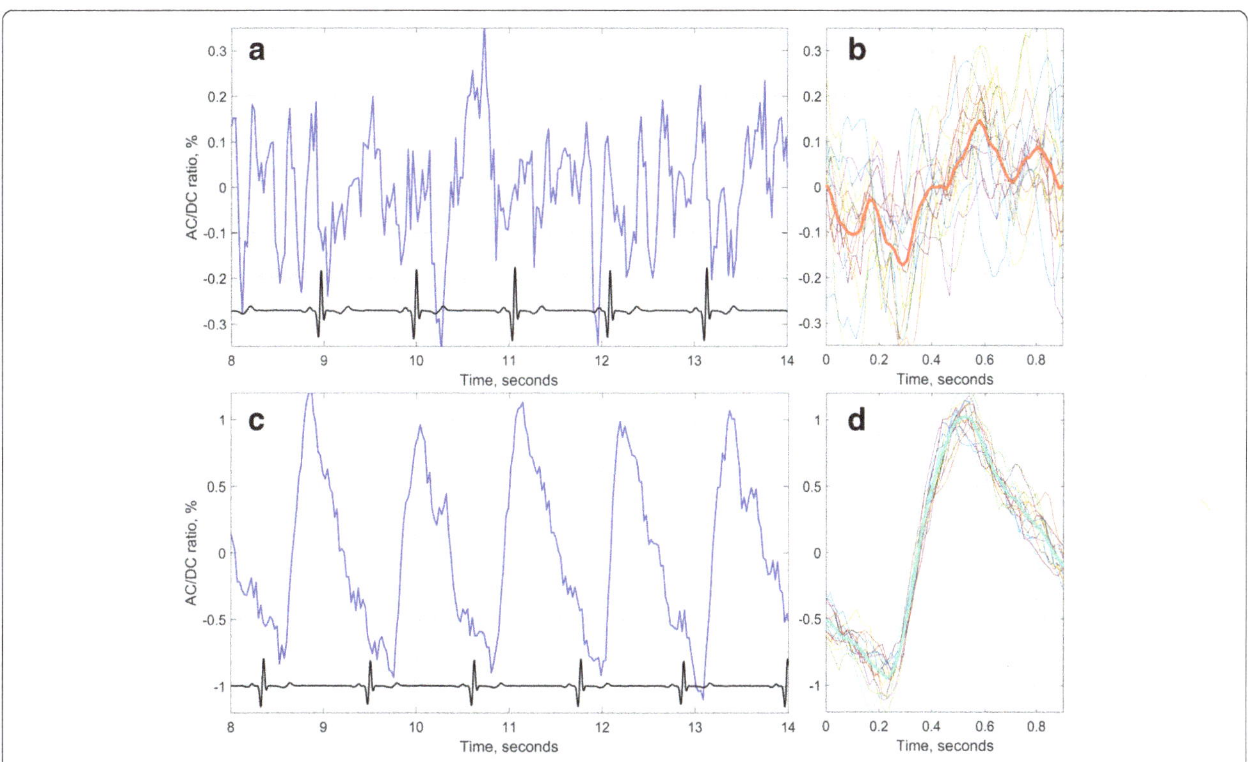

Fig. 2 Typical example of PPG waveform measured in the upper arm. Waveform shown in (**a**) was recorded before application of the capsaicin patch, whereas that in (**c**) was recorded at about 15-th minute of the patch application. Black curves in (**a**) and (**c**) show synchronously recorded ECG. Thick lines in (**b**) and (**d**) show the shape of the signal after averaging over 20 cardiac cycles

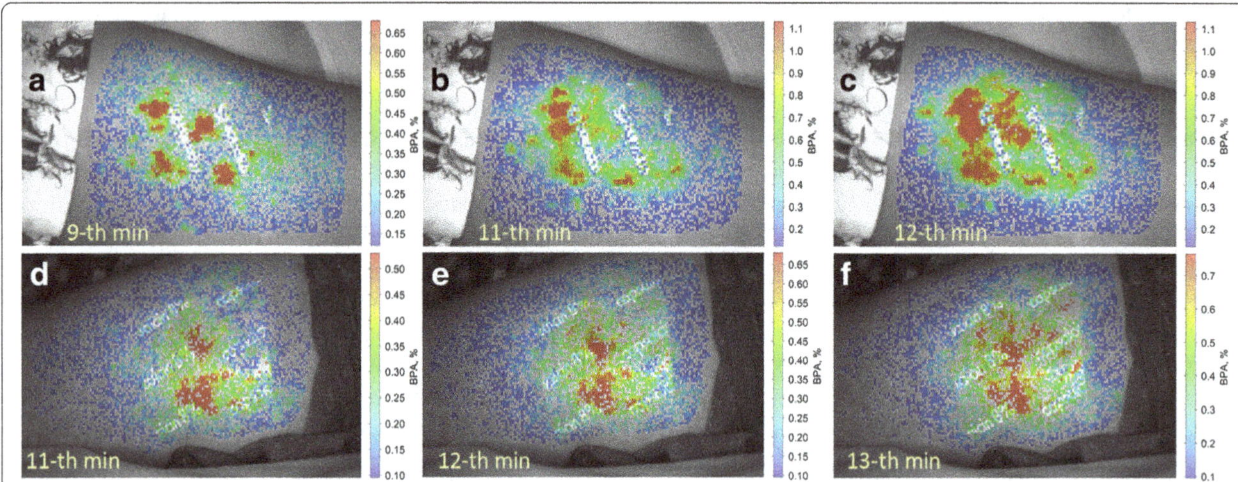

Fig. 3 Evolution of the spatial distribution of blood pulsation amplitude in the upper arm during capsaicin application. BPA maps for migraine patients are shown in the upper raw (**a-c**) whereas those for healthy subjects are in the lower raw (**d-f**). The color scale on the right of each map shows BPA as AC/DC ratio in percent for each distribution, respectively. The moment of PPG recording is shown in the left lower corner of each map with reference to the beginning of capsaicin application

(SD). The results of the comparative analysis are graphically represented as the mean, error of the mean, and SD. Non-parametric Mann - Whitney U-test was used to assess the reliability of the differences. One-variance dispersion analysis (ANOVA) with selection of the least number of significant indicators was used to assess the coupled variability of blood flow characteristics in the main and control groups. The diagnostic significance of blood flow parameters in response to capsaicin application was assessed through discriminant analysis using the lowest number of indicators. Significance was assumed when $p < 0.05$.

Results

Capsaicin-induced blood perfusion

The baseline of blood perfusion (before lidocaine application) in the capillary bed of the upper arm was at low level for majority of subjects (BPA was less than 0.3%). According to the protocol of our experiment, the lidocaine patch was applied for one hour and after its removal, the 8%-capsaicin patch was applied to the same area of the upper arm. At the beginning of capsaicin patch application the noise-like PPG waveforms (such as shown in Fig. 2a) were observed for all subjects. Similar noise-like signals were observed in the baseline recordings before lidocaine application. However, after certain delay time (DT), the modulation amplitude of PPG waveforms started to grow up. The delay time was individual for each subject with the mean value of 7.6 ± 3.5 min ranging from 1.1 to 13.9 min. The growth of BPA was accompanied by changes in the waveform shape that becomes similar to the classical PPG shape with anacrotic waves following the arterial blood pressure change. A typical example of the PPG waveform with increased BPA is shown in Fig. 2c with the mean shape of this waveform during the cardiac cycle shown in Fig. 2d. It is seen in Fig. 2d that individual signals of different cardiac cycles (thin colored lines) are well synchronized with the heartbeats defined by the R-peaks of ECG.

Blood perfusion dynamics

The transparency of the capsaicin patch for green light allowed us to measure spatial distribution of BPA an its evolution *continuously* during the whole period of patch application. First, we found that BPA was unevenly increased in all participants forming areas with elevated amplitude ("hot spots") of blood pulsations. These hot spots were clearly corresponded to the locally increased blood flow in the capillary bed. Examples of the spatial BPA distribution and its variation during capsaicin application are shown in Fig. 3 for two subjects, one from the migraine and another from the control group. Notably, there was a remarkable difference between BPA dynamics in these two subjects. Whereas the position of "hot spots" in migraine patient (Fig. 3a-c) strongly varied (providing an impression of migrating spots), there was a rather stable position of the "hot spots" in the control subject (Fig. 3d-f).

Two representative examples of BPA evolution during capsaicin application (3 for migraine patients and 3 for healthy subjects, respectively) are shown in Fig. 4. In all cases the time-course of BPA changes after capsaicin application consisted of three clearly distinguishable stages. The first stage was represented by a latent period when the heartbeat-related modulation was comparable with

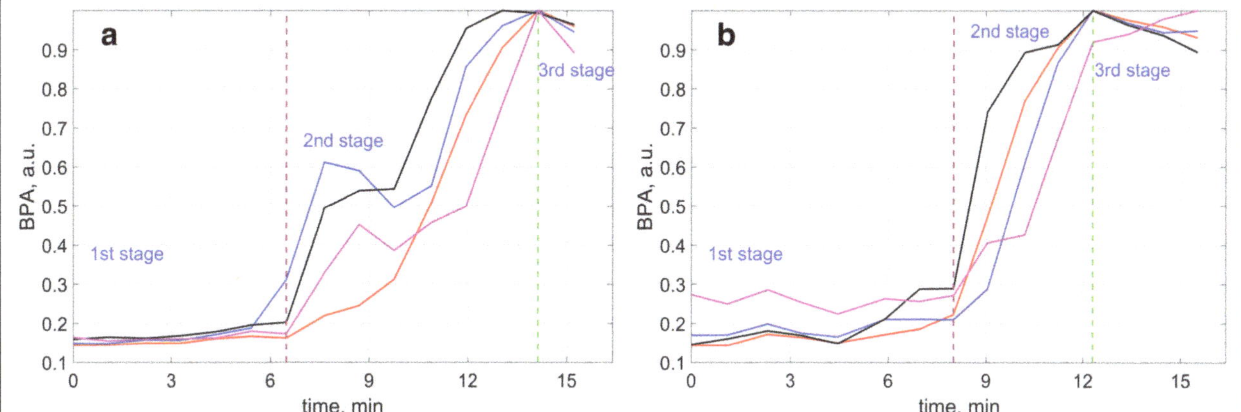

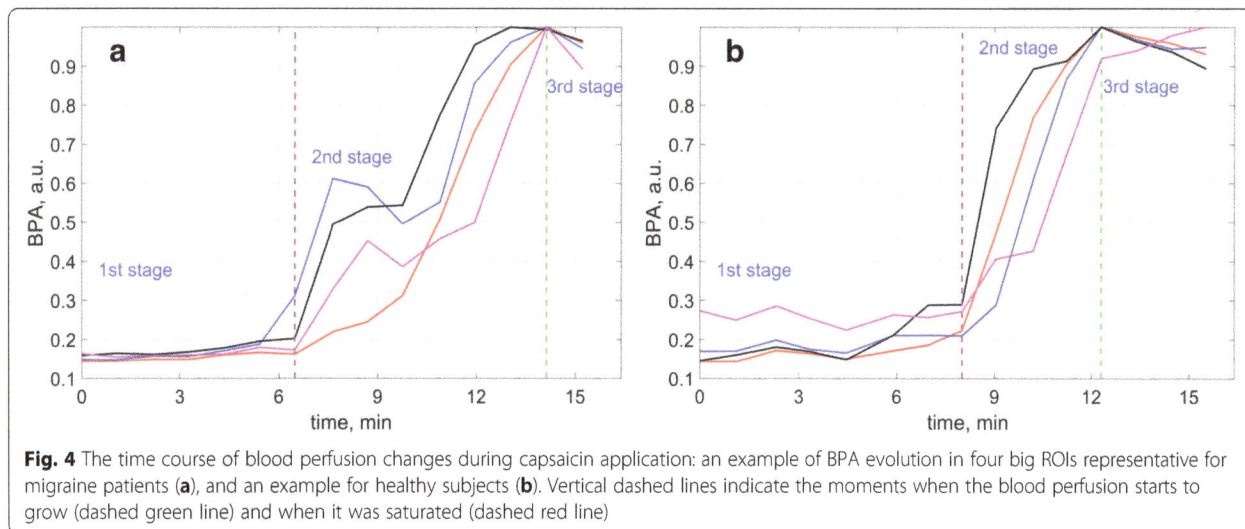

Fig. 4 The time course of blood perfusion changes during capsaicin application: an example of BPA evolution in four big ROIs representative for migraine patients (**a**), and an example for healthy subjects (**b**). Vertical dashed lines indicate the moments when the blood perfusion starts to grow (dashed green line) and when it was saturated (dashed red line)

noise (see the waveform in Fig. 2b). At the second stage a sharp increase of BPA was observed when the PPG waveform became similar to the waveform of arterial blood pressure (Fig. 2d). At the third stage, there was a saturation of the blood pulsation amplitudes. Each graph in Fig. 4 includes four curves (red, blue, black, and pink) showing BPA evolution in non-overlapping big ROIs placed in the middle of the capsaicin patch. The size of big ROIs was chosen to be 1.6×1.6 cm^2 approximately fitting the size of "hot spots" (Fig. 3). Graphs in Fig. 4a show BPA evolution for migraine patients whereas graphs in Fig.4b are of healthy subjects. One can see that there was almost synchronous increase of the blood perfusion in all ROIs for healthy subjects. In contrast, essential desynchronization of BPA growth was observed in migraine patients. Thus, there were several peaks in the growing phase of capsaicin-induced signal providing the increase of BPA in one ROI to be accompanied by the decrease in other ROI (Fig. 4a). Notably, this is another way of manifestation of the "hot spot" migration depicted in Fig. 3.

We have also found that the mean speed of the BPA growth during capsaicin application (stage 2) was different for different subjects varying from 0.04 to 0.19% per min. However, this parameter did not differ significantly between migraine and control groups: 0.11 ± 0.04 for migraine, $n = 14$ versus 0.09 ± 0.03 for control, n = 14, $p =$ 0.10. For quantitative estimation of the "hot spots" migration we used the coefficient of variation (CV) which is the ratio of the BPA-growth speed averaged over all big ROIs in the time interval between the start of growth and signal saturation (indicated by dashed lines in Fig. 4) and its standard deviation. Comparative analysis showed that the CV value in migraine group (1.24 ± 0.57) is significantly different from that in control group (0.84 ± 0.19, $p = 0.02$, Fig. 5a). This finding demonstrated for the first time essential differences in reactivity of the microcirculation to capsaicin application between migraine and control groups.

Moreover, we found that migraine patients, compared to control group, have a smaller DT of BPA growth: 6.3 ± 2.6 min versus 8.9 ± 3.9 min, $p = 0.049$, Fig. 5b, which served as a basis for studying the joint variability of the parameters CV and DT. Univariant dispersion analysis revealed that joint dispersion of the CV and DT are significantly different in migraine and control groups: $p = 0.018$ with the Fisher's criterion F = 6.37 for CV, and $p = 0.049$, F = 4.27 for DT. Distribution of CV and DT in both groups is shown in Fig. 5c. It is seen that most of migraine patients are situated within the area limited by the dashed red line. The migraine group is characterized by higher CV and lower DT of larger dispersion. In contrast, healthy subjects possess larger DT and lower CV. These parameters for the control group are located within the area limited by the dashed blue line in Fig. 5c. Discriminant analysis using parameters of CV and DT allowed us to correctly classify 23 (82%) of 28 participants ($p < 0.005$). Furthermore, a joint analysis of variance mean speed and STD also allowed detecting significant differences between patients with migraine and control groups: $p = 0.026$ with the Fisher's criterion F = 4.23.

Capsaicin-induced hyperemia

A typical reaction of the human skin to capsaicin application is progressive skin redness [10], which becomes apparent as an increase of green light absorption. Therefore, in our experiments, the skin redness (or hyperemia) could be estimated as a relative change of the DC component of the PPG waveform measured in the place of patch application. To be consistent with estimations of AC-component

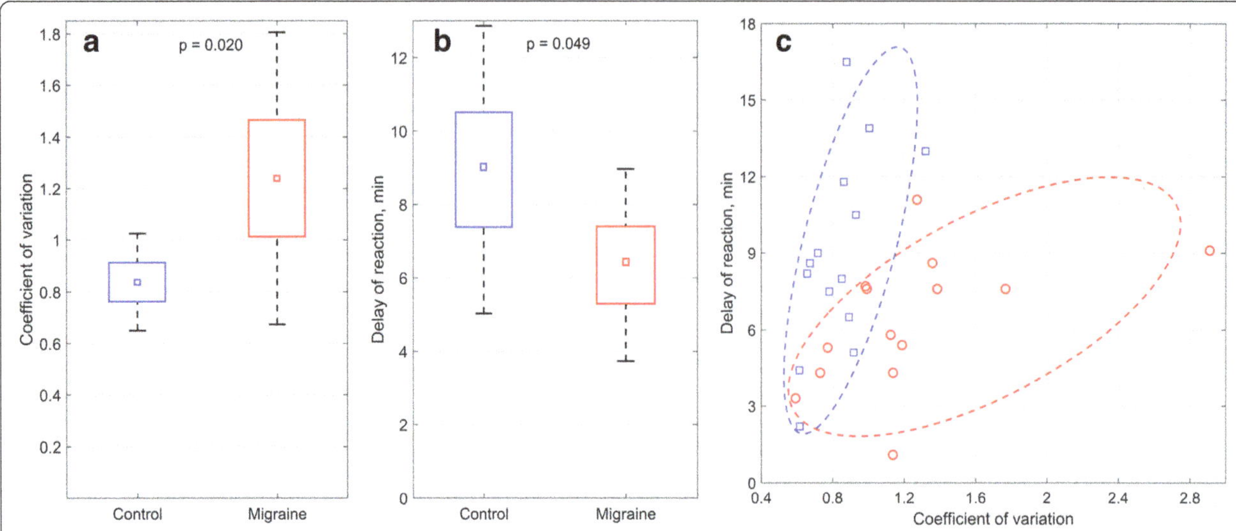

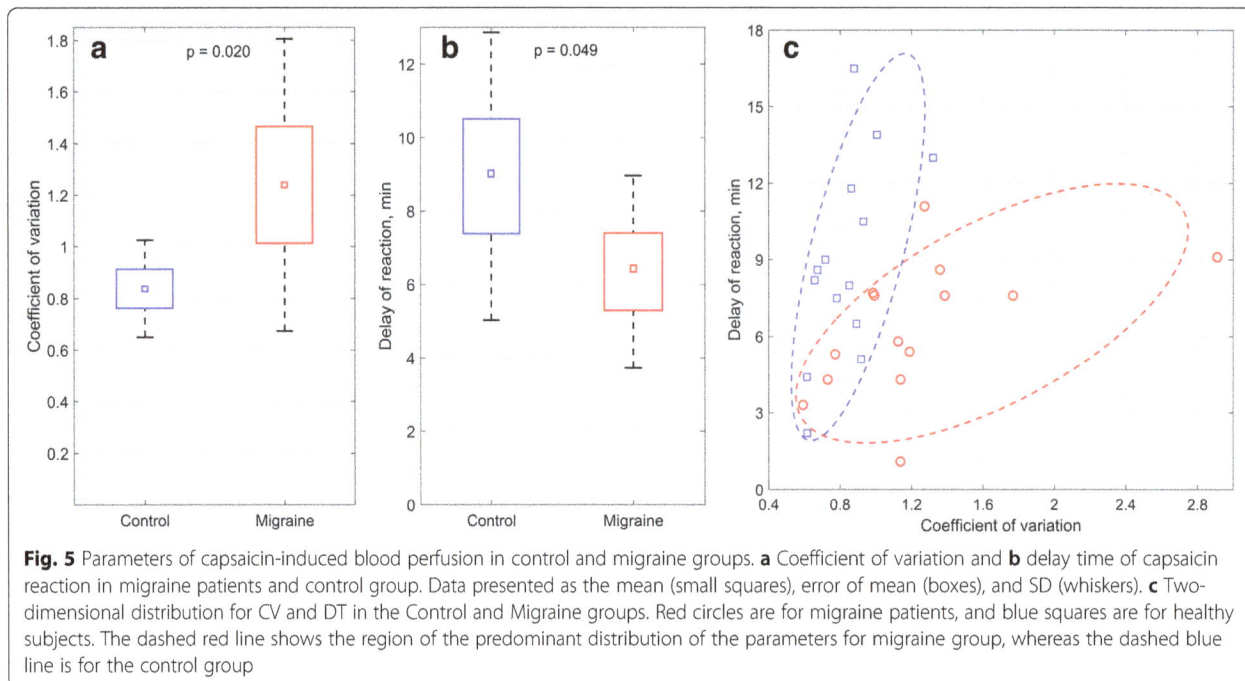

Fig. 5 Parameters of capsaicin-induced blood perfusion in control and migraine groups. **a** Coefficient of variation and **b** delay time of capsaicin reaction in migraine patients and control group. Data presented as the mean (small squares), error of mean (boxes), and SD (whiskers). **c** Two-dimensional distribution for CV and DT in the Control and Migraine groups. Red circles are for migraine patients, and blue squares are for healthy subjects. The dashed red line shows the region of the predominant distribution of the parameters for migraine group, whereas the dashed blue line is for the control group

change, we calculated the DC-component change in the time interval between the beginning of the reaction and signal saturation (indicated by dashed lines in Fig. 4). As shown in Fig. 6, we found that the degree of hyperemia was highly variable among subjects. Nevertheless, in both groups, the changes of the DC component were relatively small as they did not exceed one tenth of the initial value: 8.7 ± 4.1% and 7.8 ± 4.3% for migraine and control group, respectively. In sharp contrast, the much more pronounced increase of AC component was observed both in the control (215 ± 100%) and migraine (231 ± 110%) groups. It means that BPA increase occurs mainly because of change of AC component. No significant difference in either DC or AC change was found between the groups ($p > 0.05$).

Figure 6 shows that skin redness evaluated as changes of the DC component of PPG was twenty-fold less than changes of the amplitude of AC component. Therefore, the reaction on the capsaicin application cannot be assessed by a simple comparison of the skin redness as efficiently as by imaging photoplethysmography.

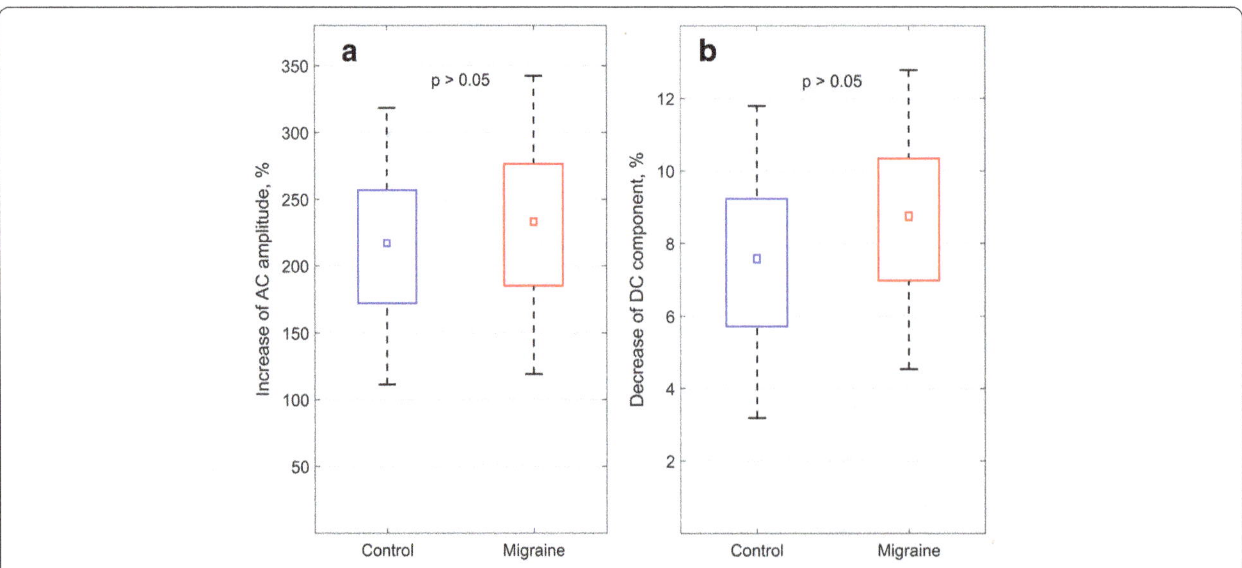

Fig. 6 Change of AC (panel **a**) and DC (panel **b**) components of the PPG waveform in control (blue) and migraine (red) groups after capsaicin application. The data are presented as the mean (small squares), error of mean (boxes), and SD (whiskers)

Discussion

Based on innovative IPPG technique, we present here the novel method for evaluation of capsaicin induced changes in peripheral blood flow that is more sensitive than the commonly used skin redness analysis. The main finding of our study is the remarkable variability (both in space and time) in skin microcirculation after capsaicin application in migraine patients. We suggest this novel phenomenon can serve as a quantitative biomarker of vascular changes in this disorder and probably as a predictive parameter for efficiency of anti-migraine CGRP-based drugs.

Despite the high prevalence of migraine, the pathogenesis of migraine pain remains unclear. However, recent animal and human studies suggested the significant role of TRPV1 receptors expressed in meningeal nerve fibers in migraine pathology [4, 5]. Accumulated evidence suggests that the neuropeptide CGRP is released upon activation of TRPV1 receptors as the main triggering factor implicated in migraine pain [6–8]. Therefore, the inhibition of the pro-nociceptive action of CGRP represents one of the most promising approaches for migraine treatment [7, 9]. For instance, the most specific agents for migraine treatment are represented by triptans which block CGRP release [21–23]. Another promising approach is neutralization of CGRP (or its receptors) by specific antibodies [24–26]. Although other treatment strategies are possible, the known contribution of CGRP to migraine pathology in the individual patients could predict the efficiency of triptans or CGRP antibodies.

Capsaicin-induced increase in DBF presented as the skin redness is a simple test to evaluate the release of CGRP in peripheral tissues and to test the efficiency of anti-migraine medicines [2]. Measuring the intensity of skin redness potentially could indirectly suggest the sensitivity to CGRP based medications. Consistent with this view, it has been shown recently that migraine patients have larger areas of skin redness after dermal application of capsaicin [10] suggesting the larger release or higher reactivity of vessels to endogenous CGRP which is one of the most powerful vasodilators. Migraine has been suggested as a systemic vasculopathy [27]. Vascular changes in migraine were suggested since the emergence of the famous Woolf's vascular theory of migraine [28]. This theory proposed the primary changes in the intracranial vessels which are hardly available. Nevertheless, the recent magnetic resonance angiography of extra- and intracranial vessels indicated the dilatation of blood vessels during migraine attack [29]. The other study reported the local asymmetry of forehead blood flow in the affected side of the migraine patient's face during an attack [30]. However, unlike most of previous studies that have addressed the functional states of large vessels, our study was focused on variability of microcirculation in migraine patients. Here we report *'local asynchronous'* reactions in certain skin areas triggered by application of capsaicin which were higher presented in migraine. One of the main findings of our study is highly heterogeneous (in time and in space) reaction of migraine patients to stimulation of TRPV1 receptors. It became possible to obtain this novel finding through the use of the advanced IPPG technique allowing us to register the pulsatile blood flow with simultaneous ECG recordings, resulting in enhanced sensitivity of this approach [18]. Another important observation is that the essential changes in BPA could develop without significant skin redness (evaluated here via calculation of the DC component of IPPG). Notably, the degree of DC changes in these relatively short period of capsaicin application was much weaker than BPA modulation. Taken together these data suggest that BPA measurement in hot spots and its variability (measured from the coefficient of BPA variations) represent the powerful biomarker of blood flow changes associated with migraine. The nature of migrating hot spots remains unclear but it could be related to the random opening and closure of precapillary sphincters which regulate blood flow in the capillaries and venules. This dynamic process could be determined by interaction of several competing mechanisms including CGRP mediated vasodilation and the opposite process of vasoconstriction based on direct activation of vascular TRPV1 receptors by capsaicin [31, 32]. It is worth noting that the local anesthetic lidocaine was applied before capsaicin due to instructions of the Quatenza plaster manufacturer. Recent study reported that lidocaine can directly stimulate TRPV1 and TRPA1 receptors and release CGRP [33] which potentially can induce vasomotor effects similar to those of capsaicin. However, in our conditions, relatively low concentrations of lidocaine did not produce measurable changes of the microcirculation.

Interestingly, the phenomenon of hot spots leading to asynchronous high intensity activation of local parts of the skin can unexpectedly slow down the global growth of the BPA masking thus the reactivity of the current individual to capsaicin. This can explain why we did not find significant changes in the speed of BPA growth in migraine patients in our small sample. Nevertheless, high variability of BPA in capsaicin test can predict the sensitivity of CGRP-specific treatments such as triptans and CGRP neutralizing antibodies.

Left-right side asymmetry (asynchronous reactions) in the sympathetic skin responses was also found in the headache-free period in unilateral migraine patients [30]. One of the key questions is whether the local reaction represented as migrating hot spots after application of capsaicin to migraine patients was mediated by pure peripheral mechanisms or operated via central sensitization [34]. The latter can potentially change the autonomous control of microcirculation via neuronal mechanisms. Indeed, we found recently that during interictal period in migraine patients a specific enhancement of the sympathetic control is observed [35].

The main limitation of the study is that it was performed in a small cohort and the data should be confirmed in a larger population. However, even in a limited number of patients we found the novel criterion for evaluation of the peripheral blood flow such as the high variability of zones in the skin with increased BPA. In addition, the trend to a shorter latency in BPA increase should be revisited in a larger population. We also used lidocaine as the obligatory component of the pre-treatment that may have partially masked the intensity of capsaicin effects. The genetic reason for asynchronous activation of microcirculation remains unclear. As TRPV1 gene polymorphism determines sensitivity to capsaicin [1] further studies are needed to explore the role of genotyping-based approaches in migraine patients. Suggested here BPA changes with IPPG technique could be used to determine the sensitivity of the particular person to capsaicin as a prognostic tool to identify the role of CGRP component in his/her vascular reactions.

Conclusion

In conclusion, in this pilot study, we suggest the novel non-invasive biomarkers of migraine such as the BPA-growth-speed variations observed during mild activation of skin TRPV1 receptors with capsaicin. This simple test performed with transparent capsaicin patch could serve for the diagnostic purposes and for the prediction of the personalized treatments of migraine patients.

Abbreviations

AC: Alternative component; BPA: Blood pulsation amplitude; CGRP: Calcitonin gene related peptide; CMOS: Complementary metal-oxide-semiconductor; CV: Coefficient of variation; DBF: Dermal blood flow; DC: Slowly varying component; DT: Delay time of the microcirculation reaction on the capsaicin application; ECG: Electrocardiogram; ICHD: the International classification of headache disorder; IPPG: Imaging photoplethysmography; LED: Light-emitted diode; NSAID: Non-steroid anti-inflammatory drugs; PNG: Portable network graphics format; PPG: Photoplethysmographic; ROI: Region of interest; SD: Standard deviation; TRPV1: Transient receptor potential vanilloid type 1

Acknowledgements

RG acknowledges support provided by the program of competitive growth of the Kazan Federal University.

Funding

The study was supported by the Russian Science Foundation (grant 15-15-20012).

Authors' contributions

AAK designed the experiment and the software for data processing, supervised the research, and wrote the manuscript. MAV performed the experiment and analyzed data. OK, DN and LB performed the experiment and contributed to patients' enrolment and data collection. AVA analyzed data and discussed the results, OVM analyzed data and wrote the manuscript, RG conceived the idea of the study, discussed the results, and wrote the manuscript. All authors read and approved the final manuscript.

Competing interests

The authors declare that they have no competing interests.

Author details

[1]Department of Computer Photonics and Videomatics, ITMO University, St. Petersburg, Russia. [2]Department of Neurology and Rehabilitation, Kazan State Medical University, Kazan, Russia. [3]Laboratory of Neurobiology, Kazan Federal University, Kazan, Russia. [4]Department of Neurobiology, University of Eastern Finland, Kuopio, Finland. [5]Department of Neurology and Neurosurgery, Pavlov First Saint Petersburg State Medical University, St. Petersburg, Russia. [6]Department of Circulation Physiology, Almazov National Medical Research Centre, St. Petersburg, Russia.

References

1. Forstenpointer J, Förster M, May D et al (2017) TRPV1-polymorphism1911 a>G alters capsaicin-induced sensory changes in healthy subjects. PLoS One 12:e0183322. https://doi.org/10.1371/journal.pone.0183322
2. Monteith D, Collins EC, Vandermeulen C et al (2017) Safety, tolerability, pharmacokinetics, and pharmacodynamics of the CGRP binding monoclonal antibody LY2951742 (Galcanezumab) in healthy volunteers. Front Pharmacol 8:740. https://doi.org/10.3389/fphar.2017.00740
3. Julius D, Basbaum AI (2001) Molecular mechanisms of nociception. Nature 413:203–210. https://doi.org/10.1038/35093019
4. Carreno O, Corominas R, Fernández-Morales J et al (2012) SNP variants within the vanilloid TRPV1 and TRPV3 receptor genes are associated with migraine in the Spanish population. Am J Med Genet B Neuropsychiatr Genet 159:94–103. https://doi.org/10.1002/ajmg.b.32007
5. Zakharov AV, Vitale K, Kilinc E et al (2015) Hunting for origins of migraine pain: cluster analysis of spontaneous and capsaicin-induced firing in meningeal trigeminal nerve fibers. Front Cell Neurosci 9:287. https://doi.org/10.3389/fncel.2015.00287
6. Karsan N, Goadsby PJ (2015) Calcitonin gene-related peptide and migraine. Curr Opin Neurol 28:250–254. https://doi.org/10.1097/WCO.0000000000000191
7. Guo S, Christensen AF, Liu ML et al (2017) Calcitonin gene-related peptide induced migraine attacks in patients with and without familial aggregation of migraine. Cephalalgia 37:114–124. https://doi.org/10.1177/0333102416639512
8. Schou WS, Ashina S, Amin FM et al (2017) Calcitonin gene-related peptide and pain: a systematic review. J Headache Pain 18:34. https://doi.org/10.1186/s10194-017-0741-2
9. Tfelt-Hansen P, Olesen J (2011) Possible site of action of CGRP antagonists in migraine. Cephalalgia 31:748–750. https://doi.org/10.1177/0333102411398403
10. You DS, Haney R, Albu S, Meagher MW (2018) Generalized pain sensitization and endogenous oxytocin in individuals with symptoms of migraine: a cross-sectional study. Headache 58:62–77. https://doi.org/10.1111/head.13213
11. Choi CM, Bennett RG (2003) Laser Dopplers to determine cutaneous blood flow. Dermatologic Surg 29:272–280. https://doi.org/10.1046/j.1524-4725.2003.29042.x
12. Opazo Saez AM, Mosel F, Nürnberger J et al (2005) Laser Doppler imager (LDI) scanner and intradermal injection for in vivo pharmacology in human skin microcirculation: responses to acetylcholine, endothelin-1 and their repeatability. Br J Clin Pharmacol 59:511–519. https://doi.org/10.1111/j.1365-2125.2004.02344.x
13. Kamshilin AA, Miridonov S, Teplov V et al (2011) Photoplethysmographic imaging of high spatial resolution. Biomed Opt Express 2:996–1006. https://doi.org/10.1364/BOE.2.000996
14. Kamshilin AA, Nippolainen E, Sidorov IS et al (2015) A new look at the essence of the imaging photoplethysmography. Sci Rep 5:10494. https://doi.org/10.1038/srep10494

15. Volkov MV, Margaryants NB, Potemkin AV et al (2017) Video capillaroscopy clarifies mechanism of the photoplethysmographic waveform appearance. Sci Rep 7:13298. https://doi.org/10.1038/s41598-017-13552-4
16. Zaproudina N, Teplov V, Nippolainen E et al (2013) Asynchronicity of facial blood perfusion in migraine. PLoS One 8:e80189. https://doi.org/10.1371/journal.pone.0080189
17. Teplov V, Shatillo A, Nippolainen E et al (2014) Fast vascular component of cortical spreading depression revealed in rats by blood pulsation imaging. J Biomed Opt 19:046011. https://doi.org/10.1117/1.JBO.19.4.046011
18. Kamshilin AA, Sidorov IS, Babayan L et al (2016) Accurate measurement of the pulse wave delay with imaging photoplethysmography. Biomed Opt Express 7:5138–5147. https://doi.org/10.1364/BOE.7.005138
19. (2013) The international classification of headache disorders, 3rd edition (beta version). Cephalalgia 33:629–808. https://doi.org/10.1177/0333102413485658
20. Sidorov IS, Volynsky MA, Kamshilin AA (2016) Influence of polarization filtration on the information readout from pulsating blood vessels. Biomed Opt Express 7:2469–2474. https://doi.org/10.1364/BOE.7.002469
21. Moore RA, Derry CJ, Derry S (2011) Sumatriptan (all routes of administration) for acute migraine attacks in adults: an overview of Cochrane reviews. Cochrane Database Syst Rev:CD009108. https://doi.org/10.1002/14651858.CD009108
22. Bird S, Derry S, Moore RA (2014) Zolmitriptan for acute migraine attacks in adults. Cochrane Database Syst Rev:CD008616. https://doi.org/10.1002/14651858.CD008616.pub2
23. Cameron C, Kelly S, Hsieh S-C et al (2015) Triptans in the acute treatment of migraine: a systematic review and network meta-analysis. Headache 55:221–235. https://doi.org/10.1111/head.12601
24. Obermann M, Holle D (2016) Recent advances in the management of migraine. F1000Research 5:2726. https://doi.org/10.12688/f1000research.9764.1
25. Khan S, Olesen A, Ashina M (2017) CGRP, a target for preventive therapy in migraine and cluster headache: systematic review of clinical data. Cephalalgia (online first). https://doi.org/10.1177/0333102417741297
26. Silberstein SD, Dodick DM, Bigal ME et al (2017) Fremanezumab for the preventive treatment of chronic migraine. N Engl J Med 377:2113–2122. https://doi.org/10.1056/NEJMoa1709038
27. Tietjen GE (2009) Migraine as a systemic vasculopathy. Cephalalgia 29:989–996. https://doi.org/10.1111/j.1468-2982.2009.01937.x
28. Wolff HG (1963) Headache and other head pain. Oxford University Press, New York
29. Amin FM, Asghar MS, de Koning PJH et al (2013) Magnetic resonance angiography of intracranial and extracranial arteries in patients with spontaneous migraine without aura: a cross-sectional study. Lancet Neurol 12:454–461. https://doi.org/10.1016/S1474-4422(13)70067-X
30. Yildiz SK, Yildiz N, Korkmaz B et al (2008) Sympathetic skin responses from frontal region in migraine headache: a pilot study. Cephalalgia 28:696–704. https://doi.org/10.1111/j.1468-2982.2008.01574.x
31. Dux M, Rosta J, Sántha P, Jancsó G (2009) Involvement of capsaicin-sensitive afferent nerves in the proteinase-activated receptor 2-mediated vasodilatation in the rat dura mater. Neuroscience 161:887–894. https://doi.org/10.1016/j.neuroscience.2009.04.010
32. Ständer S, Moormann C, Schumacher M et al (2004) Expression of vanilloid receptor subtype 1 in cutaneous sensory nerve fibers, mast cells, and epithelial cells of appendage structures. Exp Dermatol 13:129–139. https://doi.org/10.1111/j.0906-6705.2004.0178.x
33. Eberhardt MJ, Stueber T, de la Roche J et al (2017) TRPA1 and TRPV1 are required for lidocaine-evoked calcium influx and neuropeptide release but not cytotoxicity in mouse sensory neurons. PLoS One 12:e0188008. https://doi.org/10.1371/journal.pone.0188008
34. Magerl W, Wilk SH, Treede R-D (1998) Secondary hyperalgesia and perceptual wind-up following intradermal injection of capsaicin in humans. Pain 74:257–268. https://doi.org/10.1016/S0304-3959(97)00177-2
35. Mamontov OV, Babayan L, Amelin AV et al (2016) Autonomous control of cardiovascular reactivity in patients with episodic and chronic forms of migraine. J Headache Pain 17:52. https://doi.org/10.1186/s10194-016-0645-6

27

Characteristics of menstrual versus non-menstrual migraine during pregnancy: a longitudinal population-based study

Beáta Éva Petrovski[1,2*], Kjersti G. Vetvik[3], Christofer Lundqvist[1,3,4†] and Malin Eberhard-Gran[1,3,4,5†]

Abstract

Background: Migraine is a common headache disorder that affects mostly women. In half of these, migraine is menstrually associated, and ranges from completely asymptomatic to frequent pain throughout pregnancy.

Methods: The aim of the study was to define the pattern (frequency, intensity, analgesics use) of migrainous headaches among women with and without mensturai migraine (MM) during pregnancy, and define how hormonally-related factors affect its intensity.

Results: The analysis was based upon data from 280 women, 18.6% of them having a self-reported MM. Women with MM described a higher headache intensity during early pregnancy and postpartum compared those without MM, but both groups showed improvement during the second half of pregnancy and directly after delivery. Hormonal factors and pre-menstrual syndrome had no effect upon headache frequency, but may affect headache intensity.

Conclusions: Individual treatment plan is necessary for women with migrainous headaches during pregnancy, especially for those suffering highest symptoms load.

Background

Migraine is a common headache disorder that affects approximately 12% of the world's population [25]. Although the condition is very common in both genders, its post-pubescent prevalence is about two to three times greater among women than men [7, 25]. More than half of women who suffer from migraine self-report a menstrual association of the condition [17, 28].

Menstrual migraine (MM) is defined in the appendix of the International Classification of Headache Disorders 3 beta (ICHD 3 beta) [9] as attacks of migraine without aura occurring on day 1 ± 2 of the menstrual cycle in at least two out of three menstrual cycles.

The prevalence of MM varies from 4 to 70% according to previous studies [3, 10, 13, 21, 28]. This large variation can be explained by differences in the populations studied, ascertainment and the previous lack of uniform diagnostic criteria of menstrual migraine [28]. When the current diagnostic criteria are used, about one fifth of female migraineurs from the general population have MM.

According to previous population-based studies, the majority of female migraineurs experience an improvement in migraine symptoms during pregnancy, and a third of them even report complete remission [11, 14, 22]. The frequency of headaches and migraines decrease significantly during pregnancy, especially in the second and third trimester [6, 11, 22] and increase postpartum [22]. To date, few studies have reported the course of migraine during pregnancy specifically for women with MM [4, 14, 22, 23] and the results are diverging. Although some women experience decrease in the headache frequency or that migraines disappear during the pregnancy [11, 14, 22], some may suffer throughout pregnancy. Assessment of headache frequency has been either retrospective or, in a few cases, prospective either using headache diaries [11] or repeated questionnaires [14, 22]. While clinically recruited populations may give opportunities for addressing clinical, migraine-related characteristics, they may not be representative for migraine in the general population of pregnant women [11, 12, 14, 22].

* Correspondence: beata.eva.petrovski@ahus.no
Christofer Lundqvist and Malin Eberhard-Gran are senior co-authors.
†Equal contributors
[1]Health Services Research Centre, Akershus University Hospital, Post Box 1000, 1478 Lørenskog, Oslo, Norway
[2]Faculty of Dentistry, University of Oslo, Geitmyrsveien 69, 0455 Oslo, Norway
Full list of author information is available at the end of the article

The aim of the present study was to describe the changes in the frequency and intensity of migrainous headaches and analgesics use in female migraineurs with and without self-reported MM from a large and representative prospective birth cohort. In addition, we aimed to examine how hormonally-related factors such as premenstrual syndrome (PMS), menstrual pain, age at menarche, hormonal contraception, regularity of the menstrual cycle and maternal age may affect the intensity of migrainous headache during and after pregnancy.

Methods

Study population and study design

This study was part of the Akershus Birth Cohort (ABC) Study, which targeted all women scheduled to give birth at Akershus University Hospital, Norway. The hospital is located near Oslo, the capital of Norway, and serves a total population of approximately 400,000 individuals from both urban and rural areas; on average, 4000 women gave birth at the hospital each year during the study period. Women were recruited at the routine fetal ultrasound examination at pregnancy week 17, from November 2008 to April 2010. As part of the public health care program, this examination is free of charge to all women in the hospital's catchment area. Pregnant women who were able to complete a questionnaire in Norwegian were eligible for the Akershus Birth Cohort to ABC. An overview of inclusion, response rates and study sample is presented in Fig. 1. Note that the sample sizes at the different time points may deviate somewhat from previous ABC publications due to small changes in the latest quality-assured data files released for research. At enrollment, 6244 women were present, of whom 1088 (17.4%) were excluded due to language difficulties and 342 (5.5%) women were not invited due to time constraints. Of the 4814 pregnant women invited to participate, 4662 (96.8%) women gave consent and were included in the study. Data were collected by self-completed questionnaires in gestational weeks 17 (Q1) and 32 (Q2), and 8 weeks after delivery (Q3). The response rates were 80.3% (3744 of 4662), 81.1% (2931 of 3613), and 79.0% (2213 of 2801) for Q1, Q2 and Q3, respectively. In total, 1981 women returned all questionnaires and comprised our baseline sample, representing 42.5% of those included. Out of the 1981 women, 338 (17.1%) had active migraine, of which 58 were excluded due to chronic headache. This resulted in a final study sample of 280 women, of which 52 (18.6%) had self-reported MM and 228 (81.4%) had non-menstrual migraine (nMM) (Fig. 1).

Women included in the study were older (full cohort: median, IQR: 30.7 (27.2–34.2) vs. study sample: median, IQR: 31.4 (28.5–34.9); $P = 0.003$), and had a higher education (full cohort: 58.8% vs. study sample: 65.4% vs.; $P = 0.03$), compared to those in the full cohort.

Additional information was obtained by linkage to the hospital's electronic birth record. The birth record is

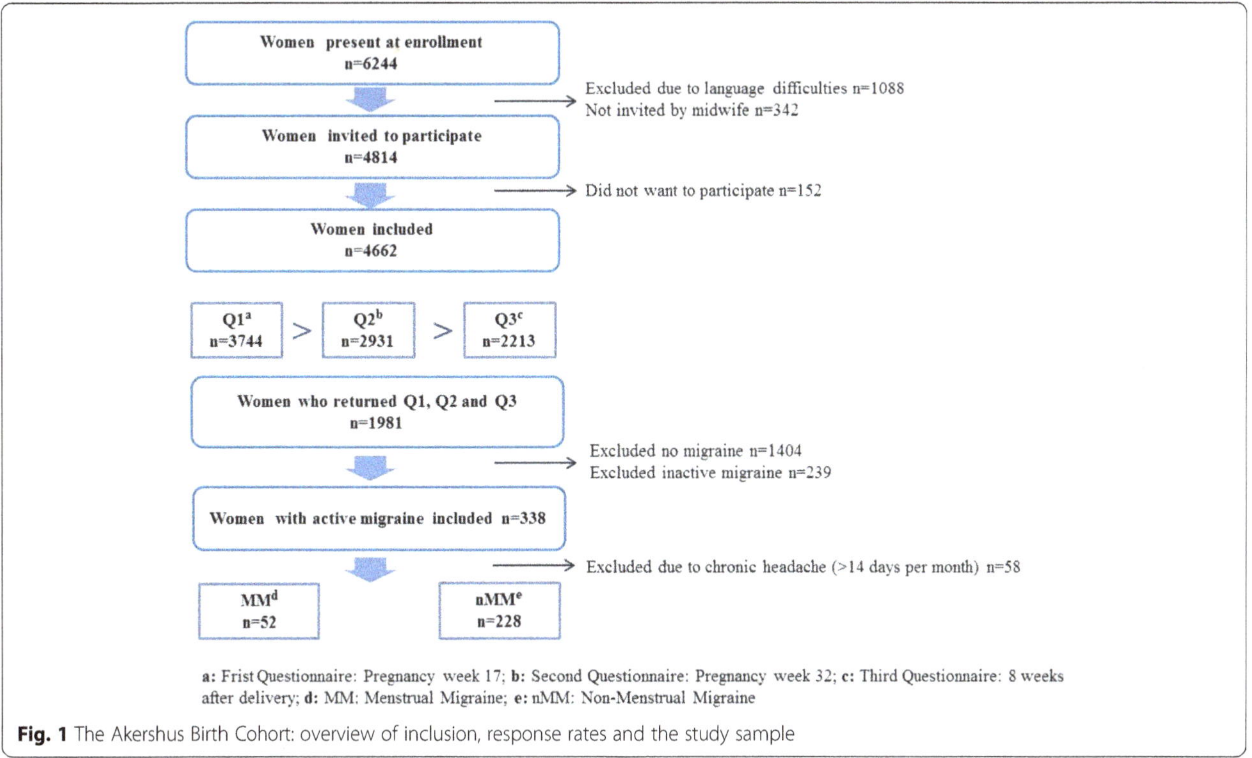

Fig. 1 The Akershus Birth Cohort: overview of inclusion, response rates and the study sample

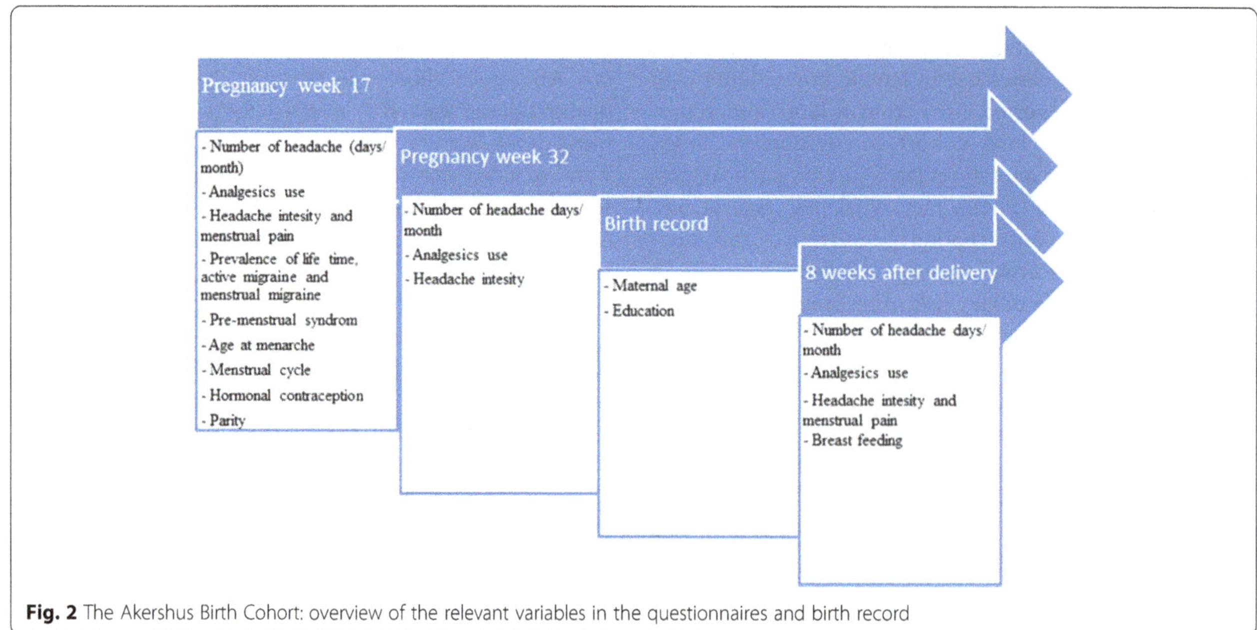

Fig. 2 The Akershus Birth Cohort: overview of the relevant variables in the questionnaires and birth record

completed by the hospital staff members and contains sociodemographic and medical information.

Maternal characteristics

An overview of the relevant variables describing maternal characteristics is presented in Fig. 2.

Migraine characteristics

The first questionnaire included specific questions about life-time ("Have you ever had migraine?") and last year-prevalence ("Have you had migraine during the past year?") of migraine. This enabled us to group the women into three mutually exclusive categories according to self-reported migraine status: no migraine history ("never had migraine"), previous history of migraine ("had migraine, but not during the past year"), migraine in the past year ("had migraine during the past year") defined as "active migraine".

Women were asked whether their migraine was menstrually-related or not. The migraine was categorized as menstrual migraine (MM), if migraine was present in at least 2/3 of menstruations [9]. The remaining cases were categorized as having nMM. Women with chronic headache, i.e. reporting more than 14 headache days per month before pregnancy, were excluded because it is impossible to judge whether their migraine attacks occurring perimenstrually occurs by chance or represents "true" menstrual migraine attacks. Information was also collected about headache frequency (days/month) in Q1, Q2, Q3 and categorized as: 0 day, 1 day/month or 2–14 days/month. Headache intensity was measured in all three questionnaires by a numeric rating scale (NRS) from 0 (no pain) to 10 (greatest pain imaginable).

Analgesic use

Women were specifically asked about use of drugs within seven categories – drugs for headache, migraine, non-headache pain, insomnia, anxiety, depression and other psychotropic medications. For each medication group, the women could tick yes or no as to whether she used a drug, and fill in the name of medication. The three questionnaires covered different periods of use – including the preceding three months before pregnancy and beginning of pregnancy until week 17 (Q1), week 17 to 32 (Q2), and the last part of pregnancy from pregnancy week 33 until 8 weeks postpartum (Q3). In the current study, use of analgesics for headache and migraine medication were combined and categorized into two categories: 'no headache analgesics use' or 'headache analgesics use'.

Other factors

Questions related to menstrual cycles and other menstrually related symptoms were asked: regularity of menstrual cycle before pregnancy (irregular/normal), menstrual pain (NRS 0–10) and age of menarche. PMS was assessed through questions of whether the participants experienced depression before menstruation (no/yes) and if it disappeared once the menstruation began (no/yes). Those women were considered as having PMS, who gave positive answer to both questions. In addition, information about hormonal contraception before pregnancy (no/yes) and breastfeeding after pregnancy (no/yes) was collected.

Included socio-demographic and life-style characteristics and some other factors that may influence migraine were as follows: maternal age, education (primary/secondary school vs. higher education) and parity (nulliparous versus multiparous).

Statistics

The analysis of the data was performed by descriptive statistical analysis; percentage distribution, mean and standard deviation (SD), median and interquartile range (IQR) are shown. The Chi-square (χ^2) test was used to test differences of the distribution of categorical variables. Normality of continuous variables was tested on Q-Q-plot and by Shapiro-Wilk and Kolmogorov-Smirnov test. The Student t-test was used to compare means of continuous, numerical variables, when the normality assumption was satisfied; otherwise Mann-Whitney U test was used.

For trend analysis, a Generalized Estimating Equations (GEE) were used. The correlation structure was assumed to be of an 'AR1' type - more details about the GEE analysis has been published before [26]. The results of the analysis regarding the relationship between pain intensity (NRS) during the pregnancy and MM, are presented as unadjusted and adjusted regression coefficients (β coefficient) and with 95% Confidence Intervals (CIs). Data are adjusted for parity, hormonal contraception and education, since education and parity were significantly associated with menstrual pain, while hormonal contraception was associated with irregularity of the menstrual cycle. The PMT and the age of menarche were not included into the full model, because none of these factors were associated with the factors included into the GEE analysis. Age was included as explanatory variable. Data analysis was based on the data of 263 participants. The effect of breast feeding on the MM and intensity of pain due to migrainous headache were analyzed separately in the last period of the study (8. weeks after delivery). Multicollinearity was detected by variance inflation factor analysis (VIF).

Significance limit was set as $P < 0.05$. All statistical analyses were performed by using the Statistical Package for STATA (Stata version 14.0; College Station, TX, USA).

Results

Characteristics of the study sample

Pregnancy-related and demographic characteristics of the studied population are shown in Table 1. There were no significant differences according to the studied factors between the two groups (MM, nMM). The average age of the participants was approximately 31 years (mean ± SD: 31.6 ± 4.6) and most of them had a higher education (65.4%). Few (8.3%) reported menstrual irregularities before pregnancy, while approximately 12% (12.2%) had used hormonal contraception before pregnancy. The occurrence of PMS was 25.0% among women and it did not differ between the MM and nMM groups (Table 1).

Table 1 Characteristics of the sample according to whether the participants had menstrual-related migraine or not

	MM *N* = 52	nMM *N* = 228	*P*-value
Parity			
Nulliparous	27 (51.9%)	134 (58.8%)	0.367
Multiparous	25 (48.1%)	94 (41.2%)	
Education[a]			
Primary/secondary school	15 (32.6%)	77 (35.0%)	0.756
Higher education	31 (67.4%)	143 (65.0%)	
Menstrual cycle[b]			
Regular	47 (90.4%)	208 (92.0%)	0.697
Irregular	5 (9.6%)	18 (8.0%)	
Hormonal contraception[c]			
No	47 (90.4%)	198 (87.2%)	0.530
Yes	5 (9.6%)	29 (12.8%)	
PMS			
No	40 (76.9%)	170 (74.6%)	0.723
Yes	12 (23.1%)	58 (25.4%)	
Breast feeding[d]			
No	7 (13.5%)	36 (15.9%)	0.657
Yes	45 (86.5%)	190 (84.1%)	
	mean ± SD		
Maternal age	32.2 ± 4.5	31.5 ± 4.6	0.281
Age of menarche	12.9 ± 1.2	12.8 ± 1.4	0.725
Menstrual pain (0–10)	3.7 ± 2.2	3.7 ± 2.3	0.901

PMS Pre-Menstrual Syndrom, *SD* Standard Deviation, *MM* Menstrual Migraine, *nMM* Non-Menstrual Migraine

[a] 14 missing values

[b] 2 missing values

[c] 1 missing value

[d] 2 missing values

Frequency of headache

Figure 3 shows the proportion of women with headache frequency of 1 day/month and 2–14 days/month. During and after pregnancy significantly fewer women had headache frequency one day/month while the proportion having 2–14 headache days/month was higher and increased in week 17. In late pregnancy, the proportion decreased from around 80% to 40% before it increased again post-partum. Proportions of headache-free patients for MM were at pre-pregnancy, early pregnancy, late pregnancy and post-partum, respectively 4.0%, 3.8%, 42.3% and 13.7%, while headache-free patients for nMM were 8.8%, 7.1%, 40.4% and 16.5% at the same time points.

No significant differences could be detected between the MM and nMM groups. However, the number of headache

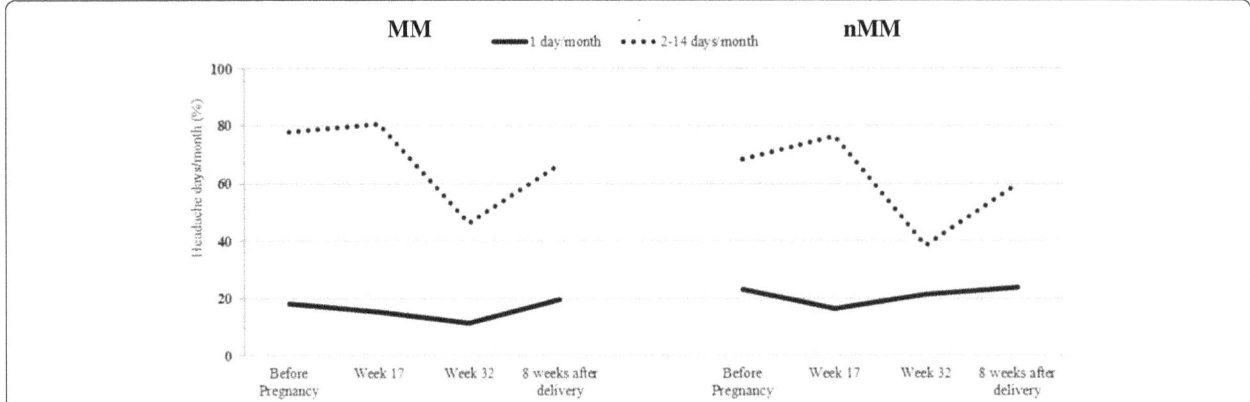

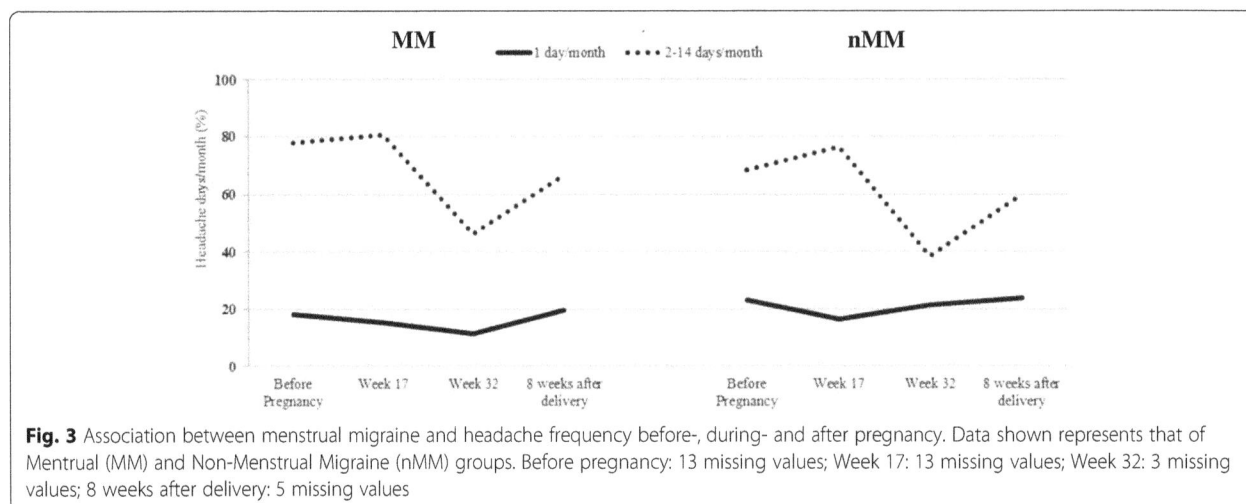

Fig. 3 Association between menstrual migraine and headache frequency before-, during- and after pregnancy. Data shown represents that of Mentrual (MM) and Non-Menstrual Migraine (nMM) groups. Before pregnancy: 13 missing values; Week 17: 13 missing values; Week 32: 3 missing values; 8 weeks after delivery: 5 missing values

days/month tended to be higher among those with MM during the whole study period than among nMM (Fig. 3).

Frequency of analgesics use

More than 80% (87.8%) of the participants used analgesics before pregnancy and this proportion decreased during pregnancy. However, more than 50% of the participants (58.4%) used analgesics up to week 17, and over 20% (23.9%) up to week 32. Analgesics use then stabilized 8 weeks after birth. There was no significant difference between MM and nMM during pregnancy with regard to analgesics use. A tendency towards a more drastic fall in analgesics use in MM was noted (Fig. 4).

Migrainous headache intensity

The headaches intensity (NRS) showed a decreasing trend during pregnancy with an increase post-partum. Significant differences between the two groups (MM vs. nMM) could be detected on pregnancy week 17, when pain intensity appeared to be higher among those with MM (MM: median: 7 (IQR: 6–8; mean ± SD.:7.02 ± 1.75) vs. nMM (nMM: median: 6 (IQR: 5–8; mean ± SD.: 6.21 ± 1.90; $P = 0.008$). A nearly significant difference in the same direction was found also post-partum (MM: median: 5 (IQR: 4–6; mean ± SD.:4.84 ± 1.24 vs. nMM: median: 4 (IQR: 4–5; mean ± SD.: 4.53 ± 1.33; $P = 0.054$) (Fig. 5).

Trend analysis

The results of the GEE analysis is shown in Table 2. The migraine status (nMM vs. MM), menstrual cycle regularity, menstrual pain and analgesics use were positively related to the pain intensity (NRS) in both, unadjusted and adjusted analysis. Conversely, the progressive time period during pregnancy was negatively correlated to the

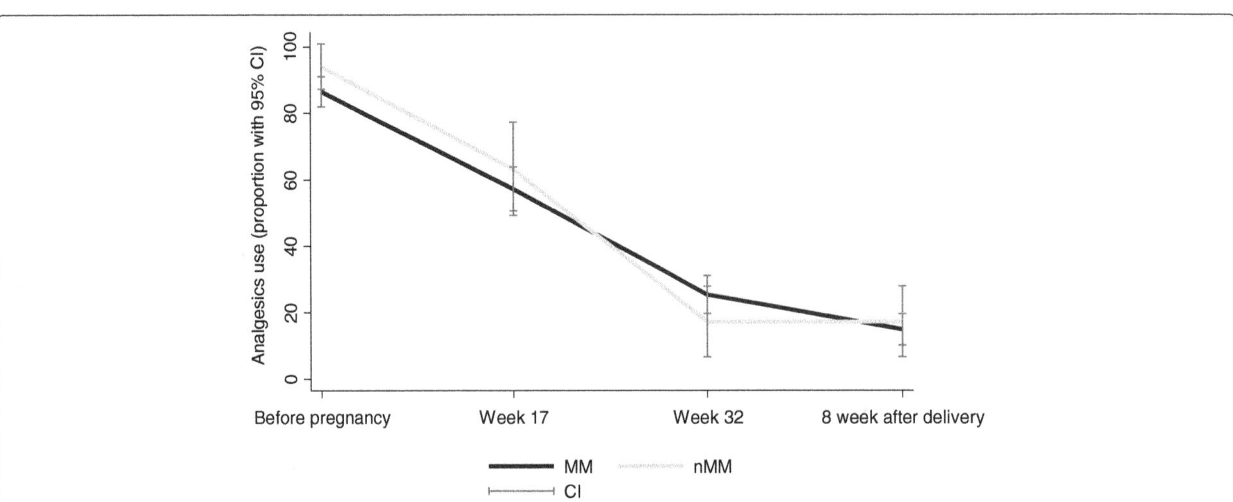

Fig. 4 Analgesics use before, during and after pregnancy. Data shown represents that of Mentrual (MM) and Non-Menstrual Migraine (nMM) groups. Before pregnancy: 9 missing values; Week 17: 11 missing values; 8 weeks after delivery: 1 missing value; % users in each group with 95% CI: Confidence Interval. Analgesics: paracetamol, NSAIDs, opioids and triptans (used for either migraine or headache)

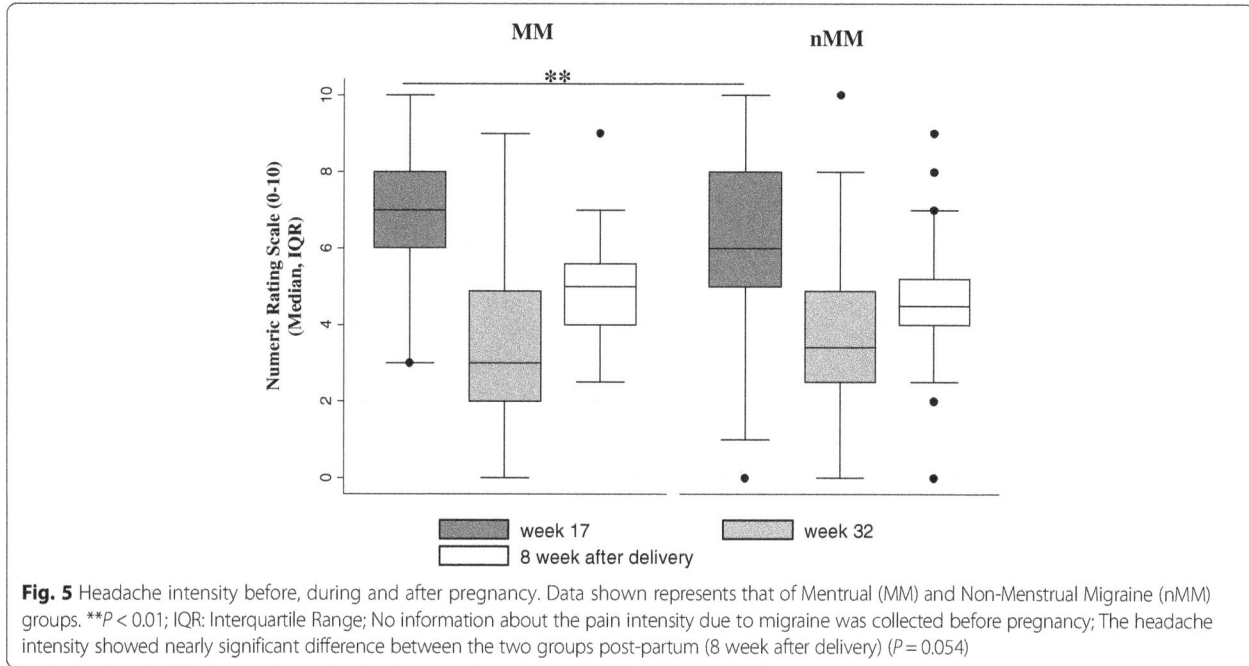

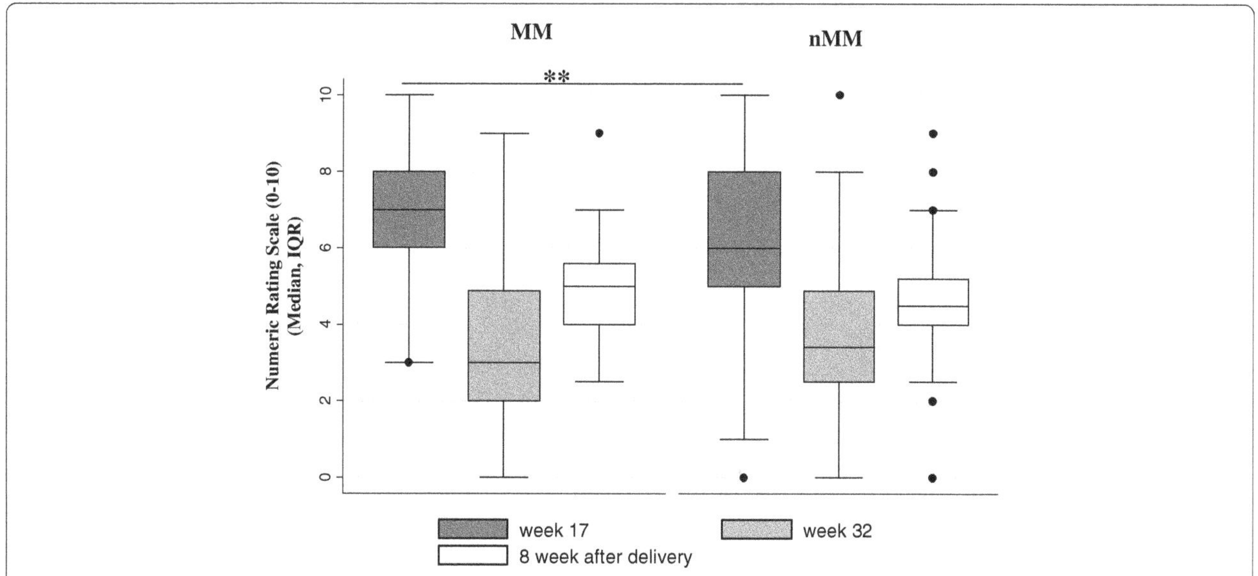

Fig. 5 Headache intensity before, during and after pregnancy. Data shown represents that of Mentrual (MM) and Non-Menstrual Migraine (nMM) groups. $^{**}P < 0.01$; IQR: Interquartile Range; No information about the pain intensity due to migraine was collected before pregnancy; The headache intensity showed nearly significant difference between the two groups post-partum (8 week after delivery) ($P = 0.054$)

pain intensity in both analyses. Maternal age, parity, education and previous use of hormonal contraception showed no significant relationship with pain intensity, either in the unadjusted or in the adjusted analysis. While education and parity showed significant association with the menstrual pain, hormonal contraception showed association with the regularity of the menstrual cycle (data not shown).

Breastfeeding showed no significant association either with the migraine status or the pain intensity due to headaches post-partum (data not shown).

Discussion

Main findings

We found a similar pre-pregnancy prevalence of MM among female migraineurs compared to other Scandinavian studies [13, 21, 28]. Headache frequency was high among both MM and nMM before pregnancy and during early pregnancy, while both groups improved during later parts of pregnancy with a slight worsening again during the post-partum period. The women with self-reported MM had more severe headache pain during first half of the pregnancy and directly post-partum, but

Table 2 Results of the Generalized Estimating Equations (GEE) analyses

	Pain intensity Unadjusted β coefficient (95% CI)	*P- value*	Pain intensity Adjusted[a] β coefficient (95% CI)	*P-* value
Migraine status				
nMM	Reference		Reference	
MM	0.37 (0.04–0.71)	0.027	0.45 (0.08–0.82)	0.017
Time period				
Pregnancy week 17	Reference		Reference	
Pregnancy week 32	−2.80 (−3.07- -2.53)	< 0.001	−2.61 (−2.91- -2.31)	< 0.001
8 week after delivery	−1.77 (− 2.01- -1.53)	< 0.001	−1.54 (−1.83- -1.26)	< 0.001
Menstrual pain	0.15 (0.09–0.20)	< 0.001	0.16 (0.10–0.23)	< 0.001
Menstrual cycle				
Normal	Reference		Reference	
Irregular	0.75 (0.11–1.40)	0.022	0.67 (0.05–1.29)	0.035
Analgesics use				
No	Reference		Reference	
Yes	1.26 (0.98–1.54)	< 0.001	0.48 (0.19–0.77)	0.001

MM Menstrual Migraine, *nMM* Non-Menstrual Migraine: [a]Adjusted for maternal age, parity, hormonal contraception, education; *P*-value< 0.05 were considered as statistically significant

headaches followed a more similar pattern during pregnancy. Other menstrual related factors such as PMS, hormonal contraception before pregnancy and age at menarche were not associated with headache intensity, while irregular menstruation was.

Strengths and limitations

The strength of this observational study is its large, prospective sample size and representative population-based cohort of pregnant women likely to be seen and treated by GPs or obstetricians. Another strength is the use of the detailed questionnaire and that self-reported migraineurs were identified using validated questions [20].

Moreover, other, menstrual- or hormone related health issues and their fate during pregnancy could be targeted. Such phenomena could thus be compared to migraine and add a dimension not previously addressed.

The ABC study had a high response rate. For the present study, however, we required women to have responded to all three questionnaires, which represent only 42.5% of all study participants. A comparison of these women with the full cohort population indicates that the women in our sample were older and had a higher education, indicating higher socioeconomic status. The aim, however, was not to estimate the occurrence of these factors in the population, but rather the strength of associations between them. This should be considered when interpreting the results.

Nevertheless, the prevalence and migraine pattern during pregnancy described here are likely to be more representative of the general population of pregnant women than samples selected from headache clinics. We did not have the possibility of performing a clinical examination and full headache interview of the women. Also, even though the study was designed as a prospective study, information about migrainous headache before pregnancy was collected retrospectively, thus making recall bias a possibility.

All women who reported migraine occurrence in at least two out of three menstruations were classified as MM. The gold standard for diagnosing MM is a prospective headache- and menstruation diary ([9, 27]. Such a diary would have enabled a more exact evaluation of the pre-pregnancy menstrual relationship. However, this study relied upon the women's self-report, as they were included only at week 17 of pregnancy. Thus, there is a lack of exact information about the timing of migraine attacks in relation to the first day of menstruation, and possibility for positive and negative misclassification within the two groups (nMM and MM). Furthermore, the differences between those with and without MM may have been clearer if such a specific diagnosis could have been made.

Interpretation

The prevalence of self-reported MM among women with migraine was 18,6% in the present study, which corresponds well with the prevalence of MM in other Scandinavian studies [13, 21], and especially with a previous study from the Norwegian general population in the same age group [28].

The characteristics of migraine through pregnancy and the immediate post-partum period which we have demonstrated here also correlates well with that from previous studies [2, 6, 10, 11, 14, 15]. We demonstrate improvement for most subjects regarding the number of headache days per month, intensity of headaches, and analgesics use. The present study, however, suggested an initial increase in the proportions of women with frequent headaches during the first half of pregnancy, although this increase was slight (Fig. 3), and thus differs from most other studies. However, the same pattern has been suggested in a previous population-based Norwegian study [1]. That general population-based study did not differentiate between MM and nMM. The present study suggests a higher headache intensity for MM in the earlier parts of pregnancy and post partum but, for both types, a high headache occurrence, especially for those with more frequent headaches, among both groups during early pregnancy. Due to the lack of detailed clinical descriptors, we cannot know whether all headaches responsible for this apparent initial increased frequency were all migrainous headaches, or if tension headaches dominated some days. Our findings of a high headache intensity during this period seem to suggest a dominating migrainous headache. No significant difference could be detected regarding the frequency of migrainous headaches during the study period between the two studied groups. A recent systematic review penetrates the literature on the presence of various headaches during pregnancy, including migraine in general, and emphasizes the importance of differential diagnosis of pregnancy headache, but does not address menstrual and non-menstrual type specifically [16].

The intensity of migrainous headaches showed a decreasing tendency during pregnancy, with a small post-partum increase, which is in line with the results from the GEE analysis. Three recent studies have described the characteristics of migrainous headaches during pregnancy and childbirth prospectively [2, 11, 15]. Melhado et al. and Allais et al described a subjective change in characteristics (improved, unchanged or worse) [15], while the diary study of Kvisvik et al described characteristics only from mid pregnancy onwards and headache intensity only during the post-partum period [11]. The pattern from these studies, however, seem to support our data with a define improvement only during later parts of pregnancy [2, 15] and a worsening again post-partum [11].

MM was positively associated with headache intensity during pregnancy, which contrasts with previous studies [4, 14, 19] There was also a positive association between pain intensity during pregnancy and self-reported menstrual pain before pregnancy. The latter was true even if results were adjusted for whether the migraine type is MM or nMM. This would seem to support a general effect on pain sensitivity over the menstrual cycle among some of the women which is associated with the intensity of migrainous headache during pregnancy. Such a general pain sensitivity mechanism affecting both migraine presumed to be hormonally related (MM) and migraines which are less hormonally influenced (nMM), would be expected to give a similar change pattern during pregnancy with other headaches such as tension type headache, as has been shown in other studies [2, 15]. The mechanisms behind such an association may be hormonally independent but remain to be explored.

According to the systematic review published by the World Health Organization (WHO, 2004) and data from some developing countries, the prevalence of irregular menstrual cycles was between 5 and 16% in the general population. Spierings and Padamsee et al. also found similar results; the prevalence of irregular menstrual cycles occurred in 16.7% of the migraine population [24], which depended on the definition used for irregular menstrual cycle. The latter study fits partly with our results, though we found a lower prevalence of irregular menstrual cycles of about 8% (47% of these women had received hormonal contraception). Though our results show irregular menstrual cycles have no significant association with MM (data not shown), the menstrual cycle was strongly associated with pain intensity due to headaches even after adjustment for hormonal contraception (Table 2). This suggests that other factors, related to the irregular menstrual cycle may affect pain intensity due to headache [18, 24].

Dean et al. reported a prevalence of PMS of 19–30% [5], which is in line with our prevalence of PMS being 25% in the studied population. In our analysis, no association could be detected between the migraine status and PMS.

Despite the importance of medication safety during pregnancy, a high proportion of women consumed analgesics due to migrainous headache during pregnancy and although this decreased during the pregnancy, it remained relatively high in the second- (60%) and third-trimesters (20%). Decreased use of headache analgesics during pregnancy may be explained either by an improvement in headache with a consequent reduced need for analgesics, or by a reduction in analgesics intake despite pain due to fear of foetal damage or based on direct advice from others. The remaining, considerable analgesics use in the early part of pregnancy may have several possible explanations. Some women may not initially have been aware of being pregnant and therefore continued their pre-pregnancy analgesic use though by at ultrasound at week 17, most would, naturally, be aware of their pregnancy status. Another possibility, which our data on headache frequency and intensity partly seems to support, is that the headache at this time point has not yet started to improve, and may for some even have worsened, leading to high requirements for analgesics. Also (or alternatively) a switch from more migraine-specific, effective medication perceived to be risky during pregnancy, to less effective, safer medications such as paracetamol could also contribute. The latter is supported by our previous data on specific analgesics use from the same material [8]. This study shows that for women afflicted by migraine during pregnancy, triptan and NSAIDs use falls drastically while paracetamol increases at the beginning of pregnancy. For women who did not experience migraine during pregnancy, this pattern was not seen [8].

Conclusions

Women with MM reported higher headache intensity during early pregnancy and postpartum compared to women with nMM. Both groups improved significantly during the second half of pregnancy and immediately post partum. Hormonal factors and PMS did not affect frequency of headaches, but may affect the headache intensity during pregnancy in female migraineurs. We suggest that an individual treatment plan for migraines during pregnancy is needed especially for those women with the highest symptoms load.

Abbreviations

ABC: Akershus Birth Cohort; CIs: Confidence Intervals; GEE: Generalized Estimating Equations; ICHD 3 beta: International Classification of Headache Disorders 3 beta; IQR: Interquartile Range; MM: Menstrual migraine; nMM: Non-menstrual migraine; NRS: Numeric Rating Scale; PMS: Premenstrual syndrome; Q1: Questionnaire in gestational weeks 17; Q2: Questionnaire in gestational weeks 32; Q3: Questionnaire 8 weeks after delivery; SD: Standard Deviation; VIF: Variance Inflation Factor; WHO: World Health Organization; χ^2: Chi-square test

Authors' contributions

All authors have read and approved the paper. The original study was designed by ME-G, CL and KGV – all experts in headache medicine and migraine research; BÉP designed and carried out the statistical analysis and put together the first draft; all authors contributed towards writing and completing the manuscript and data interpretation.

Competing interests

The authors declare that they have no competing interest related to the work presented.

Author details

[1]Health Services Research Centre, Akershus University Hospital, Post Box 1000, 1478 Lørenskog, Oslo, Norway. [2]Faculty of Dentistry, University of Oslo, Geitmyrsveien 69, 0455 Oslo, Norway. [3]Department of Neurology, Akershus University Hospital, Post Box 1000, 1478 Lørenskog, Oslo, Norway. [4]Institute of Clinical Medicine, Campus Ahus, University of Oslo, Post Box 1000, 1478 Lørenskog, Norway. [5]Domain for Mental and Physical Health, Norwegian Institute of Public Health, Lovisenberggata 6-8, 0456 Oslo, Norway.

References

1. Aegidius K, Zwart JA, Hagen K, Stovner L (2009) The effect of pregnancy and parity on headache prevalence: the head-HUNT study. Headache 49: 851–859. https://doi.org/10.1111/j.1526-4610.2009.01438.x
2. Allais G et al (2013) Migraine and pregnancy: an internet survey. Neurol Sci 34(Suppl 1):S93–S99. https://doi.org/10.1007/s10072-013-1394-9
3. Couturier EG, Bomhof MA, Neven AK, van Duijn NP (2003) Menstrual migraine in a representative Dutch population sample: prevalence, disability and treatment. Cephalalgia 23:302–308. https://doi.org/10.1046/j.1468-2982.2003.00516.x
4. Cupini LM, Matteis M, Troisi E, Calabresi P, Bernardi G, Silvestrini M (1995) Sex-hormone-related events in migrainous females. A clinical comparative study between migraine with aura and migraine without aura. Cephalalgia 15:140–144. https://doi.org/10.1046/j.1468-2982.1995.015002140.x
5. Dean BB, Borenstein JE, Knight K, Yonkers K (2006) Evaluating the criteria used for identification of PMS. J Women's Health 15:546–555. https://doi.org/10.1089/jwh.2006.15.546
6. Digre KB (2013) Headaches during pregnancy. Clin Obstet Gynecol 56:317–329. https://doi.org/10.1097/GRF.0b013e31828f25e6
7. Disease GBD, Injury I, Prevalence C (2017) Global, regional, and national incidence, prevalence, and years lived with disability for 328 diseases and injuries for 195 countries, 1990-2016: a systematic analysis for the global burden of disease study 2016. Lancet 390:1211–1259. https://doi.org/10.1016/S0140-6736(17)32154-2
8. Harris GE, Wood M, Eberhard-Gran M, Lundqvist C, Nordeng H (2017) Patterns and predictors of analgesic use in pregnancy: a longitudinal drug utilization study with special focus on women with migraine. BMC Pregnancy Childbirth 17:224. https://doi.org/10.1186/s12884-017-1399-0
9. Headache Classification Committee of the International Headache S (2013) The international classification of headache disorders, 3rd edition (beta version). Cephalalgia 33:629–808. https://doi.org/10.1177/0333102413485658
10. Karli N et al (2012) Impact of sex hormonal changes on tension-type headache and migraine: a cross-sectional population-based survey in 2,600 women. J Headache Pain 13:557–565. https://doi.org/10.1007/s10194-012-0475-0
11. Kvisvik EV, Stovner LJ, Helde G, Bovim G, Linde M (2011) Headache and migraine during pregnancy and puerperium: the MIGRA-study. J Headache Pain 12:443–451. https://doi.org/10.1007/s10194-011-0329-1
12. Marcus DA, Scharff L, Turk D (1999) Longitudinal prospective study of headache during pregnancy and postpartum. Headache 39:625–632
13. Mattsson P (2003) Hormonal factors in migraine: a population-based study of women aged 40 to 74 years. Headache 43:27–35
14. Melhado E, Maciel JA, Jr., Guerreiro CA (2005) Headaches during pregnancy in women with a prior history of menstrual headaches Arquivos de neuro-psiquiatria 63:934–940 doi:/S0004-282X2005000600006
15. Melhado EM, Maciel JA Jr, Guerreiro CA (2007) Headache during gestation: evaluation of 1101 women. J Can Sci Neurol 34:187–192
16. Negro A et al (2017) Headache and pregnancy: a systematic review. J Headache Pain 18:106. https://doi.org/10.1186/s10194-017-0816-0
17. Pavlovic JM, Stewart WF, Bruce CA, Gorman JA, Sun H, Buse DC, Lipton RB (2015) Burden of migraine related to menses: results from the AMPP study. J Headache Pain 16:24. https://doi.org/10.1186/s10194-015-0503-y
18. Popat VB, Prodanov T, Calis KA, Nelson LM (2008) The menstrual cycle: a biological marker of general health in adolescents. Ann N Y Acad Sci 1135: 43–51. https://doi.org/10.1196/annals.1429.040
19. Rasmussen BK (1993) Migraine and tension-type headache in a general population: precipitating factors, female hormones, sleep pattern and relation to lifestyle. Pain 53:65–72
20. Rasmussen BK, Jensen R, Olesen J (1991) Questionnaire versus clinical interview in the diagnosis of headache. Headache 31:290–295
21. Russell MB, Rasmussen BK, Thorvaldsen P, Olesen J (1995) Prevalence and sex-ratio of the subtypes of migraine. Int J Epidemiol 24:612–618
22. Sances G, Granella F, Nappi RE, Fignon A, Ghiotto N, Polatti F, Nappi G (2003) Course of migraine during pregnancy and postpartum: a prospective study. Cephalalgia 23:197–205. https://doi.org/10.1046/j.1468-2982.2003.00480.x
23. Serva WA et al (2011) Course of migraine during pregnancy among migraine sufferers before pregnancy. Arq Neuropsiquiatr 69:613–619
24. Spierings EL, Padamsee A (2015) Menstrual-cycle and menstruation disorders in episodic vs chronic migraine: an exploratory study. Pain Med 16:1426–1432. https://doi.org/10.1111/pme.12788
25. Stovner L et al (2007) The global burden of headache: a documentation of headache prevalence and disability worldwide. Cephalalgia 27:193–210. https://doi.org/10.1111/j.1468-2982.2007.01288.x
26. Verbeke G, Fieuws S, Molenberghs G, Davidian M (2014) The analysis of multivariate longitudinal data: a review. Stat Methods Med Res 23:42–59. https://doi.org/10.1177/0962280212445834
27. Vetvik KG, Benth JS, MacGregor EA, Lundqvist C, Russell MB (2015) Menstrual versus non-menstrual attacks of migraine without aura in women with and without menstrual migraine. Cephalalgia 35:1261–1268. https://doi.org/10.1177/0333102415575723
28. Vetvik KG, Macgregor EA, Lundqvist C, Russell MB (2014) Prevalence of menstrual migraine: a population-based study. Cephalalgia 34:280–288. https://doi.org/10.1177/0333102413507637

Permissions

All chapters in this book were first published in TJHP, by BioMed Central; hereby published with permission under the Creative Commons Attribution License or equivalent. Every chapter published in this book has been scrutinized by our experts. Their significance has been extensively debated. The topics covered herein carry significant findings which will fuel the growth of the discipline. They may even be implemented as practical applications or may be referred to as a beginning point for another development.

The contributors of this book come from diverse backgrounds, making this book a truly international effort. This book will bring forth new frontiers with its revolutionizing research information and detailed analysis of the nascent developments around the world.

We would like to thank all the contributing authors for lending their expertise to make the book truly unique. They have played a crucial role in the development of this book. Without their invaluable contributions this book wouldn't have been possible. They have made vital efforts to compile up to date information on the varied aspects of this subject to make this book a valuable addition to the collection of many professionals and students.

This book was conceptualized with the vision of imparting up-to-date information and advanced data in this field. To ensure the same, a matchless editorial board was set up. Every individual on the board went through rigorous rounds of assessment to prove their worth. After which they invested a large part of their time researching and compiling the most relevant data for our readers.

The editorial board has been involved in producing this book since its inception. They have spent rigorous hours researching and exploring the diverse topics which have resulted in the successful publishing of this book. They have passed on their knowledge of decades through this book. To expedite this challenging task, the publisher supported the team at every step. A small team of assistant editors was also appointed to further simplify the editing procedure and attain best results for the readers.

Apart from the editorial board, the designing team has also invested a significant amount of their time in understanding the subject and creating the most relevant covers. They scrutinized every image to scout for the most suitable representation of the subject and create an appropriate cover for the book.

The publishing team has been an ardent support to the editorial, designing and production team. Their endless efforts to recruit the best for this project, has resulted in the accomplishment of this book. They are a veteran in the field of academics and their pool of knowledge is as vast as their experience in printing. Their expertise and guidance has proved useful at every step. Their uncompromising quality standards have made this book an exceptional effort. Their encouragement from time to time has been an inspiration for everyone.

The publisher and the editorial board hope that this book will prove to be a valuable piece of knowledge for researchers, students, practitioners and scholars across the globe.

List of Contributors

Tamás Gyüre
Szentágothai János Doctoral School of Neurosciences, Semmelweis University, Üllői u. 26, Budapest 1085, Hungary

Éva Csépány and Máté Magyar
Szentágothai János Doctoral School of Neurosciences, Semmelweis University, Üllői u. 26, Budapest 1085, Hungary
Department of Neurology, Semmelweis University, Balassa u. 6, Budapest 1083, Hungary

Marianna Tóth
Department of Neurology, Vaszary Kolos Hospital, Petőfi Sándor u. 26-28, Esztergom 2500, Hungary

György Bozsik, Dániel Bereczki and Csaba Ertsey
Department of Neurology, Semmelweis University, Balassa u. 6, Budapest 1083, Hungary

Gabriella Juhász
SE-NAP2 Genetic Brain Imaging Migraine Research Group, Semmelweis University, Nagyvárad tér 4, Budapest 1089, Hungary
Department of Pharmacodynamics, Faculty of Pharmacy, Semmelweis University, Nagyvárad tér 4, Budapest 1089, Hungary

Jing Wang and Shengyuan Yu
School of Medicine, Nankai University, Tianjin 300071, China
Department of Neurology, Chinese PLA General Hospital, Fuxing Road 28, Haidian District, Beijing 100853, China

Weihao Xu and Shasha Sun
Department of Geriatric Cardiology, Nanlou Division, Chinese PLA General Hospital, Beijing 100853, China
National Clinical Research Center of Geriatric Diseases, Chinese PLA General Hospital, Fuxing Road 28, Haidian District, Beijing 100853, China

Li Fan
National Clinical Research Center of Geriatric Diseases, Chinese PLA General Hospital, Fuxing Road 28, Haidian District, Beijing 100853, China

Paolo Martelletti
Department of Clinical and Molecular Medicine, Sapienza University, Rome, Italy

Piero Barbanti
Headache and Pain Unit, Istituto di Ricovero e Cura a Carattere Scientifico (IRCCS) San Raffaele Pisana, Rome, Italy

Licia Grazzi
Neuroalgology Unit, Carlo Besta Neurological Institute and Foundation, Milan, Italy.

Giulia Pierangeli
IRCCS Istituto delle Scienze Neurologiche di Bologna, Bologna, Italy

Innocenzo Rainero
Department of Neuroscience, University of Turin, Turin, Italy

Pierangelo Geppetti
Headache Centre, University Hospital of Careggi, Florence, Italy

Anna Ambrosini
IRCCS Neuromed, Pozzilli, IS, Italy

Paola Sarchielli
Neurologic Clinic, Santa Maria della Misericordia Hospital, Perugia, Italy

Cristina Tassorelli
Headache Science Centre, IRCCS C. Mondino Foundation, Pavia, Italy
Department of Brain and Behavioral Sciences, University of Pavia, Pavia, Italy

Eric Liebler
electroCore, Inc., Basking Ridge, NJ, USA

Marina de Tommaso
Neurophysiology and Pain Unit, University of Bari Aldo Moro, Bari, Italy

Steffen Naegel, Josephine Biermann, Christoph Kleinschnitz, Hans-Christoph Diener and Dagny Holle
Department of Neurology, University of Duisburg-Essen, University Hospital Essen, Hufelandstr. 55, 45122 Essen, Germany

Zaza Katsarava
Department of Neurology, University of Duisburg-Essen, University Hospital Essen, Hufelandstr. 55, 45122 Essen, Germany

Department of Neurology, Evangelical Hospital Unna, Holbeinstr. 10, 59423 Unna, Germany
EVEX Medical Corporation, 40 Vazha-Pshavela Avenue, Tbilisi 0177, Georgia
Sechenov University Moscow, 8-2 Trubetskaya str., Moscow 119991, Russian Federation

Mark Obermann
Department of Neurology, University of Duisburg-Essen, University Hospital Essen, Hufelandstr. 55, 45122 Essen, Germany
Center for Neurology, Asklepios Hospitals Schildautal, Karl-Herold-Straße 1, 38723 Seesen, Germany

Nina Theysohn
Institute of Diagnostic and Interventional Radiology and Neuroradiology, University of Duisburg-Essen, University Hospital Essen, Hufelandstr. 55, 45122 Essen, Germany

Mattias Gjelset
Division of Oral Diagnostics and Rehabilitation, Department of Dental Medicine, Karolinska Institutet, SE-141 04 Huddinge, Sweden

Amal Al-Khotani
Division of Oral Diagnostics and Rehabilitation, Department of Dental Medicine, Karolinska Institutet, SE-141 04 Huddinge, Sweden
East Jeddah Hospital, Ministry of health, Jeddah, Saudi Arabia
Scandinavian Center for Orofacial Neurosciences (SCON), Huddinge, Sweden

Malin Ernberg and Nikolaos Christidis
Division of Oral Diagnostics and Rehabilitation, Department of Dental Medicine, Karolinska Institutet, SE-141 04 Huddinge, Sweden
Scandinavian Center for Orofacial Neurosciences (SCON), Huddinge, Sweden

Britt Hedenberg-Magnusson
Division of Oral Diagnostics and Rehabilitation, Department of Dental Medicine, Karolinska Institutet, SE-141 04 Huddinge, Sweden
Scandinavian Center for Orofacial Neurosciences (SCON), Huddinge, Sweden
Department of Clinical Oral Physiology at the Eastman Institute, Stockholm Public Dental Health, Stockholm, Sweden

Aron Naimi-Akbar
Oral and maxillofacial surgery, Department of Dental Medicine, Karolinska Institutet, Huddinge, Sweden

Jiyoung Kim
Department of Neurology, BioMedical Research Institute, Pusan National University Hospital, Pusan National University School of Medicine, Busan, South Korea

Soo-Jin Cho
Department of Neurology, Dongtan Sacred Heart Hospital, Hallym University College of Medicine, Hwaseong, South Korea

Won-Joo Kim
Department of Neurology, Gangnam Severance Hospital, Yonsei University College of Medicine, Seoul, South Korea

Kwang Ik Yang
Sleep Disorders Center, Department of Neurology, Soonchunhyang University College of Medicine, Cheonan Hospital, Cheonan, South Korea

Chang-Ho Yun
Clinical Neuroscience Center, Department of Neurology, Seoul National University Bundang Hospital, Seongnam, South Korea

Min Kyung Chu
Department of Neurology, Severance Hospital, Yonsei University College of Medicine, 50-1 Yonsei-ro, Seodaemoon-gu, Seoul, Republic of Korea

Daniyal J Jafree
Faculty of Medical Sciences, University College London, London, UK

Joanna M Zakrzewska, Saumya Bhatia and Carolina Venda Nova
Eastman Dental Institute, UCLH NHS Foundation Trust, London, UK

Bo Larsson, Johannes Foss Sigurdson and Anne Mari Sund
Regional Center for Child and Youth Mental Health and Child Welfare –Central Norway, NTNU, Klostergat. 46/48, N-7489 Trondheim, Norway

Chun-Yu Chen, Jong-Ling Fuh and Yen-Feng Wang
Department of Neurology, Neurological Institute, Taipei Veterans General Hospital, Taipei 112, Taiwan
Faculty of Medicine, National Yang-Ming University School of Medicine, Taipei, Taiwan

Shih-Pin Chen
Department of Neurology, Neurological Institute, Taipei Veterans General Hospital, Taipei 112, Taiwan

Faculty of Medicine, National Yang-Ming University School of Medicine, Taipei, Taiwan
Institute of Clinical Medicine, National Yang-Ming University, Taipei, Taiwan
Division of Translational Research, Department of Medical Research, Taipei Veterans General Hospital, Taipei, Taiwan

Shuu-Jiun Wang
Department of Neurology, Neurological Institute, Taipei Veterans General Hospital, Taipei 112, Taiwan
Faculty of Medicine, National Yang-Ming University School of Medicine, Taipei, Taiwan
Brain Research Center, National Yang-Ming University, Taipei, Taiwan

Jiing-Feng Lirng and Feng-Chi Chang
Faculty of Medicine, National Yang-Ming University School of Medicine, Taipei, Taiwan
Department of Radiology, Taipei Veterans General Hospital, Taipei, Taiwan

Mi Ji Lee and Soohyun Cho
Department of Neurology, Samsung Medical Center, Sungkyunkwan University School of Medicine, 81 Irwon-Ro, Gangnam-Gu, Seoul 06351, South Korea

Sook-Yeon Lee and Eun-Suk Kang
Department of Laboratory Medicine and Genetics, Samsung Medical Center, Sungkyunkwan University School of Medicine, Seoul, South Korea

Chin-Sang Chung
Department of Neurology, Samsung Medical Center, Sungkyunkwan University School of Medicine, 81 Irwon-Ro, Gangnam-Gu, Seoul 06351, South Korea
Neuroscience Center, Samsung Medical Center, Seoul, South Korea

Tae-Jin Song
Department of Neurology, College of Medicine, Ewha Womans University, Seoul, South Korea

Soo-Jin Cho
Department of Neurology, Dongtan Sacred Heart Hospital, Hallym University College of Medicine, Hwaseong, South Korea

Won-Joo Kim
Department of Neurology, Gangnam Severance Hospital, Yonsei University, College of Medicine, Seoul, South Korea

Kwang Ik Yang
Department of Neurology, Soonchunhyang University College of Medicine, Cheonan Hospital, Cheonan, South Korea

Chang-Ho Yun
Department of Neurology, Clinical Neuroscience Center, Seoul National University Bundang Hospital, Seongnam, South Korea

Min Kyung Chu
Department of Neurology, Yonsei University College of Medicine, 50-1 Yonsei-ro, Seodaemoon-gu, Seoul 03722, South Korea

Eloisa Rubio-Beltrán and Antoinette MaassenVanDenBrink
Division of Vascular Medicine and Pharmacology, Department of Internal Medicine, Erasmus University Medical Center, Rotterdam, The Netherlands

Edvige Correnti
Department of Child Neuropsychiatry, University of Palermo, Palermo, Italy

Marie Deen
Danish Headache Center, Department of Neurology, Rigshospitalet Glostrup, Glostrup, Denmark

Katharina Kamm
Department of Neurology, University Hospital, LMU Munich, Munich, Germany

Tim Kelderman
Department of Neurology, Ghent University Hospital, Ghent, Belgium

Laura Papetti
Headache Center, Bambino Gesù Children'sHospital, IRCCS, Rome, Italy

Simone Vigneri
Department of Experimental Biomedicine and Clinical Neurosciences, University of Palermo; Pain Medicine Unit, Santa Maria Maddalena Hospital, Occhiobello, Italy

Lars Edvinsson
Department of Internal Medicine, Institute of Clinical Sciences, Lund University, Lund, Sweden

Ching-I Hung and Chia-Yih Liu
Department of Psychiatry, Chang-Gung Memorial Hospital at Linkou and Chang-Gung University College of Medicine, Tao-Yuan, Taiwan

Ching-Hui Yang
Department of Nursing, Chang Gung University of Science and Technology, Tao-Yuan, Taiwan

Shuu-Jiun Wang
Faculty of Medicine and Brain Research Center, National Yang-Ming University and Neurological Institute, Taipei Veterans General Hospital, Taipei, Taiwan

Department of Neurology, Taipei Veterans General Hospital, No. 201 Shi-Pai Road, Section 2, Taipei 112, Taiwan

Lauren Schweizer, Philipp Stude, Benjamin Glaubitz and Sibel Delice
Department of Neurology, Berufsgenossenschaftliches Universitätsklinikum Bergmannsheil, Ruhr-University-Bochum, Bochum, Germany

Adina Bathel
Department of Neurology, Berufsgenossenschaftliches Universitätsklinikum Bergmannsheil, Ruhr-University-Bochum, Bochum, Germany
Department of Anesthesiology, Unfallkrankenhaus Berlin, Berlin, Germany

Niklas Wulms
Department of Neurology, St. Mauritius Therapieklinik, Meerbusch, Germany

Tobias Schmidt-Wilcke
Department of Neurology, St. Mauritius Therapieklinik, Meerbusch, Germany
Institute of Clinical Neuroscience and Medical Psychology, Universitätsklinikum Düsseldorf, Düsseldorf, Germany

Casper Emil Christensen, Samaira Younis†, Marie Deen, Sabrina Khan, Hashmat Ghanizada and Messoud Ashina
Danish Headache Center and Department of Neurology, Rigshospitalet Glostrup, Faculty of Health and Medical Sciences, University of Copenhagen, Copenhagen, Denmark

Iman Dianat and Arezou Alipour
Department of Occupational Health and Ergonomics, Tabriz University of Medical Sciences, Tabriz, Iran

Mohammad Asghari Jafarabadi
Road Traffic Injury Research Centre, Faculty of Health, Tabriz University of Medical Sciences, Tabriz, Iran
Department of Statistics and Epidemiology, Faculty of Health, Tabriz University of Medical Sciences, Tabriz 14711, Iran

Elena R. Lebedeva
Department of Neurology and Neurosurgery, The Ural State Medical University, Repina 3, Yekaterinburg 620028, Russia
International Headache Center "Europe-Asia", Yekaterinburg, Russia

Natalia M. Gurary
Medical Union "New Hospital", Yekaterinburg, Russia

Jes Olesen
Danish Headache Center, Department of Neurology, Rigshospitalet-Glostrup, University of Copenhagen, Copenhagen, Denmark

Mengmeng Ma, Ning Chen, Jian Guo, Yang Zhang and Li He
Department of Neurology, West China Hospital, Sichuan University, No. 37, Wainan Guoxue Xiang, Chengdu 610041, Sichuan, China

Junran Zhang
Department of Radiology, Huaxi MR Research Center (HMRRC), West China Hospital, Sichuan University, Chengdu, China
Department of Medical Information Engineering, School of Electrical Engineering and Information, Sichuan University, Chengdu, China

Rosaria Greco and Chiara Demartini
Laboratory of Neurophysiology of Integrative Autonomic Systems, Headache Science Centre, IRCCS Mondino Foundation, Pavia, Italy

Anna Maria Zanaboni and Cristina Tassorelli
Laboratory of Neurophysiology of Integrative Autonomic Systems, Headache Science Centre, IRCCS Mondino Foundation, Pavia, Italy
Department of Brain and Behavioral Sciences, University of Pavia, Pavia, Italy

Junpeng Liu and Xuejun Zhang
School of Medical Imaging, Tianjin Medical University, No. 1, Guangdong Road, Hexi District, Tianjin 300203, China

Jiajia Zhu
Department of Radiology, The First Affiliated Hospital of Anhui Medical University, Hefei, China

Fei Yuan and Quan Zhang
Department of Radiology, Pingjin Hospital, Logistics University of Chinese People's Armed Police Forces, No. 220, Chenglin Road, Hedong District, Tianjin 300162, China

Inken Moeller, Louisa Rosenbaum, Janine Schroeder, Christian Zimmer and Bettina Wollesen
Department of Human Movement Science, University of Hamburg, Hamburg, Germany

Kerstin Luedtke
Department of Human Movement Science, University of Hamburg, Hamburg, Germany
Academic Physiotherapy, Medical Section, Department of Orthopaedics and Trauma Surgery, University of Luebeck, Luebeck, Germany

The Jerzy Kukuczka Academy of Physical Education, Department of Physiotherapy, Katowice, Poland
Department of Systems Neuroscience, University Medical Center Hamburg-Eppendorf, Hamburg, Germany

Tibor Szikszay
Academic Physiotherapy, Medical Section, Department of Orthopaedics and Trauma Surgery, University of Luebeck, Luebeck, Germany

Waclaw Adamczyk
The Jerzy Kukuczka Academy of Physical Education, Department of Physiotherapy, Katowice, Poland
Academic Physiotherapy, Medical Section, Department of Orthopaedics and Trauma Surgery, University of Luebeck, Luebeck, Germany
Pain Research Group, Institute of Psychology, Jagiellonian University, Krakow, Poland

Katrin Mehrtens and Axel Schaefer
Faculty of Social Science, Degree Course Speech and Language Therapy and Physiotherapy, University of Applied Sciences Bremen, Bremen, Germany

Samaira Younis, Anders Hougaard, Casper Emil Christensen and Messoud Ashina
Danish Headache Center, Department of Neurology, Rigshospitalet Glostrup, University of Copenhagen, Copenhagen, Denmark

Mark Bitsch Vestergaard and Henrik Bo Wiberg Larsson
Functional Imaging Unit, Department of Clinical Physiology, Nuclear Medicine and PET, Rigshospitalet Glostrup, University of Copenhagen, Copenhagen, Denmark

Esben Thade Petersen
Danish Research Centre for Magnetic Resonance, Centre for Functional and Diagnostic Imaging and research, Copenhagen University Hospital Hvidovre, Copenhagen, Denmark

Olaf Bjarne Paulson
Neurobiology Research Unit, Department of Neurology, Rigshospitalet, University of Copenhagen, Copenhagen, Denmark

Mengyu Liu and Lin Ma
Department of Radiology, Chinese PLA General Hospital, 28 Fuxing Road, Beijing 100853, China

Mengqi Liu
Department of Radiology, Chinese PLA General Hospital, 28 Fuxing Road, Beijing 100853, China
Department of Radiology, Hainan Branch of Chinese PLA General Hospital, Beijing 100853, China

Zhiye Chen
Department of Radiology, Chinese PLA General Hospital, 28 Fuxing Road, Beijing 100853, China
Department of Radiology, Hainan Branch of Chinese PLA General Hospital, Beijing 100853, China
Department of Neurology, Chinese PLA General Hospital, 28 Fuxing Road, Beijing 100853, China

Xiaoyan Chen and Shengyuan Yu
Department of Neurology, Chinese PLA General Hospital, 28 Fuxing Road, Beijing 100853, China

Karin Zebenholzer and Christian Wöber
Department of Neurology, Medical University of Vienna, Waehringer Guertel 18-20, 1090 Vienna, Austria

Walter Gall
Center for Medical Statistics, Informatics and Intelligent Systems, Institute of Medical Information Management, Medical University of Vienna, Waehringer Guertel 18-20, 1090 Vienna, Austria

Huimin Tao, Teng Wang, Xin Dong, Qi Guo, Huan Xu and Qi Wan
Department of Neurology, The First Affiliated Hospital of Nanjing Medical University, 300 Guangzhou Road, Nanjing 210029, Jiangsu Province, China

Alexei A. Kamshilin and Maxim A. Volynsky
Department of Computer Photonics and Videomatics, ITMO University, St. Petersburg, Russia

Rashid Giniatullin
Department of Computer Photonics and Videomatics, ITMO University, St. Petersburg, Russia
Laboratory of Neurobiology, Kazan Federal University, Kazan, Russia
Department of Neurobiology, University of Eastern Finland, Kuopio, Finland

Oleg V. Mamontov
Department of Computer Photonics and Videomatics, ITMO University, St. Petersburg, Russia
Department of Circulation Physiology, Almazov National Medical Research Centre, St. Petersburg, Russia

Olga Khayrutdinova
Department of Neurology and Rehabilitation, Kazan State Medical University, Kazan, Russia

Dilyara Nurkhametova
Laboratory of Neurobiology, Kazan Federal University, Kazan, Russia

Department of Neurobiology, University of Eastern Finland, Kuopio, Finland

Laura Babayan and Alexander V. Amelin
Department of Neurology and Neurosurgery, Pavlov First Saint Petersburg State Medical University, St. Petersburg, Russia

Beáta Éva Petrovski
Health Services Research Centre, Akershus University Hospital, 1478 Lørenskog, Oslo, Norway
Faculty of Dentistry, University of Oslo, Geitmyrsveien 69, 0455 Oslo, Norway

Christofer Lundqvist
Health Services Research Centre, Akershus University Hospital, 1478 Lørenskog, Oslo, Norway
Department of Neurology, Akershus University Hospital, 1478 Lørenskog, Oslo, Norway
Institute of Clinical Medicine, Campus Ahus, University of Oslo, 1478 Lørenskog, Norway

Malin Eberhard-Gran
Health Services Research Centre, Akershus University Hospital, 1478 Lørenskog, Oslo, Norway
Department of Neurology, Akershus University Hospital, 1478 Lørenskog, Oslo, Norway
Institute of Clinical Medicine, Campus Ahus, University of Oslo, 1478 Lørenskog, Norway
Domain for Mental and Physical Health, Norwegian Institute of Public Health, Lovisenberggata 6-8, 0456 Oslo, Norway

Kjersti G. Vetvik
Department of Neurology, Akershus University Hospital, 1478 Lørenskog, Oslo, Norway

Index

www.ingramcontent.com/pod-product-compliance
Lightning Source LLC
Chambersburg PA
CBHW080249230326
41458CB00097B/4185

9781632416865